SEVERE ASTHMA

LUNG BIOLOGY IN HEALTH AND DISEASE

Executive Editor

Claude Lenfant
Director, National Heart, Lung and Blood Institute
National Institutes of Health
Bethesda, Maryland

ADDITIONAL VOLUMES IN PREPARATION

The opinions expressed in these volumes do not necessarily represent the views of the National Institutes of Health.

SEVERE ASTHMA
PATHOGENESIS AND CLINICAL MANAGEMENT
Second Edition, Revised and Expanded

Edited by

Stanley J. Szefler
Donald Y. M. Leung

National Jewish Medical and Research Center
Denver, Colorado

MARCEL DEKKER, INC.   NEW YORK · BASEL

ISBN: 0-8247-0552-1

This book is printed on acid-free paper.

Headquarters
Marcel Dekker, Inc.
270 Madison Avenue, New York, NY 10016
tel: 212-696-9000; fax: 212-685-4540

Eastern Hemisphere Distribution
Marcel Dekker AG
Hutgasse 4, Postfach 812, CH-4001 Basel, Switzerland
tel: 41-61-261-8482; fax: 41-61-261-8896

World Wide Web
http://www.dekker.com

The publisher offers discounts on this book when ordered in bulk quantities. For
more information, write to Special Sales/Professional Marketing at the headquarters address above.

Current printing (last digit):
10 9 8 7 6 5 4 3 2 1

PRINTED IN THE UNITED STATES OF AMERICA

INTRODUCTION

Since 1976, when the first volume in the Lung Biology in Health and Disease series appeared, many have been published on asthma. Actually, asthma has been the dominant topic among the 159 volumes published as of the time of this writing.

The first volume related to asthma [*Pathophysiology and Pharmacology of the Airways*, edited by J. Nadel (1980)] presented what we knew up to that point. Then, in 1987, *Drug Therapy for Asthma* (edited by J. W. Jenne and S. Murphy) was published. Those who follow the history of the modern approach to asthma will recognize 1987 as the beginning of an extraordinary movement directed toward the conquest of asthma. Indeed, in the United States, public officials, basic and clinical researchers, and voluntary and professional organizations all united, with the goal of alleviating the suffering and the public health burden of this disease.

Today there is a worldwide effort to learn more about and combat asthma. Have we been successful? In my opinion, yes! Certainly, the prevalence of this disease is very high, perhaps even increasing, at least in some parts of the world. But it is also true that many patients have their disease under control and are leading normal and productive lives. Just observe all the Olympic medalists who suffer from asthma!

What is disappointing is that not all asthma patients in the United States or elsewhere are benefiting from what we know and what we can do. Experts say that asthma can be controlled and that no one should die from it, but, unfortunately, some patients do die because asthma can become very severe.

In 1996, the first edition of *Severe Asthma: Pathogenesis and Clinical Management* (edited by S. J. Szefler and D. Y. M. Leung) appeared. Two years later, *Fatal Asthma* (edited by A. L. Sheffer) was published. Since that time, valuable data about severe asthma have been compiled. New pharmacological agents, new insight, and new approaches have emerged. For this reason, the editors, authors, publisher, and I thought that a second, revised and expanded edition of *Severe Asthma: Pathogenesis and Clinical Management* (edited by S. J. Szefler and D. Y. M. Leung) was warranted and timely.

The American writer Djuna Barnes said of her severe asthma, ''I have already died, and they brought me back. Now, I have to go through the whole horrid business again! It is terrible!'' We hope this new volume will constitute a bridge between what we know and what we must do when caring for patients, and thus will advance one more step toward decreasing the risk of severe asthma.

The editors and authors, all experts in their field, bring to the readership the latest available information and guidance. It is with great appreciation and gratitude to all of them that I introduce this new volume.

Claude Lenfant, M.D.
Bethesda, Maryland

PREFACE

Although the majority of asthmatics can be controlled with inhaled corticosteroids and an inhaled short-acting beta-adrenergic agonist or leukotriene modifier, 5 to 10% of patients are recalcitrant to the usual treatment approaches, including systemic corticosteroids. These asthmatic patients are an important group because they suffer the greatest impairment in quality of life and their illness has a profound impact on the health-care system. Physicians frequently spend a great deal of time caring for such patients, and these patients utilize the majority of health-care dollars devoted to treatment of asthma.

The first edition of this book, published in 1996, was the first to focus on this unique feature of asthma. We were already quite familiar with the concept of inflammation as a feature of chronic asthma, and our intention at that time was to gather the available literature for clinicians and to stimulate further research in this area. Attention had shifted to inhaled steroids as the cornerstone of managing persistent asthma, and so we began to ask questions regarding the measurement of inflammation and the effect that novel therapies had on airway inflammation.

This edition focuses on two major questions: (1) Can we reduce the prevalence of severe asthma by reversing its course once it is established? and (2) can we reduce the incidence of severe asthma by altering the natural course of asthma? To lay the foundation needed to address these issues, we have asked an outstanding group of investigators to review the pathophysiology, pharmacology, and management of asthma from a multidisciplinary perspective. We have focused on gathering new information that complements rather than duplicates information already presented in the first edition. This volume is organized into several sections that will allow us to approach critical questions regarding severe asthma in the next 5 years.

Part One provides an overview of the impact and pathophysiology of severe asthma. A number of important issues are addressed, including the pathology of severe asthma and the role of airway remodeling, the progressive nature of lung deterioration in asthma, the genetics and pulmonary physiology of severe asthma, and the role of inflammatory mediators and neural mechanisms. Among the important issues that are debated is whether lung deterioration can be halted by pharmacological intervention or whether it is inevitable (i.e., genetic). It is suggested that a major goal of management in established severe asthma must include the arrest of inflammation and the healing of damaged airways to enable a return to normal function.

Part Two examines the clinical pharmacology of severe asthma. It includes a review of the pharmacological management of severe asthma, as well as the use of newer drugs and controversial therapies such as herbal medications. The need to appreciate chronopharmacological principles in the management of asthma is also reviewed, along with our current understanding of the mechanisms of corticosteroid action.

Part Three focuses on the multidisciplinary approach needed for management of severe asthma. It contains discussions of confounding factors in the management of severe asthma, the role of chronic infection as a component of "treatable" severe asthma, approaches to steroid-resistant asthma, the role of sleep disorders, psychosocial factors, rhinosinusitis, and environmental triggers of severe asthma. As physicians focus more on the use of anti-inflammatory therapy in the treatment of asthma, it is critical that we develop new noninvasive tools for monitoring disease activity, which actually measure airway inflammation as opposed to surrogate markers or pulmonary physiology. Finally, the potential adverse effects of steroid therapy and strategies in the prevention of severe asthma are addressed.

In summary, *Severe Asthma: Second Edition, Revised and Expanded*, has assimilated the available information on the diagnosis, pathology, and management of severe asthma. Significant opportunities are available to reverse the course of the disease and also to prevent its development. Advances in management will require continued research on the natural history of severe asthma, pathogenesis, application of markers of inflammation, pharmacogenetics, and, most likely, continuing development of new medication to meet currently unmet needs. Success in these target areas should lead to a reduction in the incidence and prevalence of severe asthma and an overall improvement in outcomes for asthma patients.

We thank each of the authors for contributing their time and expertise, which were vital to the success of this book. We are also indebted to Dr. Claude Lenfant, who kindly agreed that a second edition on this important topic was necessary. Sandra Beberman at Marcel Dekker, Inc., provided invaluable assistance in the production of this book, and Maureen Sandoval at National Jewish Medical and Research Center was critical in the assembly of manuscripts from authors. We know this volume will provide a valuable resource for allergists, pulmonologists, internists, primary care physicians, and graduate students and investigators interested in the mechanisms and treatment of severe asthma.

Stanley J. Szefler
Donald Y. M. Leung

CONTRIBUTORS

David B. Allen, M.D. Professor of Pediatrics and Director of Endocrinology and Residency Training, Department of Pediatrics, University of Wisconsin Children's Hospital, Madison, Wisconsin

Ron Balkissoon, M.D., F.R.C.P.(C), M.Sc., D.I.H. Director, Specific Inhalation Challenge Chamber Facility, Department of Medicine, National Jewish Medical and Research Center, Denver, Colorado

Robert D. Ballard, M.D. Associate Professor; Director, Sleep Health Center, Department of Medicine, National Jewish Medical and Research Center, Denver, Colorado

Peter J. Barnes, D.M., D.Sc., F.R.C.P. Professor, Department of Thoracic Medicine, National Heart and Lung Institute, Imperial College, London, England

Bianca Beghé Southampton General Hospital and University of Southampton, Southampton, England

John W. Bloom, M.D. Associate Professor of Pharmacology and Medicine, Respiratory Sciences Center, University of Arizona College of Medicine, Tucson, Arizona

Jean Bousquet, M.D., Ph.D. Professor, Department of Respiratory Medicine, University of Montpellier, Montpellier, France

Donna L. Bratton, M.D. Associate Professor, Department of Pediatrics, National Jewish Medical and Research Center, Denver, Colorado

Pascal Chanez University of Montpellier, Montpellier, France

Qutayba Hamid, M.D., Ph.D. Professor of Medicine/Pathology, Meakins-Christie Laboratories, McGill University, Montreal, Quebec, Canada

Daniel L. Hamilos, M.D. Associate Professor of Medicine, Department of Allergy and Immunology, Washington University School of Medicine, St. Louis, Missouri

Philip D. Hanna, M.D. Director, Rocky Mountain Gastrointestinal Motility Center, Swedish Medical Center, Englewood, Colorado

Frederick E. Hargreave, M.D., F.R.C.P.C., F.R.C.P. Professor, Department of Medicine, St. Joseph's Healthcare and McMaster University, Hamilton, Ontario, Canada

Tina K. Hatley, M.D. Division of Allergy, Asthma, and Immunology, University of Virginia Health Sciences System, Charlottesville, Virginia

Stephen T. Holgate, B.Sc., M.D., D.Sc., F.R.C.P., F.R.C.Path., F.Inst.Biol., F.Med.Sci. Professor, Respiratory Cell and Molecular Biology Division, School of Medicine, Southampton General Hospital and University of Southampton, Southampton, England

John W. Holloway Southampton General Hospital and University of Southampton, Southampton, England

Charles G. Irvin, Ph.D. Professor and Director, Vermont Lung Center, University of Vermont College of Medicine, Burlington, Vermont

Steven P. Jensen, M.D. Department of Radiology, University of Colorado Health Sciences Center, Denver, Colorado

Margaret M. Kelly, M.B., Ch.B., F.C.Path(SA)   Department of Medicine, St. Joseph's Healthcare and McMaster University, Hamilton, Ontario, Canada

Gwendolyn S. Kerby, M.D.   Instructor, Section of Pediatric Pulmonary Medicine, Department of Pediatrics, University of Colorado School of Medicine and the Children's Hospital, Denver, Colorado

Monica Kraft, M.D.   Associate Professor, Department of Medicine, Pulmonary Division, National Jewish Medical and Research Center, Denver, Colorado

Esther L. Langmack, M.D.   Assistant Professor, Pulmonary Division, Department of Medicine, National Jewish Medical and Research Center, Denver, Colorado

Gary L. Larsen, M.D.   Professor and Head, Division of Pediatric Pulmonary Medicine, Department of Pediatrics, National Jewish Medical and Research Center, and University of Colorado School of Medicine, Denver, Colorado

Dennis K. Ledford, M.D.   Professor, Department of Medicine, Division of Allergy/Immunology, the Joy A. McCann Culverhouse Airway Disease Research Center, University of South Florida, and the James A. Haley VA Hospital, Tampa, Florida

Richard Leigh, M.B., M.Sc., F.C.P.(SA)   Department of Medicine, St. Joseph's Healthcare and McMaster University, Hamilton, Ontario, Canada

Donald Y. M. Leung, M.D., Ph.D.   Professor and Head, Division of Pediatric Allergy-Immunology, National Jewish Medical and Research Center, Denver, Colorado

David A. Lynch, M.D.   Professor, Department of Radiology, University of Colorado Health Sciences Center, Denver, Colorado

Richard J. Martin, M.D.   Head, Pulmonary Division and Vice-Chair, Department of Medicine, National Jewish Medical and Research Center, and Professor of Medicine, Univerity of Colorado, Denver, Colorado

Sophie Molet   INSERM U456, Université de Rennes I, Rennes, France

John D. Newell, Jr., M.D.   Professor, Department of Radiology, University of Colorado Health Sciences Center, Denver, Colorado

David N. Pham, M.D. Fellow, Pulmonary Division, Department of Medicine, National Jewish Medical and Research Center, Denver, Colorado

Thomas A. E. Platts-Mills, M.D., Ph.D. Professor of Medicine and Microbiology, and Head, Division of Asthma, Allergy, and Immunology, University of Virginia Health Sciences System, Charlottesville, Virginia

Steuart Rorke Southampton General Hospital and University of Southampton, Southampton, England

Joseph D. Spahn, M.D. Department of Pediatrics, National Jewish Medical and Research Center, Denver, Colorado

Donald D. Stevenson, M.D. Senior Consultant, Division of Allergy, Asthma and Immunology, Scripps Clinic and the Scripps Research Institute, La Jolla, California

E. Rand Sutherland, M.D. Associate Professor, Department of Medicine, National Jewish Medical and Research Center, Denver, Colorado

Stanley J. Szefler, M.D. Helen Wohlberg and Herman Lambert Chair in Pharmacokinetics, National Jewish Medical and Research Center, and Professor of Pediatrics and Pharmacology, University of Colorado Health Sciences Center, Denver, Colorado

Antonio M. Vignola University of Montpellier, Montpellier, France

Frederick S. Wamboldt, M.D. Head, Division of Psychosocial Medicine, Department of Medicine, National Jewish Medical and Research Center, and Professor of Psychiatry, University of Colorado Health Sciences Center, Denver, Colorado

Marianne Z. Wamboldt, M.D. Associate Professor, Department of Pediatrics, National Jewish Medical and Research Center, and Associate Professor of Psychiatry, University of Colorado Health Sciences Center, Denver, Colorado

George A. Ward, Jr., M.D. Associate Professor of Medicine, University of Virginia Health Sciences System, Charlottesville, Virginia

Scott T. Weiss, M.D., M.S. Professor, Channing Laboratory, Department of Medicine, Harvard Medical School, Boston, Massachusetts

Sally E. Wenzel, M.D. Associate Professor, Department of Medicine, National Jewish Medical and Research Center, and University of Colorado Health Sciences Center, Denver, Colorado

Judith A. Woodfolk, M.D. Associate Professor of Medicine, University of Virginia Health Sciences System, Charlottesville, Virginia

CONTENTS

Part Two   CLINICAL PHARMACOLOGY

SEVERE ASTHMA

1

Asthma as a Progressive Disease
Pulmonary and Epidemiological Insights

SCOTT T. WEISS

Harvard Medical School
Boston, Massachusetts

I. Introduction

The purpose of this chapter is to describe the natural history of asthma through the different stages of the life cycle. While it is clear that asthma as a disease begins very early in life, if not in utero, the clinical and phenotypic expressions of the condition change dramatically at different stages of the life cycle. This change can be seen as the interaction between environmental exposures and genetic susceptibility genes. While the number of specific genes that influence asthma is unknown at present, it is clear that the disorder aggregates in families and has measurable heritability, suggesting some genetic influence. While it may be trite to say that asthma is influenced both by genetic and environmental factors, the complex interplay of multiple genes and multiple environmental exposures creates a unique phenotype that is clearly recognizable clinically. Only 15% of the lungs' alveoli are fully formed at birth and thus the lung is an organ in that it is directly open and available to the environment and its full complement of alveoli and their development do not occur in the absence of significant environmental exposures in early childhood (1).

It is impossible to understand adult lung disease unless one clearly understands the developmental and childhood events that impact on the fully grown human organism. To this end, we begin by briefly outlining the relationship of symptoms to lung function and present a model for growth and decline of lung function throughout the life cycle. Then, we progress through each stage of human development (early childhood, later childhood and adolescence, and early adulthood and late adult life) and discuss the impact of various environmental factors and clinical conditions that impact on asthma as a disease. We conclude with a discussion of the relationship of asthma to the development of chronic obstructive pulmonary disease (COPD).

For the purposes of this chapter, asthma is defined according to the NAEP and GEENA definitions as follows: respiratory symptoms of wheeze, shortness of breath, and cough, with reversible airflow obstruction and airways responsiveness associated with a TH_2 (IL-13, IL-4, and IL-5) immune and inflammatory phenotype (2,3).

II. Relationship of Symptoms to Lung Function

Respiratory symptoms are most common at the extremes of age when lung function is lowest. It is no accident that the most common cause of death in children worldwide in the first few years of life is respiratory failure. Symptoms of wheezing are extremely common in young children, occurring in almost half of all children in the first year of life, usually in conjunction with a viral respiratory illness (4). What is less well appreciated is that symptoms are loosely correlated with lung function and are clearly less frequent if lung function (FEV_1) is higher. The relationship of symptoms to lung function, however, is not a strong correlation. In addition, symptoms have relatively low reproducibility long term. In contrast to symptoms, lung function is one of the most reproducible of all biological variables. If I know your lung function (FEV_1) today, regardless of your age, my chances of knowing your lung function in a year or 3 years is extremely high, on the order of .85–.90. This high tracking correlation for lung function makes it a very reliable index of disease severity and prognosis. This is even true for a disorder like asthma, where variation in lung function is characteristic of the disease itself. Despite the high clinical variability seen in lung function measures in asthmatics, the tracking correlations for lung function among asthmatics are not significantly different from those seen in normal people (5). It is a well-accepted truism that lung function measurements are dependent on age, height, and gender. Although this is known by all clinicians, deviation from normal and what constitutes normal variation are less well understood in the clinical community. Because of the high tracking correlation, individuals with low levels of lung function can be identified early in life and it can be shown that these individuals track along their percentile curve (Fig. 1) in such a way that individuals who begin life with low lung function tend to remain low. While environmental expo-

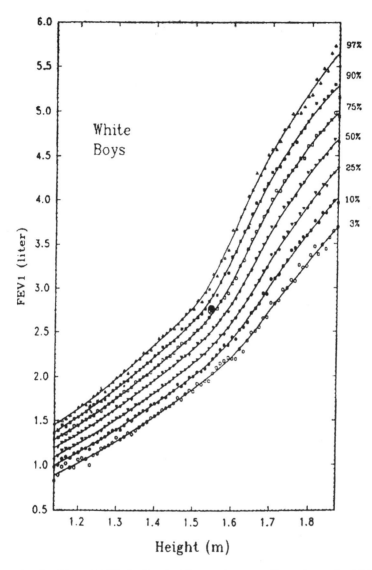

Figure 1 Tracking of FEV₁ (in liters) with growth among Caucasian male children in the Six Cities Study. Tracking curves are demonstrated for individuals starting at various percentiles of FEV₁. Extremely close tracking is demonstrated: individuals typically remain on the same tracking curve during growth and development. (From Ref. 27.)

sures will influence the variability associated with this tracking, and change it over time, their influence at any point in time will be small.

III. Growth and Decline Curve

As noted above, age, height, and gender are the three major determinants of growth of FEV_1 or lung function. Thus, there are at least three mutually independent ways that one can reach a low level of FEV_1. One can have reduced growth, premature decline, or accelerated decline in lung function. These various alternatives are presented in Fig. 2. Obviously, it is possible to combine these independent abnormal growth pathways to create even more complex patterns. For a variety of physiological reasons, airways responsiveness is strongly correlated with level of lung function. Thus, this physiological trait, which is the sine qua non of asthma, clearly impacts lung growth, premature decline, and accelerated

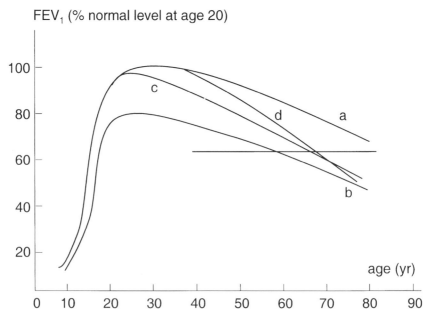

Figure 2   Hypothetical tracking curves of FEV_1 for an individual through life. The normal pattern of growth and decline in FEV_1 is shown by curve a. Significant reductions in FEV_1 can occur by (1) normal rate of decline after a reduced maximally attained FEV_1 (curve b), (2) early initiation of FEV_1 decline following normal growth (curve c); and (3) accelerated decline in FEV_1 following normal growth (curve d). (From Ref. 28.)

decline. As stated in Section II, since respiratory symptoms are correlated with level of lung function, the more symptoms one has, the lower the level of lung function, it stands to reason that with increased growth of FEV, there will be a decrease in respiratory symptoms as well as a decrease in airways responsiveness. These secular trends will contribute to a ''clinically silent period'' for asymptomatic subjects between the ages of 16 and 35 years which coincides with the plateau phase in Fig. 2. This is because the lung has tremendous physiological reserves and respiratory symptoms are only modestly correlated with lung function. The silent period will tend to obscure the importance of childhood events for adult lung disease and accentuates problems of recall bias for these early life events.

IV. Diagnosis of Asthma as a Function of Age

A. Early Childhood (Birth to Age 6)

It is now an accepted truism that asthma is first diagnosed in early childhood. It is estimated that 90% of all childhood asthma is diagnosed by the time the child reaches the age of 6. This estimate has been based on numerous population studies that have observed children prospectively (6). Perhaps the most convincing data come from Yuninger and coworkers (Fig. 3), who surveyed the population of

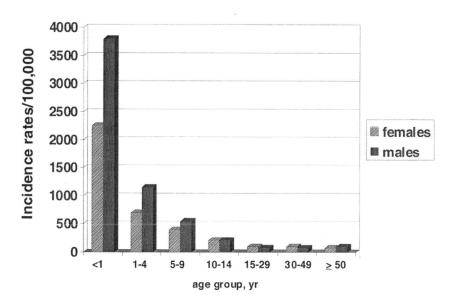

Figure 3 Annual incidence rates of asthma per 100,000 person-years, stratified by gender and age, among Rochester, Minnesota, residents between 1964 and 1983. The vast majority of asthmatic subjects are diagnosed before the age of 4 years. (From Ref. 6.)

Olmstead County, Minnesota, and asked individuals when they were diagnosed with asthma. These individual self-reports were then checked by review of the patients' medical records. Since all individuals resided in Olmstead County and received their care at the Mayo Clinic and in-migration into the county was negligible, there was an opportunity to compare prospectively collected data (the hospital records) with patient memory (self-report). It is clear that the distribution as presented in Fig. 3 from the hospital records is skewed in the direction of younger ages, and the difference between Fig. 3 and self-report can be attributed to recall bias on the part of study participants for their age of onset of disease. This suggests that in older individuals, recall bias may play a prominent role in determining when individuals report disease onset. The lack of long-term prospective studies, coupled with recall bias, creates a severely distorted picture of the natural history of asthma as a disease. To summarize this problem, 40–50% of children wheeze in the first year of life and 80–90% of all asthma is diagnosed by age 6 (7). However, respiratory symptoms are intermittent, particularly since as lung function increases, symptoms will tend to decrease. Recall of early life events before the age of 6 is relatively difficult, and hence older children and adults may not remember even significant wheezing episodes which resulted in hospitalization at an early age. Since clinicians tend to rely on symptoms rather than objective measures such as lung function, both in childhood and in adulthood, the discrepancy between symptoms and lung function can be large. Disease may appear incident in adolescence or early adulthood, when it is not truly so. The above clinical construct helps explain the relatively high prevalence of asthma intermediate phenotypes in asymptomatic adults between the ages of 16 and 35. In this age range, approximately half of all adults have skin test reactivity and about 25% will have significant methacholine airways responsiveness (8). An interaction of these intermediate phenotypes with the relevant environmental exposures will produce recrudescent (false incident) disease in the absence of knowledge of these early life events.

The magnitude of recall bias can only be assessed through longitudinal prospective studies. One such study, reported by Sears and coworkers, followed up a cohort of 713 children in Dunedin, New Zealand, who were initially seen at ages 6, 9, and 12, and looked at the presence or absence of airways responsiveness and their relationship to asthma symptoms (9). While they demonstrated a statistically significant relationship between a current diagnosis of asthma and methacholine responsiveness, what is remarkable is that almost half of the children had prior asthma that was either not reported at the current survey or was reported and had no symptoms. So roughly a quarter failed to recall their diagnosis of asthma 3 years earlier, suggesting the importance of recall bias, and in this group of prior asthmatics, which made up approximately half of all the asthma diagnoses in this preadolescent group, fully 47% of the increased airways responsiveness was seen among these individuals (Table 1). These prospective data

Table 1 Relationship Between Airways Responsiveness
and Asthma Symptoms

		Hyperresponsive	
Symptom group	*N*	*N*	%
Asymptomatic	570	21	4
Prior asthma: now			
no symptoms	28	5	14
Current wheeze	35	1	4
Prior asthma: not			
now reported	21	7	33
Current asthma	59	32	54

Note: At the initial survey, subjects were identified as having asthma
or not having asthma and were then followed up with both a questionnaire and a methacholine challenge test. At the second follow-up visit,
of 59 subjects with current asthma, 32 (54%) were also hyperresponsive
to methacholine at a PD_{20} <8 μm. Of the 49 subjects who reported
asthma at the survey 3 years earlier, 21 denied asthma in the past (43%);
significantly, 12 subjects (47%) of those without symptoms were prior
asthmatics who either did not report prior asthma or had no current
symptoms. Thus, virtually all of the increased airways responsiveness
was seen in subjects with current asthma or prior asthma.
Source: Ref. 9.

support the importance of early-childhood events and recall bias as important
factors in the natural history of asthma as a disease.

Figure 4 summarizes the dynamic nature of wheezing during the first 6
years of life and identifies a number of different groups based on symptoms that
seem to have a distinct natural history. There is a group of persistent wheezers,
who wheeze during the first year of life and also at ages 3 and 6. These persistent
wheezers are characterized by early development of allergy, cord blood eosinophilia, wheezing with lower respiratory tract infections, and a family history of
asthma and/or atopy (10). They are also characterized by lower lung function at
birth. Although this group of persistent wheezers represents a minority of the
children who wheeze in the first year of life, they represent the vast majority of
the children diagnosed with asthma at age 6, virtually all of whom are atopic
and have a parental history of asthma as a disease. Thus, certain features of
asthma and its persistence emerge, even in this early-childhood group. The
greater the duration of symptoms, the more atopy; the lower the lung function,
the more severe the disease and the more likely it is to persist. This emphasis
on the role of duration and allergies in the perpetuation of the condition seems
to be present even in early childhood. While the diagnostic label of asthma may

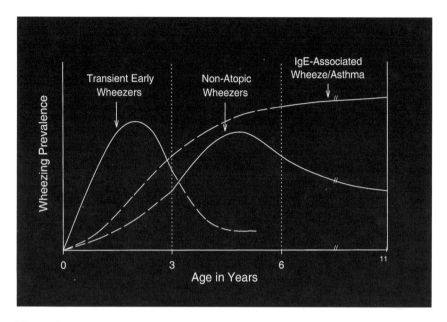

Figure 4   Histogram of wheeze prevalence vs. age. Three groups are depicted: transient early wheezers, nonatopic wheezers, and atopic wheezers. Note that these three phenotypes are not mutually exclusive. (From Ref. 29.)

be dependent on, e.g., the health care provider or health care system access, it seems clear from the epidemiological data that the atopic asthmatic can be identified at a relatively early age.

There is a second group of transient wheezers in whom the major environmental exposure seems to be in utero (e.g., tobacco smoke exposure) and who also have reduced levels of lung function (11). It is important to recognize that although this group may represent a distinct subphenotype, the exposure associated with this phenotype can also occur among asthmatics and there can be overlap between the transient early wheezer and the persistent wheezer with regard to this exposure.

Recent research has concentrated on environmental events that can influence immune system ontogeny in early life and intermediate postnatal life and may impact genetic susceptibility. In particular, interest has focused on the role of endotoxin exposure, diet, viral and bacterial infections, vaccinations, and parasitic infection and their role on immune system development (Fig. 5). It is also well known that prematurity can be a risk factor for childhood asthma, and the mechanisms by which inadequate or altered fetal lung development impacts disease is at present unclear.

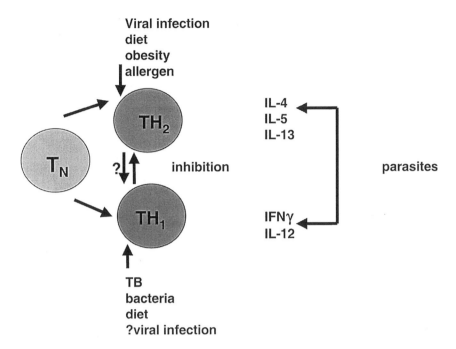

Figure 5 The importance of environmental factors in influencing immune system ontogeny. T_N cells are naive T cells that differentiate into either Th_2 or Th_1 cells in response to cytokines secreted in response to environmental exposures, as shown. (From Ref. 30.)

B. Later Childhood and Adolescence (Ages 7–16)

A significant number of children wheezing in early childhood will have their symptoms decrease or disappear in this age group. This is especially true among males. The reasons for this gender effect are unknown, but may possibly relate to the effects of female sex hormones on immune function (12). The degree of skin test reactivity and continued allergen exposure are clearly risk factors for symptom persistence in this age group (13). Allergy is one of the factors that predicts which subjects are more likely to have persistent disease. Just as in the early-childhood group, symptoms tend to beget more symptoms. It is also a clinical axiom that female asthmatics who have asthma postpuberty are unlikely to have their asthma disappear. Recently, it has been shown that obesity is one of the factors associated with asthma persistence in these young women and this may relate to increased estrogen level and hence increased effects on airways responsiveness and immune function (14).

Another important feature of this age group is experimentation with ciga-rette smoking. Active smoking at this age, even as little as one cigarette per day for as short a period of time as 3 years, can be associated with as much as a 10% reduction in maximal growth in FEV_1 (15). This very large effect of cigarette smoking during the adolescent growth spurt contrasts with much smaller effects of cigarette smoking in later adult life. Finally, the presence of other atopic dis-ease, such as atopic dermatitis or allergic rhinitis, are also factors that are associ-ated with asthma persistence in early adult life.

C. Early Adulthood (Ages 16–35)

Maximum growth in FEV_1 occurs at about age 14 in females and age 21 in males (X. Wong, personal communication, 1997). Since lung function is maximal in this period of the life cycle, symptoms are likely to be minimal and the model put forward earlier of a large group of subjects with asymptomatic airways re-sponsiveness and/or allergy who are at risk for airway inflammation with the appropriate environmental exposure is most apt. Figure 6 depicts how population

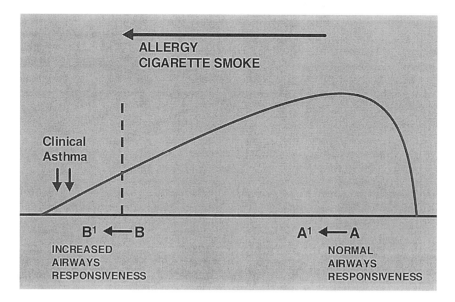

Figure 6 Schematic representation of risk for developing asthma as a function of genetic susceptibility and environmental exposures. Individuals without genetic susceptibility (A) may have some increased airways responsiveness with exposure to environmental factors such as allergic triggers and cigarette smoke (A to A[1]), but they do not cross the threshold for clinical asthma. Genetically predisposed individuals (B) can cross the threshold to develop clinical asthma (B[1]) with such environmental exposures.

distribution of airway responsiveness is log normal with individuals who could move in or out of the symptomatic range depending on their environmental exposures. Again, in this age group, the presence of persistent symptoms is associated with lower levels of lung function and more severe disease. The data from the Melbourne Study on the natural history of asthma depicted in Table 2 emphasize this (16). The symptom status at age 14 is correlated with lung function status at both ages 14 and 21, and it is clear that those people with persistent symptoms are more likely to have lower levels of lung function. This represents a progressively smaller group, as there is a secular trend for symptoms to decrease from early childhood through early adulthood as a result of lung growth. Prospective studies of individuals in this age range have demonstrated the importance of allergy, cigarette smoking, and airways responsiveness as predictors of the development of ''incident'' asthma in young adults. As noted earlier, it is likely that these are not truly ''incident'' cases and that most of these adults had symptoms and/or the development of the intermediate phenotypes at an earlier age, but now appear incident because of a long lag time since reporting prior symptoms. Dodge and coworkers studied over 1000 subjects followed for 12 years who were initially 15–19 years of age (X. Wong, personal communication, 1997). Positive skin prick tests and higher total IgE levels predicted the development of doctor's diagnosis of asthma in this cohort. Carey and coworkers studied a prospective cohort of 281 children, ages 12–18, followed for 6 years (18). Those who had a positive airway challenge test to either cold air or methacholine were almost four times more likely to wheeze at the next visit compared to nonresponsive individuals. Abramson and coworkers formed a cross-sectional study of 553 randomly selected young adults between the ages of 20 and 44 (19). A family history of asthma (OR = 2.4), current smoking (OR = 1.7), and positive skin prick test (OR = 5.9) were all independent predictors of adult asthma (19). Similar results

Table 2 Lung Function of Childhood Asthmatics at Age 21 Years

	% Predicted FEV$_1$	
Status at age 14 years	At age 14 years	At age 21 years
<5 Prior episodes of wheezing	100.2	98.4
>5 Prior episodes but none in 12 months or more	98.4	98.9
Continuing history of episodic wheezing	92.4	88.8
Very frequent or unremitting asthma	85.5	81.4

Note: Very frequent or unremitting symptoms at age 14 are associated with lower lung function both at age 14 and at follow-up (at age 21). Thus, persistent symptoms predict lower lung function, but this is not absolute.

have been found by Bodner. These data strongly support the suggestion that, in young adults, smoking is strongly associated with a diagnosis of asthma (20). In the late 1980s, Burrows reported that women with relatively little smoking history were likely to develop severe COPD (21). He noted that this fixed airflow obstruction was often associated with airways responsiveness and elevated IgE and positive skin prick tests, suggesting that fixed airflow obstruction seen in these women was a function of the asthma diathesis interacting with cigarette smoking exposure. Since there are relatively few prospective data on young adults, the relationship of smoking, airways responsiveness, and allergy in this age group is less well described than that in any other period of the life cycle.

D. Later Adult Life (Ages 37–75)

Airway responsiveness is a central feature of the asthma phenotype and is clearly associated with level of lung function. There are a number of reasons for this association. There is greater central than peripheral aerosol deposition and resistance is inversely proportional to the fourth power of the radius; thus, small changes in airway size result in large decreases in FEV_1 (22). Peripheral resistance is much greater than central resistance in asthma. At baseline, there are increases in bronchial motor tone which will be associated with lower levels of FEV_1. Finally, the methodology for expressing responsiveness is a percentage of baseline level of FEV_1 and will also accentuate these effects. Longitudinal data clearly show that increased airways responsiveness is a predictor of the occur-

Table 3 Magnitude of Effect of Increased Airways Responsiveness and Cigarette Smoking on FEV_1 Decline

Author	Airways responsiveness		Current smoking status	
	Mean (mL/year)	95% CI	Mean (mL/year)	95% CI
Frew (1989)	5.36	(0.31, 10.4)	11.6	(3.1, 19.8)
Villar (1995)	25.6	(−2.6, 53.8)	2.8	(−30.3, 35.9)
Rijcken (1995)[a]	12.5	(6.2, 18.8)	6.6[b]	(−4.7, 17.9)
O'Connor (1996)	12.8	(1.2, 24.4)	17.2	(12.54)

Note: The effect of airways responsiveness on decline in lung function varied from 5 to 25 mL/year in the different studies. In contrast, the effects of cigarette smoking on decline in lung function varied from 2.8 to 17 mL/year. Thus, both cigarette smoking and increased airways responsiveness are associated with accelerated decline in lung function in normal nonresponsive and nonsmoking subjects, and the effects between the two different factors could be deemed comparable.
[a] Males only.
[b] Current smokers of >25 cigarettes per day.

Female Smokers   Female Nonsmokers

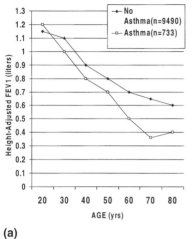
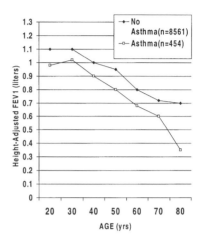

(a)

Male Smokers   Male Nonsmokers

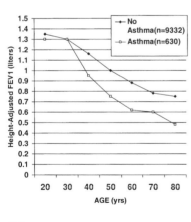
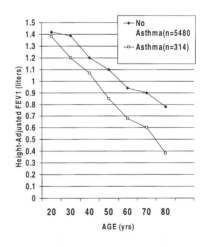

(b)

Figure 7   (a) The decline in FEV$_1$ in asthmatic and nonasthmatic female smokers and nonsmokers in the Copenhagen Heart Study. (b) The decline in FEV$_1$ in asthmatic and nonasthmatic male smokers and nonsmokers in the Copenhagen Heart Study. (From Ref. 24.)

rence of respiratory symptoms, including asthma, in adults (23). These investigators demonstrated a consistent dose/response relationship between the occurrence of asthma attacks, persistent wheezing, and shortness of breath with increased levels of airways responsiveness to histamine. A number of studies, summarized in Table 3, demonstrate that airways responsiveness antedates and precedes a decline in lung function after controlling for baseline level of FEV_1. The magnitude of these effects of increased airways responsiveness on decline in FEV_1 are comparable to the effects of current cigarette smoking. Only two studies have looked at the effects of asthma on decline in FEV_1. Lange and coworkers performed a prospective cohort study (24). They studied 17,506 subjects, who were followed for 28 years, from 1976 to 1994. Asthmatic decline in FEV_1 was 38 ml/year while the decline in FEV_1 in nonasthmatics was 22 mL/year, a difference of 16 mL/year (24). In addition, the rate of decline was greater in asthmatics who were also smokers (Fig. 7). The only other study examining the effects of adult asthma on decline in lung function was a nested case control study performed in the Busselton Cohort. Ninety-two asthma cases were matched with 186 normal controls. There was an 18-year follow-up. Asthmatic decline in FEV_1 was 50 mL/year; nonasthmatic decline was 35 mL/year, a difference of 25 mL/year. There were insufficient cigarette smokers in this study to assess the effect of cigarette smoking in addition to asthma (25). These data convincingly demonstrate that asthma is associated with an accelerated decline in FEV_1. What remains unclear is the extent to which asthma contributes to the development of chronic obstructive pulmonary disease.

V. Relationship of Asthma to Chronic Obstructive Pulmonary Disease

Existing data clearly support the relationship of asthma and airways responsiveness to accelerated decline, reduced growth, premature decline, and accelerated decline in lung function. There is also the suggestion that airways responsiveness may define the smoker who is susceptible to the development of COPD. In the Lung Health Study, airways responsiveness was demonstrated in most of the early-onset COPD cases, in both men and women, but was particularly prevalent in women. Individuals with increased airways responsiveness who continued to smoke had the most significant declines in lung function (Figs. 8A and 8B; Taskin et al.). In addition, recent population-based evidence has shown that airways responsiveness predicts mortality from COPD, as individuals with histamine airways responsiveness less than 16 mg/mL showed a 4- to 20-fold increase in COPD mortality 25 years later (26). While case series studies of COPD patients clearly show that 60–80% of COPD patients have increased airways responsiveness and that airways responsiveness clearly predicts accelerated decline in

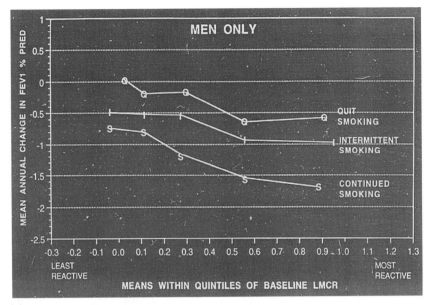

(a)

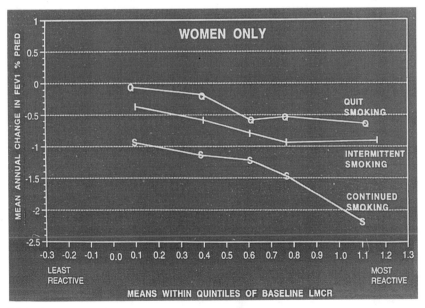

(b)

Figure 8 (a) The decline in FEV_1 plotted against the log of the methacholine challenge dose in males in the Lung Health Study stratified by smoking status. (b) Similar results for females are plotted. (From Ref. 31.)

mortality among COPD patients, these studies do not adjust for baseline level of lung function, nor do they consider a prior diagnosis of asthma as a factor influencing either FEV_1 decline or COPD mortality. Nevertheless, these data do provide increased evidence that asthma and airways responsiveness may define the phenotype of the smoker susceptible to the development of COPD.

VI. Summary

It would appear that family history of asthma, early development of atopy, other atopic diseases (e.g., allergic rhinitis and eczema), female gender, and persistent symptoms are the clinical characteristics of more severe and persistent asthma in childhood. Coupled with later cigarette smoking, there is a high risk of developing severe asthma and fixed airflow obstruction in mid-adult life. What remains to be established is how the immunological phenotype changes with aging and how this influences the development of airway wall remodeling and fixed airflow obstruction. There is the suggestion that the greater the duration and severity of childhood atopic asthma, the greater the likelihood of intrinsic asthma as an adult. This suggests that the immune phenotype of the nonsmoking asthmatic may change to develop a more autonomous type of airway inflammation, independent of allergen exposure. In order to prove this hypothesis, longitudinal data assessing immune phenotypes directly will be necessary, and as yet we still lack clear, nonevasive markers to assess airway inflammation.

The final difficulty is our inability to follow a large number of childhood asthmatics into adult life, and thus follow the natural history of airflow obstruction in this cohort, to allow us to fully predict and link childhood events to those of later adulthood. It is likely that large-scale, longitudinal studies of childhood asthma such as the Childhood Asthma Management Program (CAMP) should aid in our knowledge of the natural history of asthma and how current treatments modify that history.

References

1. Thurlbeck WM. Aspects of chronic airflow obstruction. Chest 1977; 77:341–349.
2. Expert Panel Report 2: Guidelines for the Diagnosis and Management of Asthma. US Department of Health and Human Services Report 98-4051. Washington, DC: National Asthma Education Program, 1998.
3. NHLBI/WHO Workshop Report: Global Initiative for Asthma National Institutes of Health. Report 95-3659. Geneva: WHO, 1995.
4. Martinez FD, Wright AL, Taussig LM, Holberg CJ, Halonen M, Morgen WJ. Asthma and wheezing in the first six years of life. N Engl J Med 1995; 332:133–138.

5. Rijcken B, Schouten J, Weiss ST, Rosner B, de Vries K, van der Lende R. Long-term variability of bronchial responsiveness to histamine in a random population sample of adults. Am Rev Respir Dis 1993; 148:944–949.

6. Yunginger JW, Reed CE, O'Connell EJ, Melton LJ, O'Fallon WM, Silverstein MD. A community based study of the epidemiology of asthma. Am Rev Respir Dis 1992; 146:888–894.

7. Gold DR, Burge HA, Carey V, Milton DK, Platts-Mills T, Weiss ST. Predictors of repeated wheeze in the first year of life: the relative roles of birth weight, acute lower respiratory illness, and maternal smoking. Am J Respir Crit Care Med 1999; 160:227–236.

8. Weiss ST, Sparrow D, eds. Airways Responsiveness and Atopy in the Development of the Obstructive Airways Disease. New York: Raven Press, 1989.

9. Sears MR, Burrows B, Flannery EM, Herbison GP, Hewitt CJ, Holdaway MD. Relation between airway responsiveness and serum IgE in children with asthma and apparently normal children. N Engl J Med 1991; 325:1067–1071.

10. Wright AL, Sherrill D, Holberg CJ, Halonen M, Martinez FD. Breast-feeding, maternal IgE, and total serum IgE in childhood. J Allergy Clin Immunol 1999; 104:589–594.

11. Martinez FD. Role of respiratory infection in onset of asthma and chronic obstructive pulmonary disease. Clin Exp Allergy 1999; 54(suppl 49):24–28.

12. Weiss ST, Segal MR, Tager IB, Tosteson T, Redline S, Speizer FE. Effects of asthma on pulmonary function in children: a longitudinal population-based study. Am Rev Respir Dis 1992; 145:58–64.

13. Zeiger RS, Dawson C, Weiss ST, Childhood Asthma Management Program (CAMP) Research Group. Relationship between duration of asthma and asthma severity among children in the Childhood Asthma Management Program (CAMP). J Allergy Clin Immunol 1999; 103:376–387.

14. Casto-Rodriguez JA, Holberg CJ, Morgan WJ, Martinez FD, Wright AL. Weight and early puberty are risk factors for increased wheezing in females. Am J Respir Crit Care Med 2000; 161:A498.

15. Tager IB, Munoz A, Rosner B, Weiss ST, Carey V, Speizer FE. Effect of cigarette smoking on the pulmonary function of children and adolescents. Am Rev Respir Dis 1985; 131:752–759.

16. Kelly WJW, Hudson I, et al. Childhood asthma and adult lung function. Am Rev Respir Dis 1988; 138:26–30.

17. Dodge R, Cline MG, Lebowitz MD, Burrows B. Findings before the diagnosis of asthma in young adults. J Allergy Clin Immunol 1994; 94:831–835.

18. Carey VJ, Weiss ST, Tager IB, Leeder SR, Speizer FE. Airway responsiveness, wheeze onset, and recurrent asthma episodes in young adolescents: The East Boston Childhood Respiratory Disease Cohort. Am J Respir Crit Care Med 1996; 153:356–361.

19. Abramson M, Kutin JJ, Raven J, Lanigan A, Czarny D, Walters EH. Risk factors for asthma among young adults in Melbourne, Australia. Respirology 1996; 1:291–297.

20. Bodner CH, Ross S, Little J, Douglas JG, Legge JS, Friend JA, Godden DJ. Risk factors for adult onset wheeze: a case control study. Am J Respir Crit Care Med 1998; 157:35–42.

21. Burrows B, Bloom JW, Traver GA, Cline MG. The course and prognosis of different forms of chronic airway obstruction in a sample from the general population. N Engl J Med 1987; 317:1309–1314.

22. O'Connor G, Sparrow D, Weiss ST. The role of allergy and nonspecific airway hyperresponsiveness in the pathogenesis of chronic obstructive pulmonary disease. Am Rev Respir Dis 1989; 140:225–252.

23. Xu X, Rijcken B, Schouten JP, Weiss ST. Airway responsiveness and development and remission of chronic respiratory symptoms in adults. Lancet 1997; 350:1431–1434.

24. Lange P, Parner J, Vestbo J, Schnohr P, Jensen G. A 15-year follow-up study of ventilatory function in adults with asthma. N Engl J Med 1998; 339:1194–1200.

25. Peat JK, Woolcook AJ, Cullen K. Rate of decline of lung function in subjects with asthma. Eur J Respir Dis 1987; 70:171–179.

26. Hospers JJ, Postma DS, Schouten JP, Weiss ST, Rijcken B. Histamine airway hyper-responsiveness predicts mortality from COPD in a general population sample. Lancet. In press.

27. Wang X, Dockery DW, Wypij D, Fay ME, Ferris BG Jr. Pulmonary function between 6 and 18 years of age. Pediatr Pulmonol 1993; 15:75–88.

28. Rijcken, B. Bronchial Responsiveness and COPD Risk: an Epidemiological Study. Postdoctoral dissertation.

29. Stein RT, Holberg CJ, Morgan WJ, Wright AL, Lombardi E, Taussig L, Martinez FD. Peak flow variability, methacholine responsiveness and atopy as markers for detecting different wheezing phenotypes in childhood. Thorax 1997; 52:946–952.

30. Cookson WO, Moffatt MF. Asthma: an epidemic in the absence of infection? Science 1997; 275:41–42.

31. Tashkin DP, Altose MD, Connett JE, Kanner RE, Lee WW, Wise RA. Methacholine reactivity predicts changes in lung function over time in smokers with early chronic obstructive pulmonary disease: The Lung Health Study Research Group. Am J Respir Crit Care Med 1996; 153:1802–1811.

2

Genetic Influences on Asthma Severity

JOHN W. HOLLOWAY, STEUART RORKE, BIANCA BEGHÉ,
and STEPHEN T. HOLGATE

Southampton General Hospital
University of Southampton
Southampton, England

I. Introduction

In recent years asthma-related morbidity and mortality have increased globally. In the northern area of Spain the average total annual asthma–derived cost was estimated at US$2879 per patient, with costs increasing according to the grade of severity to as much as US$6393 per patient in the case of severe asthma (1). Given the social and economic impact of severe asthma, it is essential that the underlying determinants of asthma severity are understood. It is well established that there is a strong genetic component underlying susceptibility to asthma, but few studies have addressed whether there are genetic factors that modify severity of disease. While there is some evidence that severity of asthma is heritable, and association between measures of severity and polymorphism in candidate genes have been identified, the identification of genetic factors contributing to asthma severity has been hampered by the lack of clear, easily applied, accurate phenotype definitions for asthma severity that distinguish between underlying severity and level of therapeutic control. The development of such phenotypes in conjunction with more extensive studies of the genetics of asthma severity may allow identification of at-risk individuals and targeting of prophylactic therapy.

II. Phenotypes for Measuring Asthma Severity

Diseases such as asthma that involve the interaction of multiple genetic and environmental effects are termed complex genetic diseases. Studies of the genetic basis of such diseases can be carried out using either complex phenotypes, such as affection status, or intermediate phenotypes that can be measured objectively. The advantage of using complex phenotypes is that all genes contributing to the disease susceptibility can be identified, although the contribution of each gene to the overall phenotype is small, reducing the power of any study. By using intermediate phenotypes, there are fewer genetic and environmental influences on the phenotype, and consequently power to identify genes is higher. However, genetic influences on intermediate phenotypes may not always influence the complex phenotype being considered.

Analysis of the genetic basis of any complex trait depends on accurate phenotyping. It is the lack of a clear definition of asthmatic phenotypes that presents the biggest problem when reviewing studies of the genetic basis of asthma due to multiple definitions of the same phenotype being used in different studies. The same confusion as to appropriate phenotype definition applies when considering studies of asthma severity.

Asthma is a respiratory disease characterized by recurrent respiratory symptoms, reversible variable airway obstruction, airway inflammation, and increased airway responsiveness (2). Asthma can be defined in several ways, using subjective measures (e.g., symptoms), objective measures [e.g., serum IgE level or bronchial hyperresponsiveness (BHR)], or both. In addition, the use of quantitative phenotypes, such as those developed by Lawrence et al. where all information gathered on an individual is used to derive a quantitative score, may also be useful (3). The use of such scores achieves several things: (a) all phenotypic information, including intermediate phenotypes, are used and therefore the score is more informative than a complex dichotomous trait such as affection status; (b) the problem of individuals with ''probable'' asthma is effectively dealt with, as the whole population is used; and (c) a quantitative measure such as a score allows the use of more powerful methods of quantitative trait loci (QTL) analysis for identifying disease genes.

At present there is no agreement among asthma consensus panels on methods for categorizing asthma severity. The lack of a gold standard to assess asthma severity has resulted in a failure to develop a simple severity index that could be used in both clinical and epidemiological settings as well as in genetic studies. Throughout the literature there seems to be confusion in differentiating between asthma control and asthma severity. These two concepts are not synonymous and differentiating between them is essential in categorizing patients correctly in terms of management, clinical trials, and epidemiological research. For example, most severe asthmatics may be well controlled on anti-inflammatory medication in terms of symptoms and objective physiologic measures. In contrast, patients with poorly controlled asthma having a moderate to severe exacerbation may be easy to treat with small amounts of inhaled corticosteroids and therefore their overall asthma severity would be classified as mild (4).

There are many terms used to describe the severity of asthma. Clinical severity may describe the patient with chronic persistent symptoms who experiences an impaired quality of life or may describe life-threatening asthma exacerbations. Variables that have been used traditionally include symptoms, frequency of attacks, hospitalization, glucocorticosteroid treatment, and basal FEV_1 (forced expiratory volume in 1 sec) (5). Lung function between attacks is also considered an important objective measure of severity. In the early 1980s the first classification of asthmatics into subgroups according to symptom frequency and severity was derived (6). The current UK guidelines on asthma management define severity in terms of the treatment needed to control symptoms, maintain lung function, and allow normal life (7). This definition seems plausible, as overall asthma severity in terms of treatment use can be correctly assessed under controlled conditions. The National Asthma Education and Prevention Program (NAEPP) Expert Panel II Guidelines (8) categorize asthma severity according to daytime symptoms, nocturnal asthma symptoms, and physiological measures of lung function. This set of guidelines is a significant improvement on the first set of guidelines published in 1991, as they were simplified into a severity index of only four variables that could be used for clinical and epidemiological purposes. However, this simple and widely used set of guidelines quantifies severity based solely on symptoms and physiological measures of lung function. This type of severity index makes the separation of severity from the lack of asthma control difficult, increasing the chance of incorrect categorization. Current symptoms probably reflect more the level of control and treatment efficacy rather than disease severity. Previous studies have emphasized the poor correlation between reported symptoms and objective measures of lung function (4,9–10), thereby illustrating that reported symptoms alone probably do not reflect the underlying disease severity. One phenotyping system previously reported that does show a good correlation with disease severity as assessed by specialists is the computer-based expert system (11). However, it seems far too complex and impractical for clinical practice. To determine the genetic influence, if any, on asthma severity, it is necessary to develop a phenotypic model that can comprehensively assess asthma severity. This model should be able to distinguish between severe asthma and poorly controlled asthma, thereby dissecting out the genetic contribution to severity. In addition it should be easy to implement in the context of large epidemiological and genetic studies. Recently, we have screened a large family cohort consisting of 342 families with at least two affected siblings using a health survey questionnaire including 10 questions related to severity. This detailed clinical questionnaire was based on that derived by the Medical Research Council (MRC),

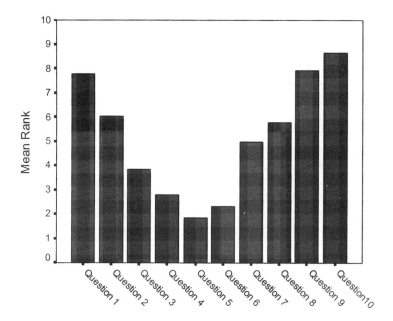

Question 1	wheezing or whistling in the chest
Question 2	wheezing or whistling in the chest in the last 12 months
Question 3	how many attacks of wheezing in the last 12 months
Question 4	sleep disturbed due to wheezing
Question 5	speech limited due to wheezing
Question 6	night in the hospital due to asthma
Question 7	chest sounded wheezy during or after exercise
Question 8	dry cough at night in the last 12 months
Question 9	cough first thing in the morning during winter
Question 10	bring phlegm from your chest during winter

Figure 1   Bar chart illustrating the expert panel response to the health survey questionnaire. Each bar represents the mean rank response for each question in terms of asthma severity.

American Thoracic Society (ATS), and International Union Against Tuberculosis and Lung Disease (IUALTD) and contained questions from the International Society of Asthma and Allergy in Children (ISAAC). In order to assess the response of the family members to the health survey in terms of asthma severity, the same questionnaire was sent to a random selection of experienced professionals in the field of asthma and allergy. They were asked to evaluate the questions as indicators of severity (a) scoring them from 1 (very important) to 4 (unimportant) and (b) ranking them in order of importance from 1 to 10 (Fig. 1).

One hundred seventy-four chest physicians, 118 general practitioners, 134 respiratory nurse specialists, and 36 pediatric respiratory consultants replied to the postal survey. The order of importance of the 10 questions was identical when analyzing both the mean score and mean rank of each question. Since these two measures were identical the expert panel illustrated consistent decision making in terms of choosing the most important severity marker. Four questions were assessed as being important indicators of severity, three of these being symptoms and the remaining question being "night spent in hospital due to asthma." By using this method we were able to assess the importance of each question asked in assessing severity, through the pooling of clinical experience. This would enable the formulation of one of the components of a severity score.

At present there is no specific phenotype to define the genetic contribution to asthma severity. Cockroft's suggestion (4) that asthma severity be defined by the minimum therapeutic intervention needed to achieve control rather than by objective measures of lung function and symptoms is a valid definition. However, the ideal asthma severity score needs to incorporate four components, namely (1) the three cardinal symptoms as assessed by our health survey (Fig. 1); (2) hospitalization; (3) objective lung function measures (FEV_1 %predicted); and (4) therapy, including current control (glucocorticosteroids) and escape therapy (β_2-agonists). This model will enable the assessment of overall asthma severity at any point during the natural course of the disease and provide the clinician and researcher with a robust phenotype to utilize in genetic studies of asthma severity.

III. Is Asthma Severity Heritable?

It is widely accepted that asthma is a heritable disease and a number of studies have shown an increased prevalence of asthma, and phenotypes associated with asthma, among the relatives of asthmatic subjects compared to nonasthmatic subjects (12–14). Numerous twin studies (15–17) have shown a significant increase in concordance of asthma among monozygotic twins compared to dizygotic twins, providing evidence for a genetic component to asthma susceptibility. However, asthma is a complex disease in which the interaction between both genetic and environmental factors plays a fundamental role both in the pathogenesis and in the development of the disease. In population-based twin studies the estimated effect of genetic factors on disease susceptibility is about 35–70%, depending on the population and the design of the study (18). In a recent study using a twin-family model, Laitinen and co-workers have reported that in families with asthma in successive generations, genetic factors alone explained as much as 87% of the development of asthma in offspring. The incidence of asthma in twins with affected parents was increased fourfold compared to the incidence in twins without affected parents, suggesting that it is more likely that asthma is recurring in families due to shared genes rather than shared environmental risk factors (19).

So while it is apparent that susceptibility to asthma has a heritable component, it is unclear whether there is a separate genetic component that modifies the severity of the disease. Very few studies of the heritability of asthma have examined phenotypes relating to asthma severity. Sarafino et al. (20) studied 39 monozygotic twin pairs and 55 same-sex dizygotic twin pairs for heritability of asthma and asthma severity. They examined asthma severity (as measured by frequency and intensity of asthmatic episodes) in twin pairs concordant for asthma. They found that severity was significantly correlated for monozygotic pairs but not for dizygotic pairs. In contrast, a more recent study by Sarafino (21) examined the family prevalence of atopy and atopic diseases, including asthma. In this study, although the prevalence of asthma in children of parents with asthma was significantly increased when compared to children whose parents did not have asthma (55% vs. 29% for the eldest child), when the severity of a child's asthma was compared to that of the parents, there was no correlation between the severity of the child's asthma and either the severity of the parents' asthma or number of parents with asthma.

There have been several other studies of familial correlation with asthma severity. A large epidemiological study (661 children and their parents) of family patterns of asthma and airways hyperresponsiveness (AHR) (22) identified a modest correlation between severity of parents' AHR and those of the child ($R = 0.51$, $P = 0.04$). Wilson et al. identified that a positive family history of asthma was the only significant predictor of asthma severity in a study of children age 5 with a history of severe wheeze in childhood (23). Togias et al., in a study of factors relating to asthma and severity in adolescents, concluded that genetic factors may contribute to severity by altering susceptibility to environmental factors, such as sensitization to allergens.

IV. Linkage and Association Studies of Asthma Severity

The concept of genes interacting to alter the effects of mutations in susceptibility genes is not unknown. A number of genetic disorders caused by mutations in single genes are known to exhibit inter- and intrafamilial variability (24). A proportion of interfamilial variability can be explained by differences in environmental factors and differences in effect of different mutations in the same gene. However, intrafamilial variability, especially in siblings, cannot be so readily accredited to these types of mechanisms. There is now increasing evidence that many genetic disorders are influenced by "modifier" genes that are distinct from the disease susceptibility locus. For example, not all individuals with insulin-dependent diabetes mellitus (IDDM) develop diabetic nephropathy, but the relative risk of this complication is increased twofold in relatives of IDDM patients with nephropathy (25).

The identification of such modifier genes in asthma is difficult due to the complex interactions between susceptibility, environment, and treatment. In addition, it is possible that disease severity is merely one end of a normal distribution, reflecting the cumulative number of disease susceptibility genes an individual has inherited along with the environmental influences they have been subjected to. If this is the case, it may be a mistake to separate studies of disease severity from susceptibility. In this situation defining asthma as a quantitative trait encompassing both affected and unaffected individuals rather than a dichotomous one may be more appropriate. By using such an asthma score, severity of disease is taken into account as well as susceptibility. Thus genes contributing to both susceptibility and severity can be identified.

Several genome-wide screens for asthma susceptibility genes have been completed which have identified a large number of loci linked to both complex

Table 1 Summary of Studies of Polymorphisms in Candidate and Association with Measures of Asthma Severity

Gene	Polymorphism	Associated phenotype	Reference
Interleukin-4 (IL-4)	C-589T	$FEV_1 < 50\%$	(41)
		Fatal/near-fatal asthma	(43)
	Intron-2 repeat	Asthma severity (NAEPP)	(42)
Interleukin-4 receptor-α (IL-4RA)	Q576R	Asthma severity (NAEPP)	(53)
		Severe airway obstruction	(43)
$β_2$-Adrenergic receptor (ADR-$β_2$)	R16G	Nocturnal asthma	(58)
		Steroid-dependent asthma	(66)
		Severe asthma	(67)
		Not associated with fatal/near-fatal asthma	(87)
Tumor necrosis factor-α (TNF-α)	A-308G	Not associated with fatal/near-fatal asthma	(76)
Leukotriene C$_4$ synthase (LTC4S)	A-444C	Aspirin-intolerant asthma (AIA)	(88)

phenotypes (asthma and atopy) as well as intermediate traits (BHR and total IgE levels) (26–31). However, the results of the genome-wide screens for asthma susceptibility genes reflect the genetic and environmental heterogeneity seen in asthma, in that while some regions have shown linkage in several studies, most show linkage in only one or two studies, even when these are undertaken in similar population groups. This illustrates the difficulty of identifying susceptibility genes for complex genetic diseases. Different genetic loci will show linkage in populations of differing ethnicity and differing environmental exposure. Identifying the gene(s) underlying the linkage observed is therefore a major challenge. Despite the huge effort that has been put into identifying susceptibility genes in these genome scans and also in linkage studies of candidate regions, none of these studies have examined linkage with measures of asthma severity. However, a number of studies of candidate genes have looked for association with measures of asthma severity (Table 1).

A. Interleukin-4 (IL-4) and the Interleukin-4 Receptor α-Chain (IL-4RA)

There are a number of genes on chromosome 5q31-33 that may be important in the development or progression of inflammation associated with atopy and atopic disease. These include the genes for the cytokines IL-3, IL-4, IL-5, IL-9, IL-12 (β-chain), IL-13, and GM-CSF. Linkage analysis of markers in 5q31–33 has provided evidence for a gene or genes that contribute to both atopy and asthma (32–37). The Collaborative Study on the Genetics of Asthma (CSGA) genomewide scan also found linkage of asthma to 5q in Caucasian families (27).

IL-4 plays an essential role in the atopic immune response, as it induces IgE synthesis in B cells and differentiation to a Th2 phenotype in T cells. This makes the IL-4 gene itself, or factors which regulate its expression, strong candidate genes for both atopy and asthma. Rosenwasser et al. identified an IL-4 promoter polymorphism (a C to T substitution at −589 bp from the open reading frame), which was in association with high serum IgE levels and was shown to increase the transcriptional levels of the IL-4 gene (38). However, Walley et al. examined two large populations, 230 nuclear families from Australia, and 124 unrelated atopic asthmatics and 59 unrelated nonatopic, nonasthmatic controls from the UK. They found only a weak association of this polymorphism to wheeze and specific IgE to house dust mite in the Australian population while no association with any measure of asthma or atopy was found in the UK population (39). In addition, Noguchi et al. studied two populations, families ascertained through an asthmatic child and a randomly ascertained population, and found no significant difference in the prevalence of the polymorphism between the two groups. They saw no difference in total or specific IgE levels, whether the individual was homozygous for the C allele or heterozygous or homozygous for the T allele. However, using the transmission disequilibrium test to look at association within families, a significant association between the T allele and asthma was found (40).

Several groups have examined the role of IL-4 polymorphisms in determining asthma severity. In a study of a large cohort of 772 asthmatic patients, Burchard et al. examined the association between IL-4 C-589T polymorphism and FEV_1 in the absence of asthma treatment as an indicator of severity (41). The subjects in the study were enrolled as part of a trial of a new asthma medication and under the study criteria were not taking oral or inhaled corticosteroids, had not been admitted to hospital for treatment of asthma for at least 6 months, and had to have a FEV_1 of 60–80% in the absence of β-agonist treatment in the previous 8 h. As such, the cohort can be considered moderate to severe asthmatics; however, by definition this cohort excludes the most severe asthmatics following a corticosteroid regimen. Usually FEV_1 represents a poor marker of severity in epidemiological studies as only a single measurement is made and the effects of treatment greatly influence it. However, in this study FEV_1 was measured in the absence of treatment for asthma; therefore it may be a more accurate reflection of asthma severity than in most cohorts recruited for epidemiological and genetic studies where treatment is not withdrawn prior to assessment. In Caucasian subjects, individuals with the TT genotype had a significantly lower mean FEV_1 and were more likely to have an FEV_1 below 50% of predicted (OR = 1.44, P = 0.013); this difference was not seen in African-American patients. However, the significance of the C-589T polymorphism in regulating asthma severity is questionable, as the authors calculated that the IL-4 C-589T polymorphism accounted for only 0.06% of the variation in FEV_1.

Couchane et al. have also investigated whether IL-4 polymorphism is associated with asthma severity (42). In a cohort of 145 Tunisian patients and 160 healthy controls, asthma severity was assessed in relation to the American Thoracic Society guidelines, with patients being divided into mild and moderate/severe groups. Mild asthmatics were characterized by a frequency of symptoms less than once a day and an FEV_1 >80%. The moderate/severe group included patients with daily or continual symptoms, frequent exacerbations, nighttime symptoms, and an FEV_1 <80%. Analysis of a microsatellite repeat in intron 2 of IL-4 showed that the A1 allele was associated with asthma. In addition the A1/A3 genotype was strongly associated with asthma severity (RR = 3.94, P < 0.001) while the A3/A3 genotype frequency was significantly reduced in the severe asthma group (RR = 0.165, P < 0.001).

Sandford and colleagues, in a study of fatal and near-fatal asthmatics, also found a weak association between the IL-4 C-589T polymorphism and asthma severity (43). In this study, the frequency of the polymorphism in 130 subjects who had had fatal asthma attacks and 27 subjects who had had near-fatal attacks was compared to that in a group of 90 mild/moderate asthmatics and 143 nonasthmatics. The frequency of the IL-5489T allele was significantly increased in subjects with fatal or near-fatal asthma ($P = 0.02$), but was not associated with asthma per se. However, unlike the study of Burchard et al., there was no association with FEV_1, although this may be due to lack of power due to the small sample size. Another possibility is that the use of asthma death or near-fatal asthma attacks as a measure of severity may identify a different subgroup of patients from those with chronic severe asthma. Fatal or near-fatal attacks may result from poor asthma control rather than chronicity and there is a subgroup of asthma patients with "brittle asthma," who are subject to repeated life-threatening attacks. The genetic factors predisposing to these phenotypes may be different from those influencing long-term chronicity.

IL-4 elicits its biological effects by binding to the IL-4 receptor (IL-4R) (44). The IL-4 receptor is composed of two subunits: an α-subunit required for IL-4 binding and signal transduction and a γ-subunit common to several cytokine receptors (45). The IL-4Rα gene is located on chromosome 16p(16p12.1) (46) and Deichmann et al., using four microsatellite markers flanking the IL-4Rα gene, found a significant linkage with specific sensitization to common inhalant allergens in atopic families, underlying the significance of IL-4Rα as a candidate gene for atopy (47).

Several polymorphisms leading to amino acid substitutions have been identified in the IL-4Rα gene (48). An extracellular variant of IL-4Rα chain consisting of a substitution of valine at amino acid 50 for isoleucine (I50V) has been shown to up-regulate receptor response to IL-4 with an increased STAT6 activation, CD23 expression, and increased IgE synthesis. The I50 allele has also been found to be associated with atopy (measured as total IgE and mite-specific IgE) and atopic asthma (49–50).

Another polymorphism in the intracellular domain of IL-4Rα, Q576R, has been shown to enhance signaling of the IL-4R, resulting in increased CD23 expression, and has been shown to be associated with hyper IgE syndrome and severe atopic eczema (51). Q576R, located in the STAT6 binding region, is adjacent to the tyrosine residue (Y575) that binds to SHP-1, a phosphotyrosine phosphatase involved in signal termination. Q576R may alter the binding of SHP-1 to phosphorylated Y575, leading to increased signaling (51). However, Krause and co-workers, investigating four polymorphisms of IL-4Rα, including Q576R, and their association with atopic phenotypes, found that Q576R is associated with lowered total IgE levels and that this effect is magnified by the simultaneous presence of another polymorphism, S503P, located in the I4R motif. While the presence of S503P alone does not influence signal transduction it is possible that the presence of both polymorphisms (S503P/Q576R) may alter the receptor's conformation and charge, abolishing the propagation of IL-4 signals leading to decreased B-cell proliferation and IgE synthesis. Conversely, a recent study showed that Q576R does not have a direct effect on IL-4 signal transduction (52). Further functional studies are required to establish the mechanisms through which these polymorphisms may alter the IL-4Rα signaling and predispose to atopy and asthma. Two studies have examined the role of the Q576R polymorphism in asthma severity. The frequency of Q576R has been examined in a cohort of 149 asthmatics categorized into mild (>80% FEV_1), moderate (60–80%), and severe (<60%) according to the NAEPP Guidelines (8). The R576 allele was shown to be associated with asthma severity as well as susceptibility to asthma when compared to nonallergic nonasthmatic controls (53). The study of fatal/near-fatal asthmatics by Sandford et al. (43) also examined association with the Q576R polymorphism. In this cohort R576 was also associated with more severe airway obstruction using the same categories, but no association was seen with fatal/near-fatal asthma.

All of these studies indicate that polymorphism of IL-4 or its signaling pathway may contribute to asthma severity. The mechanism whereby this happens, however, is still unclear. It is possible that increased susceptibility and severity of atopic immune responses may predispose to asthma severity, as atopy is a risk factor for a number of markers of asthma severity. However, it is also possible that polymorphisms of IL-4 signaling may influence airway remodeling and fibrosis and therefore directly affect the severity of asthma. Overexpression of IL-13 in the bronchial epithelium of mice causes lymphocyte and eosinophil infiltration, goblet cell metaplasia, subepithelial fibrosis, and smooth muscle proliferation associated with marked BHR (54). Conversely, when STAT6 (55) or both IL-4 and IL-13 (56) are deleted, antigen-induced BHR and goblet cell metaplasia are ablated along with the expected inhibition of Th-2 functions and IgE synthesis. Increased production of IL-4 and IL-13 may lead either directly to subepithelial fibrosis by activation of (myo-)fibroblasts or indirectly through enhanced expression of transforming growth factor (TGF-β) by the bronchial epithelium. Recent studies of primary bronchial epithelial cells from asthmatics have shown that both IL-4 and IL-13 can induce TGF-β secretion (57).

B. The β₂-Adrenergic Receptor

It has long been hypothesized that a defective β₂-adrenergic receptor (β₂AR) may be a pathogenic factor in asthma, and a linkage between BHR and markers on chromosome 5q around the β₂AR has previously been identified (34). The β₂AR is highly polymorphic, with the two most common polymorphisms being at amino acid 16 (R16G) and amino acid 27 (Q27E) (58). Studies in vitro have shown that the Gly16 variant increases down-regulation of the β₂AR after exposure to a β₂-agonist; by contrast the Glu27 polymorphism appears to protect against agonist-induced down-regulation and desensitization of the β₂-adrenoreceptor (59–60).

While it is unclear whether these polymorphisms contribute to asthma or atopy susceptibility (61–65), a number of studies have indicated that polymorphisms of the β₂AR may influence asthma severity. The frequency of the Gly16 polymorphism has been shown to be increased in patients with nocturnal asthma (66) and in steroid-dependent asthmatics (58). Furthermore, in a recent study of the frequency of the R16G and Q27E polymorphisms in 95 severe asthmatics from New Zealand, the Gly16 polymorphism was significantly associated with asthma severity, with odds ratios (95% CI) for the Gly16 allele being 1.56 (1.02–2.40, $P = 0.04$) for the severe asthma group (67). In contrast, a study by Weir et al. on the same cohort of fatal/near-fatal and mild/moderate asthmatics described above showed that neither the Gly16 or Gln27 alleles nor the Gly16/Gl27 haplotype had an increased frequency in the fatal asthma group.

When assessing asthma severity it is important to consider that apparent severity may also result from either poor treatment or poor response to treatment. Polymorphisms in genes that reduce response to a particular therapy for asthma may result in increased severity of a patient's disease by reducing control. This would then lead to such a polymorphism being associated with measures of severity. As well as in vitro studies that have shown effects of β_2AR polymorphism on agonist-induced down-regulation and desensitization of the β_2-adrenoreceptor (59–60), clinical studies have shown that β_2AR polymorphisms influence the response to bronchodilator treatment. Asthmatic patients carrying Gly16 have been shown to be more prone to develop a bronchodilator desensitization (68), while children homozygotes and heterozygotes for Arg16 are more likely to show positive responses to bronchodilators (69). However, some studies have shown that response to bronchodilator treatment is genotype independent (70–71).

In a study of 190 asthmatics, Israel et al. examined whether β_2AR genotype affects the response to regular versus as-needed albuterol use (72). During a 16-week treatment period they found that there was a small but significant decline in morning peak flow in patients homozygous for the Arg16 polymorphism who used albuterol regularly. The effect was magnified during the 4-week run-out period, when all patients returned to albuterol as needed with Arg16 homozygotes on regular albuterol having a morning peak flow 30.5 ± 12.1 L/min lower than Arg16 homozygotes who took albuterol only as needed ($P = 0.012$). These findings are difficult to explain in light of the studies above linking the Gly16 allele with BHR, β_2-agonist effectiveness, and asthma severity.

C. Tumor Necrosis Factor-α

Tumor necrosis factor-α (TNF-α) is a cytokine involved in both airway inflammation and increased airway responsiveness. The gene for TNF-α is located in the HLA class III region on chromosome 6p, which has been shown to be linked to a number of diseases with an immunological basis, including asthma, diabetes, and rheumatoid arthritis (73). Two polymorphisms of TNF-α have been identified; the first involving a guanine to adenosine substitution at position -308 of the TNF-α gene promoter (TNF1 and TNF2 alleles) and a NcoI polymorphism in the first intron of the gene (LTα*1 and LTα*2 alleles). An association between both promoter region polymorphisms and asthma has been reported, but other studies provide contrasting data (74–75). Again, Sandford and colleagues have examined the effect of the TNF-α -308 polymorphism in their cohort of fatal/near-fatal asthmatics (76). In this cohort an association between the -308 polymorphism and asthma was identified. However, no difference in allele frequency was seen between the fatal/near-fatal group and the mild/moderate asthmatics, suggesting that polymorphism of TNF-α does not contribute to asthma severity.

D. Leukotriene C₄ Synthase

Aspirin-intolerant asthma (AIA) is a syndrome of aspirin sensitivity, asthma, and nasal polyposis. Patients with AIA react to aspirin such that there is potentially life-threatening acute airway obstruction. The onset of AIA is usually beyond the 3rd decade, and these individuals commonly have severe asthma, which may require systemic corticosteroids (77). It is now recognized that AIA is not an allergic disorder, but is a cysteinyl leukotriene- (cys-LT) dependent reaction to any nonsteroidal anti-inflammatory drug that acts via inhibition of cyclooxygenase, and these reactions are superimposed upon chronically elevated cys-LT production associated with persistent severe asthma. Previously it has been unclear why such reactions are not observed in aspirin-tolerant asthma (ATA) patients or normal subjects exposed to aspirin and other NSAIDs. It has been shown that there is a fivefold overexpression of LTC₄ synthase in bronchial biopsies of AIA patients compared to ATA patients, with no significant differences in 5-LO, FLAP, or COX expression (78). The overexpression of LTC₄ synthase was the only factor that correlated with elevated cys-LT production in AIA patients, both before and after aspirin challenge, and with bronchial hyperresponsiveness to inhaled lysine-aspirin, the defining clinical measure of aspirin sensitivity. Subsequently a -444 A/C polymorphism in the LTC₄ synthase gene promoter region has been identified that creates an extra recognition site for the AP-2 transcription factor, which may lead to enhanced gene transcription (79–80). AIA patients with two variant -444 C alleles excrete more urinary LTE₄ following aspirin challenge than AIA patients with one variant allele. Genotyping by RFLP analysis showed a doubled frequency of the variant allele in AIA patients compared to ATA or normal subjects (odds ratio = 3.89) (79). However, these results have not been confirmed in subsequent studies, which have failed to show increased transcription of the -444 C allele in promoter assays (81–82) or association with aspirin-intolerant asthma (82).

V.   Genetic Influences on the Effectiveness of Therapy

As discussed above, it is important to consider that genetic variability may predispose to severe asthma by influencing the effectiveness of therapy. As well as polymorphisms of the β_2AR influencing an individual's response to β_2-agonist therapy, there are also a number of other candidate genes that may be involved in modifying the response to drug therapies for asthma. Corticosteroids are a potent and effective treatment for asthma. However, there is a small group of asthmatics in whom corticosteroids, even when given in high doses, are not effective. Polymorphisms in the receptor may influence glucocorticoid resistance; however, in a study of six steroid-sensitive and six steroid-resistant asthmatics no mutations in the GCR gene were identified (83). More recently it has been shown that there is increased expression of glucocorticoid receptor-β- (GR-β) positive cells in steroid-insensitive subjects with severe asthma (84). Insensitivity to steroids may be a major contributing factor in fatal asthma and GR-β is an alternatively spliced form of the glucocorticoid receptor that inhibits GR-α activity. It is possible that polymorphisms in splice junctions may alter the ratio of different splice forms of this receptor, leading to steroid insensitvity.

Genetic polymorphism may also play a role in regulating responses to the latest class of antiasthma drug, the antileukotrienes. A repeat-length polymorphism in the promoter of the 5-lipoxygenase enzyme (5-LO) gene has been reported to modify transcription factor binding and reporter gene expression (85). This polymorphism also seems to be associated with a reduced response to 5-LO inhibitor therapy (86).

VI. Conclusions

Although there have been few studies, the limited evidence available does tend to suggest that there may be genetic factors influencing severity as well as susceptibility to asthma. However, it remains that asthma is a complex genetic disease with multiple environmental and genetic factors interacting to determine susceptibility. Disease severity results from an equally, if not more, complex interaction of factors, including availability of medical treatment for asthma, the patient's compliance, smoking, and environmental factors, such as allergen exposure. Therefore the use of better phenotypes for disease severity in genetics studies of asthma is essential if we are to make any progress in identifying the genetic factors contributing to severe asthma.

References

1. Serra-Battles J, Plaza V, Morejon E, Comella A, Brugues J. Costs of asthma according to the degree of severity. Eur Respir J 1998; 12(6):1322–1326.
2. Sheffer A. Global Initiative for Asthma. NHLBI/WHO Workshop report, National Heart Lung and Blood Institute, 1995.
3. Lawrence S, Beasley R, Doull I, Begishvili B, Lampe F, Holgate ST, Morton NE.

Genetic analysis of atopy and asthma as quantitative traits and ordered polychotomies. Ann Hum Genet 1994; 58:359–368.

4. Cockroft DW, Swystun VA. Asthma control versus asthma severity. J Allergy Clin Immunol 1996; 98(6/1):1016–1018.

5. Kauffmann F, Dizier MH, Pin I, Paty E, Gormand F, Vervloet D, Bousquet J, Neukirch F, Annesi I, Oryszczyn MP, Lathrop M, Demenais F, Lockhart A, Feingold J. Epidemiological study of the genetics and environment of asthma, bronchial hyperresponsiveness, and atopy—phenotype issues. Am J Respir Crit Care Med 1997; 156(4):S123–S129.

6. Aas K. Heterogeneity of bronchial asthma: sub-populations—or different stages of the disease. Allergy 1981; 36:3–14.

7. The British Guidelines on Asthma Management 1995 Review and Position Statement. Thorax 1997; 52(suppl 1):2–21.

8. Expert Panel Report II: Guidelines for the Diagnosis and Management of Asthma. National Asthma Education and Prevention Program, 1997. NIH Publication No. 97-4051, National Institutes of Health, National Heart, Lung, and Blood Institute.

9. O'Connor GT, Weiss ST. Clinical and symptom measures. Am J Respir Crit Care Med 1994; 149:S21–S28.

10. Juniper EF, Kline PA, Vanzieleghem MA, Ramsdale EH, O'Byrne PM, Hargreave FE. Effect of long-term treatment with an inhaled corticosteroid (budesonide) on airway hyperresponsiveness and clinical asthma in nonsteroid-dependent asthmatics. Am Rev Respir Dis 1990; 142:832–836.

11. Redier H, Daures JP, Michel C, Proudhon H, Vervloet D, Charpin D, Marsac J, Dusser D, Brambilla C, Wallaert B, Kopferschmitt M-C, Pauli G, Taytard A, Cogis O, Michel F-B, Godard P. Assessment of the severity of asthma by an expert system: description and evaluation. Am J Respir Crit Care Med 1995; 151:345–352.

12. Sibbald B, Horn ME, Gregg I. A family study of the genetic basis of asthma and wheezy bronchitis. Arch Dis Child 1980; 55(5):354–357.

13. Sibbald B, Turner-Warwick M. Factors influencing the prevalence of asthma among first degree relatives of extrinsic and intrinsic asthmatics. Thorax 1979; 34(3):332–337.

14. Longo G, Strinati R, Poli F, Fumi F. Genetic factors in nonspecific bronchial hyperreactivity. An epidemiologic study. Am J Dis Child 1987; 141(3):331–334.

15. Hopp RJ, Bewtra AK, Watt GD, Nair NM, Townley RG. Genetic analysis of allergic disease in twins. J Allergy Clin Immunol 1984; 73(2):265–270.

16. Duffy DL, Martin NG, Battistutta D, Hopper JL, Mathews JD. Genetics of asthma and hay fever in Australian twins. Am Rev Respir Dis 1990; 142(6/1):1351–1358.

17. Harris JR, Magnus P, Samuelsen SO, Tambs K. No evidence for effects of family environment on asthma: a retrospective study of Norwegian twins. Am J Respir Crit Care Med 1997; 156(1):43–49.

18. Nieminen MM, Kaprio J, Koskenvuo M. A population-based study of bronchial asthma in adult twin pairs. Chest 1991; 100(1):70–75.

19. Laitinen T, Rasanen M, Kaprio J, Koskenvuo M, Laitinen LA. Importance of genetic factors in adolescent asthma—a population-based twin-family study. Am J Respir Crit Care Med 1998; 157(4):1073–1078.

20. Sarafino EP, Goldfedder J. Genetic factors in the presence, severity, and triggers of asthma. Arch Dis Child 1995; 73(2):112–116.

21. Sarafino EP. Connections among parent and child atopic illnesses. Pediat Allergy Immunol 2000; 11(2):80–86.

22. Gray L, Peat JK, Belousova E, Xuan W, Woolcock AJ. Family patterns of asthma, atopy and airway hyperresponsiveness: an epidemiological study. Clin Exp Allergy 2000; 30(3):393–399.

23. Wilson NM, Dore CJ, Silverman M. Factors relating to the severity of symptoms at 5 yrs in children with severe wheeze in the first 2 yrs of life. Eur Respir J 1997; 10(2):346–353.

24. Houlston RS, Tomlinson IP. Modifier genes in humans: strategies for identification. Eur J Hum Genet 1998; 6(1):80–88.

25. Quinn M, Angelico MC, Warram JH, Krolewski AS. Familial factors determine the development of diabetic nephropathy in patients with IDDM. Diabetologia 1996; 39(8):940–945.

26. Daniels SE, Bhattacharrya S, James A, Leaves NI, Young A, Hill MR, Faux JA, Ryan GF, Le Souef PN, Lathrop GM, Musk AW, Cookson WOCM. A genome-wide search for quantitative trait loci underlying asthma. Nature 1996; 383(6597): 247–250.

27. Marsh DG, Maestri NE, Freidhoff LR, et al. A genome-wide search for asthma susceptibility loci in ethnically diverse populations. Nat Genet 1997; 15(4):389–392.

28. Cox N, Beaty T, Rich S, Bleeker E, Banks-Schlegal S, Ober C, Marsh D, Blumenthal M, Meyers D. Genome screen for asthma susceptibility loci in U.S. populations. Am J Respir Crit Care Med 1998; 157(3):A855.

29. Ober C, Cox NJ, Abney M, Di Rienzo A, Lander ES, Changyaleket B, Gidley H, Kurtz B, Lee J, Nance M, Pettersson A, Prescott J, Richardson A, Schlenker E, Summerhill E, Willadsen S, Parry R. Genome-wide search for asthma susceptibility loci in a founder population. Hum Mol Genet 1998; 7(9):1393–1398.

30. Wjst M, Fischer G, Immervoll T, et al. A genome-wide search for linkage to asthma: German Asthma Genetics Group. Genomics 1999; 58(1):1–8.

31. Ober C, Tsalenko A, Parry R, Cox NJ. A second-generation genomewide screen for asthma-susceptibility alleles in a founder population. Am J Hum Genet 2000; 67(5): 1154–1162.

32. Marsh DG, Neely JD, Breazeale DR, Ghosh B, Freidhoff LR, Ehrlich KE, Schou C, Krishnaswamy G, Beaty TH. Linkage analysis of IL4 and other chromosome 5q31.1 total serum immunoglobulin E concentrations. Science 1994; 264(5162): 1152-6.

33. Meyers DA, Postma DS, Panhuysen C, Xu J, Amelung PJ, Levitt RC, Bleecker ER. Evidence for a locus regulating total serum IgE levels mapping to chromosome 5. Genomics 1994; 23(2):464–470.

34. Postma DS, Bleecker ER, Amelung PJ, Holroyd KJ, Xu JF, Panhuysen C, Meyers DA, Levitt RC. Genetic susceptibility to asthma—bronchial, hyperresponsiveness coinherited with a major gene for atopy. N Engl J Med 1995; 333(14):894–900.

35. Doull IJM, Lawrence S, Watson M, Begishivili T, Beasley RW, Lampe F, Holgate

ST, Morton NE. Allelic association of gene markers on chromosomes 5q and 11q with atopy and bronchial hyperresponsiveness. Am J Respir Crit Care Med 1996; 153(4/1):1280–1284.

36. Noguchi E, Shibasaki M, Arinami T, Takeda K, Maki T, Miyamoto T, Kawashima T, Kobayashi K, Hamaguchi H. Evidence for linkage between asthma/atopy in childhood and chromosome 5q31-q33 in a Japanese population. Am J Respir Crit Care Med 1997; 156(5):1390–1393.

37. Palmer LJ, Daniels SE, Rye PJ, Gibson NA, Tay GK, Cookson WO, Goldblatt J, Burton PR, LeSouef PN. Linkage of chromosome 5q and 11q gene markers to asthma-associated quantitative traits in Australian children. Am J Respir Crit Care Med 1998; 158(6):1825–1830.

38. Rosenwasser LJ, Klemm DJ, Dresback JK, Inamura H, Mascali JJ, Klinnert M, Borish L. Promoter polymorphisms in the chromosome 5 gene cluster in asthma and atopy. Clin Exp Allergy 1995; 25(suppl 2):74–78.

39. Walley AJ, Cookson WOCM. Investigation of an interleukin-4 promoter polymorphism for associations with asthma and atopy. J Med Genet 1996; 33(8):689–692.

40. Noguchi E, Shibasaki M, Arinami T, Takeda K, Yokouchi Y, Kawashima T, Yanagi H, Matsui A, Hamaguchi H. Association of asthma and the interleukin-4 promoter gene in Japanese. Clin Exp Allergy 1998; 28(4):449–453.

41. Burchard EG, Silverman EK, Rosenwasser LJ, Borish L, Yandava C, Pillari A, Weiss ST, Hasday J, Lilly CM, Ford JG, Drazen JM. Association between a sequence variant in the IL-4 gene promoter and FEV(1) in asthma. Am J Respir Crit Care Med 1999; 160(3):919–922.

42. Chouchane L, Sfar I, Bousaffara R, El Kamel A, Sfar MT, Ismail A. A repeat polymorphism in interleukin-4 gene is highly associated with specific clinical phenotypes of asthma. Int Arch Allergy Immunol 1999; 120(1):50–55.

43. Sandford AJ, Chagani T, Zhu S, Weir TD, Bai TR, Spinelli JJ, FitzGerald JM, Behbehani NA, Tan WC, Pare PD. Polymorphisms in the IL4, IL4RA, and FCERIB genes and asthma severity. J Allergy Clin Immunol 2000; 106(1):135–140.

44. Ohara J, Paul WE. Receptors for B-cell stimulatory factor-1 expressed on cells of haematopoietic lineage. Nature 1987; 325(6104):537–540.

45. Idzerda RL, March CJ, Mosley B, Lyman SD, Vanden Bos T, Gimpel SD, Din WS, Grabstein KH, Widmer MB, Park LS, et al. Human interleukin 4 receptor confers biological responsiveness and defines a novel receptor superfamily. J Exp Med 1990; 171(3):861–873.

46. Pritchard MA, Baker E, Whitmore SA, Sutherland GR, Idzerda RL, Park LS, Cosman D, Jenkins NA, Gilbert DJ, Copeland NG, et al. The interleukin-4 receptor gene (IL4R) maps to 16p11.2-16p12.1 in human and to the distal region of mouse chromosome 7. Genomics 1991; 10(3):801–806.

47. Deichmann KA, Heinzmann A, Forster J, Dischinger S, Mehl C, Brueggenolte E, Hildebrandt F, Moseler M, Kuehr J. Linkage and allelic association of atopy and markers flanking the IL4-receptor gene. Clin Exp Allergy 1998; 28(2):151–155.

48. Deichmann K, Bardutzky J, Forster J, Heinzmann A, Kuehr J. Common polymor-

phisms in the coding part of the IL4-receptor gene. Biochem Biophys Res Commun 1997; 231(3):696–697.

49. Mitsuyasu H, Izuhara K, Mao XQ, Gao PS, Arinobu Y, Enomoto T, Kawai M, Sasaki S, Dake Y, Hamasaki N, Shirakawa T, Hopkin JM. Ile50Val variant of IL4Rα upregulates IgE synthesis and associates with atopic asthma. Nat Genet 1998; 19(2): 119–120.

50. Mitsuyasu H, Yanagihara Y, Mao XQ, Gao PS, Arinobu Y, Ihara K, Takabayashi A, Hara T, Enomoto T, Sasaki S, Kawai M, Hamasaki N, Shirakawa T, Hopkin JM, Izuhara K. Dominant effect of Ile50Val variant of the human IL-4 receptor α-chain in IgE synthesis. J Immunol 1999; 162(3):1227–1231.

51. Khurana-Hershey GKK, Friedrich MF, Esswein LA, Thomas ML, Chatila TA. The association of atopy with a gain-of-function mutation in the α subunit of the interleukin-4 receptor. N Engl J Med 1997; 337(24):1720–1725.

52. Wang HY, Shelburne CP, Zamorano J, Kelly AE, Ryan JJ, Keegan AD. Cutting edge: effects of an allergy-associated mutation in the human IL-4Rα (Q576R) on human IL-4-induced signal transduction. J Immunol 1999; 162(8):4385–4389.

53. Rosa-Rosa L, Zimmermann N, Bernstein JA, Rothenberg ME, Khurana Hershey GK. The R576 IL-4 receptor alpha allele correlates with asthma severity. J Allergy Clin Immunol 1999; 104(5):1008–1014.

54. Zhu Z, Homer RJ, Wang Z, Chen Q, Geba GP, Wang J, Zhang Y, Elias JA. Pulmonary expression of interleukin-13 causes inflammation, mucus hypersecretion, subepithelial fibrosis, physiologic abnormalities, and eotaxin production. J Clin Invest 1999; 103(6):779–788.

55. Kuperman D, Schofield B, Wills-Karp M, Grusby MJ. Signal transducer and activator of transcription factor 6 (Stat6)-deficient mice are protected from antigen-induced airway hyperresponsiveness and mucus production. J Exp Med 1998; 187(6):939–948.

56. McKenzie GJ, Fallon PG, Emson CL, Grencis RK, McKenzie ANJ. Simultaneous disruption of interleukin (IL)-4 and IL-13 defines individual roles in T helper cell type 2-mediated responses. J Exp Med 1999; 189(10):1565–1572.

57. Richter A, Puddicombe SM, Lordan JL, Bucchieri F, Wislon SJ, Djukanovic R, Dent G, Holgate ST, Davies DE. The contribution of interleukin-4 and interleukin-13 to the epithelial-mesenchymal trpohic unit in asthma. Manuscript submitted.

58. Reihsaus E, Innis M, MacIntyre N, Liggett SB. Mutations in the gene encoding for the β₂-adrenergic receptor in normal and asthmatic subjects. Am J Respir Cell Mol Biol 1993; 8(3):334–339.

59. Green SA, Turki J, Innis M, Liggett SB. Amino-terminal polymorphisms of the human β₂-adrenergic receptor impart distinct agonist-promoted regulatory properties. Biochemistry 1994; 33(47):9414–9419.

60. Green SA, Turki J, Bejarano P, Hall IP, Liggett SB. Influence of β₂-adrenergic receptor genotypes on signal transduction in human airway smooth muscle cells. Am J Respir Cell Mol Biol 1995; 13(1):25–33.

61. Dewar JC, Wilkinson J, Wheatley A, Thomas NS, Doull I, Morton N, Lio P, Harvey JF, Liggett SB, Holgate ST, Hall IP. The glutamine 27 β₂-adrenoceptor polymorphism is associated with elevated IgE levels in asthmatic families. J Allergy Clin Immunol 1997; 100(2):261–265.

62. Dewar JC, Wheatley AP, Venn A, Morrison JFJ, Britton J, Hall IP. β_2-adrenoceptor polymorphisms are in linkage disequilibrium, but are not associated with asthma in an adult population. Clin Exp Allergy 1998; 28(4):442–448.

63. Hopes E, McDougall C, Christie G, Dewar J, Wheatley A, Hall IP, Helms PJ. Association of glutamine 27 polymorphism of β_2-adrenoceptor with reported childhood asthma: population based study. Br Med J 1998; 316(7132):664.

64. Ramsay CE, Hayden CM, Tiller KJ, Burton PR, Goldblatt J, Lesouef PN. Polymorphisms in the beta2-adrenoreceptor gene are associated with decreased airway responsiveness. Clin Exp Allergy 1999; 29(9):1195–1203.

65. Deichmann KA, Schmidt A, Heinzmann A, Kruse S, Forster J, Kuehr J. Association studies on beta2-adrenoceptor polymorphisms and enhanced IgE responsiveness in an atopic population. Clin Exp Allergy 1999; 29(6):794–799.

66. Turki J, Pak J, Green SA, Martin RJ, Liggett SB. Genetic polymorphisms of the beta 2-adrenergic receptor in nocturnal and nonnocturnal asthma. Evidence that Gly16 correlates with the nocturnal phenotype. J Clin Invest 1995; 95(4):1635–1641.

67. Holloway JW, Dunbar PR, Riley GA, Sawyer GM, Fitzharris PF, Pearce N, Le Gros GS, Beasley R. Association of $\beta2$-adrenergic receptor polymorphisms with severe asthma. Clin Exp Allergy 2000; 30(8):1097–1103.

68. Tan S, Hall IP, Dewar J, Dow E, Lipworth B. Association between β_2-adrenoceptor polymorphism and susceptibility to bronchodilator desensitisation in moderately severe stable asthmatics. Lancet 1997; 350(9083):995–999.

69. Martinez FD, Graves PE, Baldini M, Solomon S, Erickson R. Association between genetic polymorphisms of the β_2-adrenoceptor and response to albuterol in children with and without a history of wheezing. J Clin Invest 1997; 100(12):3184–3188.

70. Lipworth BJ, Hall IP, Tan S, Aziz I, Coutie W. Effects of genetic polymorphism on ex vivo and in vivo function of beta$_2$-adrenoceptors in asthmatic patients. Chest 1999; 115(2):324–328.

71. Hancox RJ, Sears MR, Taylor DR. Polymorphism of the β_2-adrenoceptor and the response to long-term β_2-agonist therapy in asthma. Eur Respir J 1998; 11(3):589–593.

72. Israel E, Drazen JM, Liggett SB, Boushey HA, Cherniack RM, Chinchilli VM, Cooper DM, Fahy JV, Fish JE, Ford JG, Kraft M, Kunselman S, Lazarus SC, Lemanske RF, Martin RJ, McLean DE, Peters SP, Silverman EK, Sorkness CA, Szefler SJ, Weiss ST, Yandava CN. The effect of polymorphisms of the β_2-adrenergic receptor on the response to regular use of albuterol in asthma. Am J Respir Crit Care Med 2000; 162(1):75–80.

73. Becker KG, Simon RM, Bailey-Wilson JE, Freidlin B, Biddison WE, McFarland HF, Trent JM. Clustering of non-major histocompatibility complex susceptibility candidate loci in human autoimmune diseases. Proc Natl Acad Sci USA 1998; 95(17):9979–9984.

74. Albuquerque RV, Hayden CM, Palmer LJ, Laing IA, Rye PJ, Gibson NA, Burton PR, Goldblatt J, LeSouef PN. Association of polymorphisms within the tumour necrosis factor (TNF) genes and childhood asthma. Clin Exp Allergy 1998; 28(5):578–584.

75. Moffatt M, Cookson W. Tumour necrosis factor haplotypes and asthma. Hum Mol Genet 1997; 6(4):551–554.

76. Chagani T, Pare PD, Zhu S, Weir TD, Bai TR, Behbehani NA, Fitzgerald JM, Sandford AJ. Prevalence of tumor necrosis factor-alpha and angiotensin converting enzyme polymorphisms in mild/moderate and fatal/near-fatal asthma. Am J Respir Crit Care Med 1999; 160(1):278–282.

77. Bigby TD. The leukotriene C(4) synthase gene and asthma. Am J Respir Cell Mol Biol 2000; 23(3):273–276.

78. Cowburn AS, Sladek K, Soja J, Adamek L, Nizankowska E, Szczeklik A, Lam BK, Penrose JF, Austen FK, Holgate ST, Sampson AP. Overexpression of leukotriene C4 synthase in bronchial biopsies from patients with aspirin-intolerant asthma. J Clin Invest 1998; 101(4):834–846.

79. Sanak M, Simon HU, Szczeklik A. Leukotriene C-4 synthase promoter polymorphism and risk of aspirin-induced asthma. Lancet 1997; 350(9091):1599–1600.

80. Sanak M, Pierzchalska M, Bazan-Socha S, Szczeklik A. Enhanced expression of the leukotriene C(4) synthase due to overactive transcription of an allelic variant associated with aspirin-intolerant asthma. Am J Respir Cell Mol Biol 2000; 23(3): 290–296.

81. Sayers I, Hayward B, Van Eerdewegh P, Keith T, Clough JB, Holloway JW, Sampson AP, Holgate ST. The role of leukotriene C4 synthase gene (LTC4S) promoter polymorphism in asthma and allied diseases. Manuscript in preparation.

82. Van Sambeek R, Stevenson DD, Baldasaro M, Lam BK, Zhao J, Yoshida S, Yandora C, Drazen JM, Penrose JF. 5′ flanking region polymorphism of the gene encoding leukotriene C4 synthase does not correlate with the aspirin-intolerant asthma phenotype in the United States. J Allergy Clin Immunol 2000; 106(1/1):72–76.

83. Lane SJ, Arm JP, Staynov DZ, Lee TH. Chemical mutational analysis of the human glucocorticoid receptor cDNA in glucocorticoid-resistant bronchial asthma. Am J Respir Cell Mol Biol 1994; 11(1):42–48.

84. Christodoulopoulos P, Leung DY, Elliott MW, Hogg JC, Muro S, Toda M, Laberge S, Hamid QA. Increased number of glucocorticoid receptor-β-expressing cells in the airways in fatal asthma. J Allergy Clin Immunol 2000; 106(3):479–484.

85. In KH, Asano K, Beier D, Grobholz J, Finn PW, Silverman EK, Silverman ES, Collins T, Fischer AR, Keith TP, Serino K, Kim SW, DeSanctis GT, Yandava C, Pillari A, Rubin P, Kemp J, Israel E, Busse W, Ledford D, Murray JJ, Segal A, Tinkleman D, Drazen JM. Naturally occurring mutations in the human 5-lipoxygenase gene promoter that modify transcription factor binding and reporter gene transcription. J Clin Invest 1997; 99(5):1130–1137.

86. Drazen JM, Yandava CN, Dube L, Szczerback N, Hippensteel R, Pillari A, Israel E, Schork N, Silverman ES, Katz DA, Drajesk J. Pharmacogenetic association between ALOX5 promoter genotype and the response to anti-asthma treatment. Nat Genet 1999; 22(2):168–170.

87. Weir TD, Mallek N, Sandford AJ, Bai TR, Awadh N, Fitzgerald JM, Cockcroft D, James A, Liggett SB, Par EP. beta$_2$-adrenergic receptor haplotypes in mild, moderate and fatal/near fatal asthma. Am J Respir Crit Care Med 1998; 158(3):787–791.

88. Sanak M, Simon HU, Szczeklik A. Leukotriene C4 synthase promoter polymorphism and risk of aspirin-induced asthma. Lancet 1997; 350(9091):1599–1600.

3

Pulmonary Physiology of Severe Asthma in Children and Adults

GARY L. LARSEN

National Jewish Medical and Research
  Center
University of Colorado School
  of Medicine
Denver, Colorado

GWENDOLYN S. KERBY

University of Colorado School of Medicine
Children's Hospital
Denver, Colorado

CHARLES G. IRVIN

Vermont Lung Center
University of Vermont College of Medicine
Burlington, Vermont

I. Introduction

Severe asthma is defined not only by airway obstruction unresponsive to adrenergic agents (status asthmaticus), but also by the difficulty of controlling the disease on a chronic basis. While tests of lung function such as the forced expiratory volume in 1 s (FEV_1) will be uniformly abnormal in patients with status asthmaticus, asymptomatic individuals with difficult-to-control chronic asthma may at times have normal conventional tests of lung function. However, as is explored in this chapter, tests of airway function that define the level of airway responsiveness will likely be abnormal in both scenarios.

Asthma can be characterized physiologically in several ways. In this chapter, we focus on three methods of characterization that best reflect altered lung function in acute and/or chronic asthma: airway responsiveness, lung mechanics, and arterial blood gases. Emphasis is placed on the results of these assessments when the disease is severe in nature. Because these measures of lung function may change with age, consideration is also given to physiological differences that reflect the age of the individual with asthma. As becomes apparent, the majority of studies assessing the pulmonary physiology of severe asthma have been performed in adults and older children. Much less is known about the physiology of severe disease in infants and small children.

II. Airway Responsiveness

A heightened airway responsiveness (hyperresponsiveness) to a variety of stimuli is considered a significant feature of asthma. A basic knowledge of the concept of airway responsiveness is important in terms of understanding current thoughts regarding asthma pathogenesis and treatment. Thus, this subject is dealt with initially since it has bearing on the discussion that follows. As noted, more conventional assessments of lung function (e.g., spirometry and arterial blood gases) may be completely within normal limits in a subject with chronic severe asthma, yet airway hyperresponsiveness may better reflect the underlying nature of the disease.

A. Definition

Airway responsiveness is commonly defined as the ease with which airways narrow in response to various nonallergic and nonsensitizing stimuli (1). The stimuli used to assess responsiveness most commonly include inhaled pharmacological agents (e.g., histamine and methacholine) as well as natural physical stimuli (e.g., exercise and exposure to cold air). In the case of the commonly used methacholine challenge, the level of responsiveness is usually defined by assessing lung function before and after inhaling increasing concentrations of methacholine. The more responsive the airways, the lower the amount of methacholine needed to decrease lung function (2; Fig. 1). What is less well appreciated is that even normal subjects may develop airway obstruction when inhaling these pharmacological agents (3–5). However, in subjects with various respiratory problems including asthma, the response to agents such as methacholine and histamine is increased in that the amount needed to produce a given decrement in lung function is much lower than that in normal subjects (6,7). Thus, the airways of these individuals are hyperresponsive to these stimuli.

In addition to giving just enough bronchoconstrictive agent to reach a target decrease in lung function (usually a 20% drop in FEV_1), more complete dose–response curves can also be obtained using agents such as histamine or methacholine. In a study of this nature, an agonist is administered to determine if a maximum response (plateau) can be defined (8,9). This provides several parameters that may be analyzed including the position, slope, and plateau of the response. The usefulness of this additional information is not fully defined. However, Woolcock and coworkers (8) described a plateau in response to high

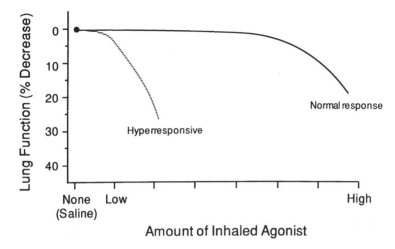

Figure 1 Airway responsiveness is commonly defined by the amount of inhaled agonist (usually histamine or methacholine) needed to reduce lung function by a defined percentage. Normal individuals (solid line) require a large amount of agonist to decrease lung function, while subjects with asthma (dashed line) require much less to reduce lung function by the same degree. A subject with asthma is "hyperresponsive" to this stimulus. (From Ref. 2.)

concentrations of agonist in normal subjects and mild asthmatics, but a loss of the plateau in moderately severe asthmatics. Thus, loss of the plateau is another indication that the severity of asthma is significant.

B. Airway Responsiveness in Normal Subjects as a Function of Age

In normal subjects, the level of airway responsiveness changes with age (3,4). For example, as part of a study of the natural history of asthma, Hopp and colleagues (3) assessed airway responsiveness to methacholine in normal nonsmoking subjects from families that had a negative family history of atopic disease for three generations. One hundred forty-eight subjects ranging in age from 5 to 86 years were studied. As shown in Fig. 2, younger and older individuals were more responsive to methacholine. The factors responsible for these normal age-related differences were not defined in this work. However, the decline in responsiveness from childhood to early adulthood may possibly reflect the increase in airway caliber seen during the growth process (4).

While the longitudinal study by Hopp et al. (3) did not assess airway responsiveness in subjects less than 5 years of age, studies by other investigators have demonstrated that normal infants bronchoconstrict when exposed to low

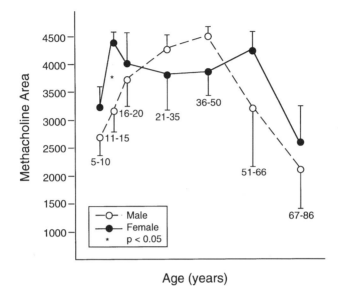

Age (years)

Figure 2   The response to methacholine in a normal population is displayed as the methacholine area vs. age for both males and females. The methacholine area is the area under the best fitting parabola of the dose–response curve. The lower the methacholine area, the more responsive the subject is to methacholine. The data demonstrate that sex was not a determinant of methacholine response in this overall population except for the 11-to-15 age group. Analysis of the age effect on the response demonstrated that younger and older individuals had lower mean methacholine areas than the mean area of the 21-to-35 and 36-to-50 age groups. (From Ref. 3.)

concentrations of bronchoreactive agents such as methacholine (5) and histamine (10) as well as the physical stimulus of cold, dry air (11). These results suggest that responsiveness in normal infants and young children (less than 5 years of age) is greater than for older children and adolescents. Furthermore, the cross-sectional and longitudinal data of Montgomery and Tepper (12) demonstrate that normal infants and young children have a decrease in airway responsiveness to methacholine as they become older. Thus, responsiveness appears to normally decrease from infancy through adulthood only to increase again at older ages. As discussed below, the normal decrease in responsiveness seen at a young age may not occur in patients with lung disease.

C. Airway Responsiveness in Asthma as Defined by Clinical Severity

Differences in airway responsiveness between normal subjects and asthmatics have been most extensively studied in adults and older children. As outlined in more detail below, subjects with asthma have heightened airways responsiveness compared to normal subjects. Less is known about infants and preschool children who have or are predisposed to develop asthma. This is in part due to the many challenges encountered in assessing lung mechanics in young infants and children. One such challenge is the need for sedation for forms of testing that assess airway mechanics in detail (5,10,11). Still, a few studies of this nature have been conducted that address important questions. One study found that airway responsiveness to histamine in recurrently wheezy infants was not greater than responsiveness found in a control group of normal infants (13). On the other hand, infants predisposed to develop asthma because of family history and/or parental smoking were more responsive than normal infants to inhaled histamine (14). Another study of infants with bronchiolitis found they did not have a decline in airway responsiveness with increasing age as occurs in otherwise normal infants (15). Thus, one hypothesis to emerge is that airway insults (e.g., viral infections, development of atopy, and exposure to tobacco smoke) during infancy may alter the decline in airway responsiveness that normally occurs with increasing age. Studies employing models have demonstrated the ability of an airway insult early in postnatal life to adversely alter the normal mechanisms that help control airway caliber (16,17).

The level of airway responsiveness has been reported to correlate with the severity of asthma symptoms (wheeze, cough, and chest tightness) and medication requirements in both adults (1,6) and children (7,18). However, there can be great variability in responsiveness seen within groups of patients classified by disease severity (19). Thus, the diagnosis of asthma as well as the classification of asthma severity in patients of all ages is based primarily on signs and symptoms of disease as well as the response to therapy monitored clinically and/or with simple tests of lung function (20). Nevertheless, the concept that the level of airway responsiveness correlates with disease severity has important implications when considering stimuli that can make an individual more responsive and their disease more severe (21).

The level of airway responsiveness in a subject with severe asthma may vary as a function of the time of day. This is demonstrated by the subset of asthmatics that have nocturnal worsening of disease associated with sleep (nocturnal asthma). This problem can be appreciated not only by monitoring symptoms that disrupt sleep, but also by recording within the home environment the overnight fall in the peak expiratory flow rates (PEFR). As the variation in normal subjects is usually less than 10%, a PEFR variability of greater than 15 to 20% has been used to define nocturnal asthma. In individuals with large overnight decrements in PEFR, Martin and colleagues (22) found that airway responsiveness at 4 A.M. was much higher than that found in the same individuals at 4 P.M. In this study of 20 asthmatic patients, the overnight fall in PEFR was related to both the severity of daytime airflow limitation and the level of airway responsiveness measured during the day. In the individuals with larger overnight decrements in PEFR, airway responsiveness at 4 A.M. was so great that they exhibited more than a 20% fall in FEV₁ upon inhalation of normal saline alone. A review of this clinically important aspect of asthma, which is associated with a greater risk of morbidity and mortality, has recently been published (23). In addition, Chapter 10 outlines in more detail the importance of nocturnal asthma as a component of severe asthma.

D. Stimuli That Increase Airway Responsiveness in Humans

The level of airway responsiveness is not static in either normal individuals or those with asthma, but may increase and decrease in response to various stimuli (2,21). This chapter concentrates on stimuli that make asthma more severe (increase responsiveness). Therapeutic maneuvers including medications that either have no effect on or decrease responsiveness are reviewed in other publications (21) and chapters within this text.

In general, stimuli that increase responsiveness are found in our environment and have the ability to produce airway inflammation (2,24). These stimuli include common viral respiratory infections, air pollutants (including cigarette smoke), allergens, and occupational agents. These stimuli are discussed separately below.

Viral Respiratory Infections

Viral respiratory infections are one of the most common clinical reasons for loss of control of asthma. This association between respiratory virus infection and symptoms of asthma has been noted for both children (25) and adults (26) with this disease. The fact that these infections can lead to increases in airway responsiveness has been recognized for over a decade and is now well established for various viral agents. Empey and coworkers (27) found that viral respiratory infections in normal subjects led to increases in airways responsiveness to histamine for as long as 6 weeks. Hall and associates (28) also found that adult subjects infected with the respiratory syncytial virus showed an exaggerated increase in airway resistance with the inhalation of carbachol, which persisted up to 8 weeks after the acute infection. Similar observations of transient increases in reactivity have been found after other viral infections including influenza A (29) and rhinovirus (30). While the consequences of this increase in responsiveness in normal subjects is minimal in terms of respiratory symptoms, the increase in a subject with asthma is of more significance in that their disease is no longer quiescent and can become much more severe in nature.

Little information is available that addresses the effect of viral infections on airway responsiveness in infants and small children. Certainly, viral respiratory infections are a common precipitant of wheezing during the preschool period. As noted above, one study suggested viral bronchiolitis may prevent the normal decrease in airway responsiveness seen with increasing age (15). If this observation is confirmed, it will suggest that increased airway responsiveness may result from failure of airways to acquire a protective mechanism early in life.

Air Pollutants

Exposure to air pollutants in normal and asthmatic subjects has been shown to increase airways responsiveness. For example, exposure to low concentrations of nitrogen dioxide in asthmatic subjects led to increased airway responsiveness to both a cholinergic agonist (31) and exercise (32). Within the laboratory, ozone caused an increase in airway responsiveness in both normal and atopic subjects (33). Under normal environmental conditions, children living in an area with high ozone concentrations were found to exhibit more frequent and severe airway hyperresponsiveness to methacholine than children from an area with low ozone concentrations (34). While the mechanisms responsible for the alterations in responsiveness are not well defined, it is known that ozone produces an inflammatory reaction within the airways of normal subjects, with generation of cyclooxygenase products of arachidonic acid metabolism (35).

Cigarette smoke must also be considered an environmental pollutant. Several studies have indicated this is a deleterious agent for infants and children in households in which there is exposure to tobacco smoke. In this respect, maternal smoking has been associated with an increased incidence of lower respiratory tract illness and diminished pulmonary function as well as higher rates of asthma, an increased likelihood of using asthma medications, and an earlier onset of disease (reviewed in Ref. 36). Exposure to passive smoke is also a risk factor for the first episode of bronchiolitis (37) as well as for recurrent wheezing later in childhood and adolescence (38). Subjects exposed to cigarette smoke through either active (39) or passive routes (40) may demonstrate an increase in airway responsiveness. In a recent study, enhanced airway responsiveness to methacholine was demonstrated as long as 3 weeks after exposure to cigarette smoke in a static test chamber (41). The observations suggest that prolonged subclinical airway inflammation might occur in the absence of a demonstrable change in airway caliber after exposure to environmental tobacco smoke. Another report suggests parental smoking may contribute to elevated levels of airway responsiveness as early as the first 2 to 10 weeks of age (14). The mechanisms by which childhood exposure to environmental tobacco smoke exerts its effects are unknown, but may include effects on the IgE immune system that can be elicited both in utero and postnatally (42).

Allergens

From both clinical and mechanistic standpoints, the best characterized stimuli that promote airway hyperresponsiveness are aeroallergens. Exposure of atopic individuals to allergens can lead to significant increases in airway responsiveness that persist for days, weeks, or even months (43,44). This heightened responsiveness has been documented not only after exposure to allergen within the laboratory, but also as a consequence of natural exposure to the offending agent (44,45). While the consequences of an increase in responsiveness may be insignificant in normal individuals, this increase may have unwanted consequences in subjects with asthma. In this respect, Cockcroft (46) proposed that a vicious cycle can develop in which continuous or repeated exposure to allergen in sensitized individuals insidiously leads to increased airway responsiveness and more severe disease in that subsequent exposure to allergen and nonallergic stimuli more easily lead to airway obstruction. As part of this scenario, frequently encountered stimuli such as cigarette smoke or normal activities such as exercise (47) usually do not cause symptoms until the level of airway responsiveness increases following exposure to allergen.

Clinical investigations in adults with asthma have documented that allergen exposure leads to an inflammatory reaction within the airways that is associated with obstruction and increased responsiveness (48). The inflammation (48) and increased responsiveness (49) may be greatest when allergen exposure leads to both immediate asthmatic responses within minutes of exposure and late asthmatic responses hours later. The association between allergen-driven late asthmatic responses and severe asthma is reviewed in detail by O'Byrne and colleagues (48).

Occupational Agents

The nature of occupational agents and the mechanisms through which they effect airway function are diverse. For example, animal dander encountered in the professional activities of veterinarians and laboratory animal workers may increase airway responsiveness through production of the IgE-initiated immediate and late asthmatic responses discussed in the previous section. For occupational agents of low molecular weight (MW < 1000 Da), including isocyanates and plicatic acid, airway obstruction and increases in airway responsiveness are produced through immunologic and other mechanisms that remain to be fully elucidated. No matter what the provocative agent, the majority of patients with symptomatic occupational asthma have been found to have airway hyperresponsiveness (50,51). Currently, most evidence suggests this hyperresponsive state is acquired as a result of exposure to the offending agent.

A strong clinical suspicion that a factor in the workplace is causing the symptoms of asthma requires investigation. To document a problem within the workplace, a practical approach is to use a peak flow meter to record several daily measures of lung function, which can then be correlated to hours of work and symptoms. If an offending agent is suspected, a challenge within the laboratory under carefully controlled conditions may also be conducted.

With removal of the affected worker from the workplace, a decrease in airway responsiveness and symptoms of asthma may be expected in many subjects. However, the proportion of workers that show clinical and laboratory-based evidence of improvement as well as the magnitude of the decrease in airway responsiveness may vary for one agent versus others. As reviewed by Chan-Yeung (51), favorable outcomes appear to be associated with shorter durations of symptoms before diagnosis, relatively normal lung function, and a lesser degree of airway hyperresponsiveness at the time of diagnosis. The workplace as a cause of severe asthma is discussed in more detail in Chapter 18.

III. Lung Mechanics

While an exact definition of asthma has eluded the best attempts to define this disease, the following is a working definition that remains useful. Asthma appears to be a syndrome characterized by the following physiological abnormalities, which may not all occur in a given individual. First, if airflow limitation exists, it should be significantly reversed by an inhaled β-adrenergic agonist. As patients with mild disease may not have baseline airflow limitation, this condition often is not met. In addition, in subjects with status asthmaticus or severe longstanding airflow obstruction, the response to inhaled bronchodilator may only be evident after therapy with a corticosteroid (52). Second, the airways are hyperresponsive to stimuli, which cause little or no change in lung function in normal subjects (see above discussion). Third, subjects with asthma exhibit variability in airflow limitation, as in the example of patients with nocturnal asthma given above. As such, asthma is a disease that is best characterized by tests of lung function. Several tests of lung mechanics have been used to characterize asthma during both symptomatic and asymptomatic phases of the disease. Abnormalities in pressure–flow, flow–volume, and pressure–volume relationships have all been described in asthma (53,54). For purposes of discussion, these abnormalities are presented in terms of lung volumes, the pressure–volume characteristics of the lung, resistance to airflow, and flow rates. Where possible, the changes that characterize the severe patient are emphasized.

A. Lung Volumes

During a severe exacerbation of asthma, all the various capacities and volumes of gas contained in the lung are altered to some extent. Typically, the residual volume (RV), functional residual capacity (FRC), and total lung capacity (TLC) are all increased (RV $\gg$ FRC $>$ TLC) while the vital capacity (VC) and its subdivision can be decreased. These alterations have been described during natural exacerbations of asthma in both adults (55) and children (56) and have also been noted within the laboratory in asthmatic subjects after exercise (57) and inhalation of either a bronchoactive substance such as histamine (58) or a relevant allergen (59). While these laboratory-induced changes in lung volumes may be immediately normalized with inhalation of a bronchodilator, it may take weeks after an episode of status asthmaticus for the RV to return to a normal range (53).

While the inflammatory changes that are found within the airway walls and lumina during an acute episode of asthma make it easier to understand how flows may be limited during an attack, the factors responsible for the increases in RV, FRC, and TLC are not as straightforward. However, several factors have been identified that may alone or in combination contribute to these alterations (53,54). First, obstruction to airflow can cause a generalized decrease in the elastic properties of the lung (60), which could contribute to the increases in lung volume. A recent report noted elastosis and fragmentation of fibers of the elastic system in fatal asthma, suggesting mechanisms via which airway recoil in asthmatic subjects can be impaired (61). Both acute and chronic changes in the pressure–volume characteristics of the lung are dealt with in more detail in the next section. Second, there may be an increase in the volume of gas trapped beyond closed airways at each of these levels of lung inflation (57,60,62). Third, tonic activity may develop in the intercostal muscles and diaphragm during episodes of obstruction in asthmatic patients such that the chest is actively held in the inspiratory position (63–65). This may be especially important when considering the increases in FRC during acute asthma.

From a practical standpoint, significant airway lability that indicates that the asthma is not well controlled can be appreciated by showing significant improvements in lung function (PEFR or FEV_1) after administration of β-adrenergic agonists. However, under certain circumstances, the response can be atypical such that lung function improves primarily through a reduction in air trapping as reflected by decreases in residual volume and the volume of thoracic gas at end-tidal respiration and increases in the forced vital capacity. This is the reverse of the isovolume shift to a higher lung volume discussed below under "Flow Rates" and may be seen in not only asthma (66,67) but also in other obstructive airway diseases (68). To detect this improvement in lung function, assessment of the response must include measurements of lung volume (69).

B. Pressure–Volume Curves

One of the major determinants of lung volume is the elastic recoil of the chest and lungs. The elastic properties of the lung are assessed with the aid of an esophageal balloon that records transpulmonary pressure [the difference between esophageal (pleural) and mouth pressures at points of no airflow] as a function of lung volume. The information generated allows the assessment of the compliance of the lung, which reflects changes in lung volume associated with changes in pressure. This can be performed under dynamic or static conditions. The former approach allows determination of frequency dependence to dynamic compliance such that at higher respiratory rates, compliance decreases, implying maldistribution of ventilation within the smaller airways (70). On the other hand, the static compliance more accurately reflects the elastic recoil properties of the lungs. Elastic recoil pressure is important in that this is a major determinant of expiratory flow rates in the more peripheral airways ("upstream" segment) during a maximum expiratory flow–volume (MEFV) maneuver (71). The normal shape of the pressure–volume (P-V) curve, based on the data of Zapletal et al. (72) for normal children, is shown in Fig. 3. An exacerbation of asthma may acutely change the shape of this curve (60,73,74). For example, Gold and associates (73) reported that in asthmatics with hyperinflation and moderate airway obstruction, there was a decrease in elastic recoil (shift of the P-V curve up and to the left). However, after 1–2 weeks of therapy with bronchodilators and corticosteroids, lung volumes as well as elastic recoil and resistance returned to a normal range of values.

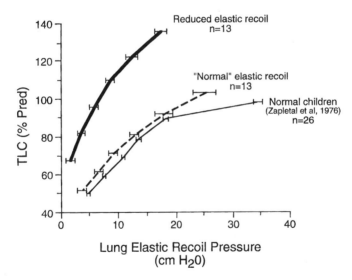

Figure 3 Pressure–volume curves are shown for two groups of age-matched children with severe asthma. For comparison, the PV curves of normal children as defined by Zapletal et al. (72) are also shown. While the FEV_1 was normal in both the group of 13 children with reduced elastic recoil and the group of 13 children with "normal" elastic recoil, the former group had a greater incidence of previous respiratory failure and a higher incidence of significant steroid requirements.

The change in lung elastic properties could not be duplicated by histamine-induced acute bronchoconstriction of either normal subjects or treated asthmatics and was likewise not reproduced in healthy subjects after 1 h in a negative-pressure suit. Thus, initially, these changes in the pressure–volume characteristics of the lung were thought to be the result of chronic airways obstruction. Subsequent studies have demonstrated that these shifts can occur rapidly when the stimulus for acute obstruction is either allergen exposure (75) or exercise (57). The factors responsible for these alterations are still unknown, but as noted above, elastosis and fragmentation of fibers of the elastic system may be present in cases of fatal asthma (61). Additional factors are likely involved.

The consequences of a shift in the pressure–volume curve up and to the left might be either advantageous or disadvantageous to the subject with asthma. Mechanically, these individuals might not have to work as hard to breathe in that the inspiratory pressures required to overcome elastic resistance in order to move a set amount of air into the lungs might be less in those with decreased elastic recoil. On the other hand, these individuals could lose the effect of increased radial traction on the airways, possibly leading to greater airways obstruction because of the loss of the tethering influence of the surrounding lung parenchyma. To the extent that elastic recoil represents the major load to smooth muscle shortening, a decrease in recoil could allow greater shortening of airways smooth muscle, leading to more narrowing and possibly airways closure. In addition, because elastic recoil is a major determinant of flows in the more distal parts of the lung (71), this would also limit flow rates. A recent report in children suggests that the latter deleterious effects of a loss of recoil outweigh any theoretical advantages. In this respect, abnormal pressure–volume curves displaying decreased lung elasticity (Fig. 3) were associated with severe childhood asthma characterized clinically by life-threatening episodes (76). In this study, 13 severely asthmatic children with hyperinflation but without airflow obstruction when their disease was under control were compared to severely asthmatic children without hyperinflation. The group with hyperinflation was found to have significantly decreased lung elasticity (Fig. 3), a greater incidence of previous respiratory failure (77% vs. 8%), and a higher incidence of significant steroid requirement as defined by the need for greater than 20 mg of prednisone every other day (77% vs. 0%). Thus, in children, loss of recoil appears to be a marker for severe, life-threatening disease.

C. Resistance to Airflow

The sine qua non of asthma is an increase in resistance to airflow that is reversible with appropriate treatment. This section deals with two different measurements that reflect resistance to airflow: airway resistance and peripheral lung resistance. The former is more commonly assessed and is discussed in terms of acute severe asthma. Measurement of peripheral lung resistance is employed as a research tool and is considered in terms of the pathogenesis of asthma.

Airway Resistance

Airway resistance (Raw) is most commonly measured with a constant-volume, variable-pressure plethysmograph using a modification of Boyle's law (77). Because Raw normally varies inversely with lung volume due to changes in airway caliber produced by traction on the outer walls of airways, it is commonly expressed as specific conductance (Sgaw, the reciprocal of resistance divided by the volume at which it was measured).

During an episode of acute asthma, the resistance to airflow increases and is reflected by increases in Raw and decreases in Sgaw (78). The magnitude of the changes correlates roughly with the severity of the episode (53). This increase in resistance is probably due to several factors. In addition to contraction of airway smooth muscle, pathology specimens from asthmatics (79,80) suggest that mucus plugging of airways as well as thickening of airways walls (e.g., smooth muscle hypertrophy, edema, goblet cell hyperplasia, and infiltration of inflammatory cells) may all contribute to the increase in resistance. Biopsy specimens from subjects not experiencing status asthmaticus demonstrate that changes seen at postmortem examination may also be present in the severe but stable patient (81). The relative contribution of these and other factors probably varies from patient to patient and will in part be determined by the precipitating factor(s) as well as the length of time that symptoms have been present.

As noted above, resistance to the flow of air is usually dependent upon lung volumes. The rise in lung volume that occurs in asthma is thought to be an important mechanism that defends airway patency via a tethering effect of the parenchymal attachments to the walls of the airways. This normal interdependence may be lost in subjects with nocturnal asthma. Irvin and colleagues (82) recently found that with sleep, there was an immediate uncoupling of the parenchyma from the airways in nocturnal asthmatics, resulting in a loss of interdependence that persisted throughout sleep. The authors speculated that the inflammatory response seen as part of nocturnal asthma together with possibly additional neural influences might explain this process. These findings suggest one explanation for the observation that many asthmatics die at night (23; Chapter 10). Uncoupling the parenchyma from the airways could result in uninhibited airway narrowing with potentially fatal consequences.

With resolution of status asthmaticus, conventional measures of airway resistance and specific conductance will approach the normal statistical range while spirometric and lung volume measurements remain grossly abnormal (78). Thus, the pressure–flow relationships reflected by body plethysmography normalize while other tests of lung function show significant abnormalities. However, as reviewed in the next section, measures of resistance that better reflect events in the more peripheral airways may remain abnormal for much longer periods of time.

Peripheral Lung Resistance

The pressure–flow relationship of the peripheral lung can also be determined in normal and asthmatic subjects (62,83,84). When peripheral lung resistance has been assessed, abnormalities have been found even in asthmatics who have normal spirometry. Wagner and colleagues (83) used a bronchoscope wedged in a subsegmental bronchus to assess the resistance of the peripheral lung in normal and asthmatic subjects. The resistance of the peripheral lung distal to the wedged bronchoscope was measured by making incremental increases in flow through a double-lumen catheter inserted through the instrument channel of the broncho-scope and recording the resultant pressures. All measurements were made at func-tional residual capacity (FRC), confirmed by a constant transpulmonary pressure, as assessed with an esophageal balloon. In these asymptomatic asthmatics with normal values for FEV_1, when expressed as a percentage of predicted, the periph-eral lung resistance for the group was more than sevenfold greater than that found in controls (0.069 ± 0.017 cm H_2O/ml/sec in asthmatics vs. 0.009 ± 0.002 in normals, $p = 0.013$). Pretreatment with a β-sympathomimetic agent did not change this assessment of resistance. In a more recent study, Kaminsky and col-leagues (62) speculated that the elevation in peripheral resistance was likely to be located in the most distal parts of the lung and to include the effects of loss of lung units as airways close. While the mechanisms responsible for these alter-ations remain to be defined, bronchial inflammation might have an important role in producing this physiological abnormality. In support of this hypothesis, a re-port employing both transbronchial as well as endobronchial biopsies suggests that both proximal and distal airways need to be evaluated to better understand the inflammatory process in asthma (85).

D. Flow Rates

The most common method of assessing the degree of airflow limitation is to measure the patient's lung function during a maximal forced exhalation. For this evaluation, the subject exhales forcibly from total lung capacity (TLC) to residual volume (RV) into either a spirometer or through a flowmeter, where flow is inte-grated to give volume. Data from this maneuver is usually expressed in one of two ways: as a time-based recording of expired volume (spirogram) or as a plot of instantaneous airflow against lung volume [maximal expiratory flow–volume (MEFV) curve]. Common tests of lung function derived from the former are the forced vital capacity (FVC), the 1-sec forced expiratory volume (FEV_1), and the forced expiratory flow 25 to 75 (FEF_{25-75}). From the flow–volume curve, the maximal expiratory flow rate (MEFR) achieved approximates the peak expiratory flow rate (PEFR) obtained from a flow meter. The flow at 50% of the vital capacity as well as flows at lower lung volumes are also generated as part of this maneuver. Since airflow is related to lung volume, plethysmography combined with the MEFV maneuver plotted as a flow–volume curve or loop (Fig. 4) allows assessment of the relationship between airflow and an absolute lung volume. In addition, combined use of plethysmography and the MEFV maneuver allows expression of the results as a percentage of the total lung capacity rather than as a percentage of the vital capacity. Assessing flow rates in this manner may be especially informative when isovolume shifts occur (see below).

Flows measured from a spirogram or MEFV curve reflect not only the resistance to airflow within airways, but also the elastic properties of the lung as well as the motivation and effort put into the maneuvers by the subject. Thus, when low flows are noted in a subject with airways disease, one must consider a loss of elastic recoil as a possible explanation for the flow limitation. This was

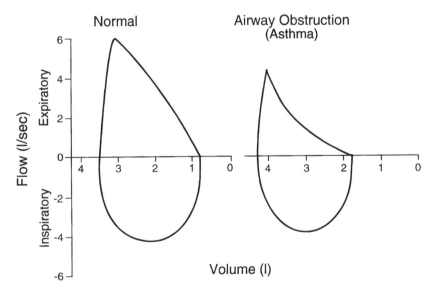

Figure 4 Maximal inspiratory and expiratory curves that constitute the flow–volume loop are shown in a patient with asthma at two points in time. The loop on the left was obtained when the disease was well controlled and is normal, while the loop on the right was obtained during an acute episode of asthma. With airway obstruction (right), an increase in total lung capacity and residual volume is seen and flow rates decrease, as manifest in the MEFV curve, which becomes concave to the volume axis. While the MEFV curve is significantly altered with moderate lower airways obstruction, the inspiratory loop is relatively preserved. (From Ref. 52.)

discussed above when considering pressure–volume curves. In addition, decreases in respiratory muscle strength due to therapy with corticosteroids may complicate asthma, leading to alterations in lung function (86).

In the asthmatic without complicating medical or psychological factors which might also influence the measurements of lung function, a typical pattern in terms of flow rates is observed during acute exacerbations. With spirometry, both the FEV_1 and FEF_{25-75} are diminished, with the former more preserved than the latter as a percentage of predicted. On the MEFV curve, the overall shape usually changes and becomes concave to the volume axis throughout the vital capacity (Fig. 4). In this respect, the MEFR is more preserved than flows obtained at lower lung volumes. In terms of flows assessed on a spirogram or MEFV curve, the most abnormal flows during acute attacks (i.e., FEF_{25-75} and flows at low lung volumes) are the last to return to the normal range.

In a minority of episodes of acute asthma, the spirogram or MEFV curve alone may not reflect a significant change in lung function. However, if these subjects are studied with both an MEFV maneuver and plethysmography, they will be noted to have a parallel displacement to a higher lung volume of the flow–volume curve without a reduction in slope of the curve itself (59). Thus, if flow is measured as a percentage of the vital capacity, no change in flow will be appreciated. However, when the same curve is plotted as a function of the absolute lung volumes present before and after onset of symptoms, substantial changes in flow become apparent at isovolumes. The factors responsible for isovolume shifts are undefined, but possibly include complete closure of some airways with subsequent loss of the contribution of these units to the flow–volume pattern.

In terms of acute severe asthma, it is important to note that the loss of symptoms and signs of asthma does not mean that lung function has returned to normal. In work by McFadden and co-workers (78), regardless of the initial presentation of the patients, when they became asymptomatic, the overall mechanical function of their lungs in terms of the FEV_1 was still between 40 and 50% of predicted normal values. When they were without signs of asthma, lung function was still only 60 to 70% of predicted.

The use of peak flow meters within the everyday environment of the patient with asthma has become one important method of monitoring for instability (87). Significant changes in the PEFR may be manifest before symptoms are evident to patients and their families. In this respect, use of these inexpensive devices may be especially helpful in defining the presence and severity of nocturnal asthma in individual patients (23). Given that excessive diurnal variations in lung function during recovery from status asthmaticus have been associated with an increased risk of sudden death (88), this vulnerable period of time should be monitored very closely with simple tests of lung function (e.g., FEV_1 and PEFR) within the hospital and home environments (89). In the more severe patients, monitoring the PEFR and FEV_1 within the home as part of their daily routine allows for earlier recognition of loss of control with more timely intervention.

IV. Arterial Blood Gases

Many studies have attempted to define arterial blood gases as a function of the severity of asthma. One of the earliest studies to present a coherent view of the abnormalities seen in this disease was by McFadden and Lyons (90). These authors were able to accomplish this by carefully choosing a large study population (101 subjects) who, because of age (14 to 45 years old) and medical history, were most likely to have mild to severe attacks of acute asthma uncomplicated by bronchitis and emphysema. Their description still provides one of the most succinct descriptions of the expected abnormalities in gas exchange. This as well as other well-designed studies are summarized below in terms of the abnormalities of blood gases most likely to be encountered in subjects with asthma.

A. Oxygen Tensions

In the study of McFadden and Lyons (90), the characteristic blood gas pattern found in patients who were experiencing acute asthmatic attacks was hypoxemia associated with respiratory alkalosis. In terms of the hypoxemia, this was the most consistently observed abnormality, found in 91 of the 101 subjects in the study. Decreasing values in FEV_1 were associated with a fall in the partial pressure of oxygen (Fig. 5, top). Patients with an FEV_1 of 50 to 85% of their predicted normal value were considered to have mild airway obstruction, those with values of 26 to 50% to have moderate obstruction, and those with values of less than 25% to have severe obstruction. The mean values of oxygen tension (mean ± SD; in mmHg as measured at sea level) ranked by disease severity were as follows: 82.8 ± 11.2, 71.3 ± 8.5, and 63.1 ± 9.1, respectively. Thus, there was an approximately 20-Torr difference in arterial oxygen tensions between the mild and severe groups. However, it was also emphasized that hypoxemia was encountered to some degree at all levels of airway obstruction. In children who were 14 months to 14 years of age, Weng et al. (91) also found that all symptomatic patients with asthma were hypoxemic, with the degree of hypoxemia correlated with the degree of airway obstruction.

In studies looking at blood gases in asthma, the primary cause of the depressed oxygen tension has been thought to be an alteration in ventilation:perfusion ratios (90,91). In severely obstructed subjects in which there were presumably atelectatic alveoli that were still perfused, anatomic shunt-like effects may have also contributed to the hypoxemia (90). In the most severely obstructed subjects, alveolar hypoventilation with hypercapnia was also observed. A de-

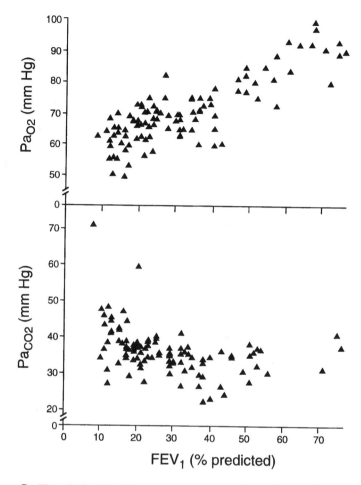

Figure 5   The relationship between arterial oxygen (in mmHg) and degree of airway obstruction (FEV_1 as a percentage of predicted) is shown in the top panel while the relationship between arterial carbon dioxide (in mmHg) and FEV_1 is shown in the bottom panel. While the level of hypoxemia correlates with the level of airway obstruction, an elevation in carbon dioxide levels is only seen when the FEV_1 is markedly compromised. (From Ref. 90.)

crease in diffusing capacity of the lung does not appear to be a significant factor in asthma (53).

The normal response of the body to a decrease in arterial oxygen tension is to increase ventilation. Kikuchi and colleagues (92) found that in patients with a history of near-fatal asthma, their respiratory responses to hypoxia were significantly lower than those found in normal subjects and in asthmatics without near-fatal attacks. Their lower hypoxic response was coupled with a blunted perception of dyspnea. Other investigators have noted that severe asthmatics with recurrent exacerbations, but not mild asthmatics, have a blunted perception of dyspnea that is related to the degree of sputum eosinophilia (93). Thus, a reduced chemosensitivity to hypoxia and a blunted perception of dyspnea are seen in subjects with more severe asthma including those in which the disease has been near-fatal.

B. Arterial Carbon Dioxide Tensions

As noted in the section above, McFadden and Lyons (90) demonstrated that the characteristic blood gas pattern found in patients experiencing acute asthmatic attacks was hypoxemia associated with respiratory alkalosis. In terms of carbon dioxide tensions, the data from the study suggested that most asthmatic attacks were associated with alveolar hyperventilation and that hypercapnia was not likely to occur until extreme degrees of obstruction were reached. In this respect, plotting increasing airways obstruction (percentage of predicted FEV_1) versus the carbon dioxide tension indicated that hypercapnia was not seen until the FEV_1 fell to less than 20% of its predicted value (Fig. 5, bottom).

C. Arterial Values of pH

In general, values of arterial pH in acute asthma have reflected the respiratory alkalosis commented upon above. In the study of McFadden and Lyons (90), the mean arterial pH was 7.44 with a standard deviation of 0.01. Seventy-three of the 101 subjects had a respiratory alkalosis (mean pH, 7.46 ± 0.03), seven had a respiratory acidosis (mean pH 7.32 ± 0.04), and 21 a normal pH. Similar results have been observed in children (91). However, one blood gas finding may be more common in younger patients with asthma. While metabolic acidosis is not common in adults, it has been noted in combination with respiratory acidosis in children with severe asthma (91,94). When this disturbance of acid/base balance is present in adults, it usually is associated with very severe airways obstruction. In a study by Appel et al. (95), all subjects had an abnormally large anion gap with venous or arterial lactate levels several times normal. While the mechanisms responsible for the development of the metabolic acidosis remain to be clarified, it is clear that subjects with this pattern on an arterial blood gas are in imminent danger of the development of respiratory failure (91,95).

D. Noninvasive Assessments

Advances have been made in the noninvasive monitoring of arterial blood gases (96,97). These advances allow for relatively quick and more easily accessible assessments in both the patient with status asthmaticus and the chronic asthmatic whose tests of lung function never completely normalize. The most widely used methods include oximetry, transcutaneous gas measurements (i.e., oxygen and carbon dioxide), and end-tidal sampling of expired gas (i.e., carbon dioxide).

Oximetry

Of all the noninvasive assessments that may be utilized, the most widely applied and clinically useful has proven to be determination of oxygen saturation. While many subjects who present to an emergency facility with acute exacerbations of asthma will have normal or nearly normal oxyhemoglobin saturations (98), oximeters offer a rapid and reliable noninvasive method of assessing one physiological consequence of the obstruction to breathing. In children, oximetry provides an assessment of acute childhood asthma that may be helpful in the decision-making process regarding the need for hospitalization. In this respect, Geelhoed and associates (99), in a study conducted in Australia, found that the initial arterial oxygen saturation was highly predictive of outcome in pediatric patients who presented to an emergency department with acute asthma. A saturation of 91% was found to discriminate between a favorable and unfavorable outcome as defined in part by the need for subsequent care after the initial visit. In addition, continuous measurements of oxygen saturation during therapy help prevent fluctuations in oxygen saturation that may be the consequence of both the disease and the therapy provided to the patient (100). The theory behind oximetry as well as the limitations of this form of monitoring are reviewed by Tobin (97).

Transcutaneous Oxygen and Carbon Dioxide

The use of transcutaneous oxygen and carbon dioxide levels to monitor the acute asthmatic state has been applied primarily to infants and children (101–103). Similarly to the patterns reviewed above regarding arterial blood gases (90,91; Fig. 5), Wennergren and associates (101) found that transcutaneous oxygen decreased with signs of even mild obstruction in infants and small children and in parallel with more severe clinical disease. Conversely, transcutaneous carbon dioxide levels were unchanged with symptoms of mild to moderate obstruction and increased only in those patients with severe symptoms.

Transcutaneous oxygen monitoring during the acute phase of asthma has demonstrated that while inhalation of bronchodilator may lead to an increase in FEV_1, oxygen levels may decrease (103). Similar observations demonstrating a deterioration in oxygenation after inhalation of bronchodilator have been made in wheezing infants (100) as well as in older children (102) and adults (104) with status asthmaticus. This phenomenon has been attributed in part to the vasodilatory effect of the drugs on the pulmonary vessels, counteracting local vasoconstrictive factors in the lung (100). Another potential explanation is that the inhaled bronchodilator causes an increase in the unevenness of the distribution of ventilation due to the uneven deposition of drug in the lung (105). Whatever the relative contribution of these and other physiological mechanisms, the important point is that in the severely obstructed patient, while some tests of lung mechanics may improve after inhalation of bronchodilator, oxygenation as assessed by either invasive or noninvasive methods may deteriorate. Patients with severe asthma should be closely observed for this paradoxical effect. Both oximetry and electrodes that assess transcutaneous oxygen provide a noninvasive method for continuous monitoring during therapy. However, one limitation of the latter method is that the electrodes are usually heated to 44°C, which necessitates frequent repositioning of the sensor to prevent cutaneous burns (97).

Capnography

Measurement of expired CO_2 provides a noninvasive method of estimating the arterial level of this gas. This is accomplished via capnography, in which the waveform of expired CO_2 is displayed so that the end-tidal plateau (alveolar) concentration of gas can be determined. Monitoring is either via an infrared absorption technique or mass spectroscopy (97). Capnography with analysis of the shape of the capnogram has also been successfully used in adults and older children with good correlations shown between the capnogram's shape and the severity of airways obstruction (106). Yet this method may not be a good reflection of arterial CO_2 when gross inequalities of ventilation and perfusion matching are present. While not currently widely employed in clinical practice, the noninvasive nature of the monitoring together with the fact that subject cooperation is not essential suggests this might be useful for monitoring selected patients with status asthmaticus or severe nocturnal asthma.

V. Conclusions

The difficulty of controlling asthma on a chronic basis, as judged by frequency of symptoms and need for medications, may be reflected in the level of airway responsiveness. In general, the more hyperresponsive the airways are to stimuli such as histamine and methacholine, the more severe the disease. Even when conventional tests of airway mechanics are normal, the severe nature of the disease may be reflected by tests that assess responsiveness. With acute flares of asthma and status asthmaticus, marked decreases in flow rates together with hyperinflation of the lungs are seen in tests of lung mechanics. In addition, hypoxemia is a common finding in subjects with wheezing with hypercapnia developing in the most severe circumstances. With resolution of the clinical signs and symptoms of airways obstruction, lung function is usually still very impaired and may not normalize for some time. In a subgroup of patients, lung function will never be completely within the normal range. In this respect, one apparent risk factor for severe episodes of airways obstruction appears to be loss of elastic recoil and the resultant uncoupling of the parenchyma and airways, allowing the latter to narrow uninhibited. In addition, reduced chemosensitivity to hypoxia and a blunted perception of dyspnea may also predispose patients to fatal asthma. A general knowledge of the pulmonary physiology of severe asthma is necessary to provide more effective treatment for patients with this life-threatening problem. Currently, our greatest deficits in terms of knowledge regarding the physiology of severe asthma are related to events in infants and younger children. This is in part due to the technical difficulties encountered in assessing airway mechanics at an early age in both normal subjects and those with asthma of varying severity. Ongoing efforts to focus on both pathologic and physiologic processes within the airways early in life when this disease commonly presents will add to our total understanding of asthma and assist us in trying to prevent the disease from becoming severe (107).

Acknowledgments

Supported in part by Grants HL 36577 and HL 56638 from the National Institutes of Health.

References

1. Hargreave FE, Dolovich J, O'Byrne PM, Ramsdale EH, Daniel EE. The origin of airway hyperresponsiveness. J Allergy Clin Immunol 1986; 78:825–832.
2. Colasurdo GN, Larsen GL. Airway hyperresponsiveness. In: Busse W, Holgate S, eds. Asthma and Rhinitis. 2d ed. Boston: Blackwell Sci. 2000:1248–1260.
3. Hopp RJ, Bewtra A, Nair NM, Townley RG. The effect of age on methacholine response. J Allergy Clin Immunol 1985; 76:609–613.
4. Ulrik CS, Backer V. Longitudinal determinants of bronchial responsiveness to inhaled histamine. Chest 1998; 113:973–979.
5. Tepper RS. Airway reactivity in infants: a positive response to methacholine and metaproterenol. J Appl Physiol 1987; 62:1155–1159.
6. Juniper EF, Frith PA, Hargreave FE. Airway responsiveness to histamine and methacholine: relationship to minimum treatment to control symptoms of asthma. Thorax 1981; 36:575–579.
7. Murray AB, Ferguson AC, Morrison B. Airway responsiveness to histamine as a test for overall severity of asthma in children. J Allergy Clin Immunol 1981; 68: 119–124.
8. Woolcock AJ, Salome CM, Yan K. The shape of the dose-response curve to histamine in asthmatic and normal subjects. Am Rev Respir Dis 1984; 130:71–75.

9. Moore BJ, King GG, D'Yachkova Y, Ahmad HR, Paré PD. Mechanisms of methacholine dose-response plateaus in normal subjects. Am J Respir Crit Care Med 1998; 158:666–669.

10. Lesouëf PN, Geelhoed GC, Turner DJ, Morgan SEG, Landau LI. Response of normal infants to inhaled histamine. Am Rev Respir Dis 1989; 139:62–66.

11. Geller DE, Morgan WJ, Cota KA, Wright AL, Taussig LM. Airway responsiveness to cold, dry air in normal infants. Pediatr Pulmonol 1988; 4:90–97.

12. Montgomery GL, Tepper RS. Changes in airway reactivity with age in normal infants and young children. Am Rev Respir Dis 1990; 142:1372–1376.

13. Stick SM, Arnott J, Turner DJ, Young S, Landau LI, Lesouëf PN. Bronchial responsiveness and lung function in recurrently wheezy infants. Am Rev Respir Dis 1991; 144:1012–1015.

14. Young S, Le Souëf PN, Geelhoed GC, Stick SM, Turner KJ, Landau LI. The influence of a family history of asthma and parental smoking on airway responsiveness in early infancy. N Engl J Med 1991; 324:1168–1173.

15. Tepper RS, Rosenberg D, Eigen H. Airway responsiveness in infants following bronchiolitis. Pediatr Pulmonol 1992; 13:6–10.

16. Colasurdo GN, Loader JE, Graves JP, Larsen GL. Maturation of nonadrenergic noncholinergic inhibitory system in normal and allergen-sensitized rabbits. Am J Physiol 267 (Lung Cell Mol Physiol 11) 1994; 267(11):L739–L744.

17. Larsen GL, Colasurdo GN. Neural control mechanisms within airways: disruption by respiratory syncytial virus. J Pediatr 1999; 135:S21–S27.

18. Avital A, Noviski N, Bar-Yishay E, Springer C, Levy M, Godfrey S. Nonspecific bronchial reactivity in asthmatic children depends on severity but not on age. Am Rev Respir Dis 1991; 144:36–38.

19. Amaro-Galvez R, McLaughlin FJ, Levison H, Rashed N, Galdes-Sebaldt M, Zimmerman B. Grading severity and treatment requirements to control symptoms in asthmatic children and their relationship with airway hyperreactivity to methacholine. Ann Allergy 1987; 59:298–302.

20. Britton J. Airway hyperresponsiveness and the clinical diagnosis of asthma: histamine or history? J Allergy Clin Immunol 1992; 89:19–22.

21. Larsen GL. Asthma in children. N Engl J Med 1992; 326:1540–1545.

22. Martin RJ, Cicutto LC, Ballard RD. Factors related to the nocturnal worsening of asthma. Am Rev Respir Dis 1990; 141:33–38.

23. Martin RJ. Nocturnal asthma: mechanistic and clinical implications. In: Holgate ST, Boushey HA, Fabbri LM, eds. Difficult Asthma. London: Martin Dunitz, 1999: 205–223.

24. Wilson MC, Irvin CG, Larsen GL. Inflammation and asthma. Semin Respir Med 1987; 8:279–286.

25. Johnston SL, Pattemore PK, Sanderson G, Smith S, Lampe F, Josephs L, Symington P, O'Toole S, Myint SH, Tyrrell DAJ, Holgate ST. Community study of role of viral infections in exacerbations of asthma in 9- to 11-year-old children. Br Med J 1995; 310:1225–1228.

26. Nicholson KG, Kent J, Ireland DC. Respiratory viruses and exacerbations of asthma in adults. Br Med J 1993; 307:982–986.

27. Empey DW, Laitenen LA, Jacobs L, Gold WM, Nadel JA. Mechanisms of bron-

chial hyperreactivity in normal subjects after upper respiratory tract infection. Am Rev Respir Dis 1976; 113:131–139.

28. Hall WJ, Hall CB, Speers DM. Respiratory syncytial virus infection in adults. Clinical, virologic, and serial pulmonary function studies. Ann Intern Med 1978; 88: 203–205.

29. Little JW, Hall WJ, Douglas RG, Mudholkar GS, Speers DM, Patel K. Airway hyperreactivity and peripheral airway dysfunction in Influenza A infection. Am Rev Respir Dis 1978; 118:295–303.

30. Lemanske RF Jr, Dick EC, Swenson CA, Vrtis RF, Busse WW. Rhinovirus upper respiratory infection increases airway hyperreactivity and late asthmatic reactions. J Clin Invest 1989; 83:1–10.

31. Orehek J, Massari JP, Gayrard P, Grimaud C, Charpin J. Effect of short-term, low-level nitrogen dioxide exposure on bronchial sensitivity of asthmatic patients. J Clin Invest 1976; 57:301–307.

32. Bauer MA, Utell MJ, Morrow PE, Speers DM, Gibb FR. Inhalation of 0.3 ppm nitrogen dioxide potentiates exercise-induced bronchospasm in asthmatics. Am Rev Respir Dis 1986; 134:1203–1208.

33. Holtzman MJ, Cunningham JH, Sheller JR, Irsigler GB, Nadel JA, Boushey HA. Effect of ozone on bronchial reactivity in atopic and nonatopic subjects. Am Rev Respir Dis 1979; 120:1059–1067.

34. Zwick H, Popp W, Wagner C, et al. Effects of ozone on the respiratory health, allergic sensitization, and cellular immune system in children. Am Rev Respir Dis 1991; 144:1075–1079.

35. Seltzer J, Bigby BG, Stulbarg M, et al. O_3-induced change in bronchial reactivity to methacholine and airway inflammation in humans. J Appl Physiol 1986; 60: 1321–1326.

36. Weitzman M, Gortmaker S, Walker DK, Sobol A. Maternal smoking and childhood asthma. Pediatrics 1990; 85:505–511.

37. McConnochie KM, Roghmann KJ. Parental smoking, presence of older siblings, and family history of asthma increase risk of bronchiolitis. Am J Dis Child 1986; 140:806–812.

38. McConnochie KM, Roghmann KJ. Wheezing at 8 and 13 years: changing importance of bronchiolitis and passive smoking. Pediatr Pulmonol 1989; 6:138–146.

39. Malo JL, Filiatrault S, Martin RR. Bronchial responsiveness to inhaled methacholine in young asymptomatic smokers. J Appl Physiol 1982; 52:1464–1470.

40. Martinez FD, Antognoni G, Macri F, et al. Parental smoking enhances bronchial responsiveness in nine-year-old children. Am Rev Respir Dis 1988; 138:518–523.

41. Menon P, Rando RJ, Stankus RP, Salvaggio JE, Lehrer SB. Passive cigarette smoke-challenge studies: increase in bronchial hyperreactivity. J Allergy Clin Immunol 1992; 89:560–566.

42. Tager IB. Passive smoking—bronchial responsiveness and atopy. Am Rev Respir Dis 1988; 138:507–509.

43. Cartier A, Thomson NC, Frith PA, Roberts R, Hargreave FE. Allergen-induced increase in bronchial responsiveness to histamine: relationship to the late asthmatic response and change in airway caliber. J Allergy Clin Immunol 1982; 70:170–177.

44. Boulet LP, Cartier A, Thomson NC, Roberts RS, Dolovich J, Hargreave FE.

Asthma and increases in nonallergic bronchial responsiveness from seasonal pollen exposure. J Allergy Clin Immunol 1983; 71:399–406.

45. Sotomayor H, Badier M, Vervloet D, Orehek J. Seasonal increase of carbachol airway responsiveness in patients allergic to grass pollen: reversal by corticosteroids. Am Rev Respir Dis 1984; 130:56–58.

46. Cockcroft DW. Mechanism of perennial allergic asthma. Lancet 1983; 2:253–256.

47. Mussaffi H, Springer C, Godfrey S. Increased bronchial responsiveness to exercise and histamine after allergen challenge in children with asthma. J Allergy Clin Immunol 1986; 77:48–52.

48. O'Byrne PM, Dolovich J, Hargreave FE. Late asthmatic responses. Am Rev Respir Dis 1987; 136:740–751.

49. Durham SR, Craddock CF, Cookson WO, Benson MK. Increases in airway responsiveness to histamine precede allergen-induced late asthmatic responses. J Allergy Clin Immunol 1988; 82:764–770.

50. Lam S, Wong R, Yeung M. Nonspecific bronchial reactivity in occupational asthma. J Allergy Clin Immunol 1979; 63:28–34.

51. Chan-Yeung MM, Malo J-L. Occupational asthma. In: Barnes PJ, Grunstein MM, Leff AR, Woolcock AJ, eds. Asthma. Philadelphia: Lippincott–Raven, 1997:2143–2155.

52. Wenzel SE, Larsen GL. Assessment of lung function: Pulmonary function testing. In: Bierman CW, Pearlmen DS, Shapiro GG, Busse WW, eds. Allergy, Asthma and Immunology from Infancy to Adulthood. 3d ed. Philadelphia: WB Saunders, 1995:157–172.

53. McFadden ER Jr. Development, structure, and physiology in the normal lung and in asthma. In: Middleton E Jr, Reed CE, Ellis EF, Adkinson NF Jr, Yunginger JW, Busse WW, eds. Allergy: Principles and Practice. 5th ed. St. Louis: Mosby, 1998: 508–519.

54. Eidelman DN, Irvin CG. Airway mechanics in asthma. In: Busse W, Holgate S, eds. Asthma and Rhinitis. 2d ed. Boston: Blackwell Scientific, 2000:1237–1247.

55. Woolcock AJ, Read J. Lung volumes in exacerbations of asthma. Am J Med 1966; 41:259–273.

56. Weng TR, Levison H. Pulmonary function in children with asthma at acute attack and symptom-free status. Am Rev Respir Dis 1969; 99:719–728.

57. Freedman S, Tattersfield AE, Pride NB. Changes in lung mechanics during asthma induced by exercise. J Appl Physiol 1975; 38:974–982.

58. Bleeker ER, Rosenthal RR, Menkes HA, Norman PS, Permutt S. Physiologic effects of inhaled histamine in asthma: reversible changes in pulmonary mechanics and total lung capacity. J Allergy Clin Immunol 1979; 64:597–602.

59. Olive JT Jr, Hyatt RE. Maximal expiratory flow and total respiratory resistance during induced bronchoconstriction in asthmatic subjects. Am Rev Respir Dis 1972; 106:366–376.

60. Finucane KE, Colebatch HJH. Elastic behavior of the lung in patients with airway obstruction. J Appl Physiol 1969; 26:330–338.

61. Mauad T, Xavier ACG, Saldiva PHN, Dolhnikoff M. Elastosis and fragmentation of fibers of the elastic system in fatal asthma. Am J Respir Crit Care Med 1999; 160:968–975.

62. Kaminsky DA, Bates JHT, Irvin CG. Effects of cool, dry air stimulation on peripheral lung mechanics in asthma. Am J Respir Crit Care Med 2000; 162:179–186.

63. Martin J, Powell E, Shore S, Emrich J, Engel LA. The role of respiratory muscles in the hyperinflation of bronchial asthma. Am Rev Respir Dis 1980; 121:441–447.

64. Muller N, Bryan AC, Zamel N. Tonic inspiratory muscle activity as a cause of hyperinflation in asthma. J Appl Physiol 1981; 50:279–282.

65. Gorini M, Iandelli I, Misuri G, Bertoli F, Filippelli M, Mancini M, Duranti R, Gigliotti F, Scano G. Chest wall hyperinflation during acute bronchoconstriction in asthma. Am J Respir Crit Care Med 1999; 160:808–816.

66. Woolcock AJ, Read J. Improvement in bronchial asthma not reflected in forced expiratory volume. Lancet 1965; ii:1323–1325.

67. Greenough A, Pool J, Price JF. Changes in functional residual capacity in response to bronchodilator therapy among young asthmatic children. Pediatr Pulmonol 1989; 7:8–11.

68. Larsen GL, Barron RJ, Landay RA, Cotton EK, Gonzalez MA, Brooks JG. Intravenous aminophylline in patients with cystic fibrosis. Am J Dis Child 1980; 134: 1143–1148.

69. Smith HR, Irvin CG, Cherniack RM. The utility of spirometry in the diagnosis of reversible airways obstruction. Chest 1992; 101:1577–1581.

70. Woolcock AJ, Vincent NJ, Macklem PT. Frequency dependence of compliance as a test for obstruction in the small airways. J Clin Invest 1969; 48:1097–1106.

71. Cherniack RM. Pulmonary Function Testing. 2d ed. Philadelphia: WB Saunders, 1992.

72. Zapletal A, Paul T, Samánek M. Pulmonary elasticity in children and adolescents. J Appl Physiol 1976; 40:953–961.

73. Gold WM, Kaufman HS, Nadel JA. Elastic recoil of the lungs in chronic asthmatic patients before and after therapy. J Appl Physiol 1967; 23:433–438.

74. Woolcock AJ, Read J. The static elastic properties of the lungs in asthma. Am Rev Respir Dis 1968; 98:788–794.

75. Mansell A, Dubrawsky C, Levison H, Bryan AC, Langer H, Collins-Williams C, Orange RP. Lung mechanics in antigen-induced asthma. J Appl Physiol 1974; 37: 297–301.

76. Liu AH, Brugman SM, Schaeffer EB, Irvin CG. Reduced lung elasticity may characterize children with severe asthma. Am Rev Respir Dis 1990; 141:A906.

77. DuBois AB, Botelho SY, Comroe JH Jr. A new method for measuring airway resistance in man using a body plethysmograph: values in normal subjects and in patients with respiratory disease. J Clin Invest 1956; 35:327–335.

78. McFadden ER Jr, Kiser R, deGroot WJ. Acute bronchial asthma. Relations between clinical and physiologic manifestations. N Engl J Med 1973; 288:221–225.

79. Dunnill MS. The pathology of asthma, with special reference to changes in the bronchial mucosa. J Clin Pathol 1960; 13:27–33.

80. Dunnill MS, Massarella GR, Anderson JA. A comparison of the quantitative anatomy of the bronchi in normal subjects, in status asthmaticus, in chronic bronchitis, and in emphysema. Thorax 1969; 24:176–179.

81. Cutz E, Levison H, Cooper DM. Ultrastructure of airways in children with asthma. Histopathology 1978; 2:407–421.

82. Irvin CG, Pak J, Martin RJ. Airway–parenchyma uncoupling in nocturnal asthma. Am J Respir Crit Care Med 2000; 161:50–56.
83. Wagner EM, Liu MC, Weinmann GG, Permutt S, Bleecker ER. Peripheral lung resistance in normal and asthmatic subjects. Am Rev Respir Dis 1990; 141:584–588.
84. Kaminsky DA, Wenzel SE, Carcano C, Gurka D, Feldsien D, Irvin CG. Hyperpnea-induced changes in parenchymal lung mechanics in normal subjects and in asthmatics. Am J Respir Crit Care Med 1997; 155:1260–1266.
85. Kraft M, Djukanovic R, Wilson S, Holgate ST, Martin RJ. Alveolar tissue inflammation in asthma. Am J Respir Crit Care Med 1996; 154:1505–1510.
86. Dekhuijzen PNR, Decramer M. Steroid-induced myopathy and its significance to respiratory disease: a known disease rediscovered. Eur Respir J 1992; 5:997–1003.
87. Expert Panel Report II: Guidelines for the Diagnosis and Management of Asthma. NIH Publication No. 97-4051. Bethesda, MD: National Asthma Education and Prevention Program, National Heart, Lung and Blood Institute, 1997.
88. Hetzel MR, Clark TJH, Branthwaite MA. Asthma: analysis of sudden deaths and ventilatory arrests in hospitals. Br Med J 1977; 1:808–811.
89. Irvin CG. Throwing the baby out with the bath water. J Asthma 1996; 33:275–276.
90. McFadden ER Jr, Lyons HA. Arterial-blood gas tension in asthma. N Engl J Med 1968; 278:1027–1032.
91. Weng TR, Langer HM, Featherby EA, Levison H. Arterial blood gas tensions and acid-base balance in symptomatic and asymptomatic asthma in childhood. Am Rev Respir Dis 1970; 101:274–282.
92. Kikuchi Y, Okabe S, Tamura G, Hida W, Homma M, Shirato K, Takishima T. Chemosensitivity and perception of dyspnea in patients with a history of near-fatal asthma. N Engl J Med 1994; 330:1329–1334.
93. in't Veen JCCM, Smits HH, Ravensberg JJ, Hiemstra PS, Sterk PJ, Bel EH. Impaired perception of dyspnea in patients with severe asthma. Am J Respir Crit Care Med 1998; 158:1134–1141.
94. Downes JJ, Wood DW, Striker TW, Pittman JC. Arterial blood gas and acid–base disorders in infants and children with status asthmaticus. Pediatrics 1968; 42:238–249.
95. Appel D, Rubenstein R, Schrager K, Williams MH Jr. Lactic acidosis in severe asthma. Am J Med 1983; 75:580–584.
96. Burki NK, Albert RK. Noninvasive monitoring of arterial blood gases: a report of the ACCP Section on Respiratory Physiology. Chest 1983; 83:666–670.
97. Tobin MJ. Respiratory monitoring. In: Bone RC, Dantzker DR, George RB, Matthay RA, Reynolds HY, eds. Pulmonary and Critical Care Medicine. St. Louis: Mosby, 1998:R6/1–R6/11.
98. McFadden ER Jr. Management of patients with acute asthma: what do we know? What do we need to know? Ann Allergy 1994; 72:385–389.
99. Geelhoed GC, Landau LI, LeSouëf PN. Predictive value of oxygen saturation in emergency evaluation of asthmatic children. Br Med J 1988; 297:395–396.
100. Prendiville A, Rose A, Maxwell DL, Silverman M. Hypoxaemia in wheezy infants after bronchodilator therapy. Arch Dis Child 1987; 62:997–1000.

Larsen et al.

101. Wennergren G, Engström I, Bjure J. Transcutaneous oxygen and carbon dioxide levels and a clinical symptom scale for monitoring the acute asthmatic state in infants and young children. Acta Paediatr Scand 1986; 75:465–469.

102. Holmgren D, Sixt R. Transcutaneous and arterial blood gas monitoring during acute asthmatic symptoms in older children. Pediatr Pulmonol 1992; 14:80–84.

103. Holmgren D, Sixt R. Effects of salbutamol inhalations on transcutaneous blood gases in children during the acute asthmatic attack: from acute deterioration to recovery. Acta Paediatr 1994; 83:515–519.

104. Palmer KNV, Diament ML. Effect of salbutamol on spirometry and blood-gas tensions in bronchial asthma. Br Med J 1969; 1:31–32.

105. Ballester E, Roca J, Ramis L, Wagner PD, Rodriguez-Roisin R. Pulmonary gas exchange in severe chronic asthma. Response to 100% oxygen and salbutamol. Am Rev Respir Dis 1990; 141:558–562.

106. You B, Peslin R, Duvivier C, Dang Vu V, Grilliat JP. Expiratory capnography in asthma: evaluation of various shape indices. Eur Respir J 1994; 7:318–323.

107. Larsen GL. Focusing on childhood asthma: the Childhood Asthma Management Program (CAMP). J Allergy Clin Immunol 1999; 103:371–373.

4

Inflammatory Mediators and Neural Mechanisms in Severe Asthma

PETER J. BARNES

National Heart and Lung Institute
Imperial College
London, England

I. Introduction

Many inflammatory mediators have been implicated in the complex inflammatory process of asthma (1). These mediators are derived from activated inflammatory and structural cells and account for the complex pathophysiology of asthma (Fig. 1). Neural mechanisms are also important through effects of airway tone and interaction with airway inflammation (2). While mediator and neural mechanisms have been extensively investigated in patients with mild asthma, there is much less information about the role of mediators in patients with more severe asthma. It is not certain whether increased amounts of mediators or different mediators are involved in more severe disease, as far fewer studies have been undertaken. Invasive procedures, such as bronchial biopsies and bronchoalveolar lavage (BAL), are much more difficult to apply in patients with severe asthma, but recently there has been increased interest in less invasive procedures to sample inflammatory mediators. These techniques include induction of sputum with hypertonic saline and measurement of mediators in the sputum supernatant and in exhaled breath (both gases and condensate). There have been important advances in the developments of new drugs for asthma, including antagonists or inhibitors of specific mediators and these have sometimes been applied to patients with

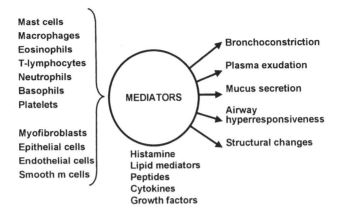

Figure 1   Inflammatory mediators may be derived from many cell types, including inflammatory and structural cells of the airway. A mixture of many mediators then results in the typical pathophysiology of asthma.

more severe asthma. However, it is often difficult to use a newly developed drug in severe asthma and if early studies in mild asthma have been unsuccessful a particular drug may not be developed.

In this chapter I emphasize the role of inflammatory mediators and neural mechanisms in severe asthma, based on the relatively few studies that have been undertaken in this important group of asthmatic patients.

II. Inflammatory Mediators

Over 50 inflammatory mediators have been implicated in asthma and reviewed in detail elsewhere (1). In this chapter I emphasize those mediators where there is relevant information on their role in severe asthma.

A. Histamine

Histamine was the first mediator implicated in asthma and it has been extensively investigated, although studies pertain mainly to patients with mild asthma. Plasma histamine levels are difficult to interpret because of release from basophils in the blood samples, but several studies have demonstrated an increase in BAL histamine in mild asthma and after allergen challenge. Histamine has many effects on airway function, but antihistamines (H_1-receptor antagonists) are without clinical benefit in asthma (3). This is particularly true in patients with severe asthma, although antihistamines may provide symptomatic improvement of rhinitis, which often accompanies severe asthma.

B. Prostanoids

There is convincing evidence for increased expression of cyclooxygenase-2 (COX-2) in asthmatic airways, suggesting that prostanoids are produced in asthmatic airways (4). Several prostanoids may be produced in asthma, including prostaglandins (PG) E_2, $PGF_{2\alpha}$, PGD_2, PGI_2, and thromboxane A_2. The role of prostanoids in asthma is difficult to determine. Nonselective COX inhibitors, such as aspirin and indomethacin, do not appear to benefit asthma. Indeed PGE_2 appears to have a protective role in asthma and it has been proposed that its production might be defective in asthma, thus predisposing to bronchoconstriction and release of inflammatory mediators (5). In the relatively rare patients with aspirin-sensitive asthma, inhibition of PGE_2 production by COX inhibitors appears to predispose to asthma through an increased release of cysteinyl leukotrienes. Whether selective COX-2 inhibitors, such as rofecoxib, also induce exacerbations in aspirin-sensitive asthma is not yet clear.

Thromboxane is a very potent bronchoconstrictor in asthmatic patients (6), but to date there is no convincing evidence that thromboxane synthesis inhibitors or antagonists are effective in asthma (7). There is no specific data on whether prostanoids are more important in severe asthma, although there are no anecdotal reports of beneficial effects of COX inhibitors in severe asthma patients. Elevated concentrations of thromboxane B_4 have been reported in severe, compared to mild, asthma, indicating that this prostanoid might be contributing to the bronchoconstriction in severe asthma. Studies of specific thromboxane inhibitors in severe asthma may therefore be warranted.

C. Leukotrienes

Leukotrienes (LT) are produced by the enzyme 5′-lipoxygenase (5-LO) from arachidonic acid and appear to play a role in asthma. LTB_4 is a potent neutrophil chemotactic factor, but its role in asthma is uncertain. An increased concentration of LTB_4 has been documented in BAL of patients with severe asthma (8). A selective LTB_4 receptor antagonist (LY293111) had no effect on the airway response to allergen in patients with mild asthma, although there was a significant reduction in the neutrophilic response in BAL during the late response (9). There is evidence for an increased neutrophilic response in airways and induced sputum of patients with severe asthma (8,10). This is consistent with data demonstrating an increase in LTB_4 in exhaled breath of patients with severe asthma (P. Montuschi et al., unpublished observations). This suggests that LTB_4 antagonists or 5-lipoxygenase inhibitors might have a useful place in severe rather than mild asthma.

Cysteinyl LTs (cys-LTs) are potent bronchoconstrictors and also cause plasma exudation and mucus secretion and may increase eosinophilic inflammation. Cys-LT receptor antagonists and a 5′-lipoxygenase inhibitor have beneficial effects in asthma, with improvement in lung function and reductions in symptoms and airway inflammation (11). However, these drugs are less effective than inhaled corticosteroids, which reflects the fact that they cover only a part of the inflammatory response in asthma. However, some patients appear to derive more benefit than others and this might be due to genetic factors relating to genetic polymorphisms in the leukotriene pathway (12). There is indirect evidence that LTs are involved in severe asthma, since there is a better clinical response to the 5-LO inhibitor zileuton in patients with moderate asthma compared to mild asthma (13). A high dose of the cys-LT antagonist zafirlukast had a beneficial effect in patients with severe asthma who were treated with oral corticosteroids (14). The concentrations of cys-LTs in exhaled breath are also increased in severe asthma compared to mild asthma (15). Patients with aspirin-sensitive asthma often have a more severe form of asthma and may show clinical benefit with antileukotriene therapy (16). Although there are anecdotal reports that patients with very severe steroid-dependent asthma respond to antileukotrienes, a double-blind controlled study showed that montelukast was apparently ineffective in this patient group (17).

D. Platelet-Activating Factor

Platelet-activating factor (PAF) was previously thought to be an important mediator in the pathophysiology of asthma, as it mimicked many features of asthma, including airway hyperresponsiveness (AHR) (18,19). However, PAF receptor antagonists that are effective in blocking the airway effects of inhaled PAF (20) are ineffective in controlling asthma symptoms, at least in patients with mild to moderate asthma (21). One possible explanation is that it is difficult to antagonize the high local concentrations of endogenous PAF with a receptor antagonist given orally. Indeed, a more potent PAF antagonist, SR27417A, has some inhibitory effect on AHR and allergen challenge, which has not been seen with less potent antagonists (22). Another possibility is that intracellular PAF, which accounts for >90% of total PAF synthesized, is playing a more important role than extracellular PAF, but its role will only be revealed when specific PAF synthase inhibitors are tested in asthma. Whether PAF antagonists may be effective in more severe asthma has not yet been determined, however. Perhaps further clinical studies with the new generation of more potent antagonists in patients with more severe asthma might be justified.

E. Adenosine

Adenosine is a potent bronchoconstrictor in asthmatic patients, acting mainly by release of bronchoconstrictor mediators from mast cells via activation of adenosine A_{2B} receptors (23). Theophylline is an antagonist of the airway effects of adenosine and is an effective therapy in severe asthma, but it is difficult to interpret this information as theophylline has other anti-asthma actions. So far no selective adenosine A_{2B} antagonist has been developed for clinical studies.

F. Endothelins

Endothelin (ET)-1 is the most potent bronchoconstrictor so far discovered and endothelins have been implicated in the pathophysiology of asthma (24,25). Inhaled ET-1 is a potent bronchoconstrictor in asthmatic patients (26). Elevated ET-1 concentrations have been demonstrated in the BAL fluid of patients with mild asthma, with increased expression of ET-1 in airway epithelial cells (27,28). BAL ET-1 levels are reduced in patients treated with inhaled corticosteroids, but no measurements have been reported in patients with severe asthma. An increase in concentration of plasma ET-1 has been reported in asthmatic children and adults and is apparently related to asthma severity (29,30). Endothelins have other properties that may be relevant in asthma and in particular stimulate fibroblast proliferation and collagen formation (31). In addition, ET potentiates the effects of growth factors on the proliferation of airway smooth muscle (32). This suggests that ET-1 may have a role in the airway remodeling that occurs in severe asthma. Although several selective ET antagonists have been developed for clinical use, they have not yet been tested in asthma. The effects of endothelins are mediated via both ET_A and ET_B receptors, so that mixed antagonists would be preferable. If a major effect of endothelins is on structural changes in the airways, then prolonged and difficult studies may be necessary to demonstrate their efficacy.

G. Nitric Oxide

Nitric oxide (NO) is derived from NO synthases, of which there are two constitutive forms, neuronal NOS (NOS1) and endothelial NOS (NOS3), and from an inducible form (iNOS or NOS2) (33). NO production is increased in asthma and this is reflected by increased concentrations of NO in exhaled air of asthmatic patients (34). This increase in exhaled NO is derived from increased expression of iNOS from epithelial cells, macrophages, and inflammatory cells, including eosinophils, in the lower respiratory tract (35). There is no simple relationship between the levels of exhaled NO and asthma severity. In patients with mild asthma who are not treated with inhaled corticosteroids there is a relationship between the levels of exhaled NO and both sputum eosinophil counts and airway responsiveness (36). However, the levels of exhaled NO are normal in patients with moderate asthma who are treated with inhaled corticosteroids, as this results in suppression of iNOS expression. However, in patients with severe asthma, who require maximal doses of inhaled corticosteroids and oral steroids, the levels of exhaled NO are again elevated (10,37). This indicates that inflammation may not be fully suppressed by corticosteroid therapy and indicates a relative corticosteroid resistance.

Whether increased production of NO in asthma contributes to its pathophysiology is not certain. NO is a potent vasodilator and may increase plasma exudation (38). There is increasing evidence that NO may increase eosinophilic inflammation by inducing chemotaxis of eosinophils and prolonging their survival (39,40). However, a nonselective inhibitor of NOS, N^G-nitro-L-arginine methyl ester (L-NAME), while reducing the levels of exhaled NO, had no effect on the early or late response to inhaled allergen (41). Selective iNOS inhibitors are now in development and will be tested in asthma.

H. Reactive Oxygen Species

Reactive oxygen species (ROS) include superoxide anions, hydrogen peroxide, and hydroxyl radicals that are generated by inflammatory cells, including macrophages and eosinophils. There is considerable evidence that ROS are generated in asthma and may contribute to its pathophysiology (42,43). In addition, there is evidence for reduced antioxidant defenses in asthma, with reduced activity of superoxide dismutase in epithelial cells of asthmatic patients (44), which is further reduced by allergen exposure (45).

Recently it has been possible to monitor oxidative stress in the airways by measurement of markers of oxidative stress in the breath. The levels of exhaled hydrogen peroxide are increased in patients with asthma (46,47) and are increased further during exacerbations (48). Isoprostanes are prostanoid mediators formed by the direct oxidation of arachidonic acid (49). The levels of 8-isoprostane are increased in patients with asthma and there is a greater increase in patients with severe asthma than with mild asthma (50). Ethane is formed by lipid peroxidation of membrane fatty acids as a result of oxidative stress. Levels of ethane in the breath are also increased in patients with asthma, and levels are greater in patients with more severe asthma (51). This suggests that oxidative stress is greater in patients with more severe asthma. Oxidative stress is a potent stimulant of the transcription factor NF-κB, which switches on the expression of multiple inflammatory genes, and therefore oxidative stress may be a mechanism for amplifying the inflammatory process in severe asthma. This suggests that antioxidants may benefit patients with severe asthma, but existing antioxidants are relatively weak and more potent antioxidants are now in clinical development.

Peroxynitrite is a potent radical formed from an interaction between superoxide anions and NO (52). Peroxynitrite is unstable and forms hydroxyl radicals but also nitrates tyrosine residues in proteins, forming 3-nitrotyrosine derivatives. Nitrotyrosine immunoreactivity is increased in the airways of asthmatic patients, indicating the probable formation of peroxynitrite in the airways (35). Nitrotyrosine is also detectable in exhaled air of patients with asthma and the levels are correlated with those of NO, indicating that it is likely to reflect increased peroxynitrite formation (15), although nitrotyrosine may also be formed by an effect of eosinophil and neutrophil peroxidases (53).

I. Bradykinin

Bradykinin has long been implicated in asthma (54). Inhaled bradykinin is a potent bronchoconstrictor in asthmatic patients (55) and acts directly on peripheral airways, but also indirectly by activating cholinergic neural reflexes and releasing tachykinins and prostanoids (56). Measurements of bradykinin are difficult, as the peptide is rapidly metabolized, particularly by neutral endopeptidase (NEP). If NEP function is impaired in asthma as a result of inflammation of oxidative stress, the effects of bradykinin may be exaggerated. Furthermore, there may be enhanced expression of bradykinin B_1 receptors in asthma in response to inflammatory signals (57). The importance of bradykinin in severe asthma is not known, as no studies have been undertaken with bradykinin antagonists in such patients. Peptide inhibitors of bradykinin receptors, such as icatibant, have been developed but have shown little beneficial effect in asthmatic patients (58). Bradykinin antagonists have not yet been studied in patients with severe asthma.

J. Proteases

The role of proteases in the pathophysiology of asthma is not yet certain. Mast cell tryptase has several relevant effects on the airways, including increasing responsiveness of airway smooth muscle, induction of plasma exudation, and stimulation of proliferation of airway smooth muscle cells and fibroblasts (59). Some of its effects are mediated via the protease-activated receptor PAR2. The role of mast cell tryptase in asthma is unknown, but a tryptase inhibitor has been shown to have some effects in an allergic sheep model (60). Its properties might suggest that mast cell tryptase may be involved in airway remodeling in asthma and therefore may be relevant in some patients with severe asthma.

Other proteases may also be involved in asthma. Mast cell chymase is a potent mucus secretagogue. Matrix metalloproteinases may play a role in airway remodeling and the levels of MMP-9 (gelatinase B) are increased in the BAL fluid of untreated asthmatic patients (61) and in induced sputum of patients with severe asthma (62).

III. Cytokines

Many cytokines have been implicated in asthma (Fig. 2) (63). Cytokines play a critical role in the perpetuation of asthmatic inflammation and certain cytokines may be important in amplifying the inflammatory process. Some cytokines are

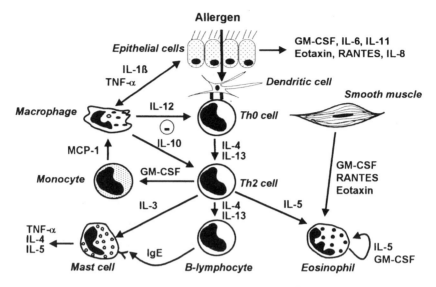

Figure 2   Many cytokines are involved in the pathophysiology of asthma and are secreted from inflammatory and structural cells.

closely linked to allergic inflammation, including IL-4, which is critical for the selection of Th2 cells and IgE formation by B lymphocytes, and IL-5, which is critical for eosinophilic inflammation. Other cytokines, such as IL-1β and TNF-α, are involved in all inflammatory diseases and appear to act as amplifying cytokines. These latter cytokines are therefore more likely to relate to asthma severity. While increased expression of many cytokines has been shown in asthmatic airways, there is little information about how specific cytokines are linked to asthma severity.

A.   TNF-α

TNF-α may act as an important amplifying cytokine of asthma through activation of NF-κB, thereby switching on the expression of multiple inflammatory genes (64,65). The concentrations of TNF-α in induced sputum are not increased in patients with mild asthma, but may be increased in severe asthma (10,66). BAL concentrations of TNF-α are also increased during exacerbations of asthma (67) and in induced sputum following the late response to allergen challenge (68). A polymorphism in the promoter of the TNF-α gene (TNF-2) that is associated with increased TNF-α secretion is more commonly associated with asthma (69,70), but is not more frequent in patients with severe asthma (71). TNF-α may also induce resistance to corticosteroids through activation of the transcription factors AP-1 and NF-κB, which oppose the effects of glucocorticoid receptor activation.

B. IL-1β

IL-1β has a similar amplifying role to TNF-α and also activates NF-κB. Patients with symptomatic asthma show increased levels of IL-1β in BAL fluid compared to patients with asymptomatic asthma (72). There is a marked increase in the concentration of IL-1β in BAL fluid from patients with status asthmaticus, with evidence that this is the most important of the proinflammatory mediators in this setting (67). Increased expression of IL-1β in asthmatic airway epithelium has been reported, together with an increased number of macrophages expressing IL-1β.

C. IL-4

IL-4 may play a critical role in the pathophysiology of asthma through its unique role in tipping the balance in favor of Th2 cells. It is also important for IgE formation. However, IL-4 is likely to be an important determinant of allergic inflammation rather than of the severity of asthma. Nevertheless IL-4 is expressed in the airways of patients with corticosteroid-resistant asthma (73) and a combination of IL-4 and IL-2 reduces the affinity of glucocorticoid receptors in T lymphocytes (74).

D. IL-13

IL-13 may play an important role in asthma. It shares many properties of IL-4 and may also be involved in IgE formation by B lymphocytes. IL-13 mimics many of the pathophysiological features of asthma, and inhibition of IL-13 with a high-affinity soluble receptor blocks many of the responses to allergen in sensitized mice (75,76). Overexpression of IL-13 in transgenic mice is associated with increased airway fibrosis, suggesting that IL-13 may be involved in airway remodeling. IL-13 expression is increased in patients with asthma (77). IL-13 also induces a reduction in glucocorticoid receptor affinity similar to that seen with IL-2 and IL-4, suggesting that IL-13 may be involved in reduced responsiveness to corticosteroids (78).

E. IL-5

IL-5 has long been associated with asthma, as it is of critical importance in the production of eosinophils from bone marrow and is also involved in recruitment of and survival of eosinophils in the airways (79). Increased circulating levels of immunoreactive IL-5 has been measured in the serum of patients with exacerbations of asthma and these levels fall with corticosteroid treatment (80). IL-5 levels are raised in induced sputum following allergen challenge of asthmatic patients (68). The levels of IL-5 in induced sputum are more likely to be raised in patients with severe asthma, despite treatment with oral corticosteroids (10). In patients who have steroid-resistant asthma there is also increased expression of IL-5 in airway T lymphocytes, consistent with the persistence of eosinophilic inflammation in these patients (73).

The role of IL-5 in the symptomatology and severity of asthma is currently uncertain. A humanized monoclonal antibody to IL-5 (mepolizumab) markedly reduces peripheral and airway eosinophilia, but has no effect on the response to allergen or on airway hyperresponsiveness in patients with mild asthma (81). Whether this antibody has any effect in patients with more severe asthma is currently being investigated in clinical studies.

F. IL-10

IL-10 has potent and widespread anti-inflammatory effects, inhibiting the expression of most inflammatory and immune cytokines and inhibiting allergen-induced responses (82). IL-10 is predominately produced by macrophages in the airways and there is evidence that macrophage secretion of IL-10 is reduced in patients with asthma and that this is correlated with increased secretion of proinflammatory cytokines (83). There is also a reduction in IL-10 secretion from monocytes in asthmatic patients (84). This suggests that IL-10 normally exerts an inhibitory effect on inflammation and that reduced IL-10 secretion may enhance inflammation (Fig. 3) (85,86). This predicts that reduction in IL-10 secretion may be linked to asthma severity. Indeed, the secretion of IL-10 from peripheral blood monocytes is significantly reduced in patients with severe asthma compared to patients with mild disease (87). This may be linked to polymorphisms of the IL-10 gene. Polymorphisms of the IL-10 gene promoter that are associated with reduced secretion of IL-10 are more frequently associated with severe asthma than with mild asthma (88).

G. IL-12

IL-12 plays a critical role in determining the balance between Th1 and Th2 cells and is protective against the development of atopic inflammation. A reduced release of IL-12 has been reported from whole blood in patients with asthma (89). A reduced expression of IL-12 has been reported in biopsies of asthmatic patients, which is normalized after corticosteroid treatment in mild asthmatic patients, but not in corticosteroid-dependent asthmatic patients (77). However, reduced expression of IL-12 has been seen in peripheral blood monocytes from patients with severe compared to mild asthma (87).

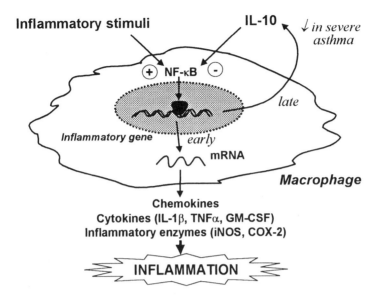

Figure 3 Defective secretion of interleukin-10 may contribute to the increase in inflammation in severe asthma. Inflammatory stimuli may activate the transcription factor nuclear factor-κB (NF-κB) in macrophages to switch on the transcription of inflammatory genes. Later the secretion of IL-10 is increased and this turns off the inflammatory process, partly by inhibiting NF-κB. The secretion of IL-10 is impaired in severe asthma, resulting in less effective suppression of immediate early genes, thus resulting in prolonged and increased inflammation.

IV. Neural Mechanisms

Neural mechanisms play an important role in the control of airway caliber, so it is likely that they contribute toward the severity of asthma (Fig. 4) (2). But, as with inflammatory mediators, little is known about the relative importance of neural mechanisms in severe, as opposed to mild, asthma.

A. Cholinergic Mechanisms

Cholinergic mechanisms are the predominant neural pathway in the control of human airways and there is considerable evidence that there is an increase in cholinergic activity in asthma. Cholinergic reflexes may be activated in asthma by stimulation of airway sensory receptors or via extrapulmonary receptors, such as esophageal and nasal receptors. Cholinergic reflexes may be enhanced in

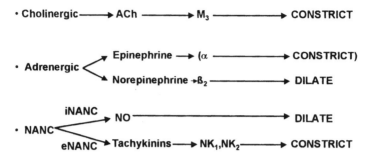

Figure 4   Autonomic regulation of airway tone. Cholinergic (parasympathetic) nerves release acetylcholine (ACh), which activates muscarinic M_3 receptors, resulting in constriction. Adrenergic (sympathetic) nerves release norepinephrine and epinephrine is released from the adrenal medulla to activate β_2-receptors, which bronchodilate. In some species α-receptors may mediate bronchoconstriction, but there is little evidence for this in humans. Nonadrenergic noncholinergic (NANC) nerves are bronchodilator (iNANC) via the release of nitric oxide (NO) or bronchoconstrictor (eNANC) via the release of tachykinins.

asthma as a result of facilitation of acetylcholine release from sensory nerves due to stimulation of various prejunctional receptors (90).

There has been much recent research into muscarinic receptors in the airways of asthmatic patients. There is no evidence for any increase in muscarinic receptors in asthmatic lung (91). However, several subtypes of muscarinic receptor have now been identified and M_1, M_2, and M_3 receptors are expressed in human airways (92). M_2 receptors are localized prejunctionally and inhibit the release of acetylcholine from cholinergic nerve terminals. There is evidence that M_2 receptors may be dysfunctional in asthmatic airways (93). There are several mechanisms that may result in M_2 receptor dysfunction, including allergen exposure and eosinophilic inflammation, oxidative stress, and certain viral infections (94). Several inflammatory cytokines also result in reduced transcription of the M_2 receptor gene or uncoupling of M_2 receptors (95,96). It is possible that in severe asthma the dysfunction of M_2 receptors may be increased, thus leading to exaggerated cholinergic tone. Some evidence in support of this is that anticholinergic drugs appear to be more effective in acute exacerbations of asthma than in control of chronic stable asthma.

Recently it has become evident that acetylcholine may be synthesized in cells other than cholinergic neurons. There is evidence for synthesis of acetylcholine in airway epithelial cells of several species, including humans (97). Since inflammatory cytokines may induce choline acetyltransferase, the enzyme that is critical to acetylcholine synthesis, this may be increased in the airways of severe asthmatic patients.

B. Inhibitory NANC Nerves

The only neural bronchodilator mechanism in human airways is nonadrenergic and noncholinergic (NANC). At first it was thought that the neurotransmitter of these nerves was the neuropeptide vasoactive intestinal peptide (VIP), as this is a potent bronchodilator of human airways and there is convincing evidence for a role as a bronchodilator neurotransmitter in some species (98). However, evidence now strongly suggests that NO is the only neurotransmitter in human airways (99). It is possible that bronchodilator NANC nerves may be defective in asthma, as superoxide anions generated by inflammatory cells such as eosinophils may inactivate NO by formation of peroxynitrite (Fig. 5). This might be expected

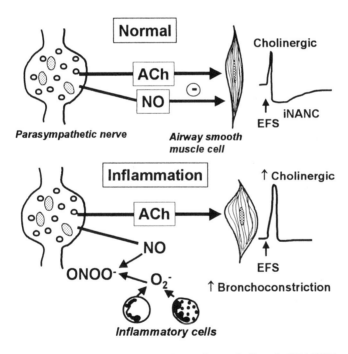

Figure 5 Possible loss of inhibitory nonadrenergic noncholinergic (iNANC) bronchodilatation and increase in cholinergic bronchoconstriction in inflamed airways. Superoxide anions (O_2^-) generated from inflammatory cells (eosinophils and neutrophils) combine with nitric oxide (NO), the neurotransmitter of iNANC nerves, to result in the formation of peroxynitrite ($ONOO^-$).

to be more prominent in severe asthma or during exacerbations. Normally, endogenous NO inhibits cholinergic bronchoconstriction (100), so that a reduction in NO released from cholinergic nerves would have the effect of increasing cholinergic neural bronchoconstriction. The intensity of inflammation and oxidative stress may be greater in severe asthma, so that this effect may be more prominent in patients with severe compared to mild asthma.

C. Neuropeptides

Many neuropeptides have been localized to nerves in human airways, although there is still very little information about their role in asthma, as there are few antagonists available for clinical use. An early report of reduced VIP expression in asthmatic airways is likely to be artifactual and has not been confirmed in subsequent studies (101,102). In patients with severe asthma treated with oral corticosteroids, there was no evidence for a decrease in VIP-immunoreactive nerves (103).

There has been particular interest in the role of tachykinins and neurogenic inflammation in asthma. Substance P-immunoreactive nerves are sparse in human airways, but an early report suggested that there might be increased expression of these nerves in the airways of patients with severe asthma (104). However, there is no evidence for an increase in the content of substance P in asthmatic lungs (101) and no evidence for increased expression of the sensory neuropeptides substance P, neurokinin A, or calcitonin gene-related peptide in the airways of patients with severe asthma (103). The expression of tachykinin NK_1 and NK_2 receptors is increased in asthmatic airways (105,106). Whether this increase is greater in patients with severe asthma has not yet been determined. It has recently been demonstrated that tachykinins may also be expressed in inflammatory cells, such as macrophages and eosinophils, so that nonneuronal production of tachykinins is a possibility (107). Tachykinin antagonists have now been developed for clinical use. To date these NK_1-receptor antagonists have shown little effect in patients with mild asthma (108,109), but there have been no studies in patients with more severe asthma.

Neuropeptide Y (NPY) is colocalized with norepinephrine in sympathetic nerves, which are sparse in human airways. There is some increase in NPY-immunoreactive nerves in patients with asthma, but this is not correlated with disease severity (103).

V. Conclusions

There is little concrete information about the role of specific inflammatory mediators, cytokines, or neural mechanisms in patients with severe asthma. This is largely because most studies have concentrated on patients with mild asthma, who are much easier to study with invasive techniques, such as bronchial biopsies. Recently, the availability of specific mediator antagonists has made it feasible to study patients with more severe asthma, but this may not be possible if the specific inhibitor is not developed because it is ineffective in mild asthma. It is possible that some patients with severe asthma have a specific abnormality in a particular mediator or its receptor and that these patients will respond to a specific drug therapy. These abnormalities may only become apparent when we understand more about the genetic polymorphisms that affect these mediator systems, but this is an area that will expand in the future.

References

1. Barnes PJ, Chung KF, Page CP. Inflammatory mediators of asthma: an update. Pharmacol Rev 1998; 50:515–596.
2. Barnes PJ. Is asthma a nervous disease? Chest 1995; 107:119S–124S.
3. van Ganse E, Kaufman L, Derde MP, Yernault JC, Delaunois L. Effects of antihistamines in adult asthma: a meta-analysis of clinical trials. Eur Respir J 1997; 10: 2216–2224.
4. Taha R, Olivenstein R, Utsumi T, Ernst P, Barnes PJ, Rodger IW, et al. Prostaglandin H synthase 2 expression in airway cells from patients with asthma and chronic obstructive pulmonary disease. Am J Respir Crit Care Med 2000; 161:636–640.
5. Pavord ID, Tattersfield AE. Bronchoprotective role for endogenous prostaglandin E_2. Lancet 1995; 344:436–438.
6. Saroca HG, Inman MD, O'Byrne PM. U46619-induced bronchoconstriction in asthmatic subjects is mediated by acetylcholine release. Am J Respir Crit Care Med 1995; 151:321–324.
7. O'Byrne PM, Fuller RW. The role of thromboxane A_2 in the pathogenesis of airway hyperresponsiveness. Eur Resp J 1989; 2:782–786.
8. Wenzel SE, Szefler SJ, Leung DY, Sloan SI, Rex MD, Martin RJ. Bronchoscopic evaluation of severe asthma: persistent inflammation associated with high dose glucocorticoids. Am J Respir Crit Care Med 1997; 156:737–743.
9. Evans DJ, Barnes PJ, Coulby LJ, Spaethe SM, van Alstyne EC, Pechous PA, et al. The effect of a leukotriene B_4 antagonist LY293111 on allergen-induced responses in asthma. Thorax 1996; 51:1178–1184.
10. Jatakanon A, Uasaf C, Maziak W, Lim S, Chung KF, Barnes PJ. Neutrophilic inflammation in severe persistent asthma. Am J Respir Crit Care Med 1999; 160: 1532–1539.
11. Drazen JM, Israel E, O'Byrne PM. Treatment of asthma with drugs modifying the leukotriene pathway. N Engl J Med 1999; 340:197–206.
12. Drazen JM, Yandava CN, Dube L, Szczerback N, Hippensteel R, Pillari A, et al. Pharmacogenetic association between ALOX5 promoter genotype and the response to anti-asthma treatment. Nat Genet 1999; 22:168–170.

13. Israel E, Rubin P, Kemp JP, Grossman J, Pierson W, Siegel SC, et al. The effect of inhibition of 5-lipoxygenase by zileuton in mild-to-moderate asthma. Ann Int Med 1993; 119:1059–1066.

14. Virchow J-C, Hassall SM, Summerton L, Klim J, Harris A. Reduction of asthma exacerbations with zafirlukast in patients on inhaled corticosteroids. Eur Respir J 1997; 10(suppl 25):420S.

15. Hanazawa T, Kharitonov SA, Barnes PJ. Increased nitrotyrosine in exhaled breath condensate of patients with asthma. Am J Resp Crit Care Med 2000; 162:1273–1276.

16. Dahlen B, Nizankowska E, Szezeklik A, Zetterstrom O, Bochenek G, Kumlin M, et al. Benefits from adding the 5-lipoxygenase inhibitor zileuton to conventional therapy in aspirin-intolerant asthmatics. Am J Respir Crit Care Med 1998; 157:1187–1194.

17. Robinson DS, Campbell DA, Barnes PJ. Montelukast sodium has minimal effect as add-on therapy in moderate to severe asthma. Am J Resp Crit Care Med 2000; 161:A198.

18. Spence DPS, Johnston SL, Calverley PMA, Dhillon P, Higgins C, Ramhamadany E, et al. The effect of the orally active platelet-activating factor antagonist WEB 2086 in the treatment of asthma. Am J Resp Crit Care Med 1994; 149:1142–1148.

19. Chung KF. Platelet-activating factor in inflammation and pulmonary disorders. Clin Sci 1992; 83:127–138.

20. O'Connor BJ, Uden S, Carty TJ, Eskra D, Barnes PJ, Chung KF. Effect of a potent and specific platelet activating factor (PAF) receptor antagonist on airway and systemic responses to PAF in man. Am J Resp Crit Care Med 1994; 150:35–40.

21. Kuitert LM, Angus RM, Barnes NC, Bone MF, Chung KF, Fairfax AJ, et al. The effect of a novel potent PAF antagonist, modipafant, in chronic asthma. Am J Respir Crit Care Med 1995; 151:1331–1335.

22. Evans DJ, Barnes PJ, Cluzel M, O'Connor BJ. Effects of a potent platelet activating factor antagonist, SR27417A, on allergen-induced asthmatic responses. Am J Respir Crit Care Med 1997; 156:11–16.

23. Feoktistov I, Biaggioni I. Pharmacological characterization of adenosine A_{2B} receptors: studies in human mast cells co-expressing A_{2A} and A_{2B} adenosine receptor subtypes. Biochem Pharmacol 1998; 55:627–633.

24. Hay DWP, Henry PJ, Goldic RG. Is endothelin-1 a mediator in asthma? Am J Respir Crit Care Med 1996; 155:1994–1997.

25. Goldie RG, Henry PJ. Endothelins and asthma. Life Sci 1999; 65:1–15.

26. Chalmers GW, Little SA, Patel KR, Thomson NC. Endothelin-1-induced bronchoconstriction in asthma. Am J Respir Crit Care Med 1997; 156:382–388.

27. Redington AE, Springall DR, Ghatei MA, Lau LC, Bloom SR, Holgate ST, et al. Endothelin in bronchoalveolar lavage fluid and its relation to airflow obstruction in asthma. Am J Respir Crit Care Med 1995; 151:1034–1039.

28. Redington AE, Springall DR, Meng QH, Tuck AB, Holgate ST, Polak JM, et al. Immunoreactive endothelin in bronchial biopsy specimens: increased expression in asthma and modulation by corticosteroid therapy. J Allergy Clin Immunol 1997; 100:544–552.

29. Aoki T, Kojima T, Ono A, Unishi G, Yoshijima S, Kameda Hayashi N, et al. Circulating endothelin-1 levels in patients with bronchial asthma. Ann Allergy 1994; 73: 365–369.

30. Chen WY, Yu J, Wang JY. Decreased production of endothelin-1 in asthmatic children after immunotherapy. J Asthma 1995; 32:29–35.

31. Peacock AJ, Dawes KE, Shock A, Gray AJ, Reeves JT, Laurent GJ. Endothelin-1 and endothelin-3 induces chemotaxis and replication of pulmonary artery fibroblasts. Am J Respir Cell Mol Biol 1992; 7:492–499.

32. Panettieri RA, Jr., Goldie RG, Rigby PJ, Eszterhas AJ, Hay DW. Endothelin-1-induced potentiation of human airway smooth muscle proliferation: an ETA receptor-mediated phenomenon. Br J Pharmacol 1996; 118:191–197.

33. Nathan C, Xie Q-W. Regulation of biosynthesis of nitric oxide. J Biol Chem 1994; 269:13725–13728.

34. Barnes PJ, Kharitonov SA. Exhaled nitric oxide: a new lung function test. Thorax 1996; 51:218–220.

35. Salch D, Ernst P, Lim S, Barnes PJ, Giaid A. Increased formation of the potent oxidant peroxynitrite in the airways of asthmatic patients is associated with induction of nitric oxide synthase: effect of inhaled glucocorticoid. FASEB J 1998; 12: 929–937.

36. Jatakanon A, Lim S, Kharitonov SA, Chung KF, Barnes PJ. Correlation between exhaled nitric oxide, sputum eosinophils and methacholine responsiveness. Thorax 1998; 53:91–95.

37. Stirling RG, Kharitonov SA, Campbell D, Robinson D, Durham SR, Chung KF, et al. Increase in exhaled nitric oxide levels in patients with difficult asthma and correlation with symptoms and disease severity despite treatment with oral and inhaled and corticosteroids. Thorax 1998; 53:1030–1034.

38. Bernareggi M, Mitchell JA, Barnes PJ, Belvisi MG. Dual action of nitric oxide on airway plasma leakage. Am J Respir Crit Care Med 1997; 155:869–874.

39. Ferreira HHA, Medeiros MV, Lima CSP, Flores CA, Sannomiya P, Antunes E, et al. Inhibition of eosinophil chemotaxis by chronic blockade of nitric oxide biosynthesis. Eur J Pharmacol 1996; 310:201–207.

40. Hebestreit H, Dibbert B, Balatti I, Braun D, Schapowal A, Blaser K, et al. Disruption of Fas receptor signalling by nitric oxide in eosinophils. J Exp Med 1998; 187: 415–425.

41. Taylor DA, McGrath JL, Orr LM, Barnes PJ, O'Connor BJ. Effect of endogenous nitric oxide inhibition on airway responsiveness to histamine and adenosine-5'-monophosphate in asthma. Thorax 1998; 53:483–489.

42. Barnes PJ. Reactive oxygen species and airway inflammation. Free Rad Biol Med 1990; 9:235–243.

43. Repine JE, Bast A, Lankhorst I. Oxidative stress in chronic obstructive pulmonary disease. Am J Respir Crit Care Med 1997; 156:341–357.

44. de Raeve HR, Thunnissen FB, Kaneko FT, Guo FH, Lewis M, Kavuru MS, et al. Decreased Cu,Zn-SOD activity in asthmatic airway epithelium: correction by inhaled corticosteroid in vivo. Am J Physiol 1997; 272:L148–154.

45. Comhair SA, Bhathena PR, Dweik RA, Kavuru M, Erzurum SC. Rapid loss of superoxide dismutase activity during antigen-induced asthmatic response [letter]. Lancet 2000; 355:624.

46. Antczak A, Nowak D, Shariati B, Krol M, Piasecka G, Kurmanowska Z. Increased hydrogen peroxide and thiobarbituric acid-reactive products in expired breath condensate of asthmatic patients. Eur Respir J 1997; 10:1235–1241.

47. Horvath I, Donnelly LE, Kiss A, Kharitonov SA, Lim S, Chung KF, et al. Combined use of exhaled hydrogen peroxide and nitric oxide in monitoring asthma. Am J Respir Crit Care Med 1998; 1046–1048.

48. Dohlman AW, Black HR, Royall JA. Expired breath hydrogen peroxide is a marker of acute airway inflammation in pediatric patients with asthma. Am Rev Respir Dis 1993; 148:955–960.

49. Morrow JD, Roberts LJ. The isoprostanes: current knowledge and directions for future research. Biochem Pharmacol 1996; 51:1–9.

50. Montuschi P, Ciabattoni G, Corradi M, Nightingale JA, Collins JV, Kharitonov SA, et al. Increased 8-isoprostane, a marker of oxidative stress, in exhaled condensates of asthmatic patients. Am J Respir Crit Care Med 1999; 160:216–220.

51. Paredi P, Leak D, Ward S, Cramer D, Kharitonov SA, Barnes PJ. Increased exhaled ethane in exhaled air of asthmatic patients. Am J Respir Crit Care Med 1999; 159: A97.

52. van der Vliet A, Eiserich JP, Shigenaga MK, Cross CE. Reactive nitrogen species and tyrosine nitration in the respiratory tract: epiphenomena or a pathobiologic mechanism of disease? Am J Respir Crit Care Med 1999; 160:1–9.

53. Wu W, Chen Y, Hazen SL. Eosinophil peroxidase nitrates protein tyrosyl residues: implications for oxidative damage by nitrating intermediates in eosinophilic inflammatory disorders. J Biol Chem 1999; 274:25933–25944.

54. Barnes PJ. Bradykinin and asthma. Thorax 1992; 47:979–983.

55. Fuller RW, Dixon CMS, Cuss FMC, Barnes PJ. Bradykinin-induced bronchoconstriction in man: mode of action. Am Rev Respir Dis 1987; 135:176–180.

56. Hulsmann AR, Raatgep R, Saxena PR, Kerrebijn KF, de Jongste JC. Bradykinin-induced contraction of human peripheral airways mediated by both bradykinin B_2 and thromboxane receptors. Am J Respir Crit Care Med 1994; 150:1012–1018.

57. Trevisani M, Schmidlin F, Tognetto M, Nijkamp FP, Gies JP, Frossard N, et al. Evidence for in vitro expression of B_1 receptor in the mouse trachea and urinary bladder. Br J Pharmacol 1999; 126:1293–1300.

58. Akbary AM, Wirth KJ, Scholkens BA. Efficacy and tolerability of Icatibant (Hoe 140) in patients with moderately severe chronic bronchial asthma. Immunopharmacology 1996; 33:238–242.

59. Caughey GH. Of mites and men: trypsin-like proteases in the lungs. Am J Respir Cell Mol Biol 1997; 16:621–628.

60. Clark JM, Abraham WM, Fishman CE, Forteza R, Ahmed A, Cortes A, et al. Tryptase inhibitors block allergen-induced airway and inflammatory responses in allergic sheep. Am J Respir Crit Care Med 1995;152:2076–2083.

61. Mautino G, Oliver N, Chanez P, Bousquet J, Capony F. Increased release of matrix metalloproteinase-9 in bronchoalveolar lavage fluid and by alveolar macrophages of asthmatics. Am J Respir Cell Mol Biol 1997; 17:583–591.

62. Vignola AM, Riccobono L, Mirabella A, Profita M, Chanez P, Bellia V, et al. Sputum metalloproteinase-9/tissue inhibitor of metalloproteinase-1 ratio correlates

with airflow obstruction in asthma and chronic bronchitis. Am J Respir Crit Care Med 1998; 158:1945–1950.

63. Chung KF, Barnes PJ. Cytokines in asthma. Thorax 1999; 54:825–857.
64. Kips JC, Tavernier JH, Joos GF, Peleman RA, Pauwels RA. The potential role of tumor necrosis factor a in asthma. Clin Exp Allergy 1993; 23:247–250.
65. Barnes PJ, Karin M. Nuclear factor-κB: a pivotal transcription factor in chronic inflammatory diseases. N Engl J Med 1997; 336:1066–1071.
66. Keatings VM, Collins PD, Scott DM, Barnes PJ. Differences in interleukin-8 and tumor necrosis factor-α in induced sputum from patients with chronic obstructive pulmonary disease or asthma. Am J Respir Crit Care Med 1996; 153:530–534.
67. Tillie-Leblond I, Pugin J, Marquette CH, Lamblin C, Saulnier F, Brichet A, et al. Balance between proinflammatory cytokines and their inhibitors in bronchial lavage from patients with status asthmaticus. Am J Respir Crit Care Med 1999; 159:487–494.
68. Keatings VM, O'Connor BJ, Wright LG, Huston DP, Corrigan CJ, Barnes PJ. Late response to allergen is associated with increased concentrations of TNF-α and interleukin-5 in induced sputum. J Allergy Clin Immunol 1997; 99:693–698.
69. Moffatt MF, Cookson WO. Linkage and candidate gene studies in asthma. Am J Respir Crit Care Med 1997; 156:S110–S112.
70. Albuquerque RV, Hayden CM, Palmer LJ, Laing IA, Rye PJ, Gibson NA, et al. Association of polymorphisms within the tumour necrosis factor (TNF) genes and childhood asthma. Clin Exp Allergy 1998; 28:578–584.
71. Chagani T, Pare PD, Zhu S, Weir TD, Bai TR, Behbehani NA, et al. Prevalence of tumor necrosis factor-α and angiotensin converting enzyme polymorphisms in mild/moderate and fatal/near-fatal asthma. Am J Respir Crit Care Med 1999; 160:278–282.
72. Sousa AR, Lane SJ, Nakhosteen JA, Lee TH, Poston RN. Expression of interleukin-1 beta (IL-1b) and interleukin-1 receptor antagonist (IL-1ra) on asthmatic bronchial epithelium. Am J Respir Crit Care Med 1996; 154:1061–1066.
73. Leung DYM, Martin RJ, Szefler SJ, Sher ER, Ying S, Kay AB, et al. Dysregulation of interleukin 4, interleukin 5, and interferon-γ gene expression in steroid-resistant asthma. J Exp Med 1995; 181:33–40.
74. Kam JC, Szefler SJ, Surs W, Sher FR, Leung DYM. Combination IL-2 and IL-4 reduces glucocorticoid-receptor binding affinity and T cell response to glucocorticoids. J Immunol 1993; 151:3460–3466.
75. Wills-Karp M, Luyimbazi J, Xu X, Schofield B, Neben TY, Karp CL, et al. Interleukin-13: central mediator of allergic asthma. Science 1998; 282:2258–2261.
76. Grunig G, Warnock M, Wakil AE, Venkayya R, Brombacher F, Rennick DM, et al. Requirement for IL-13 independently of IL-4 in experimental asthma. Science 1998; 282:2261–2263.
77. Naseer T, Minshall EM, Leung DY, Laberge S, Ernst P, Martin RJ, et al. Expression of IL-12 and IL-13 mRNA in asthma and their modulation in response to steroids. Am J Resp Crit Care Med 1997; 155:845–851.
78. Spahn JD, Szefler SJ, Surs W, Doherty DE, Nimmagadda SR, Leung DY. A novel action of IL-13: induction of diminished monocyte glucocorticoid receptor-binding affinity. J Immunol 1996; 157:2654–2659.

79. Egan RW, Umland SP, Cuss FM, Chapman RW. Biology of interleukin-5 and its relevance to allergic disease. Allergy 1996; 51:71–81.

80. Corrigan CJ, Hamid Q, North J, Barkans J, Moqbel R, Durham S, et al. Peripheral blood CD4 but not CD8 T-lymphocytes in patients with exacerbations of asthma transcribe and translate messenger RNA encoding cytokines which prolong eosinophil survival in the context of a Th2 pattern: effect of glucocorticoid therapy. Am J Respir Cell Mol Biol 1995; 12:567–578.

81. Leckie MJ, ten Brincke A, Lordan J, Khan J, Diamant Z, Walls CM, et al. SB 240563, a humanized anti-IL-5 monoclonal antibody: initial single dose safety and activity in patients with asthma. Am J Respir Crit Care Med 1999; 159:A624.

82. Pretolani M, Goldman M. IL-10: a potential therapy for allergic inflammation? Immunol Today 1997; 18:277–280.

83. John M, Lim S, Seybold J, Robichaud A, O'Connor B, Barnes PJ, et al. Inhaled corticosteroids increase IL-10 but reduce MIP-1a, GM-CSF and IFN-γ release from alveolar macrophages in asthma. Am J Respir Crit Care Med 1998; 157:256–262.

84. Borish L, Aarons A, Rumbyrt J, Cvietusa P, Negri J, Wenzel S. Interleukin-10 regulation in normal subjects and patients with asthma. J Allergy Clin Immunol 1996; 97:1288–1296.

85. Barnes PJ, Lim S. Inhibitory cytokines in asthma. Mol Medicine Today 1998; 4: 452–458.

86. Barnes PJ. Endogenous inhibitory mechanisms in asthma. Am J Respir Crit Care Med 2000; 161:S176–S181.

87. Tomita K, Lim S, Hanazawa T, Stirling RG, Adcock IM, Chung KF, et al. Attenuated production of intracellular IL-12 in monocytes from patients with severe asthma. Am J Resp Crit Care Med 2000; 161:A923.

88. Lim S, Crawley E, Woo P, Barnes PJ. Haplotype associated with low interleukin-10 production in patients with severe asthma. Lancet 1998; 352:113.

89. van der Pouw Kraan Tc, Boeije LC, de Groot ER, Stapel SO, Snijders A, Kapsenberg ML, et al. Reduced production of IL-12 and IL-12-dependent IFN-γ release in patients with allergic asthma. J Immunol 1997; 158:5560–5565.

90. Barnes PJ. Modulation of neurotransmission in airways. Physiol Rev 1992; 72: 699–729.

91. Haddad E-B, Mak JCW, Barnes PJ. Expression of β-adrenergic and muscarinic receptors in human lung. Am J Physiol 1996; 270:L947–L953.

92. Mak JCW, Baraniuk JN, Barnes PJ. Localization of muscarinic receptor subtype mRNAs in human lung. Am J Respir Cell Mol Biol 1992; 7:344–348.

93. Minette PAH, Lammers J, Dixon CMS, McCusker MT, Barnes PJ. A muscarinic agonist inhibits reflex bronchoconstriction in normal but not in asthmatic subjects. J Appl Physiol 1989; 67:2461–2465.

94. Fryer AD, Adamko DJ, Yost BL, Jacoby DB. Effects of inflammatory cells on neuronal M_2 muscarinic receptor function in the lung. Life Sci 1999; 64:449–455.

95. Haddad E-B, Rousell J, Lindsay MA, Barnes PJ. Synergy between TNF-α and IL-1β in inducing down-regulation of muscarinic M_2 receptor gene expression. J Biol Chem 1996; 271:32586–32592.

96. Rousell J, Haddad E-B, Barnes PJ. Down-regulation of M_2 muscarinic receptor mRNA by PDGF in a human lung cell line. Mol Pharmacol 1997; 52:966–973.

97. Wessler I, Kirkpatrick CJ, Racke K. Non-neuronal acetylcholine, a locally acting molecule, widely distributed in biological systems: expression and function in humans. Pharmacol Ther 1998; 77:59–79.
98. Belvisi MG, Stretton CD, Miura M, Verleden GM, Tadjarimi S, Yacoub MH, et al. Inhibitory NANC nerves in human tracheal smooth muscle: a quest for the neurotransmitter. J Appl Physiol 1992; 73:2505–2510.
99. Belvisi MG, Stretton CD, Barnes PJ. Nitric oxide is the endogenous neurotransmitter of bronchodilator nerves in human airways. Eur J Pharmacol 1992; 210:221–222.
100. Ward JK, Belvisi MG, Fox AJ, Miura M, Tadjkarimi S, Yacoub MH, et al. Modulation of cholinergic neural bronchoconstriction by endogenous nitric oxide and vasoactive intestinal peptide in human airways in vitro. J Clin Invest 1993; 92:736–743.
101. Lilly CM, Bai TR, Shore SA, Hall AE, Drazen JM. Neuropeptide content of lungs from asthmatic and nonasthmatic patients. Am J Respir Crit Care Med 1995; 151:548–553.
102. Howarth PH, Springall DR, Redington AE, Djukanovic R, Holgate ST, Polak JM. Neuropeptide-containing nerves in bronchial biopsies from asthmatic and non-asthmatic subjects. Am J Respir Cell Mol Biol 1995; 13:288–296.
103. Chanez P, Springall D, Vignola AM, Moradoghi-Hattvani A, Polak JM, Godard P, et al. Bronchial mucosal immunoreactivity of sensory neuropeptides in severe airway diseases. Am J Respir Crit Care Med 1998; 158:985–990.
104. Ollerenshaw SL, Jarvis D, Sullivan CE, Woolcock AJ. Substance P immunoreactive nerves in airways from asthmatics and non-asthmatics. Eur Resp J 1991; 4:673–682.
105. Adcock IM, Peters M, Gelder C, Shirasaki H, Brown CR, Barnes PJ. Increased tachykinin receptor gene expression in asthmatic lung and its modulation by steroids. J Mol Endocrinol 1993; 11:1–7.
106. Bai TR, Zhou D, Weir T, Walker B, Hegele R, Hayashi S, et al. Substance P (NK_1)- and neurokinin A (NK_2)-receptor gene expression in inflammatory airway diseases. Am J Physiol 1995; 269:L309–L317.
107. Joos GF, Germonpre PR, Pauwels RA. Role of tachykinins in asthma. Allergy 2000; 55:321–337.
108. Fahy J, Wong HH, Geppetti P, Reiss JM, Harris SC, MacLean DB, et al. Effect of an NK_1 receptor antagonist (CP-99,994) on hypertonic saline-induced broncho-constriction and cough in male asthmatic subjects. Am J Resp Crit Care Med 1995; 152:879–884.
109. Ichinose M, Miura M, Yamauchi H, Kageyama N, Tomaki M, Oyake T, et al. A neurokinin 1-receptor antagonist improves exercise-induced airway narrowing in asthmatic patients. Am J Respir Crit Care Med 1996; 153:936–941.

5

Role of Airway Remodeling in Severe Asthma

SOPHIE MOLET

INSERM U456
Université de Rennes I
Rennes, France

QUTAYBA HAMID

Meakins-Christie Laboratories
McGill University
Montreal, Quebec, Canada

I. Introduction

Despite advances in our understanding of the pathophysiology and immunobiology of asthma, death rate from this illness appears to be increasing. There is also increased incidence of patients with severe intractable disease with considerable impairment of lung function and a requirement for oral corticosteroids. Airway obstruction in asthma is not a completely reversible disorder and is presumed to be the result of inflammation-induced structural changes—or remodeling—of the airways (1). These structural changes include epithelial detachment and regeneration, goblet cell hyperplasia, submucosal glands hypertrophy, subepithelial fibrosis (thickening of the basement membrane), inflammatory cell infiltration, hyperplasia and hypertrophy of the bronchial smooth muscle, and vascular changes. Increase in subepithelial and submucosal collagen depositions was found in asthmatic airway (2,3). Asthmatics are classified as severe if they are steroid-dependent, need frequent hospital administrations, have a long history of persistent asthma, and require time away from work (4,5). In contrast, mild asthmatics occasionally use bronchodilators and/or inhaled steroids. Structural changes in mild asthma are less prominent than those observed in airways of severe or fatal asthma. This suggests that there is a progression in the degree of inflammation from mild to severe asthma with alterations in epithelial cell integrity and basement membrane, bronchial smooth muscle, and mucous gland. Patients with long-standing disease and altered airway structure are more likely to die from asthma.

Although the remodeling process has been invoked to explain the development of chronic airflow obstruction and airway hyperresponsiveness (6,7), the cause of remodeling and its reversibility in response to treatment remain to be clarified. In this chapter, we focus on the different components of the airway remodeling process and their contribution to severe asthma.

II. Somatic Components of Asthma

A. Epithelial Damage/Desquamation

Histological shedding and damage of airway epithelium are prominent features of asthma (8). Support for epithelial desquamation comes from the finding of epithelial cells in mucus plugs in the airways of patients who died from asthma (9). Epithelial shedding could be caused by weakened attachment of columnar epithelial cells to each other or to basal cells, possibly reflecting a reaction to irritation or a cell maturation defect (10). Another feature of epithelial changes in asthma is squamous metaplasia, which could result in epithelial regeneration. Soderberg et al. have suggested that epithelial desquamation may be an artifact in all bronchial biopsies obtained by fiberoptic bronchoscopy (11). Moreover, Caroll et al. have demonstrated that epithelial desquamation did not differ significantly in fatal asthma compared to non-asthma-related death or nonfatal asthma (12).

Increase in epithelial desquamation leads to an augmentation in airway responsiveness (8). However, epithelial desquamation is not restricted to asthma: Epithelial cell shedding has been observed in nonasthmatic subjects with chronic cough and in subjects with allergic rhinitis (13).

B. Goblet Cells, Submucosal Glands, and Mucus Production

Goblet cells are the principal mucus-secreting cells of the surface epithelium and as such contribute to "first line" defense of the airways (14). Submucosal glands are a complex network of tubules and ducts opening on to the airway lumen (15). In normal human airways, the ratio of submucosal glands to goblet cells has been calculated as 40:1 (16), indicating that goblet cells might not play a significant role in secretion. However, bronchial goblet cell hyperplasia, submucosal gland hyperplasia, and metaplasia have been reported in asthma and are associated with reduced numbers of serous and ciliated cells and possibly Clara cells. This may contribute to the excessive production of mucus and the plugging of airways (17). Goblet cell and submucosal gland hyperplasia are described in both small and large airways of asthmatics (12,18,19) and could be the cause of death (9,18). Goblet cell hyperplasia is not only seen in fatal asthma, since Laitinen et al. have demonstrated these changes in newly diagnosed asthmatics (20). Moreover, in some sudden fatal asthma, this feature is not prominent and these patients seem to die from bronchial constriction of empty or dry airways (21). Goblet cell changes in the peripheral small airways could contribute to a larger extent of the disease because the clearance of mucus from small airways appears to be more difficult compared to that in larger airways.

The primary role of airway mucus is to form a protective barrier between the external environment and the body's sterile internal environment. The visco-elastic properties of airway mucus are attributed largely to high-molecular-weight glycoproteins known as mucins (22), which are secreted by specialized cells in the epithelium and submucosa (23). Mucins are expressed in goblet cells and glandular mucous cells. Currently nine mucin genes are recognized, namely MUC1–MUC4, MUC5AC, MUC5B, and MUC6–MUC8 (24–28). The predominant mucins in adult respiratory secretions appear to be MUC5AC and MUC5B (29–30). MUC4 is also expressed in airway and may contribute to respiratory secretion (31). The surface epithelial goblet cells and the mucous cells of the submucosal glands could also act as a reservoir, releasing large amounts of mucus into the lumen in response to stimuli. Other secretory cells in the airways are the surface epithelial serous cells (32), Clara cells, and possibly ciliated cells. Several secretagogues are involved in mucus production in asthma. These include mediators released by mast cells (leukotrienes, prostaglandins, and histamine) (33), eosinophils (MBP and EPO) (34–35), macrophages (macrophage-derived mucous secretagogue, or MMS) (36), or nerves (substance P) (37). Neutrophil elastase has been also reported to be a potential inducer of goblet cell hyperplasia and mucin production (38).

The increased amount of mucus in the airways could also be attributed partially to a disturbance in mucociliary clearance, particularly in severe asthma (39). A number of factors can reduce clearance including epithelial shedding (with consequent loss of cilia) and mediators that slow mucociliary clearance directly, e.g., leukotriene D4 (40). The major basic protein (MBP) in eosinophils has also been reported to cause epithelium damage and loss of ciliary epithelium (41,42).

C. Smooth Muscle Hypertrophy/Hyperplasia

Airway smooth muscle (ASM) hypertrophy and hyperplasia are not constant observations in asthmatics (43). However, they are believed to be two of the principal contributors to airway wall thickening and obstruction in asthma (44). It was originally believed that smooth muscle hyperplasia is the main pathological change in the airways of asthmatics (45–46) (Fig. 1) but Ebina et al. have suggested that while hyperplasia is seen predominantly in the large airways, hyper-

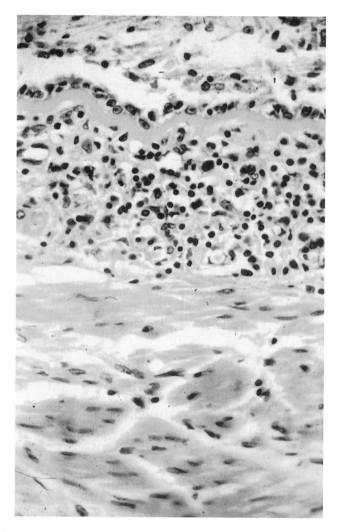

Figure 1 Hematoxylin–eosin staining of a bronchial biopsy recovered from a severe asthmatic patient showing smooth muscle hyperplasia and hypertrophy.

trophy is the main pathological feature of the smaller airways (44). However, the increase in smooth muscle mass in asthma does not appear to extend to airways of less than 2 mm in diameter (47).

Recent data from Thomson et al. suggest that the hyperreactivity associated with asthma is not a consequence of increased ASM in airways since no difference in the smooth muscle mass was observed between asthmatic and nonasthmatic subjects (48). However, the airway wall was shown to be thicker in cases of fatal asthma than in cases of nonfatal asthma and cases without asthma (12). The fact that patients with mild asthma had thickening of the airway wall supports the hypothesis that chronic inflammatory changes lead to airway wall thickening. Changes in the smaller airways, which have smooth muscle that completely encircles the airway lumen, will have a much greater effect than similar changes in the more central airways (49). As a consequence of airway wall thickness, less muscle shortening is required to close the airways of asthmatics as compared to nonasthmatics (50). Furthermore, an increase in the amount of ASM will allow greater shortening in response to a bronchoconstrictor stimulus. In addition, the stiffness of the remodeled airway wall has been shown to be the cause of loss of airway distensibility (7). It seems very likely that excess muscle shortening due to extensive remodeling of airway walls is the cause of death in some cases of asthma where mucus plugging or submucosal edema are absent. The magnitude of airway wall thickening that is observed in the airways of subjects with asthma may contribute substantially to airway hyperresponsiveness in addition to airflow obstruction.

Classically ASM cells were considered the major end-effector cells mediating bronchomotor tone in health and disease. Recent evidence, however, suggests that in addition to their contractile properties, ASM cells can potentially contribute to the pathogenesis of asthma by participating in and coordinating the inflammation. ASM cells have the ability to produce proinflammatory and profibrotic cytokines including IL-6 and IL-11 (51), chemokines (eotaxin, IL-8, LIF, MIP-1α, MCP-1, and RANTES) (51–55), and growth factors (GM-CSF) (56). They can also express cell adhesion molecules such as ICAM-1 and VCAM-1, particularly upon TNF-α stimulation (57). ASM cells may be also a source of extracellular matrix (ECM)-related products including types I and IV collagen, elastin, biglycan, decorin, fibronectin, and MMP-1 (68,59), which are capable of perpetuating and increasing the severity of airway wall thickening.

D. Subepithelial Fibrosis (Thickening of the BM)

In normal subjects, laminin and type IV collagen are the components of a thin basement membrane. One feature of airway remodeling in asthma is subepithelial fibrosis, which could be due to deposition of different types of collagen (types I, III, and V) (Fig. 2) as well as fibronectin and laminin beneath the basement membrane (2,60). This subepithelial fibrosis contributes to asthma pathology and correlates with the disease severity (61,62). It has been suggested that these proteins are produced by myofibroblasts, which are reported to be increased in asthma and are shown to be correlated with the basement membrane thickness (2,63,64). Multiple factors have been associated with subepithelial fibrosis, including frequency of asthma episodes (65), duration of symptoms (66), T-lym-

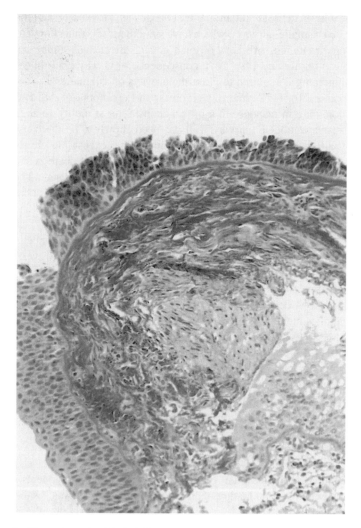

Figure 2   Extensive subepithelial fibrosis evaluated by Van Gieson staining in a bronchial biopsy recovered from a severe asthmatic patient. Total collagen deposition is seen. (From Ref. 87.)

phocyte activity (67), epithelial damage (2), fibroblast activity (63), and mast cell and eosinophil infiltration (68).

Basement Membrane

In asthmatics and normal subjects, examination of the ultrastructure of the basement membrane has shown that the organization of the lamina rara and lamina densa of the true basement membrane are of normal appearance. Beneath these, in normal subjects there is a loose array of collagen fibrils forming a well-preserved reticular layer. In contrast in asthmatics, the lamina reticularis is increased in depth (2), which was previously described as "basement membrane thickening" (65,69), and is a consistent feature of asthma deaths. However, some data suggest that such a structural alteration is also present in the early phases of airway inflammation in asthma and that airway remodeling can occur even in patients suffering from mild forms of the disease (70). Most studies on "basement membrane thickening" have been done at the level of the large airways and almost nothing has been described in the more distal airways, which are more and more described as potent key players in the pathology of asthma (71–76).

Extracellular Matrix

The extracellular matrix (ECM) is composed of a mixture of macromolecules such as polysaccharides glycosaminoglycans (GAG), proteoglycans (PG), and fibrous proteins of two functional types: structural (collagen and elastin) and adhesive (fibronectin and laminin). The GAG and PG molecules form a highly hydrated, gel-like "ground substance" in which the fibrous proteins are embedded. The pulmonary ECM, classically thought to be inert, is subjected to a continuous turnover of >10% of the total ECM per day (77–78). A dynamic equilibrium between synthesis and degradation of the pulmonary ECM is required to maintain the physiological balance. This balance is tightly controlled by three regulatory mechanisms: (1) de novo synthesis and deposition of ECM components such as collagens; (2) proteolytic degradation of existing ECM by matrix metalloproteinases (MMPs); and (3) inhibition of MMP activity by specific endogenous antiproteases, the tissue inhibitors of metalloproteinases (TIMPs) (77–80). The ECM plays a profound role in providing the mechanical support and properties for tissue and in particular during reorganization and repair of damaged tissues. Moreover, the extracellular components of this matrix can influence many functions including structural support; compartmentalization, separating epithelium and endothelium from interstitium; mechanical characteristics; and cellular function such as adhesion, spreading, and growth differentiation. These processes are key in organogenesis, angiogenesis, injury, and repair. During the pathogenesis of lung fibrosis, the homeostasis deteriorates, resulting in a net increase in deposited ECM and collagen content of the lung. This altered ECM is responsible for the severe loss of lung function associated with lung fibrosis (77,81). The net deposition of ECM material in the bronchial subepithelial area can be the result of an increased synthesis and/or decreased degradation. The processes of ECM disassembly, renewal, restructuring, and assembly of ECM are highly regulated, especially by activated myofibroblasts, which are the main cells synthesizing and degrading matrix components. In this regard, fibroblasts produce many MMPs, which can cleave most of the ECM components (80).

Collagens

In the lung, collagen deposition is strictly regulated to ensure a balance between the rate of biosynthesis and degradation. Imbalance of this control leads to increased collagen deposition and consequently fibrosis. Subepithelial fibrosis in asthma is partly due to increased expression of various types of collagens. Immunohistochemical analysis suggests that this thickening is largely composed of collagen types III, V, and, to a lesser extent, I (2). Collagen types I, III, and V were localized in the interstitial submucosal tissue while a strong immunoreactivity for collagen type IV was shown within the bronchial smooth muscle (2). However, the distribution of collagen type IV was reported to be unaltered in asthma (2). Collagens are synthesized in the lung predominantly by fibroblasts, although other cell types are also capable of synthesizing collagens including type II pneumocytes and epithelial and endothelial cells (82–86). We have reported a relationship between the extent of subepithelial collagen deposition and the severity of asthma (87), suggesting a role for collagen deposition in the irreversible airway narrowing that can occur in this disease. However, this area is a subject of debate since others have not found a correlation between the subepithelial fibrosis in large bronchi and clinical or physiological indicators of asthma severity (2,88). This could be due to differences in the methods used for measuring the extent of collagen deposition, sampling error, and low population numbers. It has been suggested that the structural properties of collagens and the actual amount of these proteins are more relevant to clinical features than the extent of their deposition.

Fibronectin

Fibronectin is the earliest known and by far the best studied adhesive protein component of ECM involved in cell attachment and chemotaxis as well as in repair processes (89). Fibronectin is produced by a variety of cell types including airway epithelial cells. This production is increased in asthmatics compared to that in normal subjects (90). The bronchoalveolar lavage (BAL) level of fibronectin is higher in asthmatics compared to that in normal subjects (91). Increased accumulation of fibronectin within the bronchial mucosa has been identified as an important factor of the thickening of the basal membrane (2,60). Concentrations of fibronectin also increased after antigen challenge and correlated with increased presence of inflammatory cells (lymphocytes, eosinophils, neutrophils, and macrophages) (92). The release and expression of fibronectin are directly modulated by TGF-β. Moreover, it has been found that increased TGF-β production precedes the synthesis of fibronectin, suggesting a role for TGF-β in airway repair through modulation of FN production.

Tenascin

Tenascin is a protein produced in response to injury and repair. Molecular interactions of tenascin with other components of ECM are restricted to chondroitin sulfate proteoglycans. Asthmatic bronchi showed accumulation of tenascin in the basement membrane zone beneath the basal lamina (93). This could be due to either increased production or decreased degradation.

Proteoglycans

Proteoglycans are the most abundant, and perhaps functionally the most versatile, nonfibrillar components of ECM (94,95). These complex macromolecules are made up of a core polypeptide to which linear heteropolysaccharides, glycosaminoglycans (GAG), are covalently attached. These GAGs may be heparan sulfate (HSPG), chondroitin sulfate (CSPG), dermatan sulfate (DSPG), or keratan sulfate (KSPG). Perlecan is one major component of basement membrane. Additional members of the family of ECM, PG are represented by three well-known members: decorin, biglycan, and fibromodulin. We have recently demonstrated the increased deposition of both small (lumican and biglycan) and large (versican) PG in the airway wall of mild atopic asthmatics (96). Although the functional role of increased PG deposition in the airway wall of asthmatics is unknown, this change correlates with airway hyperresponsiveness, suggesting that PG may play a role in airway remodeling.

Matrix Metalloproteinases

Matrix metalloproteinases (MMPs or matrixins) consist of a family of highly homologous endopeptidases, which are capable of cleaving most, if not all, protein constituents of the extracellular matrix including collagen, proteoglycan, laminin, fibronectin, and elastin. Organogenesis, cell migration, inflammation, angiogenesis, wound healing, and tissue remodeling are some of the physiological processes in which MMPs play a crucial part (97). With regard to the lung, MMPs have been implicated in the pathophysiology of lung cancer and acute and chronic inflammatory diseases including adult respiratory distress syndrome, interstitial lung fibrosis, bronchiectasis, and cystic fibrosis (80,98–100). In lung MMPs are involved in normal ECM turnover and also participate in the wound healing response following injury (77,101). MMPs can participate in the fibrotic process at two stages: (1) at the injury stage by degrading BM and ECM constituents; and (2) at the "attempted repair" stage, where modulation of the production or action of MMPs may contribute to tissue remodeling. According to their substrate specificity and structure, members of the MMP gene family can be classified into the following subgroups:

1. *Collagenases* (MMP-1, MMP-8, and MMP-13), which degrade connective tissue collagens.
2. *Matrilysin and stromelysins* (MMP-3, MMP-10, MMP-11, and MMP-7), which have the broadest substrate range and specificity in degrading matrix PG, laminin, FN, elastin, and the globular portion of collagens (102).
3. *Gelatinases* (MMP-2 and MMP-9), formerly known as type IV collagenases, which have activity against BM collagens and matrix PG as well as gelatinolytic activity. Although the substrate specificities of MMP-2 (gelatinase A/72-kDA gelatinase) and MMP-9 (gelatinase B/92-kDA gelatinase) seem similar, the two enzymes are known to be synthesized by different cells in vitro. Principally fibroblasts, endothelial cells, and osteoblasts synthesize the 72-kDa form, whereas the 92-kDa form is produced mainly by inflammatory cells including polymorphonuclear leukocytes, macrophages, eosinophils (103), and lymphocytes (104). MMP-9 is able to degrade type IV collagen, native type V collagen, denatured collagens, and fibronectin and has also elastolytic properties (105,106). The release of MMP-9, the major MMP secreted by alveolar macrophages (107), is increased in BAL from asthmatics compared to that from controls (110). Eosinophil is also reported to be a source of MMP-9 mRNA in bronchial tissues of asthmatics (109). MMP-9 has also been found to be highly expressed in epithelium and submucosa of asthmatics compared to those in controls (110). Types II and V collagen as well as tenascin deposition in the BM in asthmatics are associated with increased expression of MMP-9.
4. *Elastase*, of which the major source in human lung is neutrophil (111). Other sources include macrophage (112) and eosinophil (113). Neutrophil elastase can reproduce many of the pathologic features of asthma, including mucous gland hyperplasia (114), excess mucus secretion (115), epithelial damage (116), and connective tissue destruction (117). Elastase exposure has also been found to increase directed fibroblast migration through the ECM (118). In induced sputum from asthmatics, the level of elastase is increased (119). This level correlated with the number of neutrophils and is inversely correlated with FEV1 values. The expression of α_1-anti-trypsin or α_1-proteinase inhibitor (α_1-PI), which is the main inhibitor of elastase (120), is also increased in sputum from asthmatics compared to controls; however, this may not be sufficient to counterbalance the increased level of elastase.

5. *Membrane-type MMPs* (MT-MMP-1 to -4), which are localized to the cell surface.

Moreover, we anticipate the discovery of many more new MMPs, which will introduce further complexity in tissue matrix catabolism.

The MMPs are produced by virtually all resident lung cells including fibroblasts (predominant source), alveolar macrophages, and epithelial and endothelial cells, but they could also be produced by phagocytic and inflammatory cells (neutrophils, macrophages, and eosinophils). Normal tissue does not store MMPs and constitutive expression is minimal. With the exception of neutrophil MMPs (collagenase and MMP-9), which are stored in secondary and tertiary granules poised for rapid release, MMP production and activity are highly regulated. In stromal cells MMP production is regulated at the transcriptional level by a range of cytokines and growth factors (e.g., IL-1β, TNF-α, PDGF, EGF, TGF-β, bFGF, NGF, IL-10, IFN-γ, and IL-4), hormones, and cellular transformations which all influence the production and stability of MMP mRNAs (121). Many of these cytokines also enhance the production of TIMP-1.

Most MMPs are secreted as inactive or latent precursors (zymogens) and are proteolytically activated in the extracellular space (122,123). In serum and in extracellular space there are a number of specific inhibitors of MMPs, including α_2-macroglobulin and tissue inhibitor of metalloproteinases or TIMPs (123). The TIMP gene family consists of four structurally related members, TIMP-1, -2, -3, and -4 (124). TIMP-1, -2, and -4 are secreted in soluble form, whereas TIMP-3 is associated with ECM. TIMPs have biological effects that extend beyond their roles as inhibitors of MMP activity including stimulation of the growth of several cell types (124). TIMP-1, a major member of the TIMP family, inhibits MMP-1, MMP-2, MMP-3, and MMP-9 (125). Interestingly, TIMP-1 and TIMP-2 can also bind the latent form of both MMP-9 and MMP-2, respectively (107,126). TIMP-1 is found in high proportions in epithelium and submucosa of subjects with asthma (110). TIMP-1 levels in asthmatics are found to be significantly correlated with the number of alveolar macrophages, but not with eosinophils, lymphocytes, or neutrophils (127). The TIMP-1 level was significantly higher in stable asthmatics than in glucocorticoid-treated subjects or in controls, while TIMP-2 was undetectable (127). The level of TIMP-1 was found to be positively correlated with IL-6 (127). Whereas IL-6 modulated TIMP-1 expression, TNF-α and, to a lesser extent, IL-1β and IL-6 modulated that of MMP-9 in asthmatics (128). There is a tendency for TIMP-1 to increase with the severity of asthma (127). In normal subjects, TIMP-1 and MMP-9 were found to be coreleased by alveolar macrophages (128). Similar results were found in corticosteroid-treated asthmatics, with a stronger correlation between TIMP-1 and MMP-9 (128). The baseline serum MMP-9:TIMP-1 ratio correlates strongly with airflow obstruction improvement following oral corticosteroid therapy in severe asthma (129). It has been shown that the higher the MMP-9:TIMP-1 ratio, the better the FEV_1 improvement. However, enhanced release of TIMP-1 was not correlated with that of MMP-9 in mild asthmatics, suggesting an altered balance between enzyme and inhibitor production (128). Dosage of MMPs and TIMPs in serum may be a novel potential noninvasive tool to evaluate the pathological profile of asthma and help to predict its response to corticosteroid. TIMP-1 may also act through its cell-growth-promoting activity by increasing myofibroblast proliferation (130) and TGF-β production (131). This in turn may amplify TIMP-1 production (132). The fibrotic effect of TGF-β1 and -β3 in lung fibroblasts results from (1) an increase in the secretion and deposition of total ECM and collagens, (2) a decrease in MMP-1 secretion, and (3) an increase of TIMP-1 expression (133). However, TIMP-1 was previously shown to enhance fibroblasts to produce MMP-1 (134).

Because matrix metabolism is a balance between synthesis and lysis, an increase in inhibitor production would prevent proteolytic degradation and repair and would hence result in the accumulation of collagen types I, III, and V and fibronectin (2). The coordinated production of MMPs and their specific tissue inhibitors in a range of developing and remodeling situations suggest that TIMPs play a significant role in the regulation of MMP activation in vivo (122). Not only soluble fators but also cell–matrix and cell–cell interations may be some other keys in gene expression of MMPs as follows: induction of MMP-2 in T cells through very late antigen-4 vascular cell adhesion molecule-1-mediated adhesion to endothelial cells (135), MMP-9 expression in monocytes by activated T cells through gp39–CD40 interactions (136), and $\alpha_5\beta_1$-integrin–fibronectin interactions for MMP-9 expression during macrophage differentiation (137).

Myofibroblasts

Myofibroblasts are identified as an important source of ECM proteins (63,79) and are present in large numbers beneath the bronchial epithelium (63). Myofibroblasts contribute to tissue repair by assembling newly secreted matrix proteins into more complex structures such as fibrils. Myofibroblasts possess fibroblast morphology and contain contractile elements, which are best seen on examination by electron microscopy. In some cases, the contractile elements may contain an actin filament that is normally found in smooth muscle cells (smooth muscle actin, or SMA) (138). Although myofibroblasts are found in both normal and asthmatic subjects, their numbers were increased in atopic asthma and found to correlate positively with the extent of collagen below the bronchial epithelium, suggesting that these cells might be responsible for the deposition of collagen (63,64). Brewster et al. have demonstrated a relationship between the number of myofibroblasts and the duration of asthma (63). In contrast, Roche et al. (2) found no correlation between the subepithelial fibrosis in large bronchi and clinical or physiological indicators of asthma severity. Jeffery et al. showed that the response to corticosteroids is not associated with the decrease in subepithelial fibrosis, suggesting dissociation between this process and the severity of the disease (139). Cytokines such as GM-CSF and TGF-β have been shown to be capable of inducing fibroblast differentiation to myofibroblasts with expression of SMA in vitro and to some extent in vivo in human cells (140). In addition to producing matrix molecules, fibroblasts are important immune-effector cells that produce, in an antigen-independent fashion, a variety of mediators and cytokines that can serve to amplify and/or perpetuate tissue inflammation (54,141).

E. Inflammation (Inflammatory Cells and Mediators)

Asthma is recognized as an inflammatory condition of the airways in which there is tissue eosinophilia and a predominance of T lymphocytes of the CD4 (helper) subset. In fatal asthma there is a marked inflammatory cell infiltrate throughout the airway wall and also in the occluding plugs (9,142).

Eosinophils are considered to be the prominent effector inflammatory cells in asthma (143). Eosinophils release a number of mediators thought to be the major cause of airway inflammation. Recent evidence suggests that eosinophils may also play a key role in airway remodeling since they were shown to express some mediators that are profibrotic or associated with fibrosis, including TGF-β (87,144–147), IL-6 (148), IL-11 (149), IL-17 (150), and MMP-9 (109) as well as other metalloproteinases. All these mediators regulate the proliferation and matrix production of fibroblasts and other stromal cells. In contrast to observations in biopsy specimens obtained from patients with mild asthma after treatment with inhaled corticosteroids (151), in the patients with severe asthma, corticosteroids failed to deplete the bronchial mucosa of eosinophils (152).

Mast cell hyperplasia has also been reported in asthmatic airways and is a frequent pathologic finding in tissue fibrosis and remodeling responses (153). Their participation in the development of airway remodeling in asthma is still not well understood. However, β-tryptase, which constitutes the major protein component of the mast cell secretory granules, has been shown to stimulate in vitro fibroblast proliferation and collagen production (154).

Th2-type lymphocytes are implicated in allergic responses since they are the primary source of IL-5 (155,156), which contributes to eosinophil differentiation and survival (159,160). However, since activated T lymphocytes adhere to and stimulate DNA synthesis in cultures of human airway smooth muscle cells (57), this suggests that cell adhesion molecule/T-lymphocyte-mediated adhesion may partly contribute to airway remodeling in vivo.

Increased numbers of activated human alveolar macrophages are present in the airways inflammatory infiltrate and have been detected in biopsies in the submucosa and among epithelial cells (161). Alveolar macrophages play an important role in inflammatory processes and regulate healing and repair processes by releasing several growth factors and/or ECM components, which include TGF-β and FN (162,163). AM can also modulate the turnover of ECM by their capacity to regulate the production of MMPs and TIMPs (107,164).

The role of neutrophils in asthma is controversial. Although they have not been demonstrated to play a key role in mild asthma, this may not be so in more severe cases of the disease. The mucosa of patients who have died from status asthmaticus contains mixed cellular infiltrates consisting of eosinophils, neutrophils, macrophages, lymphocytes, and plasma cells (165). In fatal asthma, the length of the attack preceding death seems to be related to the presence or absence of neutrophils. Patients who have died from sudden-onset asthma (crises lasting less than 1 h) had significantly more neutrophils in the airway submucosa and fewer eosinophils compared to those in patients who have died from slow-onset asthma (crises lasting longer than 2.5 h) (166). This is in agreement with other data from Carroll et al. in patients who had severe asthma requiring constant treatment and at least one hospital admission for asthma (167). They showed increases in the number of neutrophils and of the area of mucous glands in cases of fatal asthma attacks of short duration compared to those of long duration. Synek et al. found no difference between the number of neutrophils in fatal and mild to moderate asthma (168). Recently Wenzel et al. showed high numbers and percentages of neutrophils in BAL, endobronchial, and transbronchial biopsy specimens of severe, oral glucocorticoid-dependent asthmatics (172). Some reports have suggested that corticosteroids may enhance neutrophil number and functions while effectively eliminating eosinophils (152,170–171). Another way for inflammatory cells to contribute to asthma pathology is through the secretion of mediators that can induce structural cells (airway epithelial cells, smooth muscle cells, and fibroblasts) to secrete cytokines (173–176).

Cytokines are important in asthma because they play a central role in the amplification, specificity, and persistence of inflammation (177). Similarly, liberation and activation of potent cytokines during the inflammatory phase of tissue repair are important to the overall process of regeneration and remodeling. During the pathogenesis of lung fibrosis, local overexpression of cytokines and/or growth factors stimulates resident lung fibroblasts to synthesize increased amounts of ECM. Many growth factors and other mediators have the potential to be implicated in the airway wall remodeling on the basis of their in vitro biological properties. These include TGF-β (178); PDGF (179); bFGF (180), cytokines such as TNF-α (181), IL-4 (182), IL-6 (183), IL-11 (51), and IL-17 (150); endothelin (184); histamine (185); and tryptase (186). All of these factors are able to elicit a mitogenic response on fibroblasts and/or airway smooth muscle cells, to promote connective tissue synthesis, or to stimulate the release of profibrotic mediators. In vivo a number of profibrotic cytokines have been identified in asthmatic airways (Fig. 3A) (87,149–150,187–190). TGF-β is considered to be a major fibrogenic cytokine (191,192) and considerable evidence suggests that TGF-β iso-

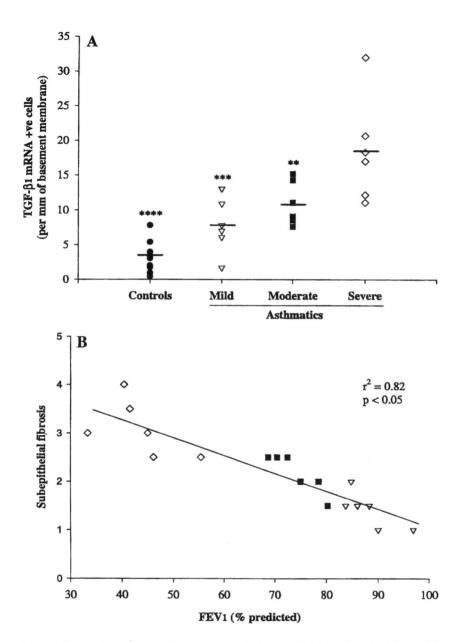

Figure 3 (A) TGF-β1 mRNA expression within bronchial biopsies of subjects with mild, moderate, and severe asthma and that of nonasthmatic control subjects. There was a significant increase in numbers of cells expressing TGF-β1 mRNA in severe asthma ($n = 6$) compared with those in moderate ($n = 6$) and mild asthma ($n = 6$) and non-asthmatic control subjects ($n = 8$), (**$p < 0.05$, ***$p < 0.01$, and ****$p < 0.001$, respectively). (B) Correlational relationships between percentage predicted FEV$_1$ values and sub-epithelial fibrosis. There was significant correlation between subepithelial fibrosis and this index of pulmonary function ($p < 0.05$). (From Ref. 87.)

forms are key mediators responsible for ECM changes seen in lung fibrosis (Fig. 3B) (78,81,191–194). In normal human lung, TGF-β isoforms are frequently expressed in bronchiolar epithelial cells and interstitial fibroblasts (195,196). Immunoreactive TGF-β1 in human airways is principally extracellular and matrix-associated TGF-β1 is likely to be bound, at least in part, by decorin. This interaction, which neutralizes the biological activity of the cytokine, may provide a reservoir of TGF-β1 that can be released in an active form in response to appropriate stimuli (197). Basal levels of TGF-β1 are increased in BAL fluids in asthma and these levels are further increased in response to allergen exposure (198). TGF-β leads to angiogenic and fibrotic responses. The response to TGF-β may be reversible to some extent (199). In vitro TGF-β increases the synthesis of many components of the ECM by fibroblasts, including collagen types I and III, FN, vitronectin, tenascin, and proteoglycans (178). TGF-β acts by increasing both the rate of transcription of procollagen genes (200) and mRNA stability (201) as well as decreasing the degradation of newly synthesized collagen, thereby augmenting the increase in collagen deposition (202). In addition TGF-β decreases the synthesis of enzymes that degrade the ECM, such as collagenase and stromelysin, and increases the synthesis of antiproteases (131,203,204), including tissue inhibitor of metalloproteinase-1 (TIMP-1) and plasminogen activator type-1 (PAI-1) (178). Based on their ability to synthesize TGF-β1 in vitro, most cellular constituents of the airway wall have the potential to contribute to expression of this cytokine in the airways, including bronchial epithelial cells (205), vascular endothelial cells (206), macrophages (207), lymphocytes (208), fibroblasts (209), and eosinophils (87,144–146).

IL-11 is produced by human lung fibroblasts, alveolar and airway epithelial cell lines in response to cytokines (210–212), histamine (213), MBP (176), and respiratory viruses (212). Overexpression of IL-11 within the lungs results in subepithelial fibrosis (214,215) and promotes the accumulation of myocytes and myofibroblasts (215). We have recently demonstrated that IL-11 is expressed in asthma and is associated with increasing severity of the disease (Figs. 4 and 5) (149). We have also shown that IL-11 is localized to eosinophils within the bronchial tissues (149). Studies from Elias et al. raised the intriguing possibility of a positive feedback loop in the airway, with TGF-β1 stimulating local epithelial cells, human airway smooth muscle cells, and fibroblasts to produce IL-11, which in turn induces smooth muscle hyperplasia and fibroblast proliferation (51).

There are other inflammatory mediators that are involved in airway remodeling to a lesser extent including IL-4, TNF-α, IL-1β, IL-6, and EGF. IL-4 is capable of inducing the expression of MUC2 gene and mucous glycoconjugate in a human airway epithelial cell line (NCI-H292) (216). However, Jayawickreme et al. demonstrated that IL-4 has an inhibitory effect on other mucin genes, e.g., MUC5AC and MUC5B (217). TNF-α and IL-1β have been shown to stimulate expression of MMP-9 (218) and IL-6 was shown to stimulate TIMP-1 production

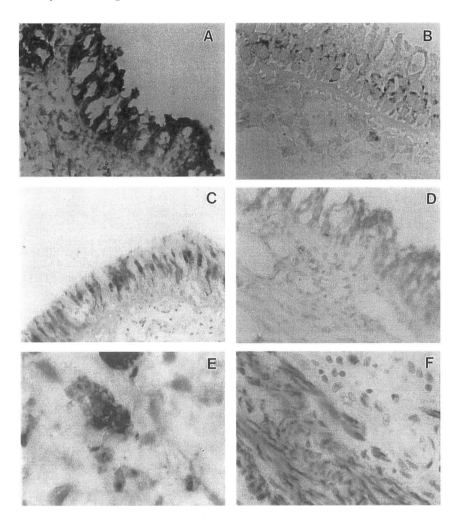

Figure 4 In situ hybridization with digoxigenin for IL-11 mRNA in bronchial biopsy specimens from (A) a patient with severe asthma and (B) a nonasthmatic control subject. In the original, note dark brown/purple staining, indicative of IL-11 mRNA within airways epithelium and associated with individual cells in subepithelium. (C) Immunostaining for IL-11 in individual with severe asthma. (D) Primary antibody isotype control for IL-11 immunoreactivity. (E) Colocalization of IL-11 immunoreactivity and eosinophil-specific marker (MBP) in individual with severe asthma. IL-11 immunoreactivity localizes to MBP-positive cells. (F) Type III collagen immunoreactivity, as determined by avidin–biotin–peroxidase method, in individual with severe asthma. (From Ref. 149.)

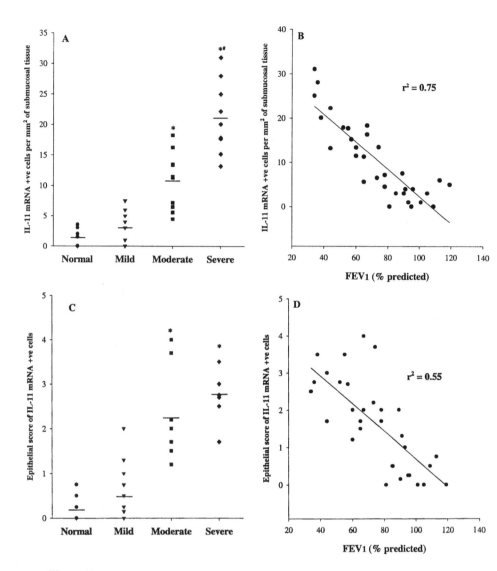

Figure 5 IL-11 mRNA expression within (A) subepithelium and (C) epithelial cell layers of subjects with mild, moderate, and severe asthma and that of nonasthmatic control subjects. There was significant increase in numbers of cells expressing IL-11 mRNA in moderate ($n = 9$) and severe ($n = 9$) asthma compared to those with mild asthma ($n = 13$) and those of nonasthmatic control subjects ($n = 9$, *$p < 0.001$, controls vs. mild asthmatics). Within submucosa, patients with severe asthma had significantly increased numbers of IL-11 mRNA-positive cells compared with those with moderate asthma (#$p < 0.05$). Correlational relationships between percentage predicted FEV$_1$ values and numbers of cells expressing IL-11 mRNA within (B) subepithelium and (C) epithelial layer are shown. There were significant correlations between numbers of IL-11 mRNA-positive cells in both airway epithelium and subepithelial regions and this index of pulmonary function ($p < 0.05$). (From Ref. 149.)

in human alveolar macrophages (219,220). EGF does not stimulate collagen production but has an inhibitory effect on TGF-β (219). However, following the induction of EGF receptor (EGFR) on the human airway epithelial cell line by TNF-α, subsequent stimulation of EGFR by EGF or TGF-α resulted in MUC5AC production at the gene and protein levels (221). In addition, similarly to PDGF, EGF has been shown to induce human airway smooth muscle cell proliferation (222,223).

F. Vascular Changes

The contribution of the vascular bed to airway wall remodeling has not been fully investigated. However, dilatation of bronchial mucosal blood vessels with swollen endothelial cells, congestion, and wall edema have been demonstrated to be features of fatal asthma (9). Similarly, in the peripheral airways of asthmatic subjects who died suddenly during an asthma attack, the muscular pulmonary arteries adjacent to occluded and inflamed bronchioles were shown to have an inflammation in their wall (142). Vascular permeability is known to be increased in asthma. Inflammatory mediators known to be released in asthma, such as histamine (224), bradykinin (225), leukotrienes (226), and neuropeptides (227), may contribute to bronchial vascular dilatation. Capillary engorgement and/or leakage in the circulatory bed could directly alter airway wall thickness. A model of airway wall thickening proposed by Moreno et al. (228) suggests that a small increase in thickness, such as that caused by edema or vascular engorgement, might account for the increased airway resistance seen with bronchial provocation (229).

Not only is the vascularity of the airways increased in asthmatics as compared to that in controls, but also more large vessels (>300 μm^2) have been identified (230). Li et al. (230) suggested that angiogenesis is a component of the chronic inflammatory response even in mild-to-moderate asthma. Possible factors responsible for angiogenesis in airway inflammation include basic fibroblast growth factor (231), tumor necrosis factor-α (232), and vascular endothelial growth factor (233). Any release of angiogenic growth factors in the bronchial wall may be either secondary to an inflammatory response or part of the remodeling response to intramural mechanical forces (234).

G. Cartilage Changes

The cartilage is primarily responsible for maintaining the stability of the airways. There are few data concerning the structural modifications of airway cartilage in asthma. Nevertheless, cartilage remodeling, including PG degradation, has been described in the 1- to 5-mm-diameter airways of those who have died from asthma (60). A recent study showed that the proportion of degenerated cartilage and peribronchial fibrosis to total cartilage in bronchi (3 to 8 mm in diameter) was significantly higher in asthmatics compared to that in controls (235). Peribronchial fibrosis correlated with number of eosinophils in the bronchial walls, thickness of basement membrane, bronchial gland area, and goblet cell area (235). These data indicate that airways in those patients with bronchial asthma have degenerative changes in the cartilage (chondrocytes) (235). Loss of cartilage PGs may be an indicator of a much more general process of extracellular matrix degradation in asthma since one mechanism for cartilage degradation is due to the secretion of matrix metalloproteinases from chondrocytes (236). Numerous enzymes, such as the neutrophil elastase, mast cell tryptase, or cysteine proteinases, are also able to degrade collagen, elastin, and PGs. Degradation of airway cartilage could contribute to airflow obstruction by decreasing airway wall stiffness, which would decrease maximal expiratory flow rates from the lung. Cartilage degradation could also decrease the force required for smooth muscle to constrict the airways.

III. Effect of Treatment on Airway Remodeling

The effect of current treatments on structural changes in the asthmatic airways is not well understood. Corticosteroids (CSs) act on every cell involved in airway inflammation and have been shown to decrease the airway cellular infiltrate in asthma (139) and to reduce airway smooth muscle cell proliferation (238). One study suggested that inhaled steroid treatment is associated with a reduction in goblet cell numbers in the airways (239). Dexamethasone has been shown to suppress MUC2 and MUC5AC mucin gene expression in a human pulmonary mucoepidermoid carcinoma cell line (240). CSs reduce ''bronchorrhea'' sputum in hospitalized severe asthmatic patients (241). Regarding the effect of CSs on collagen synthesis, the data are more controversial. Cockayne et al. (241) showed that CSs inhibit collagen production, whereas others demonstrated that CSs have no effect on collagen deposition (139). CSs might reduce other ECM components including tenascin (93). By inhibiting MMP-9 and TIMP-1 (108,242), CSs are capable of maintaining the balance between the enzyme and its inhibitor.

More studies are needed to establish the effects of steroids in preventing airway remodeling and in investigating the effects of steroids on different components of the airway remodeling process.

IV. Conclusion   .

Our knowledge in airway remodeling relies mostly on descriptive histopathological studies or on mathematical models. Further studies should be conducted to better understand the in vivo mechanisms leading to airway remodeling. We need to define when this process starts and if there is any heterogeneity among the asthmatic population. Future studies should also assess and analyze airway remodeling more quantitatively. It is more likely that the amount of extracellular matrix rather than the extent of its distribution is the major factor. We need also to establish the role of steroids and other anti-inflammatory drugs in regulating processes associated with airway remodeling.

References

1. Redington AE, Howarth PH. Airway wall remodeling in asthma. Thorax 1997; 52: 310–312.
2. Roche WR, Beasley R, Williams JH, Holgate ST. Subepithelial fibrosis in the bronchi of asthmatics. Lancet 1989; 1:520–523.
3. Wilson JW, Li X. The measurement of reticular basement membrane and submucosal collagen in the asthmatic airway. Clin Exp Allergy 1997; 27:363–371.
4. Strunk RC. Identification of the fatality-prone subject with asthma. J Allergy Clin Immunol 1989; 83:477–485.
5. Rea HH, Sears MR, Beaglehole R, Fenwick J, Jackson RT, Gillies AJ, O'Donnell TV, Holst PE, Rothwell RP. Lessons from the national asthma mortality study: circumstances surrounding death. NZ Med J 1987; 100:10–13.
6. Wiggs BR, Bosken C, Pare PD, Hogg JC. A model of airway narrowing in asthma and in chronic obstructive pulmonary disease. Am Rev Respir Dis 1992; 145:1251–1258.
7. Wilson JW, Li X, Pain MCF. The lack of distensibility of asthmatic airways. Am Rev Respir Dis 1993; 148:806–809.
8. Jeffery PK, Wardlaw AJ, Nelson FC, Collins JV, Kay AB. Bronchial biopsies in asthma. An ultrastructural, quantitative study and correlation with hyperreactivity. Am Rev Respir Dis 1989; 140:1745–1753.
9. Dunnill MS. The pathology of asthma with special reference to changes in the bronchial mucosa. J Clin Pathol 1960; 13:27–33.
10. Johnson NF, Hubbs AF. Epithelial progenitor cells in the rat trachea. Am J Respir Cell Mol Biol 1990; 3:579–584.
11. Soderberg M, Hellstrom S, Sandstrom T, Lundgren R, Bergh A. Structural characterization of bronchial mucosal biopsies from healthy volunteers: a light and electron microscopical study. Eur Respir J 1990; 3:261–266.
12. Carroll N, Elliot J, Morton A, James A. The structure of large and small airways in nonfatal and fatal asthma. Am Rev Respir Dis 1993; 147:405–410.
13. Boulet LP, Turcotte H, Boutet M, Montminy L, Laviolette M. Influence of natural antigenic exposure on expiratory flows, methacholine responsiveness, and airway inflammation in mild allergic asthma. J Allergy Clin Immunol 1993; 91:883–893.
14. Rogers DF. Airway goblet cells: responsive and adaptable front-line defenders. Eur Respir J 1994; 7:1690–1706.
15. Fung DCK, and Rogers DF. Airway submucosal glands: physiology and pharmacology. In Rogers DF, Lethem MI, eds. Airway Mucus: Basic Mechanisms and Clinical Perspectives. Basel: Birkhäuser, 1997:179–210.

16. Reid L. Pathology of chronic bronchitis. Lancet 1954; 1:275–279.
17. Aikawa T, Shimura S, Sasaki H, Ebina M, Takishima T. Marked goblet cell hyperplasia with mucus accumulation in the airways of patients who died of severe acute asthma attack. Chest 1992; 101:916–921.
18. Dunnill MS, Massarella GR, Anderson JA. A comparison of the quantitative anatomy of the bronchi in normal subjects, in status asthmaticus, in chronic bronchitis and in emphysema. Thorax 1969; 24:176–179.
19. Shimura S, Andoh Y, Haraguchi M, Shirato K. Continuity of airway goblet cells and intraluminal mucus in the airways of patients with bronchial asthma. Eur Respir J 1996; 9:1395–1401.
20. Laitinen L, Laitinen A, Haahtela TA. Airway mucosal inflammation even in patients with newly diagnosed asthma. Am Rev Respir Dis 1993; 147:697–704.
21. Kay AB. Pathology of mild, severe, and fatal asthma. Am J Respir Crit Care Med 1996; 154:S66–S69.
22. King M. Rheological requirements for optimal clearance of secretions: ciliary transport versus cough. Eur J Respir Dis 1980; 61(suppl. 110):39–45.
23. Hovenberg HW, Carlstedt I, Davies JR. Mucus glycoproteins in bovine trachea: identification of the major mucin populations in respiratory secretions and investigation of their tissue origins. Biochem J 1997; 321:117–123.
24. Porchet N, Nguyen VC, Dufosse J, Audie JP, Guyonnet-Duperat V, Gross MS, Denis C, Degand P, Bernheim A, Aubert JP. Molecular cloning and chromosomal localization of a novel human tracheo-bronchial mucin cDNA containing tandemly repeated sequences of 48 base pairs. Biochem Biophys Res Commun 1991; 175: 414–422.
25. Dufosse J, Porchet N, Audie J-P, Guyonnet-Duperat V, Laine A, Van-Seuningen I, Marrakchi S, Degand P, Aubert J-P. Degenerate 87-base-pair tandem repeats create hydrophilic/hydrophobic alternating domains in human mucin peptides mapped to 11p15. Biochem J 1993; 293:329–337.
26. Meerzaman D, Charles P, Daskal E, Polymeropoulos MH, Martin BM, Rose MC. Cloning and analysis of cDNA encoding a major airway glycoprotein, human tracheobronchial mucin (MUC5). J Biol Chem 1994; 269:12932–12939.
27. Shankar V, Pichan P, Eddy RL Jr, Tonk V, Nowak N, Sait SN, Shows TB, Schultz RE, Gotway G, Elkins RC, Gilmore MS, Sachdev GP. Chromosomal localization of a human mucin gene (MUC8) and cloning of the cDNA corresponding to the carboxy terminus. Am J Respir Cell Mol Biol 1997; 16:232–241.
28. Rose MC, Gendler SJ. Airway mucin genes and gene products. In Rogers DF, Lethem MI, eds. Airway Mucus: Basic Mechanisms and Clinical Perspectives. Basel: Birkhäser Verlag, 1997:41–66.
29. Hovenberg HW, Davies JR, Herrmann A, Linden CJ, Carlstedt I. MUC5AC, but not MUC2, is a prominent mucin in respiratory secretions. Glycoconj J 1996; 13: 839–847.
30. Thornton DJ, Howard M, Khan N, Sheehan JK. Identification of two glycoforms of the MUC5B mucin in human respiratory mucus: evidence for a cysteine-rich sequence repeated within the molecule. J Biol Chem 1997; 272:9561–9566.
31. Reid CJ, Gould S, Harris A. Developmental expression of mucin genes in the human respiratory tract. Am J Respir Cell Mol Biol 1997; 17:592–598.

32. Rogers AV, Dewar A, Corrin B, Jeffery PK. Identification of serous-like cells in the surface epithelium of human bronchioles. Eur Respir J 1993; 6:498–504.

33. Marom Z, Shelhamer JH, Sun F, Kaliner M. Human airway monohydroxyeicosatetraenoic acid generation and mucus release. J Clin Invest 1983; 72:122–127.

34. Zheutlin LM, Ackerman SJ, Gleich GJ, Thomas LL. Donor sensitivity to basophil activation by eosinophil granule major basic protein. Int Arch Allergy Appl Immunol 1985; 77:216–217.

35. Davis WB, Fells GA, Sun XH, Gadek JE, Venet A, Crystal RG. Eosinophil-mediated injury to lung parenchymal cells and interstitial matrix: a possible role for eosinophils in chronic inflammatory disorders of the lower respiratory tract. J Clin Invest 1984; 74:269–278.

36. Marom Z, Shelhamer JH, Kaliner M. Human monocyte-derived mucus secretagogue. J Clin Invest 1985; 75:191–198.

37. Shelhamer JH, Marom Z, Kaliner M. Immunologic and neuropharmacologic stimulation of mucous glycoprotein release from human airways in vitro. J Clin Invest 1980; 66:1400–1408.

38. Lou YP, Takeyama, K, Grattan KM, Lausier JA, Ueki IF, Agusti C, Nadel JA. Platelet-activating factor induces goblet cell hyperplasia and mucin gene expression in airways. Am J Respir Crit Care Med 1998; 157:1927–1934.

39. O'Riordan TG, Zwang J, Smaldone GC. Mucociliary clearance in adult in asthma. Am Rev Respir Dis 1992; 146:598–603.

40. Russi EW, Abraham WM, Chapman GA, Stephenson JS, Codias E, Wanner A. Effects of leukotriene D4 on mucociliary and respiratory function in allergic and nonallergic sheep. J Appl Physiol 1985; 59:1416–1422.

41. Frigas E, Loegering DA, Gleich GJ. Cytotoxic effects of the guinea pig eosinophil major basic protein on tracheal epithelium. Lab Invest 1980; 42:35–43.

42. Ayers MM, Jeffery PK. Proliferation and differentiation in mammalian airway epithelium. Eur Respir J 1988; 1:58–80.

43. Thomson RJ, Bramley AM, Schellenberg RR. Airway smooth muscle stereology: implications for increased shortening in asthma. Am J Respir Crit Care Med 1996; 154:749–757.

44. Ebina M, Takahashi T, Chiba T, Motomiya M. Cellular hypertrophy and hyperplasia of airway smooth muscles underlying bronchial asthma: a 3-D morphometric study. Am Rev Respir Dis 1993; 148:720–726.

45. Heard BE, Hossain S. Hyperplasia of bronchial smooth muscle in asthma. J Pathol 1971; 110:319–331.

46. Hossain S. Quantitative measurement of bronchial muscle in men with asthma. Am Rev Respir Dis 1973; 107:99–109.

47. Huber HL, Koessler K. The pathology of bronchial asthma. Arch Intern Med 1922; 30:689–760.

48. Thomson RJ, Schellenberg RR. Increased amount of airway smooth muscle does not account for excessive bronchoconstriction in asthma. Can Respir J 1998; 5:61–62.

49. Wiggs BR, Moreno R, Hogg JC, Hilliam C, Paré PD. A model of the mechanics of airway narrowing. J Appl Physiol 1990; 69:849–860.

50. James AL, Paré PD, Hogg JC. The mechanics of airway narrowing in asthma. Am Rev Respir Dis 1989; 139:242–246.

51. Elias JA, Wu Y, Zheng T, R Panettieri. Cytokine- and virus-stimulated airway smooth muscle cells produce IL-11 and other IL-6-type cytokines. Am J Physiol 1997; 273(3Pt1):L648–L655.

52. Sousa AR, Lane SJ, Nakhosteen JA, Yoshimura T, Lee TH, Poston RN. Increased expression of the monocyte chemoattractant protein-1 in bronchial tissue from asthmatic subjects. Am J Respir Cell Mol Biol 1994; 10:142–147.

53. Lukacs NW, Kunkel SL, Allen R, Evanoff HL, Shaklee CL, Sherman JS, Burdick MD, Strieter RM. Stimulus and cell-specific expression of C-X-C and C-C chemokines by pulmonary stromal cell populations. Am J Physiol 1995; 268(5Pt1):L856–L861.

54. Ghaffar O, Hamid Q, Renzi PM, Allakhverdi Z, Molet S, Hogg JC, Shore SA, Luster AD, Lamkhioued B. Constitutive and cytokine-stimulated expression of eotaxin by human airway smooth muscle cells. Am J Respir Crit Care Med 1999; 159:1933–1942.

55. John M, Hirst SJ, Jose PJ, Robichaud A, Berkman N, Witt C, Twort CHC, Barnes PJ, Chung K. Human airway smooth muscle cells express and release RANTES in response to T helper 1 cytokines: regulation by T helper 2 cytokines and corticosteroids. J Immunol 1997; 158:1841–1847.

56. Hallsworth MP, Soh CPC, Twort CHC, Lee TH, Hirst SJ. Cultured human airway smooth muscle cells stimulated by IL-1β enhance eosinophil survival. Am J Respir Cell Mol Biol 1998; 19:910–919.

57. Lazaar AL, Albelda SM, Pilewski JM, Brennan B, Pure E, Panettieri RA Jr. T lymphocytes adhere to airway smooth muscle cells via integrins and CD44 and induce smooth muscle cell DNA synthesis. J Exp Med 1994; 180:807–816.

58. Panettieri RA Jr, Tan EML, Ciocca V, Luttmann MA, Leonard TB, Hay DW. Effects of LTD_4 on human airway smooth muscle cell proliferation, matrix expression, and contraction in vitro: differential sensitivity to cysteinyl leukotriene receptor antagonists. Am J Respir Cell Mol Biol 1998; 19:453–461.

59. Rajah R, Nunn SE, Herrick DJ, Grunstein MM, Cohen P. Leukotriene D4 induces MMP-1, which functions as an IGFBP protease in human airway smooth muscle cells. Am J Physiol 1996; 271 (Lung Cell Mol Physiol 15):L1014–L1022.

60. Roberts CR. Is asthma a fibrotic disease? Chest 1995; 107(suppl 3):111S–117S.

61. Boulet LP, Laviolette M, Turcotte H, Cartier A, Dugas M, Malo J-L, Boutet M. Bronchial subepithelial fibrosis correlates with airway responsiveness to methacholine. Chest 1997; 112:45–52.

62. Chetta A, Foresi A, Del Donno M, Bertorelli G, Pesci A, Olivieri D. Airways remodeling is a distinctive feature of asthma and is related to severity of disease. Chest 1997; 111:852–857.

63. Brewster CEP, Howarth PH, Djukanovic R, Wilson J, Holgate ST, Roche WR. Myofibroblasts and subepithelial fibrosis in bronchial asthma. Am J Respir Cell Mol Biol 1990; 3:507–511.

64. Roche WR. Fibroblasts and asthma. Clin Exp Allergy 1991; 21:545–548.

65. McCarter JH, Vazques JJ, Durham NC. The bronchial basement membrane in asthma. Arch Path 1966; 82:328–335.

66. Meinl M, Brunner P. Alterations in the structure of bronchial basement membrane in relation to textural changes in bronchial mucosa. Pathol Res Pract 1980; 169: 21–28.

67. Holgate ST, Djukanovic R, Howarth PM, Montefort S, Roche W. The T cell and the airway's fibrotic response in asthma. Chest 1993; 103(suppl):125S–128S.

68. Djukanovic R, Wilson JW, Britten KM, Wilson SJ, Walls AF, Roche WR, Howarth PH, Holgate ST. Quantitation of mast cells and eosinophils in the bronchial mucosa of symptomatic atopic asthmatics and healthy control subjects using immunohistochemistry. Am Rev Respir Dis 1990; 142:863–871.

69. Molina C, Brun J, Coulet M, Betail G, Delage J. Immunopathology of the bronchial mucosa in "late-onset" asthma. Clin Allergy 1977; 7:137–145.

70. Vignola AM, Chanez P, Campbell AM, Souques F, Lebel B, Enander I, Bousquet J. Airway inflammation in mild intermittent and in persistent asthma. Am J Respir Crit Care Med 1998; 157:403–409.

71. Sekisawa K, Sasaki H, Shimizu Y, Takishima T. Dose-response effects of methacholine in normal and in asthmatic subjects. Relationship between the site of airway response and overall airway hyperresponsiveness. Am Rev Respir Dis 1986; 133: 593–599.

72. Yanai M, Sekisawa K, Ohrui T, Sasaki H, Takishima T. Site of airway obstruction in pulmonary disease: direct measurement of intrabronchial pressure. J Appl Physiol 1992; 72:1016–1023.

73. Kuwano K, Bosken CH, Pare PD, Bai TR, Wiggs BR, Hogg JC. Small airways dimensions in asthma and in chronic obstructive pulmonary disease. Am Rev Respir Dis 1993; 148:1220–1225.

74. Hamid Q, Song Y, Kotsimbos TC, Minshall E, Bai TR, Hegele RG, Hogg JC. Inflammation of small airways in asthma. J Allergy Clin Immunol 1997; 100:44–51.

75. Minshall EM, Hogg JC, Hamid QA. Cytokine mRNA expression in asthma is not restricted to the large airways. J Allergy Clin Immunol 1998; 101:386–390.

76. Wagner EM, Bleecker ER, Permutt S, Liu MC. Direct assessment of small airways reactivity in human subjects. Am J Respir Crit Care Med 1998; 157:447–452.

77. Davidson JM. Biochemistry and turnover of lung interstitium. Eur Respir J 1990; 3:1048–1068.

78. Laurent GJ. Dynamic state of collagen: pathways of collagen degradation in vivo and their possible role in regulation of collagen mass. Am J Physiol 1987; 252(1Pt1):C1–C9.

79. Dunsmore SE, Rannels DE. Extracellular matrix biology in the lung. Am J Physiol 1996; 270(1Pt1):L3–L27.

80. O'Connor CM, FitzGerald MX. Matrix metalloproteases and lung disease. Thorax 1994; 49:602–609.

81. McAnulthy RJ, Laurent GJ. Pathogenesis of lung fibrosis and potential new therapeutic strategies. Exp Nephrol 1995; 3:96–107.

82. Berrih S, Savino W, Cohen S. Extracellular matrix of the human thymus: immunofluorescence studies on frozen sections and cultured epithelial cells. J Histochem Cytochem 1985; 33:655–664.

83. Sage H, Bornstein P. Endothelial cells from umbilical vein and a hemangioendothelioma secrete basement membrane largely to the exclusion of interstitial procollagens. Arteriosclerosis 1982; 2:27–36.

84. Madri JA, Dreyer B, Pitlick FA, Furthmayr H. The collagenous components of the subendothelium: correlation of structure and function. Lab Invest 1980; 43:303–315.

85. Scheinman JI, Tanaka H, Haralson M, Wang SL, Brown O. Specialized collagen mRNA and secreted collagens in human glomerular epithelial, mesanglial, and tubular cells. J Am Soc Nephrol 1992; 2:1475–1483.

86. Stampfer MR, Yaswen P, Alhadeff M, Hosoda J. TGF beta induction of extracellular matrix associated proteins in normal and transformed human mammary epithelial cells in culture is independent of growth effects. J Cell Physiol 1993; 155:210–221.

87. Minshall EM, Leung DYM, Martin RJ, Song YL, Cameron L, Ernst P, Hamid Q. Eosinophil-associated TGF-β1 mRNA expression and airway fibrosis in bronchial asthma. Am J Respir Cell Mol Biol 1997; 17:326–333.

88. Chu HW, Halliday JL, Martin RJ, Leung DYM, Szefler S, Wenzel SE. Collagen deposition in large airways may not differentiate severe asthma from milder forms of the disease. Am J Respir Crit Care Med 1998; 158:1936–1944.

89. Limper AH, Roman J. Fibronectin. A versatile matrix protein with roles in thoracic development, repair and infection. Chest 1992; 101:1663–1673.

90. Mattoli S, Mattoso VL, Soloperto M, Allegra L, Fasoli A. Cellular and biochemical characteristics of bronchoalveolar lavage fluid in symptomatic nonallergic asthma. J Allergy Clin Immunol 1991; 87:794–802.

91. Campbell AM, Chanez P, Vignola AM, Bousquet J, Couret I, Michel FB, Godard P. Functional characteristics of bronchial epithelium obtained by brushing from asthmatic and normal subjects. Am Rev Respir Dis 1993; 147:529–534.

92. Meerschaert J, Kelly EA, Mosher DF, Busse WW, Jarjour NN. Segmental antigen challenge increases fibronectin in bronchoalveolar lavage fluid. Am J Respir Crit Care Med 1999; 159:619–625.

93. Laitinen A, Altraja A, Kämpe M, Linden M, Virtanen I, Laitinen LA. Tenascin is increased in airway basement membrane of asthmatics and decreased by an inhaled steroid. Am J Respir Crit Care Med 1997; 156:951–958.

94. Jackson RL, Busch SJ, Cardin AD. Glycosaminoglycans: molecular properties, protein interactions, and role in physiological processes. Physiol Rev 1991; 71:481–539.

95. Wight TN, Kinsella MG, Qwarnstrom EE. The role of proteoglycans in cell adhesion, migration and proliferation. Curr Opin Cell Biol 1992; 4:793–801.

96. Huang J, Olivenstein R, Taha R, Hamid Q, Ludwig M. Enhanced proteoglycan deposition in the airway wall of atopic asthmatics. Am J Respir Crit Care Med 1999; 160:725–729.

97. Murphy G, Docherty AJP. The matrix metalloproteinases and their inhibitors. Am J Respir Cell Mol Biol 1992; 7:120–125.

98. Sepper R, Konttinen YT, Sorsa T, Koski H. Gelatinolytic and type IV collagenolytic activity in bronchiectasis. Chest 1994; 106:1129–1133.

99. Sepper R, Konttinen YT, Ding Y, Takagi M, Sorsa T. Human neutrophil collage-

nase (MMP-8), identified in bronchiectasis BAL fluid, correlates with severity of disease. Chest 1995; 107:1641–1647.

100. Power C, O'Connor CM, MacFarlane D, O'Mahoney S, Gaffney K, Hayes J, Fitz-Gerald MX. Neutrophil collagenase in sputum from patients with cystic fibrosis. Am J Respir Crit Care Med 1994; 150:818–822.

101. Hammar H. Wound healing. Int J Dermatol 1993; 32:6–15.

102. Nagase H, Ogata Y, Suzuki K, Enghild JJ, Salvesen G. Substrate specificities and activation mechanisms of matrix metalloproteinases. Biochem Soc Trans 1991; 19: 715–718.

103. Stahle-Backdahl M, Inoue M, Guidice GJ, Parks WC. 92-kD gelatinase is produced by eosinophils at the site of blister formation in bullous pemphigoid and cleaves the extracellular domain of recombinant 180-kD bullous pemphigoid autoantigen. J Clin Invest 1994; 93:2022–2030.

104. Montgomery AMP, Sabzevari H, Reisfeld RA. Production and regulation of gelatinase B by human T-cells. Biochem Biophys Acta 1993; 1176:265–268.

105. Murphy G, Cockett MI, Ward RV, Docherty AJP. Matrix metalloproteinase degradation of elastin, type IV collagen and proteoglycan: a quantitative comparison of the activities of 95 kDa and 75 kDa gelatinases, stromelysine-1 and -2 and punctuated metalloproteinase (PUMP). Biochem J 1991; 277:277–279.

106. Senior RM, Griffin GL, Fliszar CJ, Shapiro SD, Goldberg GI, Welgus HG. Human 92- and 72-kilodalton type IV collagenases are elastases. J Biol Chem 1991; 266: 7870–7875.

107. Welgus HG, Campbell EJ, Cury JD, Eisen AZ, Senior RM, Wilhelm SM, Goldberg GI. Neutral metalloproteinases produced by human mononuclear phagocytes: enzyme profile, regulation, and expression during cellular development. J Clin Invest 1990; 86:1496–1502.

108. Mautino G, Oliver N, Chanez P, Bousquet J, Capony F. Increased release of matrix metalloproteinase-9 in bronchoalveolar lavage fluid and by alveolar macrophages of asthmatics. Am J Respir Cell Mol Biol 1997; 17:583–591.

109. Ohno I, Ohtani H, Nitta Y, Suzuki J, Hoshi H, Honna M, Isoyama S, Tanno Y, Tamura G, Yamauchi K, Nagura H, Shirato K. Eosinophils as a source of matrix metalloproteinase-9 in asthmatic airway inflammation. Am J Respir Cell Mol Biol 1997; 16:212–219.

110. Hoshino M, Nakamura Y, Sim J-J, Shimojo J, Isogai S. Bronchial subepithelial fibrosis and expression of matrix metalloproteinase-9 in asthmatic airway inflammation. J Allergy Clin Immunol 1998; 102:783–788.

111. Cohen AB, Rossi M. Neutrophils in normal lungs. Am Rev Respir Dis 1983; 127: S3–S9.

112. Senior RM, Connolly NL, Cury JD, Welgus HG, Campbell EJ. Elastin degradation by human alveolar macrophages: a prominent role of metalloproteinase activity. Am Rev Respir Dis 1989; 139:1251–1256.

113. Lungarella G, Menegazzi R, Gardi C, Spessotto P, de Santi MM, Bertoncin P, Patriarca P, Calzoni P, Zabucchi G. Identification of elastase in human eosinophils: immunolocalization, isolation, and partial characterization. Arch Biochem Biophys 1992; 292:128–135.

114. Snider GL. Distinguishing among asthma, chronic bronchitis, and emphysema. Chest 1985; 87:35S–39S.

115. Sommerhoff CP, Finkbeiner WE. Human tracheobronchial submucosal gland cells in culture. Am J Respir Cell Mol Biol 1990; 2:41–50.

116. Amitani R, Wilson R, Rutman A, Read R, Ward C, Burnett D, Stockley RA, Cole PJ. Effects of human neutrophil elastase and *Pseudomonas aeruginosa* proteinases on human respiratory epithelium. Am J Respir Cell Mol Biol 1991; 4:26–32.

117. Janoff A. Elastases and emphysema. Current assessment of the protease-antiprotease hypothesis. Am Rev Respir Dis 1985; 132:417–433.

118. Chetty A, Davis P, Infeld M. Effect of elastase on the directional migration of lung fibroblasts within a three-dimensional collagen matrix. Exp Lung Res 1995; 21: 889–899.

119. Vignola AM, Bonanno A, Mirabella A, Riccobono L, Mirabella F, Profita M, Bellia V, Bousquet J, Bonsignore G. Increased levels of elastase and α_1-antitrypsin in sputum of asthmatic patients. Am J Respir Crit Care Med 1998; 157:505–511.

120. Travis J, Salvesen GS. Human plasma proteinase inhibitors. Annu Rev Biochem 1983; 52:655–709.

121. Mauviel A. Cytokine regulation of metalloproteinase gene expression. J Cell Biochem 1993; 53:288–295.

122. Matrisian LM. Metalloproteinases and their inhibitor in matrix remodeling. Trends Genet 1990; 6:121–125.

123. Woessner JF. Matrix metalloproteinases and their inhibitors in connective tissue remodelling. FASEB J 1991; 5:2145–2154.

124. Gomez DE, Alonso DF, Yoshiji H, Thorgeirsson UP. Tissue inhibitors of metalloproteinases: structure, regulation and biological functions. Eur J Cell Biol 1997; 74:111–122.

125. Birkedal-Hansen H. Proteolytic remodeling of extracelluar matrix. Curr Opin Cell Biol 1995; 7:728–735.

126. Stetler-Stevenson WG, Krutzsch HC, Liotta LA. Tissue inhibitor of metalloproteinase (TIMP-2). A new member of the metalloproteinase inhibitor family. J Biol Chem 1989; 264:17374–17378.

127. Mautino G, Henriquet C, Jaffuel D, Bousquet J, Capony F. Tissue inhibitor of metalloproteinase-1 levels in bronchoalveolar lavage fluid from asthmatic subjects. Am J Respir Crit Care Med 1999; 160:324–330.

128. Mautino G, Henriquet C, Gougat C, Le Cam A, Dayer J-M, Bousquet J, Capony F. Increased expression of tissue inhibitor of metalloproteinase-1 and loss of correlation with matrix metalloproteinase-9 by macrophages in asthma. Lab Invest 1999; 79:39–47.

129. Bossé M, Chakir J, Rouabhia M, Boulet L-P, Audette M, Laviolette M. Serum matrix metalloproteinase-9:tissue inhibitor of metalloproteinase-1 ratio correlates with steroid responsiveness in moderate to severe asthma. Am J Respir Crit Care Med 1999; 159:596–602.

130. Hayakawa T. Tissue inhibitors of metalloproteinase and their cell growth-promoting activity. Cell Struct Funct 1994; 19:109–114.

131. Edwards DR, Murphy G, Reynolds JJ, Whitham SE, Docherty AJ, Angel P, Heath

JK. Transforming growth factor-beta modulates the expression of collagenase and metalloproteinase inhibitor. EMBO J 1987; 6:1899–1904.

132. Overall CM, Wrana JL, Sodek J. Transforming growth factor-beta regulation of collagenase, 72kDa-progelatinase, TIMP and PAI-1 expression in rat bone cell populations and human fibroblasts. Connect Tissue Res 1989; 20:289–294.

133. Eickelberg O, Köhler E, Reichenberger F, Bertschin S, Woodtli T, Erne P, Perruchoud AP, Roth M. Extracelluar matrix deposition by primary human lung fibroblasts in response to TGF-β1 and TGF-β3. Am J Physiol 1999; 276(5Pt1):L814–L824.

134. Clark IM, Powell LK, Cawston TE. Tissue inhibitor of metalloproteinases (TIMP-1) stimulates the secretion of collagenase from human skin fibroblasts. Biochem Biophys Res Commun 1994; 203:874–880.

135. Romanic AM, Madri JA. The induction of 72-kD gelatinase in T cells upon adhesion to endothelial cells is VCAM-1 dependent. J Cell Biol 1994; 125:1165–1178.

136. Malik N, Greenfield BW, Wahl AF, Kiener PA. Activation of human monocytes through CD40 induces matrix metalloproteinases. J Immunol 1996; 156:3952–3960.

137. Xie B, Laouar A, Huberman E. Fibronectin-mediated cell adhesion is required for induction of 92-kDa type IV collagenase/gelatinase (MMP-9) gene expression during macrophage differentiation: the signaling role of protein kinase c-β. J Biol Chem 1998; 273:11576–11582.

138. Skalli O, Schurch W, Seemayer T, Lagace R, Montandon D, Pittet B, Gabbiani G. Myofibroblasts from diverse pathologic settings are heterogenous in their content of actin isoforms and intermediate filament proteins. Lab Invest 1989; 60:275–285.

139. Jeffery PK, Godfrey RW, Ädelroth E, Nelson F, Rogers A, Johansson SA. Effects of treatment on airway inflammation and thickening of basement membrane reticular collagen in asthma. A quantitative light and electron microscopic study. Am Rev Respir Dis 1992; 145:890–899.

140. Verbeek MM, Otte-Höller I, Wesseling P, Ruiter DJ, de Waal RM. Induction of α-smooth muscle actin expression in cultured human brain pericytes by transforming growth factor-β1. Am J Pathol 1994; 144:372–382.

141. Gauldie J, Jordana M, Cox G, Ohtoshi T, Dolovitch J, Denburg J. Fibroblasts and other structural cells in airway inflammation. Am Rev Respir Dis 1992; 145:S14–S17.

142. Saetta M, Di Stefano A, Rosina C, Thiene G, Fabbri LM. Quantitative structural analysis of peripheral airways and arteries in sudden fatal asthma. Am Rev Respir Dis 1991; 143:138–143.

143. Weller PF. The immunobiology of eosinophils. N Engl J Med 1991; 324:1110–1118.

144. Ohno I, Lea RG, Flanders KC, Clark DA, Banwatt D, Dolovich J, Denburg J, Harley CB, Gauldie J, Jordana M. Eosinophils in chronically inflamed human upper airway tissues express transforming growth factor β1 gene (TGFβ1). J Clin Invest 1992; 89:1662–1668.

145. Elovic A, Wong DTW, Weller PF, Matossian K, Galli SJ. Expression of transforming factors-α and β1 messenger RNA and product by eosinophils in nasal polyps. J Allergy Clin Immunol 1994; 93:864–869.

146. Wong DTW, Elovic A, Matossian K, Nagura N, McBride J, Chou MY, Gordon JR, Rand TH, Galli SJ, Weller PF. Eosinophils from patients with blood eosinophilia express transforming growth factor β1. Blood 1991; 78:2702–2707.

147. Levi-Schaffer F, Garbuzenko E, Rubin A, Reich R, Pickholz D, Gillery P, Emonard H, Negler A, Maquart FX. Human eosinophils regulate human lung- and skin-derived fibroblast properties in vitro: a role for transforming growth factor β (TGF-β). Proc Natl Acad Sci USA 1999; 96:9660–9665.

148. Hamid Q, Barkans J, Meng Q, Ying S, Abrams JS, Kay AB, Moqbel, R. Human eosinophils synthesize and secrete interleukin-6, in vitro. Blood 1992; 80:1496–1501.

149. Minshall E, Chakir J, Laviolette M, Molet S, Zhu Z, Olivenstein R, Elias J, Hamid Q. Interleukin-11 expression is increased in severe asthma: association with epithelial cells and eosinophils. J Allergy Clin Immunol 2000; 105:232–238.

150. Molet S, Hamid Q, Pagé N, Taha R, Nutku E, Davoine F, Olivenstein R, Elias J, Chakir J. Interleukin-17, a new eosinophil-associated cytokine increased in asthmatic airways (abstr). Eur Respir J 1999; 14(suppl. 30):1939.

151. Djukanovic R, Wilson JW, Britten KM, Wilson SJ, Walls AF, Roche WR, Howarth PH, Holgate ST. Effect of an inhaled corticosteroid on airway inflammation and symptoms in asthma. Am Rev Respir Dis 1992; 145:669–674.

152. Wenzel SE, Schwartz LB, Langmack EL, Halliday JL, Trudeau JB, Gibbs RL, Chu HW. Evidence that severe asthma can be divided pathologically into two inflammatory subtypes with distinct physiologic and clinical characteristics. Am J Respir Crit Care Med 1999; 160:1001–1008.

153. Inoue Y, King TE Jr, Tinkle SS, Dockstader K, Newman LSW. Human mast cell basic fibroblast growth factor in pulmonary fibrotic disorders. Am J Pathol 1996; 149:2037–2054.

154. Cairns JA, Walls AF. Mast cell tryptase stimulates the synthesis of type I collagen in human lung fibroblasts. J Clin Invest 1997; 99:1313–1321.

155. Hamid Q, Azzawi M, Ying S, Moqbel R, Wardlaw AJ, Corrigan CJ, Bradley B, Durham SR, Collins JV, Jeffery PK, Quint DJ, Kay AB. Expression of mRNA of interleukin-5 in mucosal bronchial biopsies from asthma. J Clin Invest 1991; 87:1541–1546.

156. Robinson DS, Hamid Q, Ying S, Tsicopoulos A, Barkans J, Bentley AM, Corrigan C, Durham SR, Kay AB. Evidence for a predominant "Th2-type" bronchoalveolar lavage T-lymphocyte population in atopic asthma. N Engl J Med 1992; 326:298–304.

157. Clutterbuck EJ, Sanderson CJ. Human eosinophil hematopoiesis studied in vitro by means of murine eosinophil differentiation factor (IL5): production of functionally active eosinophils from normal human bone marrow. Blood 1988; 71:646–651.

158. Rothenberg ME, Petersen J, Stevens RL, Silberstein DS, McKenzie DT, Austen KF, Owen WF Jr. IL-5-dependent conversion of normodense human eosinophils to the hypodense phenotype using 3T3 fibroblasts for enhanced viability, accelerated hypodensity and sustained antibody-dependent cytotoxicity. J Immunol 1989; 143:2311–2316.

159. Yamaguchi Y, Suda T, Ohta S, Tominaga K, Miura Y, Kasahara T. Analysis of the survival of mature human eosinophils: interleukin-5 prevents apoptosis in mature human eosinophils. Blood 1991; 78:2542–2547.

160. Tai PC, Sun L, Spry CJ. Effects of IL-5, granulocyte/macrophage colony-stimulating factor (GM-CSF) and IL-3 on the survival of human blood eosinophils in vitro. Clin Exp Immunol 1991; 85:312–316.

161. Poston RN, Chanez P, Lacoste JY, Litchfield T, Lee TH, Bousquet J. Immunohistochemical characterization of the cellular infiltration in asthmatic bronchi. Am Rev Respir Dis 1992; 145:918–921.

162. Rennard SI, Hunninghake GW, Bitterman PB, Crystal RG. Production of fibronectin by the human alveolar macrophage: mechanism for the recruitment of fibroblasts to sites of tissue injury in interstitial lung diseases. Proc Natl Acad Sci USA 1981; 78:7147–7151.

163. Vignola AM, Chanez P, Chiappara G, Merendino A, Zinnanti E, Bousquet J, Bellia V, Bonsignore G. Release of transforming growth factor-beta (TGF-β) and fibronectin by alveolar macrophages in airway diseases. Clin Exp Immunol 1996; 106: 114–119.

164. Hibbs MS, Hoidal JR, Kang AH. Expression of a metalloproteinase that degrades native type V collagen and denatured collagens by cultured human alveolar macrophages. J Clin Invest 1987; 80:1644–1650.

165. Kaliner MA, Blennerhasset J, and Austen KF. Bronchial asthma. In: Meischer PA, Muller-Eberhard HJ, eds. Textbook of Immunopathology. New York: Grune & Stratton, 1976:387.

166. Sur S, Crotty TB, Kephart GM, Hyma BA, Colby TV, Reed CE, Hunt LW, Gleich GJ. Sudden-onset fatal asthma. A distinct entity with few eosinophils and relatively more neutrophils in the airway submucosa? Am Rev Respir Dis 1993; 148:713–719.

167. Carroll N, Carello S, Cooke C, James A. Airway structure and inflammatory cells in fatal attacks of asthma. Eur Respir J 1996; 9:709–715.

168. Synek M, Beasley R, Frew AJ, Goulding D, Holloway L, Lampe FC, Roche WR, Holgate ST. Cellular infiltration of the airways in asthma of varying severity. Am J Respir Crit Care Med 1996; 154:224–230.

169. Wenzel SE, Szefler SJ, Leung DYM, Sloan SI, Rex MD, Martin RJ. Bronchoscopic evaluation of severe asthma: persistent inflammation associated with high dose glucocorticoids. Am J Respir Crit Care Med 1997; 156:737–743.

170. Schleimer RP, Freeland HS, Peters SP, Brown KE, Derse CP. An assessment of the effects of glucocorticoids on degranulation, chemotaxis, binding to vascular endothelium and formation of leukotriene B4 by purified human neutrophils. J Pharmacol Exp Ther 1989; 250:598–605.

171. Cox G. Glucocorticoid treatment inhibits apoptosis in human neutrophils: separation of survival and activation outcomes. J Immunol 1995; 154:4719–4725.

172. Chanez P, Paradis L, Vignola AM, Vachier I, Vic P, Godard P, Bousquet J. Changes in bronchial inflammation of steroid (GCs) dependent asthmatics (abstr). Am J Respir Crit Care Med 1996; 153:212.

173. Levine SJ. Bronchial epithelial cell-cytokine interactions in airway epithelium. J Invest Med 1995; 43:241–249.

174. Johnson SR, Knox AJ. Synthetic functions of airway smooth muscle in asthma. Trends Pharmacol Sci 1997; 18:288–292.

175. Bombara MP, Webb DL, Conrad P, Marlor CW, Sarr T, Ranges GE, Aune TM, Greve JM, Blue ML. Cell contact between T cells and synovial fibroblasts causes induction of adhesion molecules and cytokines. J Leukoc Biol 1993; 54:399–406.

176. Rochester CL, Ackerman SJ, Zheng T, Elias JA. Eosinophil-fibroblast interactions: granule major basic protein interacts with IL-1 and transforming growth factor-β in the stimulation of lung fibroblast IL-6-type cytokine production. J Immunol 1996; 156:4449–4456.

177. Barnes PJ. Cytokines as mediators of chronic asthma. Am J Respir Crit Care Med 1994; 150:S42–S49.

178. Massagué J. The transforming growth factor-β family. Annu Rev Cell Biol 1990; 6:597–641.

179. Raines EW, Bowen-Pope DF, Ross R. Platelet-derived growth factor. In: Sporn MB, Roberts AB, ed. Handbook of Experimental Pharmacology: Peptide Growth Factors and Their Receptors. Heidelberg: Springer-Verlag, 1990:173–262.

180. Burgess WH, Maciag T. The heparin-binding (fibroblast) growth factor family of proteins. Ann Rev Biochem 1989; 58:575–606.

181. Vilcek J, Palombella VJ, Henriksen-DeStefano D, Swenson C, Feinman R, Hirai M, Tsujimoto M. Fibroblast growth enhancing activity of tumor necrosis factor and its relationship to other polypeptide growth factors. J Exp Med 1986; 163:632–643.

182. Postlethwaite AE, Holness MA, Katai H, Raghow R. Human fibroblasts synthesize elevated levels of extracellular matrix proteins in response to interleukin 4. J Clin Invest 1992; 90:1479–1485.

183. DiCosmo EB, Geba GP, Picarella D, Elias J, Rankin JA, Stripp BR, Whitsett JA, Flavell RA. Airway targeted interleukin-6 in transgenic mice: uncoupling of airway inflammation and bronchial hyperreactivity. J Clin Invest 1994; 94:2028–2035.

184. Doherty AM. Endothelin: a new challenge. J Med Chem 1992; 35:1493–1508.

185. Panettieri RA, Yadvish PA, Kelly AM, Rubinstein NA, Kotlikoff MI. Histamine stimulates proliferation of airway smooth muscle and induces c-fos expression. Am J Physiol 1990; 259(6Pt1):L365–L371.

186. Ruoss SJ, Hartmann T, Caughey GH. Mast cell tryptase is a mitogen for cultured fibroblasts. J Clin Invest 1991; 88:493–499.

187. Marini M, Avoni E, Hollemborg J, Mattoli S. Cytokine mRNA profile and cell activation in bronchoalveolar lavage fluid from nonatopic patients with symptomatic asthma. Chest 1992; 102:661–669.

188. Molet S, Chakir J, Laviolette M, Zhu Z, Elias JA, Hamid Q. Response of remodeling-associated cytokines to steroids in bronchial biopsies of asthmatic patients (abstr). Am J Respir Crit Care Med 2000; 161:686.

189. Jarjour NN, Calhoun WJ, Schwartz LB, Busse WW. Elevated bronchoalveolar lavage fluid histamine levels in allergic asthmatics are associated with increased airway obstruction. Am Rev Respir Dis 1991; 144:83–87.

190. Redington AE, Springall DR, Ghatei MA, Lau LC, Bloom SR, Holgate ST, Polak JM, Howarth PH. Endothelin in bronchoalveolar lavage fluid and its relation to airflow obstruction in asthma. Am J Respir Crit Care Med 1995; 151:1034–1039.

191. Border WA, Noble NA. Transforming growth factor β in tissue fibrosis. N Engl J Med 1994; 331:1286–1292.

192. Kovacs EJ, DiPietro LA. Fibrogenic cytokines and connective tissue production. FASEB J 1994; 8:854–861.

193. Grande JP. Role of transforming growth factor-β in tissue injury and repair. Proc Soc Exp Biol Med 1997; 214:27–40.

194. Ignotz RA, Massagué J. Transforming growth factor-β stimulates the expression of fibronectin and collagen and their incorporation into the extracellular matrix. J Biol Chem 1986; 261:4337–4345.

195. Aubert JD, Dalal BI, Bai TR, Roberts CR, Hayashi S, Hogg JC. Transforming growth factor β1 gene expression in human airways. Thorax 1994; 49:225–232.

196. Coker RK, Laurent GJ, Shahzeidi S, Hernández-Rodríguez NA, Pantelidis P, du-Bois RM, Jeffery PK, McAnulty RJ. Diverse cellular TGF-β1 and TGF-β3 gene expression in normal human and murine lung. Eur J Respir J 1996; 9:2501–2507.

197. Redington AE, Roche WR, Holgate ST, Howarth PH. Co-localization of immuno-reactive transforming growth factor-beta-1 and decorin in bronchial biopsies from asthmatic and normal subjects. J Pathol 1998; 186:410–415.

198. Redington AE, Madden J, Frew AJ, Djukanovic R, Roche WR, Holgate ST, Howarth PH. Transforming growth factor-β1 in asthma: measurement in broncho-alveolar lavage fluid. Am J Respir Crit Care Med 1997; 156:642–647.

199. Roberts AB, Sporn MB, Assoian RK, Smith JM, Roche NS, Wakefield LM, Heine UI, Liotta LA, Falanga V, Hehrl JH, Fauci AS. Transforming growth factor type β: rapid induction of fibrosis and angiogenesis in vivo and stimulation of collagen formation in vitro. Proc Natl Acad Sci USA 1986; 83:4167–4171.

200. Rossi P, Karsenty G, Roberts AB, Roche NS, Sporn MB, de Crombrugghe B. A nuclear factor 1 binding site mediates the transcriptional activation of a type I colla-gen promoter by transforming growth factor-β. Cell 1988; 52:405–414.

201. Raghow R, Postlethwaite AE, Keski-Oja J, Moses HL, Kang AH. Transforming growth factor-β increases steady-state levels of type I procollagen and fibronectin messenger RNAs posttranscriptionally in cultured human dermal fibroblasts. J Clin Invest 1987; 79:1285–1288.

202. McAnulty RJ, Campa JS, Cambrey AD, Laurent GJ. The effect of transforming growth factor β on rates of procollagen synthesis and degradation in vitro. Biochem Biophys Acta 1991; 1091:231–235.

203. Edwards DR, Leco KJ, Beaudry PP, Atadja PW, Veillette C, Riabowol KT. Differ-ential effects of transforming growth factor beta 1 on the expression of matrix metalloproteinases and tissue inhibitors of metalloproteinases in young and old hu-man fibroblasts. Exp Gerontol 1996; 31:207–223.

204. Zeng G, McCue HM, Mastrangelo L, Millis AJT. Endogenous TGF-β activity is modified during cellular aging: effects on metalloproteinase and TIMP-1 expres-sion. Exp Cell Res 1996; 228:271–276.

205. Sacco O, Romberger D, Rizzino A, Beckmann JD, Rennard SI, Spurzem JR. Spon-taneous production of transforming growth factor-β2 by primary cultures of bron-chial epithelial cells: effects on cell behavior in vitro. J Clin Invest 1992; 90:1379–1385.

206. Phan SH, Gharaee-Kermani M, Wolber F, Ryan US. Stimulation of rat endothelial

cell transforming growth factor-β production by bleomycin. J Clin Invest 1991; 87:148–154.

207. Assoian RK, Fleurdelys BE, Stevenson HC, Miller PJ, Matdes DK, Raines EW, Ross R, Sporn MB. Expression and secretion of type β transforming growth factor by activated human macrophages. Proc Natl Acad Sci USA 1987; 84:6020–6024.

208. Kehrl JH, Wakefield LM, Roberts AB, Jakowlew S, Alvarez-Mon M, Derynck R, Sporn MB, Fauci AS. Production of transforming growth factor β by human T lymphocytes and its potential role in the regulation of T cell growth. J Exp Med 1986; 163:1037–1050.

209. Kelley J, Fabisiak JP, Hawes K, Absher M. Cytokine signaling in the lung: transforming growth factor-β secretion by lung fibroblasts. Am J Physiol 1991; 260(2Pt1):L123–L128.

210. Elias JA, Zheng T, Einarsson O, Landry M, Trow T, Rebert N, Panuska J. Epithelial interleukin-11: regulation by cytokines, respiratory syncytial virus, and retinoic acid. J Biol Chem 1994; 269:22261–22268.

211. Elias JA, Zheng T, Whiting NL, Trow TK, Merrill WW, Zitnik R, Ray P, Alderman EM. IL-1 and transforming growth factor-β regulation of fibroblast-derived IL-11. J Immunol 1994; 152:2421–2429.

212. Einarsson O, Geba GP, Zhu Z, Landry M, Elias JA. Interleukin-11: stimulation in vivo and in vitro by respiratory viruses and induction of airways hyperresponsiveness. J Clin Invest 1996; 97:915–924.

213. Zheng T, Nathanson MH, Elias JA. Histamine augments cytokine-stimulated IL-11 production by human lung fibroblasts. J Immunol 1994; 153:4742–4752.

214. Ray P, Tang W, Wang P, Homer R, Kuhn C 3rd, Flavell RA, Elias JA. Regulated overexpression of interleukin-11 in the lung. Use to dissociate development-dependent and -independent phenotypes. J Clin Invest 1997; 100:2501–2511.

215. Tang W, Geba GP, Zheng T, Ray P, Homer RJ, Kuhn C 3rd, Flavell RA, Elias JA. Targeted expression of IL-11 in the murine airway causes lymphocytic inflammation, bronchial remodeling, and airways obstruction. J Clin Invest 1996; 98: 2845–2853.

216. Dabbagh K, Takeyama K, Lee H-M, Ueki IF, Lausier JA, Nadel JA. IL-4 induces mucin gene expression and Goblet cell metaplasia in vitro and in vivo. J Immunol 1999; 162:6233–6237.

217. Jayawickreme SP, Gray T, Nettesheim P, Eling T. Regulation of 15-lipoxygenase expression and mucus secretion by IL-4 in human bronchial epithelial cells. Am J Physiol 1999; 276(4Pt1):L596–L603.

218. Sarén P, Welgus HG, Konaven PT. TNF-α and IL-1β selectively induce expression of 92-kDa gelatinase by human macrophages. J Immunol 1996; 156:4159–4165.

219. Lacraz S, Nicod L, Galve-de-Rochemonteix B, Baumberger C, Dayer JM, Welgus HG. Suppression of metalloproteinase biosynthesis in human alveolar macrophages by interleukin-4. J Clin Invest 1992; 90:382–388.

220. Bugno M, Graeve L, Gatsios P, Koj A, Heinrich PC, Travis J, Kordula T. Identification of the interleukin-6/oncostatin M response element in the rat tissue inhibitor of metalloproteinases-1 (TIMP-1) promoter. Nucleic Acids Res 1995; 23:5041–5047.

221. Takeyama K, Dabbagh K, Lee H-M, Agustí C, Lausier JA, Ueki IF, Grattan KM,

Nadel JA. Epidermal growth factor system regulates mucin production in airways. Proc Natl Acad Sci USA 1999; 96:3081–3086.

222. Stewart AG, Grigoriadis G, Harris T. Mitogenic actions of endothelin-1 and epidermal growth factor in cultured airway smooth muscle. Clin Exp Pharmacol Physiol 1994; 21:277–285.

223. Hirst SJ, Barnes PJ, Twort CHC. Quantifying proliferation of cultured human and rabbit airway smooth muscle cells in response to serum and platelet-derived growth factor. Am J Respir Cell Mol Biol 1992; 7:574–581.

224. Chediak AD, Elsasser S, Csete ME, Gazeroglu H, Wanner A. Effects of histamine on tracheal mucosal perfusion, water content and airway smooth muscle in sheep. Respir Physiol 1991; 84:231–242.

225. Laitinen LA, Laitinen A, Widdicombe J. Effects of inflammatory and other mediators on airway vascular beds. Am Rev Respir Dis 1987; 135:S67–S70.

226. Laitinen LA, Laitinen AM, Widdicombe JG. Dose-related effects of pharmacological mediators on tracheal vascular resistance in dogs. Br J Pharmacol 1987; 92: 703–709.

227. McDonald DM. Neurogenic inflammation in the respiratory tract: actions of sensory nerve mediators on blood vessels and epithelium of the airway mucosa. Am Rev Respir Dis 1987; 136:S65–S72.

228. Moreno RH, Hogg JC, Pare PD. Mechanics of airway narrowing. Am Rev Respir Dis 1986; 133:1171–1180.

229. Hogg JC, Pare PD, Moreno R. The effects of submucosal edema on airways resistance. Am Rev Respir Dis 1987; 135:S54–S56.

230. Li X, Wilson JW. Increased vascularity of the bronchial mucosa in mild asthma. Am J Respir Crit Care Med 1997; 156:229–233.

231. Tsuboi R, Sato Y, Rifkin DB. Correlation of cell migration, cell invasion, receptor number, proteinase production, and basic fibroblast growth factor levels in endothelial cells. J Cell Biol 1990; 110:511–517.

232. Bradding P, Roberts JA, Britten KM, Montefort S, Djukanovic R, Mueller R, Heusser CH, Howarth PH, Holgate ST. Interleukin-4, -5, and -6 and tumor necrosis factor-α in normal and asthmatic airways: evidence for the human mast cell as a source of these cytokines. Am J Respir Cell Mol Biol 1994; 10:471–480.

233. Connolly DT, Heuvelman DM, Nelson R, Olander JV, Eppley BL, Delfino JJ, Siegel NR, Leimgrumber RM, Feder J. Tumor vascular permeability factor stimulates endothelial cell growth and angiogenesis. J Clin Invest 1989; 84:1470–1478.

234. Sumpio BE, Banes AJ, Levin JG, Johnson G Jr. Mechanical stress stimulates aortic endothelial cells to proliferate. J Vasc Surg 1987; 6:252–256.

235. Haraguchi M, Shimura S, Shirato K. Morphometric analysis of bronchial cartilage in chronic obstructive pulmonary disease and bronchial asthma. Am J Respir Crit Care Med 1999; 159:1005–1013.

236. Saklatvala J, Sarsfield SJ. How do interleukin 1 and tumor necrosis factor induce degradation of proteoglycan in cartilage? In: Glauert AM, ed. The control of tissue damage. New York: Elsevier, 1988:97–108.

237. Stewart AG, Fernandes D, Tomlinson PR. The effect of glucocorticoids on proliferation of human cultured airway smooth muscle. Br J Pharmacol 1995; 116:3219–3226.

238. Laitinen LA, Laitinen A, Haahtela TA. A comparative study of the effects of an inhaled corticosteroid, budesonide, and a β2-agonist, terbutaline, on airway inflammation in newly diagnosed asthma: a randomized, double-blind, parallel-group controlled trial. J Allergy Clin Immunol 1992; 90:32–42.

239. Kai H, Yoshitake K, Hisatsune A, Kido T, Isohama Y, Takahama K, Miyata T. Dexamethasone suppresses mucus production and MUC-2 and MUC-5AC gene expression by NCI-H292 cells. Am J Physiol 1996; 271(3Pt1):L484–L488.

240. Shimura S, Sasaki T, Sasaki H, Takishima T. Chemical properties of bronchorrhea sputum in bronchial asthma. Chest 1988; 94:1211–1215.

241. Cockayne D, Sterling KM Jr, Shull S, Mintz KP, Illeyne S, Cutroneo KR. Glucocorticoids decrease the synthesis of type I procollagen mRNAs. Biochemistry 1986; 25:3202–3209.

242. Shapiro SD, Campbell EJ, Kobayashi DK, Welgus HG. Dexamethasone selectively modulates basal and lipopolysaccharide-induced metalloproteinase and tissue inhibitor of metalloproteinase production by human alveolar macrophages. J Immunol 1991; 146:2724–2729.

6

Pharmacological Management of Severe Asthma

STANLEY J. SZEFLER

National Jewish Medical and Research Center
University of Colorado Health Science Center
Denver, Colorado

I. Introduction

In *Severe Asthma: Pathogenesis and Clinical Management*, prepared over 5 years ago for the Lung Biology in Health and Diseases series, Dr. Kamada and I provided a comprehensive review of information on the asthma medications available for the management of severe asthma (1). Since that time, new medications and new insights related to the pathogenesis of asthma and the mechanisms of action of these medications have been introduced. The purpose of this chapter is to summarize new insights on the role of available medications and to organize these medications into a framework for the management of severe asthma.

II. What Are the Goals of Management for the Patient with Severe Asthma?

Since the 1995 publication of *Severe Asthma*, several sets of guidelines have been published on the management of asthma including severe asthma. A "Global Initiative for Asthma" has been published, along with revised guidelines in indi-

Table 1 Classification and Goals of Therapy for Severe Persistent Asthma[a]

Clinical features of severe persistent asthma before treatment

Symptoms	Nighttime symptoms	Lung function
Continual symptoms	Frequent	FEV_1 or PEF $\leq 60\%$
Limited physical activity		predicted
Frequent exacerbations		PEF variability $>30\%$

Goals of therapy

Prevent chronic and troublesome symptoms (e.g., coughing or breathlessness in the night, in the early morning, or after exertion)

Maintain (near-) normal pulmonary function

Maintain normal activity levels (including exercise and other physical activity)

Prevent recurrent exacerbations of asthma and minimize the need for emergency care visits or hospitalizations

Provide optimal pharmacotherapy with minimal or no adverse effects

Meet patients' and families' expectations of and satisfaction with asthma care

[a] From Ref. 3.

vidual countries, such as the United States, as well as a third revision of the international guidelines for the management of childhood asthma (2–4). Specifically regarding severe asthma, classification, goals of therapy, and management principles have been summarized (Tables 1 and 2). There is an implicit message in these guidelines suggesting that a careful approach to early recognition and early intervention for overall asthma management could provide benefits in preventing severe asthma. Therefore, we should keep in mind management principles that seek to reverse the course of patients who have established severe asthma and also look to identify patients at risk for severe asthma utilizing management principles that will alter the course of the disease, so-called "disease modification." The chapter focuses on the management of established asthma of a severe level. The topic of prevention and disease modification is addressed in Chapter 25.

III. What Do We Know?

To improve the management of severe asthma, it is important to understand the natural history of asthma. We know that asthma can occur early in life. Current therapy, even in children, is based on the concept that chronic inflammation is a key feature of asthma, but there is very little information on the time of onset of inflammation and the mechanism for its initiation, progression, and persistence. Asthma presentation can be broken down into four broad categories of asthma control measures, as summarized in Table 3. These measures of control include

Table 2 Management of Severe Persistent Asthma[a]

Adults and children over 5 years of age
  Long-term control
    Anti-inflammatory: inhaled corticosteroids (high dose)
    High-dose inhaled steroids (mcg per day)—adults
      Fluticasone: >660 mcg
      Budesonide Turbuhaler: >600 mcg
      Beclomethasone dipropionate: >840 mcg
      Flunisolide: >2000 mcg
      Triamcinolone acetonide: >2000 mcg
    High-dose inhaled steroids (mcg per day)—children
      Fluticasone: >440 mcg
      Budesonide Turbuhaler: >400 mcg
      Beclomethasone dipropionate: >672 mcg
      Flunisolide: >1250 mcg
      Triamcinolone acetonide: >1200 mcg
    Long-acting bronchodilator: long-acting inhaled β2-agonists, sustained-release theophylline, or long-acting β2-agonist tablets AND
    Corticosteroid tablets or syrup long term (2 mg/kg/day, generally not to exceed 60 mg per day)
  Quick Relief
    Short-acting bronchodilator: inhaled β2-agonists as needed for symptoms
    Intensity of treatment depends on severity of exacerbation
    Use of short-acting inhaled β2-agonists on a daily basis; increasing use indicates the need for additional long-term-control therapy

Infants and young children
  Long-term control
    Daily anti-inflammatory medicine
      High-dose inhaled corticosteroid with spacer/holding chamber and face mask
      If needed, add systemic corticosteroids 2 mg/kg/day and reduce to lowest daily or alternate-day dose that stabilizes asthma
  Quick relief
    Bronchodilator as needed for symptoms up to three times a day

[a] From Ref. 3.

clinical, pulmonary function, progression, and inflammation parameters. Each of these features can be measured in individual patients and followed over time (5,6).

Given the paucity of published information on severe asthma in children, we recently performed a retrospective review of 164 consecutive adolescents admitted to our institution with the diagnosis of severe asthma (7). Several features of this study have implications for the pharmacologic management of severe

Table 3 Indicators of Asthma Control[a]

Clinical measures
  Mortality
  Hospitalizations
  Acute exacerbations
    Emergency department visits
    Courses of prednisone or high-dose inhaled steroids
  Nocturnal symptoms
  Breakthrough symptoms
    β-agonist use for symptom relief
    Wheezing or symptomatic (including chest tightness, cough, shortness of breath)
      episodes affecting activity

Pulmonary function measures
  Peak expiratory flow
  Pulmonary function (spirometry)
    $FEV_1\%$ predicted
    FEV_1/FVC or RV/TLC
  Pulmonary function (bronchial hyperresponsiveness to the following)
    Exercise
    Methacholine or histamine
  Body plethysmography
    Residual volume
    Total lung volume

Progression
  Increasing medication requirement
  Decline in pulmonary function
  Increasing airway hyperresponsiveness
  Serial biopsy (limited application at present)
    Cytology
      Eosinophils, mast cells, lymphocytes, and neutrophils
    Features of airway remodeling
      Collagen, elastin, and tenascin tissue deposition
    Alteration in markers of inflammation

Markers of inflammation
  Blood
    Total eosinophils, activated eosinophils
  Exhaled nitric oxide
  Plasma
    Eosinophilic cationic protein
  Induced sputum
    Cytology, especially eosinophils, or mediators
  Bronchoalveolar lavage
    Cytology and mediators

[a] Reprinted with permission from Szefler SJ, Martin RJ, National Heart, Lung and Blood Institute Asthma Clinical Research Network. Evaluation and comparison of inhaled steroids. In: Schleimer RP, O'Byrne PM, Szefler SJ, Brattsand R, eds, Airway Activity and Selectivity of Inhaled Steroids in Asthma: Optimizing Effects in the Airways. New York: Marcel Dekker, 2001 (in press).

asthma. The median age of the study population was 14.0 years, with a median duration of asthma of 11.9 years. All were on high-dose inhaled corticosteroid therapy (1500 µg/day) and roughly 50% also required maintenance oral corticosteroid therapy. Despite high-dose inhaled and oral corticosteroid therapy, these children had evidence for ongoing airway inflammation as evidenced by elevated eosinophil cationic protein (ECP) levels (median: 14.0 ng/mL, normal range: 0–10) and airflow obstruction with an admission FEV_1 of 77% of predicted. In addition, nearly three-fourths of the children were atopic. Of some surprise, nearly 25% of the children were found to be corticosteroid insensitive as defined by a less than 15% improvement in their morning prebronchodilator FEV_1 following a course of high-dose oral prednisone therapy. Corticosteroid-insensitive asthmatics required a larger maintenance oral corticosteroid dose, required oral corticosteroid therapy at an earlier age, and were more likely to be African American than those adolescents with steroid-sensitive asthma. In summary, our data would suggest that children with severe asthma had asthma for much of their lives and had evidence for ongoing disease activity despite aggressive inhaled and oftentimes oral corticosteroid therapy. In addition, a higher than expected number of these adolescents had a less than expected response to oral corticosteroid therapy and were termed corticosteroid insensitive.

The management of severe asthma poses some unique challenges. The available literature on the management of severe asthma in children is a fraction of that published from research in adult patients. While some of the principles can be extrapolated from experience in managing adult patients, additional research is needed to determine if the pathogenesis of severe asthma is similar in children with severe asthma. Similar to adults with severe asthma, the cornerstone of management for severe asthma in children includes high-dose inhaled corticosteroids. Dosage guidelines are available in the *National Asthma Education and Prevention Program Expert Panel Report* for the various inhaled corticosteroids and available delivery devices (3, Table 2). This treatment is combined with a long-acting nonsteroid controller medication (long-acting inhaled β2-agonist, sustained-release theophylline, or long-acting β2-agonist tablets) and, if necessary, corticosteroid tablets or syrup long term. It is recommended to make repeated attempts to reduce systemic corticosteroid and to maintain control with high-dose inhaled corticosteroid therapy (2,3). It is extremely important to monitor adherence to the treatment program.

A. General Approach

Before approaching a course of aggressive pharmacologic therapy, especially high-dose, long-term inhaled and oral corticosteroids, it is essential to perform a careful evaluation for diseases that can be mistaken as asthma, for example, vocal cord dysfunction, cystic fibrosis, and congenital heart disease. In addition, it is important that concomitant disorders, such as sinusitis and gastroesophageal reflux, are evaluated, as these disorders can contribute to poor asthma control (8,9; also see Chapters 11 and 18). The clinician should be sure that an action plan is developed and that the patient is carefully following this plan. This along with frequent visits to review asthma control are key elements in reducing the oral and inhaled corticosteroid requirement, a necessity for minimizing the risk of significant adverse corticosteroid effects (10). This method of close follow-up is strengthened if the patient can maintain records on daily peak flow measurement, medication requirement, need for rescue bronchodilator therapy, and severe exacerbations. Using this information to assess the benefits of various methods of therapeutic intervention can help the physician determine the most cost-effective method of treatment for the individual patient.

B. Inhaled Steroid Therapy

Although a preferred inhaled corticosteroid has not been defined to date, it seems reasonable that patients with severe asthma should be treated with a high-potency inhaled corticosteroid, such as fluticasone propionate, to minimize the number of actuations administered. An inhaled corticosteroid administered with a delivery device that improves delivery to the lung, such as budesonide with the Turbuhaler device or beclomethasone dipropionate with the hydrofluorocarbon propellent, are reasonable alternatives (3,6,11,12). This strategy has the benefit of minimizing the dose frequency and the number of actuations per treatment. Both features help improve medication adherence.

To minimize the dose of inhaled corticosteroid, long-term noncorticosteroid controllers can be added, as mentioned above. The options include frequent quick relief, such as rapid-acting β-adrenergic agonists and anticholinergic agents, and nonsteroid long-term control medications, such as long-acting β-adrenergic agonists, leukotriene modifiers, theophylline, nedocromil, cromolyn, and allergen immunotherapy. The relative benefits and disadvantages of each medication are summarized in Tables 4 and 5.

A recent study by Sont et al. (13) evaluated the level of asthma control resulting from inhaled steroid dose adjustments using airway hyperresponsiveness (AHR) as an additional guide to long-term treatment. This study used, in one group (reference group), the approach of adjusting inhaled steroid dosage according to levels of clinical symptoms, bronchodilator use, peak expiratory flow variability, and FEV_1 and, in another group (AHR-strategy group), same criteria plus airway responsiveness (Table 6). Based on the score determined at 3-month intervals, the dose could be adjusted to no inhaled steroid or to low-, medium-, or high-dose inhaled steroid.

After a 2-year follow-up, the investigators made several interesting observations. First, they observed greater improvements in asthma control and pulmo-

Table 4 Benefits and Risks of Available Quick Relief Medications for the Treatment of Severe Asthma

β-Adrenergic agonists
  Advantages (preferably albuterol, terbutaline, or pirbuterol due to longer duration of effect and high specificity for β2-adrenergic agonist effect)
    Most effective bronchodilator
    Rapid onset of effect contributes to immediate symptom relief
    Most effective medication in preventing or relieving exercise-induced bronchospasm
  Disadvantages
    Limited duration of effect, usually less then 6 h
    Requires frequent administration to maintain pulmonary function
    Desensitization with frequent and prolonged administration reduces duration of effect
    Undesirable systemic effects including tachycardia and anxiety due to sympathomimetic effect, especially with frequent administration and high doses

Anticholinergics (preferably ipratropium bromide due to low systemic absorption)
  Advantages
    Relatively slow onset of effect as compared to β-adrenergic agonists
    Additive effect with β-adrenergic agonist
    May be useful for psychogenic-induced bronchospasm
  Disadvantages
    Selective activity on cholinergic mechanisms associated with airway obstruction
    Limited duration of effect, approximately 6 h

nary function with the AHR strategy. Second, biopsy samples obtained before and after 2 years' treatment showed significant reductions in reticular layer thickness and reduced eosinophil infiltration only in the AHR-strategy group. Finally, they observed that a higher proportion of patients in the AHR-strategy group required high- and moderate-dose inhaled steroid therapy (Fig. 1). These observations suggest that patients with persistent asthma would receive better control and better resolution of inflammation, and the consequences of chronic inflammation, such as airway remodeling, if treatment were based on periodic measures of AHR. However, this strategy would result in treatment with higher doses of inhaled steroids, at least temporarily. On a cautionary note, clinical experience and available literature suggest that with aggressive therapy, AHR rarely normalizes and usually changes the provocative dose of methacholine and histamine by no more than twofold. Therefore, attempting to normalize AHR could result in protracted therapy and incur risk for adverse effects with little gain in response. Therefore, the application of measures of AHR needs careful consideration. Perhaps other measures, such as sputum eosinophils, or an alternative measure of

Table 5 Benefits and Risks of Available Nonsteroid Long-Term Control Medications for the Treatment of Severe Asthma

Long-acting β-adrenergic agonists
  At present limited to inhaled salmeterol (and formoterol pending approval) and controlled-release oral β2-adrenergic agents (several albuterol controlled-release formulations)
  Advantages
    Effective bronchodilator with long duration of action, approximately 12 h
    Bronchoprotective effect for exercise-induced bronchospasm
      Longer duration of action (for example, 4 to 8 h) than quick relief inhaled albuterol (efficacy is limited to several hours, especially in severe asthma), which is a benefit for those patients engaging in competitive sports, such as basketball, soccer, and football
    May prevent the pulmonary early- and late-phase reaction to an allergen challenge in a sensitized patient; however, will not prevent the consequent airway hyperresponsiveness
    Additive effect with inhaled steroids in reducing the frequency of severe exacerbations
  Disadvantages
    Potential for desensitization with regular administration; could result in reduction of duration of effect by 1 to 2 h
    No evidence of reduction of chronic airway inflammation or airway hyperresponsiveness with continuous treatment
    Reduction of symptoms and improvement of pulmonary function could mask ongoing airway inflammation

Leukotriene modifiers
  Leukotriene receptor antagonists (LTRA) (montelukast, zafirlukast, and pranlukast)
  Advantages
    Easy administration
    Can prevent or at least attenuate pulmonary and airway inflammatory response when administered prior to an allergen challenge in sensitized patients.
    May have benefit for aspirin-sensitive asthmatics
    Feasibility of once- (montelukast) or twice- (zafirlukast) daily administration favors medication adherence
    For montelukast there are dosage guidelines and formulations for children as young as 2 years; for zafirlukast guidelines go down to 6 years
    No evidence for drug interactions with montelukast
  Disadvantages
    No evidence for reduction of airway inflammation or airway hyperresponsiveness with continued administration
    For zafirlukast, there is potential for drug interaction with warfarin and recommendation to administer on an empty stomach due to food effects on absorption
    Concern regarding risk, although rare, for Churg–Strauss syndrome (Growing evidence suggests that this is likely a preexisting disease, especially in patients presenting with severe asthma)
    Limited spectrum of activity in selective blocking of LTD_4

Table 5 Continued

5-lipoxygenase inhibitors (zileuton)
  Advantages
    Easy administration
    Effect on an array of leukotriene mediators offers an advantage over LTRAs; specifically, inhibition of LTB_4 synthesis could influence neutrophil infiltration but not specifically studied in severe asthma
    Similar efficacy as demonstrated for LTRAs
    May have benefit for aspirin-sensitive asthmatics
  Disadvantages
    Requires administration four times per day
    Must monitor for potential hepatotoxicity
    Drug interaction with theophylline, warfarin, and terfenadine
    No dosage guidelines for children less than 12 years of age
Theophylline
  Advantages
    Bronchodilator effect
    Long duration of effect (as long as 12 to 24 h depending on product administered)
    Once-daily administration for certain products
    Effective in controlling nocturnal asthma
    Reduction of airway lymphocytes associated with inflammation
  Disadvantages
    Increased gastric acidity may exacerbate symptoms or inflammation associated with gastroesophageal reflux
    Undesirable adverse effects associated with doses needed to achieve high serum theophylline concentrations, such as nausea, gastrointestinal distress, and caffeinelike behavioral effects (e.g., anxiety)
    Variable absorption, specifically decreased absorption at night, for certain products when administered twice daily; this may result in low serum theophylline concentrations at night in patients with rapid metabolism
    Certain products may have significant variability in absorption in relation to food intake
    Potential for significant drug interactions with medications that induce (e.g., phenytoin, carbamazepine, rifampin, and phenobarbital) or inhibit (e.g., zileuton, macrolide antibiotics, and ketoconazole) enzymes necessary for theophylline metabolism
Nedocromil
  Advantages
    Extremely safe
    Can prevent immediate, late-phase, and airway hyperresponsiveness when administered prior to an allergen exposure in sensitized patients
    Can be effective in attenuating exercise-induced bronchospasm, especially when combined with inhaled β-adrenergic agonists
    Some evidence of inhaled steroid sparing effect, approximately 25% of total daily dose, when added to treatment of patients with moderate to severe asthma

Table 5 Continued

Disadvantages
  Greatest efficacy is in patients with mild persistent asthma
  No evidence of reduction of chronic airway inflammation or airway hyperrespon-
    siveness with continuous treatment
  Some patients complain of bad taste
  Requires administration four times per day when initiating therapy
  Cost and inconvenience of additional inhaler administrations may not offset the
    limited beneficial effect

Cromolyn
  Advantages
    Extremely safe
    Can prevent immediate, late-phase, and airway hyperresponsiveness when adminis-
      tered prior to an allergen exposure in sensitized patients
    Can be effective in attenuating exercise-induced bronchospasm, especially when
      combined with inhaled β-adrenergic agonists
  Disadvantages
    Greatest efficacy is in patients with mild persistent asthma
    No evidence of reduction of chronic airway inflammation or airway hyperrespon-
      siveness with continuous treatment
    No evidence of steroid sparing effect when added to treatment of moderate to se-
      vere asthma
    Requires administration four times per day when initiating therapy
    Cost and inconvenience of additional inhaler administrations may not offset the
      limited beneficial effect

Immunotherapy
  Advantages
    Could help control allergen-induced inflammation
    Environmental control is practically difficult in patients who maintain an active
      lifestyle; immunotherapy for a limited allergen panel increases likelihood of
      beneficial effect
    Evidence for efficacy in asthma is limited to a few allergens
  Disadvantages
    High risk for severe adverse effects; anaphylaxis, especially in the setting of vari-
      able pulmonary function inherent in patients with severe asthma
    Requires frequent visits early in course to initiate therapy
    Patients with severe asthma often have an extensive array of allergen sensitivity
      [i.e., environmental (pollen, house dust, pets, and insects), food, and medica-
      tions], which necessitates careful determination of the most relevant allergens
      for the specific patient to design an immunotherapy regimen most likely to
      provide benefit

Table 6 Severity Classes of Symptoms, Bronchodilator Usage, Diurnal Variability in PEF, FEV$_1$, and Airway Hyperresponsiveness with Corresponding Treatment Steps[a]

Treatment step	Both strategies				AHR strategy only
	Symptoms >3 day/2 weeks	Bronchodilator use	PEF variability (%)	FEV$_1$ (% pred)	Airway hyper-responsiveness: methacholine PC$_{20}$ (mg/ml)
4	Disturbed sleep/early wake-up/limited physical activities	>4 hourly	>50	<50	<0.25
3	Nighttime symptoms/ early wake-up/affect activities	>6 hourly	30–50	50–60	0.25–1.0
2	Mild nighttime/morn-ing symptoms/may affect activities	1–4×/day	20–30	60–70	1.0–4.0
1	<3 day/2 week	<Daily	<20	>70	>4.0

[a] From Ref. 13.

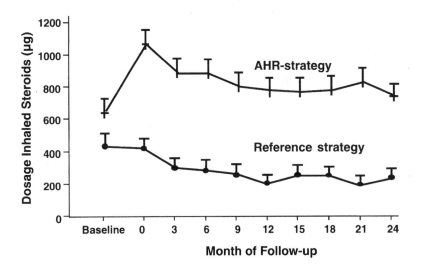

Figure 1 Actual daily doses of inhaled steroids (µg; mean ± SEM) according to the AHR strategy and the reference strategy. The median difference in treatment with inhaled steroids was ±400 µg during the 2-year follow-up. Treatment requirement decreased with both strategies. However, the decrease with the AHR strategy was somewhat greater than with the reference strategy. (Reprinted with permission from Sont JK, et al. Am J Respir Crit Care Med 1999; 159:1043–1051, Fig. 1.)

ongoing inflammation could be included as indicators for the adjustment of inhaled steroid therapy.

C. Long-Acting β-Adrenergic Agonist Therapy

It should be noted that the studies demonstrating an additive effect between inhaled corticosteroids and long-acting β-adrenergic agonists have been performed on adults with moderate to severe asthma (14–17). There has only been one study that evaluated this issue in childhood asthma. Verberne et al. (16) studied the effect of beclomethasone dipropionate (BDP) at 400 μg/day vs. BDP 800 μg/day vs. BDP 400 μg/day plus salmeterol 100 μg/day in a group of 177 asthmatic children already on inhaled corticosteroid therapy. After 1 year, no significant differences in FEV_1, methacholine PD_{20} values, or symptom scores were noted. Each treatment resulted in improved baseline lung function (~5%) and reduced airway responsiveness (0.60 to 1.3 doubling doses). Of note, those on BDP 800 μg/day grew at a slower rate than those of the other two groups (mean height: 3.6 cm for BDP 800 vs. 5.1 cm for BDP 400 + salmeterol vs. 4.5 cm in the BDP 400 group). Of significance, BDP at a dose of 400 μg/day was as effective as either doubling the dose of BDP or adding salmeterol to the regimen. The results of this study differ from those performed in adults with asthma. The authors suggest that the adult studies recruited asthmatics with more severe and unstable disease, as evidenced by their lower baseline lung function and greater symptoms upon entry into the study. Also of note, the improvement in airway responsiveness in the BDP 800 μg/day group was much greater than that seen in the adult studies where the dose of BDP was doubled. This would suggest that BHR can be altered to a greater extent in children than in adults.

For the combination of inhaled steroids and long-acting β-adrenergic agonist therapy, the strategy of high-dose inhaled steroid therapy plus long-acting β-adrenergic agonist may offer the most advantages. Pauwels et al. (17) compared four different treatment strategies in a study of patients with persistent asthma including twice-daily administration of a dry-powder budesonide inhaler (Turbuhaler) preparation of 100 μg of budesonide plus 12 μg of formoterol, 100 μg of budesonide plus placebo, 400 μg of budesonide plus 12 μg of formoterol, or 400 μg of budesonide plus placebo. They found that the rates of severe and mild exacerbations were reduced by 26 and 40%, respectively, when formoterol was added to the lower dose of budesonide therapy. The higher dose of budesonide alone reduced the rates of severe and mild exacerbations by 49 and 37%, respectively. Patients treated with formoterol and the higher dose of budesonide had the greatest reductions, 63 and 62% respectively. Symptoms of asthma and lung function improved with both formoterol and higher dose budesonide, but the improvement with formoterol was greater (Fig. 2).

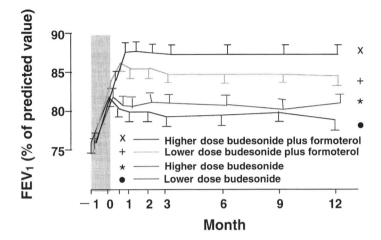

Figure 2 Forced expiratory volume in 1 sec (FEV₁) during the study. FEV₁ is shown as a mean percentage of the predicted value during the run-in period (shaded area) and the treatment period. The bars indicate 2 SE. During the run-in period, all patients received 800 μg of budesonide twice daily. Patients were then randomly assigned to twice-daily treatment with 100 μg of budesonide, 100 μg of budesonide plus 12 μg of formoterol, 400 μg of budesonide, or 400 μg of budesonide plus 12 μg of formoterol. (Reprinted with permission from Pauwels RA, et al. N Engl J Med 1997; 337: 1409, Fig. 1.)

D. Leukotriene Modifiers

Beyond high-dose, high-potency, or increased pulmonary delivery of inhaled corticosteroids combined with a long-acting bronchodilator, it is not clear what the preferred additional long-term controller medication should be. The introduction of a product that combines an inhaled steroid, fluticasone propionate, and a long-acting β-adrenergic agonist, salmeterol, in one inhaled delivery device (Advair Diskus, GlaxoWellcome) now reduces the number of inhalations necessary to administer these medications. There are no studies that evaluate the combination of high-dose inhaled corticosteroids with a long-acting inhaled β2-agonist together with another long-term controller medication, for example, a leukotriene modifier, theophylline, or nedocromil. Therefore, it is not known which combination is most effective in enhancing asthma control, resolving inflammation, and perhaps contributing to normalization of the airway. Studies are needed in this area to assist the clinician. In the absence of this information, the clinician should follow clinical parameters carefully in assessing the best combination of medications. There is increasing information on the role of leukotriene antagonists as well as of theophylline in preventing the inflammatory response to allergen challenge and reducing the number of inflammatory cells in the airways (see Chapter 7 for a detailed review). This could be beneficial in reducing inflammation in patients with severe asthma; however, no studies are available to document this proposed feature of asthma control in patients with severe asthma. There is information available indicating that the addition of a leukotriene antagonist to inhaled steroid therapy permits the reduction of the inhaled steroid dose, suggesting a steroid sparing effect (18,19).

E. Corticosteroid-Insensitive Asthma

While environmental control can be helpful in the sensitized patient, immunotherapy should not be considered in severe asthma since it may incur a significant risk for adverse effects (20) and the beneficial effect, if any, is small. If a patient fails to respond or is unable to tolerate oral corticosteroid doses lower than 20 mg every other day with either prednisone or methylprednisolone, evaluation of corticosteroid pharmacokinetics, if available, could be helpful. This procedure can identify patients with incomplete corticosteroid absorption, failure to convert an inactive form (prednisone) to an active form (prednisolone), or rapid elimination (1,21,22). However, this is not a reason for poor response in all severe asthmatics since less than 25% of severe asthmatics show significantly increased clearance of either prednisolone or methylprednisolone. Most of the patients, both adults and children, with increased clearance have a specific reason for rapid elimination, such as a drug interaction with a medication that induces corticosteroid metabolism, for example, the anticonvulsants phenytoin, carbamazepine or phenobarbital, or rifampin (1) (Table 7).

Several recent observations help to explain the limitations in response to conventional therapy in patients with severe asthma. Certain patients have been termed "corticosteroid-resistant" or "corticosteroid-insensitive" asthmatics (see Chapter 24). These patients are characterized by having a prebronchodilator FEV_1 less than 70% predicted while maintaining a bronchodilator response. Corticosteroid insensitivity is defined clinically by administering a course of oral prednisone [e.g., 40 mg per day (divided doses) for a minimum of 7 days, preferably 2 weeks] and observing the effect on morning prebronchodilator FEV_1 (23). If the FEV_1 fails to increase by 15% or more, then the patient is considered corticosteroid insensitive.

It is not clear which corticosteroid dose should be administered in patients who are already receiving high-dose oral and inhaled corticosteroid therapy. A trial of prednisone at 40 mg per day for 2 weeks is usually given to assess the possibility of poor adherence to the maintenance regimen. If the patient fails to respond, the dose is generally doubled and the patient is monitored for an additional 2 weeks. If the patient responds to this high corticosteroid dose, then the

Table 7 Glucocorticoid Interactions with Other Medications[a]

Glucocorticoid	Drug	Effect	Mechanism
Cortisol	β-adrenergic agonist	Enhanced β-agonist response	Alteration of β-adrenergic receptor affinity
	Phenobarbital, phenytoin	Increased elimination of cortisol	Increased cytochrome P450 activity
	Rifampicin	Decreased steroid effect	Increased elimination of cortisol
Prednisolone	Ketoconazole	Enhanced steroid effect	Impaired elimination
	Oral contraceptives	Increased steroid availability	Impaired elimination, increased protein binding
	Phenobarbital, phenytoin, carbamazepine	Decreased steroid effect	Increased cytochrome P450 activity
	Rifampicin	Decreased steroid effect	Increased steroid elimination
	Troleandomycin	No effect	
	Clarithromycin	No effect	
Methyl-prednisolone	Erythromycin	Enhanced steroid effect	Impaired MP[b] elimination
	Ketoconazole	Enhanced steroid effect	Impaired MP elimination
	Phenobarbital, phenytoin, carbamazepine	Probable diminished steroid effect	Increased cytochrome P450 activity
	Rifampicin	Decreased steroid effect	Probable increased cytochrome P450 activity
	Troleandomycin	Enhanced steroid effect	Partially related to impaired MP elimination
	Clarithromycin	Probable enhanced steroid effect	Impaired MP elimination
Dexamethasone	Ephedrine	Enhanced elimination	Possible increased metabolism
	Phenobarbital, phenytoin	Increased dexamethasone elimination	Increased cytochrome P450 activity

[a] Modified from Ref. 63.
[b] MP, Methylprednisolone.

dose is gradually decreased while monitoring daily PEF to determine a threshold dose.

Studies of the corticosteroid-insensitive patient population show that they have reduced glucocorticoid receptor (GCR) binding affinity, increased GCRβ concentrations (an inactive form of the GR), and failure to reduce inflammatory cells in bronchoalveolar lavage (BAL) fluid following a 2-week course of high-dose oral prednisone therapy (23–27). These abnormalities appear to be related to persistent inflammation despite high-dose oral and inhaled corticosteroid therapy (24,28–31). Their course of treatment is often complicated by adverse effects of corticosteroid therapy, such as growth impairment, corticosteroid-induced osteoporosis, hypertension, and obesity. In addition, some of these patients with severe asthma appear to have a neutrophil predominance (28,30), and additional studies are needed to determine if the neutrophils play a role in refractoriness to corticosteroid therapy and if a specific approach to altering neutrophil chemotaxis or activity would be an effective form of therapy. To date, clinical trials with the alternative anti-inflammatory and immunomodulator therapies are based on the symptom complex of severe asthma patients, not on specific pathologies.

While examining corticosteroid-insensitive asthma patients, it was also noted that a small proportion have a low GCR number (24). This may be related to a genetic abnormality in the constitution of the receptor number. Other genetic abnormalities have been observed in the asthma population such as β-adrenergic receptor polymorphism (32) and 5-lipoxygenase polymorphism (33). The prevalence of these abnormalities and clinical significance in the pathogenesis of severe asthma and refractoriness to treatment remains to be defined.

F. Chronopharmacology

Chronopharmacologic principles can be applied to optimize response to theophylline and corticosteroids (34–36). Patients with nocturnal exacerbations may do much better with a single dose of a once-daily sustained-release theophylline preparation administered in the evening rather than with a standard twice-daily preparation (34). Children and rapid theophylline metabolizers appear to be prone to a reduction in serum theophylline concentrations with twice-daily theophylline preparations during the night, when the rate of elimination may exceed the rate of absorption (35). An oral corticosteroid may also be more effective when administered in the late afternoon rather than in the morning (36). Although this strategy may increase the risk of steroid adverse effects, the priority is to regain asthma control. The steroid dose can then be tapered as tolerated.

G. Markers of Inflammation

As discussed above, studies in patients with severe asthma suggest that inflammation is still persistent despite treatment with high-dose inhaled steroids (28–

31). Markers of inflammation, for example, plasma eosinophil cationic protein levels and circulating eosinophil counts, may be helpful in examining medication response in children with severe asthma when they are detectable. In patients with severe asthma, the marker can be measured before and after a 1- to 2-week course of oral corticosteroid therapy (37). A significant reduction in the marker should be noted following a course of prednisone therapy. Failure to respond to high-dose corticosteroid therapy provides a strong base for incorporating trials of alternative anti-inflammatory or immunomodulator therapies, such as intravenous gammaglobulin, oral gold, or cyclosporine.

Furthermore, clinical studies suggest that clinical indicators, such as symptoms and pulmonary function, are inadequate predictors of breakdown in asthma control (38,39). Measurements of exhaled nitric oxide may also be useful as a measure of inflammation and response to therapeutic intervention (40), but even this measure has not been regularly incorporated in studies of severe asthma in children (see Chapter 19 for a detailed review of markers of inflammation in severe asthma). Finally, in occasional circumstances a tissue biopsy approach may be considered in the evaluation of highly refractory patients. These studies should only be done in centers with experience in performing and interpreting biopsies from asthma patients. By the identification of tissue pathology, these studies could provide insight into the design of treatment options specifically suited to the pathology identified (28,30). This could also lead to a differentiation of the disease among this patient population to guide the selection of individual patient treatment courses.

H. Adverse Effects of Steroid Therapy

In addition, the clinician managing severe asthma must keep in mind the complicating effects of corticosteroids, especially those of high-dose systemic corticosteroid therapy, such as growth impairment, osteoporosis, hypertension, and reduced neuromuscular function. The latter complication contributes to respiratory muscle weakness and may interfere with the pulmonary assessment of the beneficial effects of anti-inflammatory and immunomodulating medications. Additional pharmacologic therapy may be indicated to manage or prevent adverse effects, such as steroid-induced osteoporosis (41,42).

I. Alternative Anti-Inflammatory and Immunomodulator Therapy

In patients with severe persistent asthma who remain symptomatic despite optimal application of conventional therapy and management of concomitant disorders, studies are available primarily in adults demonstrating modest and inconsistent efficacy of alternative anti-inflammatory and immunomodulating drugs, such as methotrexate, gold, cyclosporine, and intravenous γ-globulin and macrolide antibiotics (43,44). In general, these studies indicate an ability to reduce oral corticosteroid requirements by approximately 50%, but with limited effect on improving pulmonary function and BHR.

Most of the studies with the alternative anti-inflammatory and immunomodulating drugs were conducted at a time when it was not customary to utilize high-dose, high-potency, or enhanced-delivery inhaled corticosteroids. In the presence of this form of treatment and especially in combination with other long-term controllers, these immunomodulator and alternative anti-inflammatory treatments are not very impressive. Intravenous γ-globulin can be effective in certain patients but its high cost is prohibitive, and while some studies have suggested a significant effect, others have shown little or no benefit (45,46). Significant benefit with regard to oral steroid reduction is noted especially in patients requiring high-dose oral steroids (Fig. 3) (46). This steroid sparing effect, despite an improvement in clinical features, could play a significant

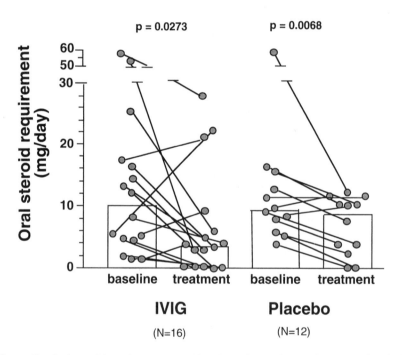

Figure 3 Oral steroid requirements (mg/day) in patients who required more than 2000 mg/year oral steroid therapy in the preceding year. Solid circles indicate average values in each patient during phases I (baseline) and IV (treatment). Median values for each group are indicated by open bars. (Reprinted with permission from Salmun LM, et al. J Allergy Clin Immunol 1999; 103:813, Fig. 2.)

role in reducing the risk of adverse effects to high-dose systemic glucocorticoid therapy.

Methotrexate has limited efficacy and carries a risk for liver toxicity and immunosuppression (10,47). Cyclosporine has only been utilized in a limited study population and carries a significant risk for renal disease and hypertension (48,49). Oral gold has limited efficacy and gastrointestinal adverse effects can limit its use (50). In the limited number of studies where a placebo control is incorporated, there are responders and nonresponders to each treatment arm including placebo, but there is no methodology to predict who will respond favorably. These protocols have almost uniformly failed to incorporate methods to measure resolution of inflammation, specifically with bronchial biopsy and bronchoalveolar lavage techniques (43,44).

In studies where an indirect measure of resolving inflammation was incorporated, i.e., BHR, no change was observed following treatment with methotrexate or intravenous γ-globulin (10,45). Biopsy studies in adults with severe asthma have stimulated a resurgence of interest in the use of macrolide antibiotics in the treatment of asthma, with the recognition of mycoplasma and chlamydialike organisms as a complicating feature of severe asthma (51–54). The beneficial effects of macrolide antibiotics could be related to their effect on reducing chlamydial infection in these patients or an intrinsic anti-inflammatory effect (55). Two new medications that could be useful in a therapeutic trial in patients with severe steroid-dependent asthma include nebulized budesonide (Fig. 4) and anti-IgE therapy (Fig. 5) (56–58). Both of these medications provide the potential for significant steroid reduction in oral-steroid-dependent severe asthma patients; however, anti-IgE is undergoing formulation changes and the anticipated availability is not known. Studies are needed with all of these agents to carefully define their benefits and risks as well as the patients most likely to respond to the selected treatment. Therefore, all patients who require this form of alternative treatment should be directed to sites of clinical research with organized protocols.

IV. What Do We Need to Know?

In order to effectively design treatment strategies for severe asthma in both children and adults it is obviously important to understand the pathophysiology of the disease. Several questions must be addressed to improve our approach to management, including but not limited to the following: If severe asthma is a manifestation of persistent inflammation or different types of inflammation, what is the key driving force for this inflammatory response? If there are different types of persistent inflammation, can we match effective treatments to specific

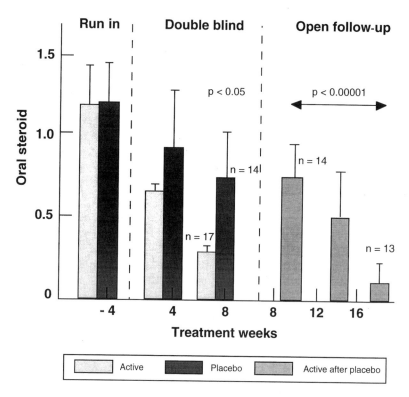

Figure 4   Dose of prednisolone by mouth (mg/kg/alternate day) showing a significant reduction for the group treated with nebulized budesonide during the double-blind period and an open follow-up period. The bar indicates SEM. (Reprinted with permission from Ilangovan P, et al. Arch Dis Child 1993; 68:357, Fig. 2.)

types of inflammation? Are there patients in whom steroid therapy may conceivably be disadvantageous? What diagnostic tests can be used to select those patients who will respond to alternative anti-inflammatory or immunomodulator therapies?

Besides the available immunomodulator, anti-inflammatory, and antibiotic therapies, there are some new medications on the horizon that could be useful in altering the course of inflammation associated with severe persistent and refractory asthma. These medications include anti-IgE, cytokine antagonists, soluble cytokine receptors, adhesion molecule antagonists, selective agonists and antagonists of the neurogenic pathways, metalloproteinases, low-molecular-weight heparin, respiratory anti-sense oligonucleotides, and DNA vaccines. To find their appropriate place in asthma management, studies are needed to determine their

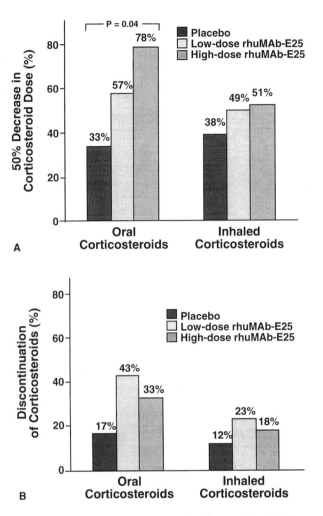

Figure 5 Results of efforts to taper the dose of corticosteroids. (A) The percentage of subjects in each group who were able to reduce their daily corticosteroid dose by at least 50% at 20 weeks. (B) The percentage of subjects in each group who were able to discontinue corticosteroid therapy. In the placebo, low-dose, and high-dose groups, 12, 14, and 9 subjects, respectively, used oral corticosteroids and 93, 92, and 97 subjects, respectively, used inhaled corticosteroids. Subjects who left the study had their last recorded dose carried forward. (Reprinted with permission from Milgrom H, et al. N Engl J Med 1999; 341:1970, Fig. 2.)

overall effect on the various asthma control measures, which include clinical, pulmonary, progression, and inflammation parameters (Table 3).

V. How Do We Get the Answers?

Clinical studies in severe asthma in adults and children should incorporate a standardized approach with all attempts made to obtain as much information as possible to address specific questions without compromising safety. As many available tools as possible should be used to understand the disease and evaluate response to treatment including pulmonary physiology (spirometry; bronchial challenge to methacholine, histamine, or exercise; and body plethysmography), biopsy, bronchoalveolar lavage, induced sputum, exhaled nitric oxide, and peripheral blood cell and plasma markers. Some, but not all, could be used in pediatric clinical studies.

If at all possible, more information is needed on the pathology of severe asthma in adults as well as children to define the nature of the ultrastructural abnormalities. It is possible that aggressive courses of anti-inflammatory or immunomodulator therapy can suppress active inflammation, but airway remodeling may predispose the patient to residual symptoms secondary to persistent BHR or, possibly, a noninflammatory based BHR. Obviously, more effort must be placed on understanding the pathophysiology of severe asthma to refine the selection of pharmacotherapy for this challenging group of patients. It is important to assess the effect of age, gender, duration of disease, and race on response to medications as well as risks of adverse effects (59–62).

The core structure of a medication trial in severe asthma should consist of a multicenter, placebo-controlled, randomized, parallel design. Objective measures of response, such as pulmonary function measures and measures of airway inflammation, should be incorporated to carefully evaluate responders and nonresponders within the treatment groups.

Clinical trials in individual patients or studies with selected interventions should consist of two phases. Upon initiating therapy, the selected medication (or corresponding placebo in a clinical research study) should be added with no change in concomitant therapy. The purpose of this phase is to assess the direct benefit of study medication. The minimum time period to assess efficacy is usually 6 weeks; however, this can be modified based on preliminary open label trials directly designed to evaluate the time of onset of effect. The second phase is where medication reduction can be evaluated, specifically oral corticosteroid therapy. The purpose is to assess the oral corticosteroid sparing effect of the trial medication. This phase usually takes a minimum of 3 months. Comprehensive measurements of pulmonary function and airway inflammation could be obtained prior to randomization and upon completion of each of the two study phases.

This type of design would permit pharmacologic trials to assess the effect of treatment on active inflammation vs. arrested progression, to identify major inflammatory cells and thus focus selection of treatment to correlate clinical response to alteration of inflammation, to assess the role of infection, and to assess the role of individual and combination therapy. The combination of careful clinical studies in children with established severe asthma and the coordination of programs to identify patients at risk and an appropriate intervention would go a long way toward reducing the risks of this life-threatening disease.

VI. Conclusions

Since the first edition of *Severe Asthma* in 1995, new medications and new insights into the pathogenesis have increased our ability to alleviate much of the morbidity of severe asthma. Additional chapters in this second edition focus on specific components of severe asthma and their medical management. Further insight and advances in therapy should provide greater benefit in managing patients with severe asthma and with hope could also alter the natural history of asthma and thus reduce the incidence of patients with this level of severity.

Acknowledgments

Supported in part by Public Health Services Research Grants 1NO1-HR-16048, HL36577, and HL 51834; General Clinical Research Center Grant 5 MO1 RR00051 from the Division of Research Resources; and NICHHD Pediatric Pharmacology Research Unit Network Grant 1-U01-HD37237.

References

1. Kamada AK, Szefler SJ. Pharmacologic management of severe asthma. In: Szefler SJ, Leung DYM, eds. Severe Asthma: Pathogenesis and Clinical Management. New York: Marcel Dekker, 1995:165–205.
2. NHLBI/NIH Workshop Report: Global Initiative for Asthma. Global Strategy for Asthma Management and Prevention. National Institutes of Health, National Heart, Lung, and Blood Institute Publication No. 95-3659. Bethesda, MD: National Institutes of Health, 1995.
3. National Asthma Education and Prevention Program Expert Panel Report 2: Guidelines for the Diagnosis and Management of Asthma. National Institutes of Health, National Heart, Lung, and Blood Institute Publication No. 97-4051. Bethesda, MD: National Institutes of Health, 1997.

4. Warner JO, Naspitz CK. Third International Pediatric Consensus Statement on the Management of Childhood Asthma: International Pediatric Asthma Consensus Group. Pediatr Pulmonol 1998; 25(1):1–17.

5. Szefler SJ. Asthma—the new advances. Adv Ped 2000; 47:273–308.

6. Szefler S, Martin RJ. National Heart, Lung and Blood Institute Asthma Clinical Research Network: evaluation and comparison of inhaled steroids. In: Schleimer RP, O'Byrne PM, Szefler SJ, Brattsand R, eds. Airway Activity and Selectivity of Inhaled Steroids in Asthma—Mechanisms, Models of Evaluation and Clinical Impacts. New York: Marcel Dekker, 2001, in press.

7. Chan MT, Leung DYM, Szefler SJ, Spahn JD. Difficult-to-control asthma: clinical characteristics of steroid-insensitive asthma. J Allergy Clin Immunol 1998; 101(5): 594–601.

8. Szefler SJ, Leung DYM. Severe persistent and corticosteroid insensitive asthma. In: Neffenand H, Baebna-Cagnani C. Asthma: A Link Between Environment, Immunology and the Airways. Proceedings of the XVI World Congress of Asthma. Seattle: Hogrefe & Huber, 1999:177–185.

9. Irwin RS, Curley FJ, French CL. Difficult-to-control asthma. Contributing factors and outcome of a systematic management protocol. Chest 1993; 103(6):1662–1669.

10. Erzurum SC, Leff JA, Cochran JE, Ackerson LM, Szefler SJ, Martin RJ, Cott GR. Lack of benefit of methotrexate in severe, steroid-dependent asthma: a double-blind, placebo-controlled study. Ann Intern Med 1991; 114(5):353–360.

11. Thorsson L, Edsbacker S, Conradson TB. Lung deposition of budesonide from Turbuhaler is twice that from a pressurized metered-dose inhaler P-MDI. Eur Respir J 1994; 7(10):1839–1844.

12. Seale JP, Harrison LI. Effect of changing the fine particle mass of inhaled beclomethasone dipropionate on intrapulmonary deposition and pharmacokinetics. Respir Med 1998; 92(suppl A):9–15.

13. Sont JK, Willems LN, Bel EH, van Krieken JH, Vandenbroucke JP, Sterk PJ. Clinical control and histopathologic outcome of asthma when using airway hyperresponsiveness as an additional guide to long-term treatment: The AMPUL Study Group. Am J Respir Crit Care Med 1999; 159(4 Pt 1):1043–1051.

14. Greening AP, Ind PW, Northfield M, Shaw G. Added salmeterol versus higher-dose corticosteroid in asthma patients with symptoms on existing inhaled corticosteroid. Allen & Hanburys Limited UK Study Group. Lancet 1994; 344(8917):219–224.

15. Woolcock A, Lundback B, Ringdal N, Jacques LA. Comparison of addition of salmeterol to inhaled steroids with doubling of the dose of inhaled steroids. Am J Respir Crit Care Med 1996; 153(5):1481–1488.

16. Verberne AA, Frost C, Duiverman EJ, Grol MH, Kerrebijn KF. Addition of salmeterol versus doubling the dose of beclomethasone in children with asthma: The Dutch Asthma Study Group. Am J Respir Crit Care Med 1998; 158(1):213–219.

17. Pauwels RA, Löfdahl CG, Postma DS, Tattersfield AE, O'Byrne P, Barnes PJ, Ullman A. Effect of inhaled formoterol and budesonide on exacerbations of asthma: Formoterol and Corticosteroids Establishing Therapy (FACET) International Study Group. N Engl J Med 1997; 337(20):1405–1411.

18. Tamaoki J, Kondo M, Sakai N, Nakata J, Takemura H, Nagai A, Takizawa T, Konno K. Leukotriene antagonist prevents exacerbation of asthma during reduction of high-

dose inhaled corticosteroid: The Tokyo Joshi-Idai Asthma Research Group. Am J Respir Crit Care Med 1997; 155(4):1235–1240.

19. Laviolette M, Malmstrom K, Lu S, Chervinsky P, Pujet JC, Peszek I, Zhang J, Reiss TF. Montelukast added to inhaled beclomethasone in treatment of asthma: Montelukast/Beclomethasone Additivity Group. Am J Respir Crit Care Med 1999; 160(6):1862–1868.

20. Bousquet J, Michel FB. Specific immunotherapy in asthma: is it effective? J Allergy Clin Immunol 1994; 94(1):1–11.

21. Spahn JD, Leung DYM, Szefler SJ. Difficult to control asthma: New insights and implications for management. In: Szefler SJ, Leung DYM, eds. Severe Asthma: Pathogenesis and Clinical Management. New York: Marcel Dekker, 1996:497–535.

22. Hill MR, Szefler SJ, Ball BD, Bartoszek M, Brenner AM. Monitoring glucocorticoid therapy: a pharmacokinetic approach. Clin Pharmacol Ther 1990; 48(4):390–398.

23. Lee TH, Brattsand R, Leung DYM. Corticosteroid action and resistance in asthma. Am J Respir Cell Mol Biol Supplement 1996; 154:S1–S79.

24. Sher ER, Leung DYM, Surs W, Kam JC, Zieg G, Kamada AK, Szefler SJ. Steroid-resistant asthma: Cellular mechanisms contributing to inadequate response to glucocorticoid therapy. J Clin Invest 1994; 93(1):33–39.

25. Leung DYM, Martin RJ, Szefler SJ, Sher ER, Ying S, Kay AB, Hamid Q. Dysregulation of interleukin 4, interleukin 5, and interferon gamma gene expression in steroid-resistant asthma. J Exp Med 1995; 181(1):33–40.

26. Lane SJ, Adcock IM, Richards D, Hawrylowicz C, Barnes PJ, Lee TH. Corticosteroid-resistant bronchial asthma is associated with increased c-fos expression in monocytes and T lymphocytes. J Clin Invest 1998; 102(12):2156–2164.

27. Leung DYM, Hamid Q, Vottero A, Szefler SJ, Surs W, Minshall E, Chrousos GP, Klemm DJ. Association of glucocorticoid insensitivity with increased expression of glucocorticoid receptor beta. J Exp Med 1997; 186(9):1567–1574.

28. Wenzel SE, Szefler SJ, Leung DYM, Sloan SI, Rex MD, Martin RJ. Bronchoscopic evaluation of severe asthma: Persistent inflammation associated with high dose glucocorticoids. Am J Respir Crit Care Med 1997; 156(3 Pt 1):737–743.

29. Louis R, Lau LC, Bron AO, Roldaan AC, Radermecker M, Djukanovic R. The relationship between airways inflammation and asthma severity. Am J Respir Crit Care Med 2000; 161(1):9–16.

30. Wenzel SE, Schwartz LB, Langmack EL, Halliday JL, Trudeau JB, Gibbs RL, Chu HW. Evidence that severe asthma can be divided pathologically into two inflammatory subtypes with distinct physiologic and clinical characteristics. Am J Respir Crit Care Med 1999; 160(3):1001–1008.

31. Vrugt B, Wilson S, Underwood J, Bron A, de Bruyn R, Bradding P, Holgate ST, Djukanovic R, Aalbers R. Mucosal inflammation in severe glucocorticoid-dependent asthma. Eur Respir J 1999; 13(6):1245–1252.

32. Turki J, Pak J, Green SA, Martin RJ, Liggett SB. Genetic polymorphisms of the beta 2-adrenergic receptor in nocturnal and nonnocturnal asthma: evidence that Gly16 correlates with the nocturnal phenotype. J Clin Invest 1995; 95(4):1635–1641.

33. In KH, Asano K, Beier D, Grobholz J, Finn PW, Silverman EK, Silverman ES, Collins T, Fischer AR, Keith TP, Serino K, Kim SW, De Sanctis GT, Yandava C, Pillari A, Rubin P, Kemp J, Israel E, Busse W, Ledford D, Murray JJ, Segal A,

Tinkleman D, Drazen JM. Naturally occurring mutations in the human 5-lipoxygenase gene promoter that modify transcription factor binding and reporter gene transcription. J Clin Invest 1997; 99(5):1130–1137.

34. Martin RJ, Cicutto LC, Ballard RD, Goldenheim PD, Cherniack RM. Circadian variations in theophylline concentrations and the treatment of nocturnal asthma. Am Rev Respir Dis 1989; 139(2):475–478.

35. Kossoy AF, Hill M, Lin FL, Szefler SJ. Are theophylline "levels" a reliable indicator of compliance? J Allergy Clin Immunol 1989; 84(1):60–65.

36. Beam WR, Weiner DE, Martin RJ. Timing of prednisone and alterations of airways inflammation in nocturnal asthma. Am Rev Respir Dis 1992; 146(6):1524–1530.

37. Spahn JD, Leung DYM, Surs W, Harbeck RJ, Nimmagadda S, Szefler SJ. Reduced glucocorticoid binding affinity in asthma is related to ongoing allergic inflammation. Am J Respir Crit Care Med 1995; 151(6):1709–1714.

38. Jatakanon A, Lim S, Barnes PJ. Changes in sputum eosinophils predict loss of asthma control. Am J Respir Crit Care Med 2000; 161(1):64–72.

39. Parameswaran K, Pizzichini E, Pizzichini MM, Hussack P, Efthimiadis A, Hargreave FE. Clinical judgement of airway inflammation versus sputum cell counts in patients with asthma. Eur Respir J 2000; 15(3):486–490.

40. Mattes J, Storm van's Gravesande K, Reining U, Alving K, Ihorst G, Henschen M, Kuehr J. NO in exhaled air is correlated with markers of eosinophilic airway inflammation in corticosteroid-dependent childhood asthma. Eur Respir J 1999; 13(6):1391–1395.

41. Wang WQ, Ip MS, Tsang KW, Lam KS. Antiresorptive therapy in asthmatic patients receiving high-dose inhaled steroids: a prospective study for 18 months. J Allergy Clin Immunol 1998; 101(4 Pt 1):445–450.

42. Herrala J, Puolijoki H, Liippo K, Raitio M, Impivaara O, Tala E, Nieminen MM. Clodronate is effective in preventing corticosteroid-induced bone loss among asthmatic patients. Bone 1998; 22(5):577–582.

43. Jarjour N, McGill K, Busse WW, Gelfand EW. Alternative anti-inflammatory and immunomodulatory therapy. In: Szefler SJ, Leung DYM, eds. Severe Asthma: Pathogenesis and Clinical Management. New York: Marcel Dekker, 1996:333–369.

44. Spector SL. Treatment of the unusually difficult asthmatic patient. Allergy Asthma Proc 1997; 18(3):153–155.

45. Mazer BD, Gelfand EW. An open-label study of high-dose intravenous immunoglobulin in severe childhood asthma. J Allergy Clin Immunol 1991; 87(5):976–983.

46. Salmun LM, Barlan I, Wolf HM, Eibl M, Twarog FJ, Geha RS, Schneider LC. Effect of intravenous immunoglobulin on steroid consumption in patients with severe asthma: a double-blind, placebo-controlled, randomized trial. J Allergy Clin Immunol 1999; 103(5 Pt 1):810–815.

47. Marin MG. Low-dose methotrexate spares steroid usage in steroid-dependent asthmatic patients: a meta-analysis. Chest 1997; 112(1):29–33.

48. Alexander AG, Barnes NC, Kay AB. Trial of cyclosporin in corticosteroid-dependent chronic severe asthma. Lancet 1992; 339(8789):324–328.

49. Lock SH, Barnes NC, Kay AB. Cyclosporin (CsA) as a corticosteroid sparing agent in corticosteroid-dependent asthma. Eur Respir J 1994; 7(suppl 18):282s.

50. Bernstein IL, Bernstein DI, Dubb JW, Faiferman I, Wallin B. A placebo-controlled

multicenter study of auranofin in the treatment of patients with corticosteroid-dependent asthma: Auranofin Multicenter Drug Trial. J Allergy Clin Immunol 1996; 98(2): 317–324.

51. Hahn DL. Intracellular pathogens and their role in asthma: Chlamydia pneumonia in adult patients. Eur Respir Rev 1996; 6(38):224–230.

52. Black PN. The use of macrolides in the treatment of asthma. Eur Respir Rev 1996; 6(38):240–243.

53. Kraft M, Cassell GH, Henson JE, Watson H, Williamson J, Marmion BP, Gaydos CA, Martin RJ. Detection of Mycoplasma pneumoniae in the airways of adults with chronic asthma. Am J Respir Crit Care Med 1998; 158(3):998–1001.

54. Hahn DL, Bukstein D, Luskin A, Zeitz H. Evidence for Chlamydia pneumoniae infection in steroid-dependent asthma. Ann Allergy Asthma Immunol 1998; 80(1): 45–49.

55. Ianaro A, Ialenti A, Maffia P, Sautebin L, Rombola L, Carnuccio R, Iuvone T, D'Acquisto F, Di Rosa M. Anti-inflammatory activity of macrolide antibiotics. J Pharmacol Exp Ther 2000; 292(1):156–163.

56. Ilangovan P, Pedersen S, Godfrey S, Nikander K, Noviski N, Warner JO. Treatment of severe steroid dependent preschool asthma with nebulised budesonide suspension. Arch Dis Child 1993; 68(3):356–359.

57. Szefler SJ. Meeting needs of infants and young children with asthma: new developments in nebulized corticosteroid therapy. Introduction. J Allergy Clin Immunol 1999; 104(4 Pt 2):159–161.

58. Milgrom H, Fick RB, Jr., Su JQ, Reimann JD, Bush RK, Watrous ML, Metzger WJ. Treatment of allergic asthma with monoclonal anti-IgE antibody: rhuMAb- E25 Study Group. N Engl J Med 1999; 341(26):1966–1973.

59. Covar R, Leung DYM, Chan MTS, Spahn JD. Risk factors associated with glucocorticoid (GC) side effects in adolescents with severe asthma-revisited. J Allergy Clin Immunol 1999; 103(1 Pt 2):S261.

60. Spahn JD, Brown EE, Covar R, Leung DYM. Do African Americans display a diminished response to glucocorticoids? J Allergy Clin Immunol 1999; 102 (1 Pt 2): S262–S263.

61. Alward WL, Fingert JH, Coote MA, Johnson AT, Lerner SF, Junqua D, Durcan FJ, McCartney PJ, Mackey DA, Sheffield VC, Stone EM. Clinical features associated with mutations in the chromosome 1 open-angle glaucoma gene (GLC1A). N Engl J Med 1998; 338(15):1022–1027.

62. Uitterlinden AG, Burger H, Huang Q, Yue F, McGuigan FE, Grant SF, Hofman A, van Leeuwen JP, Pols HA, Ralston SH. Relation of alleles of the collagen type I alpha-1 gene to bone density and the risk of osteoporotic fractures in postmenopausal women. N Engl J Med 1998; 338(15):1016–1021.

63. Szefler, SJ. In: Schleimer RP, Claman HN, Oronsky A, eds. Anti-Inflammatory Steroid Action. San Diego: Academic Press, 1989:365–366.

7

Leukotrienes and Antileukotriene Therapy in Severe Asthma

SALLY E. WENZEL

National Jewish Medical and Research Center
University of Colorado Health Sciences Center
Denver, Colorado

I. Introduction

Inflammation is likely the most significant contributing factor to the symptoms and physiologic changes of asthma. As part of this inflammatory process, activation of the arachidonic acid cascade leads to production of lipid mediators known as leukotrienes (LT). These leukotrienes are thought to play a central role in the bronchoconstriction, edema formation, and increase in mucus associated with the symptoms of asthma, all of which can be prominently associated with severe asthma. Drugs have recently become available which will specifically interfere with that pathway, namely leukotriene receptor antagonists (LTRAs) and 5-lipoxygenase (5-LO) inhibitors. This chapter reviews the evidence that leukotrienes (both cysteinyl and LTB4) are important mediators in severe asthma and whether blocking their production or effects will improve outcomes in severe asthma.

II. The Leukotriene Pathway

Leukotrienes are potent lipid mediators implicated in the pathogenesis of asthma. They are products of the metabolism of arachidonic acid formed from phospholipids, which are ubiquitous elements of cellular membranes. Phospholipids in the cell or nuclear membrane can be metabolized by enzymes known as phospholipases, leading to the production of arachidonic acid. This arachidonic acid can then be further metabolized down a variety of pathways, including the cyclooxygenase pathway, which leads to production of prostaglandins and thromboxane and the 5-LO pathway, which leads to the production of leukotrienes (1). Activation of 5-LO is thought to require generalized cellular activation and the availability of arachidonic acid as a substrate. It is presumed to require interactions with a protein known as 5-LO activating protein, which may channel arachidonic acid to the enzyme 5-LO (1). In certain inflammatory cells (macrophages and likely mast cells) this process is felt to occur at the nuclear (rather than the cytoplasmic) membrane (2,3). 5-LO activation then leads to the production of an intermediate known as LTA4, which can be further metabolized, depending on cell type, to LTB4 or the cysteinyl LTs (cLTs) LTC4, D4, and E4 (formerly known as slow-reacting substance of anaphylaxis).

Leukotrienes are produced almost exclusively by cells of the myeloid lineage. LTC4 is produced primarily by mast cells, basophils, and eosinophils, cells commonly associated with mild asthma (1). LTB4 is produced primarily by neutrophils and monocyte/macrophages, cells which have only recently been described to be increased in severe asthma (4–7).

The physiological properties of the LTs are outlined in Table 1. Cysteinyl LTs are potent bronchoconstrictors (100 to 1000 times more potent than histamine) which enhance membrane permeability and decrease mucociliary clearance (8). In addition, inhalation of LTE4 has recently been shown to lead to the chemoattraction of eosinophils into the lungs of asthmatics (9). Some of this chemoattractant activity may occur through secondary activation of the eosinophil chemoattractant and activator interleukin-5 (10). LTB4 is a potent chemoattractant for neutrophils and eosinophils as well as an activator of neutrophils, which appears to enhance adhesion and migration of the cells through the endothelium (8). It has also been suggested to augment production of other inflammatory cytokines, such as tumor necrosis factor-α and interleukin-8 (11–13). Recently, both

Table 1 Relevant Physiological Effects of Leukotrienes to Severe Asthma

Cysteinyl LTs	LTB4
Bronchoconstriction	Neutrophil and eosinophil chemoattraction
Vasodilation/edema formation	Neutrophil activation
Mucous production	Augmentation of IL-8/TNF-α inflammation
Eosinophilic inflammation	
Augmentation of smooth muscle proliferation	

LTRAs and 5-LO inhibitors have been shown to decrease airway eosinophils, supporting the chemoattractant qualities of these leukotrienes (14–16). Both cysteinyl LTs and LTB4 have been measured in body fluids of asthmatics, including bronchoalveolar lavage (BAL) fluid, urine, and blood (14,17–19). The cysteinyl LTs have also been shown to be increased in urine from patients in status asthmaticus, decreasing with treatment (17,18).

Cysteinyl LTs in humans appear to activate cells predominantly through a single receptor, known as the cysLT1 receptor, although there appears to be at least one other receptor present in humans. The cysLT1 receptor has recently been cloned and mRNA for the receptor has been localized in airway smooth muscle cells and perhaps macrophages (20). Whether there are differences in the distribution or amounts of the receptor in different disease states or whether the second LT receptor, the cysLT2 receptor, will prove to be important in human diseases await further study. LTB4 functions solely through the LTB4 receptor, which was also recently cloned (21). An extensive overview of the location of this receptor in the airways has not been performed.

III. Evidence for Leukotriene Involvement in Severe Asthma

Only a limited number of studies have addressed the issue of the presence of LTs in asthma patients with more severe disease. These few studies have suggested that both LTB4 and the cysteinyl LTs may be elevated, at least in some severe asthma patients. These findings were perhaps initially unexpected, as it had been believed that corticosteroids would effectively eliminate activation of the 5-lipoxygenase pathway by limiting arachidonic metabolism through production of lipocortins (22). However, studies have now evaluated the effect of in vivo corticosteroids, often in high doses, on both lung and urinary cysteinyl LT levels in patients with mild asthma (23,24). These studies have failed to demonstrate that LT production is diminished in the face of high doses of corticosteroids. This would suggest that severe asthma patients, who are treated with high doses of corticosteroids, may not have adequate suppression of the LT-associated components of inflammation.

There are three types of severe asthma in which increased LT levels have been measured: acute severe asthma, asthma associated with aspirin sensitivity, and chronic severe asthma. The first type includes patients with acute severe asthma. Early studies measured increased excretion of LTE4 (as a marker of total body cLT production) in the urine of patients with acute asthma exacerbations. These increased levels decreased over time, with treatment and improvement in the exacerbation (17,18). Although LT levels have not been reported in the airway fluids from patients intubated with status asthmaticus, there have been several reports documenting the increased numbers and activation of neutrophils (and eosinophils) in these patients (25,26). Along with these neutrophils, increased levels of the chemokines, including both TNF-α and interleukin-8 (a potent neutrophil chemoattractant) have also been reported (25). Both TNF-α and IL-8 have been reported to upregulate LTB4 (or to be upregulated by it), suggesting that LTB4 might be increased in these cases as well (11–13).

The second group of severe asthmatics are those with aspirin-sensitive asthma (ASA). Although ASA makes up a small portion (5–10%) of the general asthma population, this group appears to be overrepresented at the level of severe asthma. In a group of nearly 100 severe asthmatics studied at National Jewish, nearly 30% of these severe asthmatics expressed a historical sensitivity to aspirin (27). ASA has recently been associated with increased basal levels of cLTs and markedly increased cLT levels following challenge with aspirin (see Chapter 16). These increased levels have been reported in both bronchoalveolar lavage fluid and in urine (28–30). The amount excreted in the urine has been reported to be associated with the severity of the aspirin reaction (31). Additionally, severe asthmatics with a history of aspirin sensitivity were reported to have higher basal urinary LTE4 levels than those of a control group of asthmatics well matched for age and steroid dose (27). The role of LTB4 in ASA is not clear. LTB4 has been reported to increase in BAL fluid following airway challenge with indomethacin, although the increase is not of the magnitude seen with the cLTs (32).

There have also been reports of abnormalities in a particular enzyme in the 5-LO pathway, namely LTC4 synthase, which metabolizes LTA4 into LTC4. A genetic mutation in the promoter of the LTC4 synthase gene has been reported in ASA but the number of individuals evaluated was small (33). Increased expression of this enzyme by eosinophils has also been described in the airways of aspirin-sensitive asthmatics compared to those not sensitive to aspirin (34).

The third group of severe asthmatics are those with severe, chronic airflow limitation; on high doses of corticosteroids; and without a history of aspirin sensitivity. There are only two studies which have looked at LT levels in the lungs of these severe patients. In a study which evaluated a single group of severe asthmatics compared to mild asthmatics and normal controls, higher levels of LTB4 were recorded in the severe asthmatics than in the control groups (4). This study also reported an increase in the numbers of tissue neutrophils in severe asthmatics. In a second study by the same group, which classified severe asthmatics into two groups on the basis of the presence or absence of eosinophils in the endobronchial biopsies, increased levels of cLTs were measured in severe asthmatics who had evidence for increases in tissue eosinophils (5). LTB4 levels were not increased in the second study, although neutrophils were increased in both groups of severe asthmatics. Interestingly, increased levels of endotoxin in house dust have been reported to be associated with more severe asthma (35).

Endotoxin, a potent stimulator of LTB4 production from alveolar macrophages, could contribute to increased neutrophilic inflammation and chronically elevated LTB4 levels (12).

IV. Usefulness of Antileukotriene Therapy in Severe Asthma

Anti-LT drugs include four different agents, as listed in Table 2. Anti-LT therapy has been reported to have therapeutic effects in all three severe asthma categories described above. In the first reported study of the usefulness of anti-LT therapy in acute exacerbations of asthma, the leukotriene receptor antagonist zafirlukast, given once at a high dose (160 mg orally) and followed by 20 mg bid in conjunction with "usual care," was shown to improve the increase in FEV_1 in the emergency room and decrease hospital admissions and exacerbation rates in the short term (36). A second trial using an intravenous formulation of a receptor antagonist (montelukast) is currently underway.

Aspirin-sensitive asthmatics were one of the first groups of asthmatics targeted for treatment with anti-LT drugs. Aspirin-sensitive asthmatics generally have more severe symptoms and greater medication needs than non-aspirin-sensitive asthmatics. Bronchoconstriction associated with aspirin challenge has been nearly completely prevented by LTRAs and 5-LO inhibitors, confirming the importance of leukotrienes in the bronchospasm associated with the aspirin reaction (28,37,38). Studies utilizing 5-LO inhibitors in this population have demonstrated an associated reduction in urinary LTE4 excretion and, intriguingly, a reduction in nasal tryptase levels as well (37,39). All of these studies, however, were done using a threshold dose of aspirin (that dose of aspirin required to produce a 15–20% fall in FEV_1). In fact, aspirin-sensitive asthmatics who have mistakenly taken full doses of aspirin while on an anti-LT drug have not been adequately protected against the bronchospastic reaction (40).

Table 2 Leukotriene Receptor Antagonists and Pathway Inhibitors

Receptor antagonists	Pathway inhibitors
Action	Action
Block the actions of cysteinyl leukotrienes	Block the production of LTB4 *and* cysteinyl leukotrienes
Drug names	Drug name
Zafirlukast (Accolate)	Zileuton (Zyflo)
Montelukast (Singulair)	
Pranlukast (Onon)	

Longer term placebo-controlled studies of aspirin-sensitive asthmatics support the efficacy of chronic dosing in this population as well (41,42). These populations of severe asthmatics showed incremental improvements in FEV_1 and symptoms upon the addition of a 5-LO inhibitor or a LT receptor antagonist to the treatment regimen, despite concomitant treatment with inhaled as well as oral corticosteroids. Studies with the 5-LO inhibitor zileuton demonstrated improvement in associated nasal/sinus symptoms as well (41). Although in theory one might assume that all aspirin-sensitive asthmatics would respond to anti-LT therapy, experience suggests otherwise. It is currently unknown whether the percentage of ASAs responding to anti-LT therapy is any different from that of the general asthmatic population ($\sim$50% responders).

The third group of severe asthmatics has not been adequately studied with the addition of anti-LT therapy in placebo-controlled trials. There are currently no studies which have evaluated oral steroid sparing in patients with more severe disease. There have been three placebo-controlled studies done in patients with moderately severe asthma on high doses of inhaled corticosteroids. Two published studies have confirmed the ability of LT receptor antagonists to allow clinically successful reduction in high inhaled corticosteroid (ICS) doses beyond that seen with placebo. The first double-blind, placebo-controlled study demonstrated that the concomitant use of pranlukast allowed the starting inhaled corticosteroid dose (1600 µg/day) to be cut to 800 µg/day in moderate asthmatics without compromising asthma control (43). The addition of pranlukast maintained morning and evening peak flows, despite the reduced beclomethasone dose (Fig. 1). Similarly, while patients receiving the reduced dose of beclomethasone (with placebo) had increases in peripheral blood eosinophilic cationic protein levels and exhaled nitric oxide, there were no increases in these parameters in those patients in whom pranlukast was added to the reduced ICS dose. The second study was done with montelukast. In that study, ICS doses were tapered to a point where subjects began to show evidence for exacerbation of their asthma in a single-blind placebo run-in period. Doses were reduced from 1600 to $\sim$1000 µg/day. At that point, subjects were treated with montelukast 10 mg qd or placebo. The group treated with montelukast was able to reduce their dose another 47% before demonstrating signs of an exacerbation, while the group on placebo reduced 30% (44). Perhaps most importantly, a study published in abstract form suggested that a leukotriene receptor antagonist (zafirlukast) added at 80 mg bid to high doses ($\sim$1300 µg/day) of inhaled corticosteroids, in patients still symptomatic on those doses, could improve both symptoms and pulmonary function (45). Although these studies in more severe patients have never been analyzed for the percentage of patients "responding" to the therapy, it is likely that the percentage of individuals doing well on this therapy is not different from patients with milder disease. As in patients with milder disease, it is imperative that

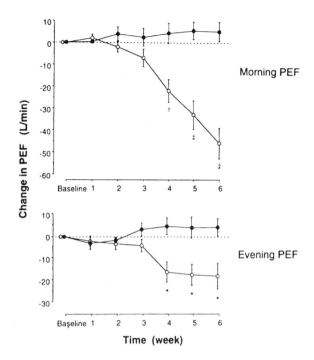

Figure 1 The anti-LT drug, pranlukast, maintained starting AM peak expiratory flow rates as compared to placebo following a 50% reduction in inhaled corticosteroid dose. (—●—● = pranlukast, —○—○ = placebo). Weeks 4–6 all significantly different compared to placebo. (Reprinted by permission from Am J Respir Crit Care Med 1997; 155: 1235–40.)

follow-up of the patients is scheduled to determine the efficacy of therapy. As FEV_1 may not change dramatically in these patients following treatment, it is important to evaluate symptoms and β-agonist use, as these may be more likely to be affected by the treatment (46).

There are no studies which have adequately compared the efficacy of LT receptor antagonists vs. 5-LO inhibitors in severe asthmatics. In theory, a 5-LO inhibitor which blocks both the cLTs and LTB4 might be expected to be more efficacious, especially in patients with more severe disease, where neutrophils and LTB4 may play a greater role. However, the currently used 5-LO inhibitor, zileuton, is limited by four-times-daily dosing, which may discourage compliance and limit efficacy in that manner. Further studies with better 5-LO inhibitors are needed.

V. Antileukotriene Therapy and the Prevention of Disease Progression

Nothing is known at present regarding the long-term, disease-modifying nature of these drugs or the impact on existing or developing "airway remodeling." Although not completely clear, it has been assumed that remodeling is associated with long-term, uncontrolled inflammation. Recent studies with anti-LT drugs do support a modest effect on "classic" eosinophilic inflammation. Both LTRAs and 5-LO inhibitors may decrease the inflammatory cell influx into the airways after instillation of allergen (47,48). Administration of zafirlukast for 1 week prior to instillation of allergen directly into the airways of asthmatics significantly decreased the influx of basophils and lymphocytes into the airways 48 h after allergen exposure when compared to placebo. Zafirlukast also tended to decrease the numbers of eosinophils migrating into the airways (48). There was an associated decrease in airway histamine and tumor necrosis factor-α levels, although the mechanisms behind these reductions are not clear. In contrast, however, in an *inhaled* allergen challenge model, no effect on late-phase sputum eosinophils was seen with the LTRA montelukast (49).

Using a nocturnal asthma model, the 5-LO inhibitor zileuton was found to decrease urinary and BAL LT levels while improving pulmonary function and symptoms in patients with nocturnal asthma. The improvement in FEV_1 correlated with the levels of LTB4 in the airways. Additionally, the eosinophils in the BAL and peripheral blood decreased significantly, supporting a cellular-level anti-inflammatory effect (14).

Studies of the anti-inflammatory effect in chronic asthma are also beginning to emerge. The LTRA pranlukast was shown to decrease airway eosinophils in endobronchial biopsy samples after 6 weeks of therapy. However, there was no significant improvement in FEV_1 during the course of therapy (16). A second study, utilizing sputum analysis, demonstrated a significant decrease in sputum eosinophils following 6 weeks of therapy with montelukast (15). Finally, virtually all published studies of LT modulating drugs have demonstrated a significant decrease in circulating eosinophil numbers (14,46,50,51).

Whether these modest anti-inflammatory effects will have any impact on airway remodeling is not known. However, there are additional studies in animals and in vitro which suggest that anti-LT therapy may impact smooth muscle proliferation (52,53). If, as many have suggested, smooth muscle hypertrophy and/or hyperplasia in the airways is an element of airway remodeling in asthma, then the long-term reduction of this increase in smooth muscle mass by anti-LT therapy could have beneficial effects. Unfortunately, this effect may be impossible to determine in humans at the present time due to our limited ability to evaluate airway smooth muscle in vivo.

VI. Suggestions for the Use of Antileukotriene Therapy in Patients with Severe Asthma

Severe asthma remains a difficult disease to treat. Other chapters of this book present the many issues which may influence the state of severe asthma, including compliance issues. Anti-LT therapy is given orally, and therefore, in some asthmatics, where compliance/adherence are critical issues, giving an oral drug may enhance compliance and therefore outcomes. As with all severe asthmatics, however, therapy should be individualized. If anti-LT therapy is initiated, patients should be followed at regular intervals. Experience suggests that the treatment trial should consist of a 2- to 3-month period of time rather than the 2- to 4-week trials used to study mild asthmatics. Symptoms, β-agonist use, and pulmonary function should be monitored for improvement. If zafirlukast is used, it may be beneficial to utilize higher doses, e.g., 40 mg bid. Experience suggests that some severe patients (especially aspirin-sensitive patients) may respond to a 5-LO inhibitor better than to a receptor antagonist. Therefore, in patients in whom adequate improvement has not been seen with a receptor antagonist, a trial with a 5-LO inhibitor should also be undertaken. There are further anecdotal reports of patients who have done best in the presence of both subclasses of anti-LT therapy, but this approach is not generally recommended.

Children with severe asthma can also be treated with anti-LT drugs. Montelukast is approved for children 2 years old and above, zafirlukast for children 6 years old and above, and zileuton in children 12 years old and above.

Although the use of anti-LT drugs for severe asthmatics is generally much safer than alternatives, such as methotrexate or cyclosporin, patients with severe disease may be at greater risk for the development of Churg–Strauss syndrome, an eosinophilic vasculitis, when corticosteroids are withdrawn. The initial report of Churg–Strauss syndrome was of eight patients treated with zafirlukast who had previously been on oral steroids and had since had their oral steroids tapered. Since that report, further reports of Churg–Strauss syndrome have been received with both montelukast and pranlukast (54). Whether this effect is due to the steroid withdrawal in patients whose disease was previously masked by the high doses of steroids or whether the anti-LT therapy had any effect on the development of the disease is not fully understood. More information is needed before conclusions can definitively be drawn, but physicians should seriously consider complaints regarding new rashes and neurological or worsening respiratory symptoms (55). All of these symptoms require assessment with at least a chest X-ray and an eosinophil count.

References

1. Henderson WR Jr. The role of leukotrienes in inflammation. Ann Intern Med 1994; 121:684–697.

2. Woods JW, Coffey MJ, Brock TG, Singer II, Peters-Golden M. 5-Lipoxygenase is located in the euchromatin of the nucleus in resting human alveolar macrophages and translocates to the nuclear envelope upon cell activation. J Clin Invest 1995; 95:2035–2046.

3. Brock TG, Paine RI, Peters-Golden M. Localization of 5-lipoxygenase to the nucleus of unstimulated rat basophilic leukemia cells. J Biol Chem 1994; 269:22059–22066.

4. Wenzel SE, Szefler SJ, Leung DYM, Sloan SI, Rex MD, Martin RJ. Bronchoscopic evaluation of severe asthma: persistent inflammation associated with high dose glucocorticoids. Am J Respir Crit Care Med 1997; 156:737–743.

5. Wenzel SE, Schwartz LB, Langmack EL, Halliday JL, Trudeau JB, Gibbs RL, Chu HW. Evidence that severe asthma can be divided pathologically into two inflammatory subtypes with distinct physiologic and clinical characteristics. Am J Respir Crit Care Med 1999; 160:1001–1008.

6. Jatakanon A, Uasuf C, Maziak W, Lim S, Chung KF, Barnes PJ. Neutrophilic inflammation in severe persistent asthma. Am J Respir Crit Care Med 1999; 160: 1532–1539.

7. Louis R, Lau LCK, Bron AO, Roldaan AC, Radermecker M, Djukanovic R. The relationship between airways inflammation and asthma severity. Am J Respir Crit Care Med 2000; 161:9–16.

8. Lewis RA, Austen F, Soberman RJ. Leukotrienes and other products of the 5-lipoxygenase pathway. N Engl J Med 1990; 323:645–655.

9. Laitinen LA, Laitinen A, Haahtela T, Vikka V, Spur BW, Lee TH. Leukotriene E4 and granulocytic infiltration into asthmatic airways. Lancet 1993; 341:989–990.

10. Underwood DC, Osborn RR, Newsholme SJ, Torphy TJ, Hay DW. Persistent airway eosinophilia after leukotriene (LT) D4 administration in the guinea pig: modulation by the LTD4 receptor antagonist, pranlukast, or an interleukin-5 monoclonal antibody. Am J Respir Crit Care Med 1996; 154:850–857.

11. Schade UF, Ernst M, Reinke M, Wolter DT. Lipoxygenase inhibitors suppress formation of tumor necrosis factor in vitro and in vivo. Biochem Biophys Res Commun 1989; 159:748–754.

12. Rankin J, Harris P. The effect of inhibition of leukotriene B4 release on lipopolysaccharide-induced production of neutrophil attractant/activation protein-1 (interleukin-8) by human alveolar macrophages. Prostaglandins 1993; 45:77–84.

13. McCain RW, Holden EP, Blackwell TR, Christman JW. Leukotriene B4 stimulates human polymorphonuclear leukocytes to synthesize and release interleukin-8 in vitro. Am J Respir Cell Mol Biol 1994; 10:651–657.

14. Wenzel S, Trudeau J, Kaminsky D, Cohn J, Martin R, Westcott J. Effect of 5-lipoxygenase inhibition on bronchocontraction and airway inflammation in nocturnal asthma. Am J Respir Crit Care Med 1995; 152:897–905.

15. Pizzichini E, Leff JA, Reiss TF, Hendeles L, Boulet L-P, Wei LX, Efthimiadis AE, Zhang J, Hargreave, FE. Montelukast reduces airway eosinophilic inflammation in asthma: a randomized, controlled trial. Eur Respir J 1999; 14:12–18.

16. Nakamura Y, Hoshino M, Sim JJ, Ishii K, Hosaka K, Sakamoto T. Effect of the leukotriene receptor antagonist pranlukast on cellular infiltration in the bronchial mucosa of patients with asthma. Thorax 1998; 53:835–841.

17. Taylor GW, Black P, Turner N, Taylor I, Maltby NH, Fuller RW, Dollery CT. Uri-

nary leukotriene E4 after antigen challenge and in acute asthma and allergic rhinitis. Lancet 1989; 1:584–587.

18. Westcott JY, Johnston K, Batt RA, Wenzel SE, Voelkel NF. Measurement of peptidoleukotrienes in biologic fluid. J Appl Physiol 1990; 68:2640–2648.

19. Wenzel SE, Larsen GL, Johnston K, Voelkel NF, Westcott JY. Elevated levels of leukotriene C4 in bronchoalveolar lavage fluid from atopic asthmatics after endobronchial allergen challenge. Am Rev Respir Dis 1990; 142:112–119.

20. Lynch KR, O'Neill GP, Liu Q, et al. Characterization of the human cysteinyl leukotriene CysLT1 receptor. Nature 1999; 399:789–793.

21. Yokomizo T, Izumi T, Chang K, Takuwa Y, Shimizu T. A G-protein-coupled receptor for leukotriene B4 that mediates chemotaxis. Nature 1997; 387:620–624.

22. De Caterina R, Sicari R, Giannessi D, Paggiaro PL, Paoletti P, Lazzerini G, Bernini W, Solito E, Parente L. Macrophage-specific eicosanoid synthesis inhibition and lipocortin-1 induction by glucocorticoids. J Appl Physiol 1993; 75:2368–2375.

23. Balter MS, Eschenbacher WL, Peters-Golden M. Arachidonic acid metabolism in cultured alveolar macrophages from normal, atopic, and asthmatic subjects. Am Rev Respir Dis 1988; 138:1134–1142.

24. Dworski R, Fitzgerald GA, Oates JA, Sheller JR. Effect of oral prednisone on airway inflammatory mediators in atopic asthma. Am J Respir Crit Care Med 1994; 149: 953–959.

25. Lamblin C, Gosset P, Tillie-Leblond I, Saulnier F, Marquette C-H, Wallaert B, Tonnel AB. Bronchial neutrophilia in patients with noninfectious status asthmaticus. Am J Respir Crit Care Med 1998; 157:394–402.

26. Tillie-Leblond I, Pugin J, Marquette C-H, Lamblin C, Saulnier F, Brichet A, Wallaert B, Tonnel A-B, Gosset P. Balance between proinflammatory cytokines and their inhibitors in bronchial lavage from patients with status asthmaticus. Am J Respir Crit Care Med 1999; 159:487–494.

27. Langmack EL, Gibbs RL, Halliday JL, Trudeau JB, Wenzel SE. Airway inflammation in severe aspirin-intolerant asthmatics (S-AIA) compared to severe aspirin-tolerant asthmatics (S-ATA) and mild aspirin-intolerant asthmatics (M-AIA) (abstract). Am J Respir Crit Care Med 1999; 159:A125.

28. Christie PE, Tagari P, Ford-Hutchinson AW, Charlesson S, Chee P, Arm JP, Lee TH. Urinary leukotriene E4 concentrations increase after aspirin challenge in aspirin-sensitive asthmatic subjects. Am Rev Respir Dis 1991; 143:1025–1029.

29. Sladek K, Dworski R, Soja J, Sheller JR, Nizankowska E, Oates JA, Szczeklik A. Eicosanoids in bronchoalveolar lavage fluid of aspirin-intolerant patients with asthma after aspirin challenge. Am J Respir Crit Care Med 1994; 149:940–946.

30. Szczeklik A, Sladek K, Dworski R, Nizankowska E, Soja J, Sheller J, Oates J. Bronchial aspirin challenge causes specific eicosanoid response in aspirin-sensitive asthmatics. Am J Respir Crit Care Med 1996; 154:1608–1614.

31. Daffern PJ, Muilenburg D, Hugli TE, Stevenson DD. Association of urinary leukotriene E_4 excretion during aspirin challenges with severity of respiratory responses. J Allergy Clin Immunol 1999; 104:559–564.

32. Langmack EL, Wenzel SE. Mast cell and eosinophil responses after indomethacin in asthmatics tolerant and intolerant to aspirin. In: Szczeklik A, Gryglewski RJ, Vane

JR, eds. Eicosanoids, Aspirin, and Asthma. Vol. 114. New York: Marcel Dekker, 1998:337–350.

33. Sanak M, Simon H-U, Szczeklik A. Leukotriene C$_4$ synthase promoter polymorphism and risk of aspirin-induced asthma. Lancet 1997; 350:1599–1600.

34. Cowburn AS, Sladek K, Soja J, Adamek L, Nizankowska E, Szczeklik A, Lam BK, Penrose JF, Austen KF, Holgate ST, Sampson AP. Overexpression of leukotriene C$_4$ synthase in bronchial biopsies from patients with aspirin-intolerant asthma. J Clin Invest 1998; 101:834–846.

35. Michel O, Kips J, Duchateau J, Vertongen F, Robert L, Collet H, Pauwels R, Sergysels R. Severity of asthma is related to endotoxin in house dust. Am J Respir Crit Care Med 1996; 154:1641–1646.

36. Silverman RA, Miller CJ, Chen Y, Bonuccelli CM, Simonson SG. Zafirlukast reduces relapses and treatment failures after an acute asthma episode. Chest 1999; 116:296S.

37. Israel E, Fischer AR, Rosenberg MA, Lilly CM, Callery JC, Shapiro J, Cohn J, Rubin P, Drazen JM. The pivotal role of 5-lipoxygenase products in the reaction of aspirin-sensitive asthmatics to aspirin. Am Rev Respir Dis 1993; 148:1447–1451.

38. Dahlen B, Kumlin M, Margolskee D. The leukotriene receptor antagonist MK-0679 blocks airway obstruction induced by inhaled lysine aspirin in aspirin sensitive asthmatics. Eur Respir J 1993; 6:1018–1026.

39. Fischer AR, Rosenberg MA, Lilly CM, et al. Direct evidence for a role of the mast cell in the nasal response to aspirin in aspirin-sensitive asthma. J Allergy Clin Immunol 1994; 94:1046–1056.

40. Menendez R, Venzor J, Ortiz G. Failure of zafirlukast to prevent ibuprofen-induced anaphylaxis. Ann Allergy Asthma Immunol 1998; 80:225–226.

41. Dahlen B, Nizankowska E, Szczeklik A, Zetterstrom O, Bochenek G, Kumlin M, Mastalerz L, Pinis G, Swanson LJ, Boodhoo TI, Wright S, Dube LM, Dahlen S.-E. Benefits from adding the 5-lipoxygenase inhibitor Zileuton to conventional therapy in aspirin-intolerant asthmatics. Am J Respir Crit Care Med 1998; 157:1187–1194.

42. Kuna P, Malmstrom K, Dahlen SE, Nizankowska E, Kowalski M, Stevenson D, Bousquet J, Dahlen B, Picado C, Lumry W, Holgate S, Pauwels R, Szczeklik A, Shahane A, Reiss TF. Montelukast (MK-0476), a CysLT1 receptor antagonist, improves asthma control in aspirin-intolerant asthmatic patients. Am J Respir Crit Care Med 1997; 155:975.

43. Tamaoki J, Kondo M, Sakai N. Leukotriene antagonist prevents exacerbation of asthma during reduction of high-dose inhaled corticosteroid. Am J Respir Crit Care Med 1997; 155:1235–1240.

44. Lofdahl C-G, Reiss TF, Leff JA, Israel E, Noonan MJ, Finn AF, Seidenberg BC, Capizzi T, Kundu S, Godard P. Randomised, placebo controlled trial of effect of a leukotriene receptor antagonist, montelukast, on tapering inhaled corticosteroids in asthmatic patients. Br Med J 1999; 319:87–90.

45. Virchow J, Hassall SM, Summerton L, Harris A. Improved asthma control over 6 weeks in patients on high dose inhaled corticosteroids. Eur Respir J 1997; 10(suppl 25):437.

46. Reiss TF, Chervinsky P, Dockhorn RJ, Shingo S, Seidenberg B, Edwards TB. Mon-

telukast, a once-daily leukotriene receptor antagonist, in the treatment of chronic asthma. Arch Intern Med 1998; 158:1213–1220.

47. Kane GC, Pollice M, Kim C-J, Cohn J, Dworski RT, Murray JJ, Sheller JR, Fish JE, Peters SP. A controlled trial of the effect of the 5-lipoxygenase inhibitor, zileuton, on lung inflammation produced by segmental antigen challenge in human beings. J Allergy Clin Immunol 1996; 97:646–654.

48. Calhoun WJ, Lavins BJ, Minkwitz MC, Evans R, Gleich GJ, Cohn J. Effect of zafirlukast (Accolate) on cellular mediators of inflammation. Am J Respir Crit Care Med 1998; 157:1381–1389.

49. Diamant Z, Grootendorst DC, Veselic-Charvat M, Timmers MC, De Smet M, Leff JA, Seidenberg BC, Zwinderman AH, Peszek I, Sterk PJ. The effect of montelukast (MK-0476), a cysteinyl leukotriene receptor antagonist, on allergen-induced airway responses and sputum cell counts in asthma. Clin Exp Allergy 1999; 29:42–51.

50. Malmstrom K, Rodriguez-Gomez G, Guerra J, Villaran C, Pineiro A, Wei LX, Seidenberg BC, Reiss TF. Oral montelukast, inhaled beclomethasone, and placebo for chronic asthma. Ann Int Med 1999; 130:487–495.

51. Liu MC, Dube LM, Lancaster J, Group ZS. Acute and chronic effects of a 5-lipoxygenase inhibitor in asthma: a 6-month randomized multicenter trial. J Allergy Clin Immunol 1996; 98:859–871.

52. Panettieri RA, Tan EML, Ciocca V, Luttmann MA, Leonard TB, Hay DWP. Effects of LTD4 on human airway smooth muscle cell proliferation, matrix expression, and contraction in vitro: Differential sensitivity to cysteinyl leukotriene receptor antagonists. Am J Respir Cell Mol Biol 1998; 19:453–461.

53. Wang CG, Du T, Xu LJ, Martin JG. Role of leukotriene D_4 in allergen-induced increases in airway smooth muscle in the rat. Am Rev Respir Dis 1993; 148:413–417.

54. Wechsler ME, Pauwels R, Drazen JM. Leukotriene modifiers and Churg–Strauss syndrome. Drug Safety 1999; 21:241–251.

55. Wechsler ME, Garpestad E, Flier SR, Kocher O, Weiland DA, Polito AJ, Klinek MM, Bigby TD, Wong GA, Helmers RA, Drazen JM. Pulmonary infiltrates, eosinophilia, and cardiomyopathy following corticosteroid withdrawal in patients with asthma receiving zafirlukast. J Am Med Assoc 1998; 279:455–457.

8

Molecular Mechanisms of Glucocorticoid Action

JOHN W. BLOOM

Respiratory Sciences Center
University of Arizona College of Medicine
Tucson, Arizona

I. Introduction

Airway inflammation plays a central role in the pathogenesis of asthma, and glucocorticoids (also referred to as corticosteroids or glucocorticosteroids) are the most effective agents in the management of this chronic disease (1). The anti-inflammatory effectiveness of inhaled glucocorticoids in asthma is the result of actions on multiple inflammatory and structural cells in the lung. Glucocorticoids inhibit expression of many inflammatory proteins, and the anti-inflammatory effects of glucocorticoids are mediated through receptors that function by modulation of gene expression. Glucocorticoid receptors (GR) are members of the large steroid/nuclear receptor family that includes more than 25 subfamilies of receptors that act primarily as ligand-activated transcription factors (2). The nuclear receptor family includes receptors for estrogen, progesterone, mineralocorticoids, androgens, vitamin D, thyroid hormone, and retinoic acid as well as a large group of "orphan" receptors for which endogenous and synthetic ligands have recently been identified (3).

In recent years, there has been a tremendous growth in the knowledge of the mechanisms by which glucocorticoids regulate gene expression. Much is known about how glucocorticoids enhance activation of gene expression, but an important part of the anti-inflammatory effects of glucocorticoids in asthma involves repression of the expression of inflammatory mediators. Less is known about the mechanisms through which glucocorticoids repress gene expression, but this is an intensive area of research. Recent studies have demonstrated a significant role for steroid/nuclear receptor coactivators, chromatin structure, and histone acetylation/deacetylation in gene regulation. This chapter opens with an overview of glucocorticoid receptor structure and glucocorticoid-induced transcriptional activation and then focuses on mechanisms of glucocorticoid-mediated gene repression.

II. Glucocorticoid Receptors

A. Structure of the Glucocorticoid Receptor Gene

The effects of glucocorticoids are mediated through a single receptor that is expressed in nearly all cell types. Although GR is widely expressed, GR levels vary somewhat in different cells (4). Control of GR expression is a complicated process that is affected by a number of conditions and involves both transcriptional and posttranscriptional mechanisms (5). Data from a number of studies demonstrate a correlation between GR number and glucocorticoid responsiveness. For example, in transgenic mice engineered to express antisense GR mRNA, a twofold reduction in GR levels produces a variety of abnormalities, including an increase in circulating glucocorticoid levels and obesity (6).

The GR gene is situated on chromosome 5 in the region 5q31-q32 (7,8). Interestingly, this region includes many genes with presumed roles in allergy and asthma, including the IL-3, IL-4, IL-5, IL-9, IL-13, granulocyte macrophage colony stimulating factor (GM-CSF), CD14, and β_2-adrenergic receptor genes. The genomic structure (Fig. 1) of the gene for GR includes nine exons spanning approximately 80 kb of the human genome (9). The exon boundaries correlate with functional domains in the receptor, indicating an evolutionary association between structure and function. Although there is evidence for three distinct promoters in the mouse GR gene (10), to date only a single promoter has been identified for the human GR gene (9,11). Recent studies have demonstrated putative cAMP-responsive elements in the human GR promoter, and cAMP appears to enhance transcriptional activation of the promoter, at least in some cell types (12). An enhanced understanding of the tissue-specific transcriptional regulation of human GR could lead to the development of improved strategies for glucocorticoid therapy.

Although there is no evidence for glucocorticoid receptor subtypes with differing affinities for glucocorticoid hormone, a GR receptor isoform, GR-β, has been characterized that is distinct from the classic ligand-activated GR (GR-α) (13–16). Alternative splicing of exon 9 of the GR gene results in the synthesis

Receptor Protein

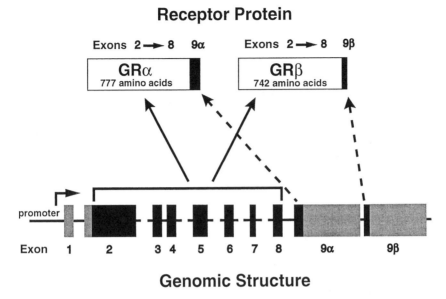

Genomic Structure

Figure 1 Structure of the glucocorticoid receptor gene and receptor protein isoforms, GRα and GRβ. The genomic organization of the GR gene is shown at the bottom of the figure. The translated sequences in each of the nine exons are shown in black, and the 5′-untranslated and 3′-untranslated sequences in exons 1 and 2 and in exon 9α/9β, respectively, are shown in gray. The spaces between exons represent intronic sequences. The expressed proteins for the GRα and GRβ isoforms are identical for amino acids 1–727 and differ only in the carboxyl terminal region (amino acids 727–777 for GRα; amino acids 727–742 for GRβ) as the result of alternative splicing for the 9α/9β exon.

of two homologous mRNAs and protein isoforms (17). GR-β differs from GR-α only in the carboxyl terminus, with replacement of the last 50 amino acids of GRα with a unique 15-amino-acid sequence (Fig. 1). This is the region of the hormone binding domain, and GR-β does not bind ligand, but has been identified in human tissues. Expression of GR-β is induced by cytokines (18), and a role for GR-β has been proposed in modulating transcriptional activities of GR-α by competing for rate-limiting protein factors or by forming nonfunctional GR-α/GR-β heterodimers (14,16,18). The GR-β isoform may play an important role in steroid resistance in asthma (17,19,20) (see Chap. 24).

B. Structural Domains of the Glucocorticoid Receptor

A structure–function map of the GR protein has been created through biochemical and genetic analyses (Fig. 2). The deduced amino acid sequence for human

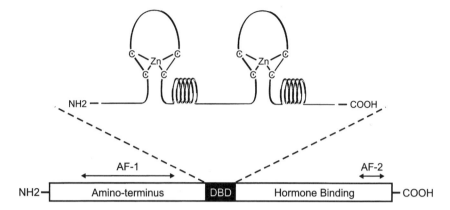

Figure 2 Glucocorticoid receptor domains. The receptor protein consists of three struc-ture–function domains designated the amino-terminus, the DNA binding domain (DBD), and the hormone binding domain. For the DBD, the "zinc-finger" structure and α-helical regions are depicted. Each zinc finger structure consists of a molecule of Zn tetrahedrally coordinated by four cysteine amino acids. The locations of the ligand-dependent (AF-2) and ligand-independent (AF-1) transcriptional activation functions are indicated.

GR consists of 777 residues and has greater than 90% sequence homology with GR sequences of other species (reviewed in Ref. 21). GR has a modular structure such that different functions are performed by discrete domains within the recep-tor protein. The major domains are a carboxyl terminal ligand binding domain, an amino-terminal transcriptional activation domain, and a small central DNA binding domain that comprises two repeats of a protein motif termed a "zinc finger."

In the hormone binding domain, a "core" region of ~135 amino acids has been shown to interact with ligand during hormone binding (reviewed in Ref. 22). Point mutations outside as well as inside this core binding area have been shown to cause either a total loss of hormone binding or a significant decrease in binding affinity. These data suggest a model of a ligand binding cavity for the receptor in which multiple amino acids are necessary for proper folding of the cavity. Heat shock protein 90 (hsp90) also binds sequences in the hormone bind-ing domain, and this interaction with hsp90 may mask nuclear localization signals located in this region. Thus, GR translocation to the nucleus is only possible after ligand binding and the resulting dissociation of heat shock proteins from GR. A conserved motif within the hormone binding domain, referred to as AF-2, appears to be important in GR transcriptional function. Several lines of evidence suggest that GR and other nuclear receptors must interact with additional factors via an intact AF-2 domain to mediate transcriptional activities (23–26). The AF-2 domain appears to be the interaction site for GR with coactivators (described below), and hormone binding to GR greatly stimulates this interaction with coactivator proteins (27,28). The AF-2 function in the GR hormone binding domain has been mapped to four putative α-helical regions that are thought to make direct contacts with coactivator proteins (29).

The DNA binding domain, a short (66-amino-acid) segment situated in the middle of GR, mediates the interaction of GR with DNA (Fig. 2). Transcriptional activation by GR at specific target genes is regulated by binding of GR as a homodimer to specific glucocorticoid response elements (GREs). The consensus GRE is a partial palindromic 15-bp sequence (reviewed in Refs. 30 and 31). In the DNA binding domain, eight cysteine residues tetrahedrally coordinate two zinc atoms in two "zinc fingers." The structure and interaction of the DNA binding domains of two GR monomers with DNA has been determined from crystallographic analysis (32). An α-helix structure is located at the carboxy-terminal end of each zinc finger (Fig. 2). Each half-site of the GRE binds one monomer of GR, with the major GR–DNA interaction occurring between the α-helix of the first or amino-terminal zinc finger and the major groove of the DNA. Amino acids in this region determine the response element specificity of the GR binding to DNA sequences. Although the first zinc finger is the main determinant of binding specificity, the carboxy-terminal finger is necessary for dimerization and overall binding affinity (Fig. 2).

The large ~400-amino-acid domain located at the amino-terminus of GR contains a 200-amino-acid region, termed AF-1, that includes a hormone-independent transcriptional activation function (33,34). The transcriptional activity of AF-1 appears to lie in a core region of 41 negatively charged acidic amino acids similar to transcriptional activation domains in viral and yeast transcription proteins (35). Several major sites of phosphorylation have been identified in the glucocorticoid receptor amino-terminus through work done primarily in the mouse and rat receptors. Treatment of cells with activators and inhibitors of protein kinases and phosphatases affects the transcriptional activity of steroid receptors, suggesting that these receptors are regulated by phosphorylation. The glucocorticoid receptor is phosphorylated in the absence of hormone; however, additional phosphorylation occurs in conjunction with agonist (36). The mechanisms by which phosphorylation alters steroid receptor function are unclear, but phosphorylation may modulate hormone binding, influence nucleocytoplasmic shuttling of the protein, or affect transcription by altering DNA binding or interaction with the basal transcription machinery (36,37).

A recently identified nucleotide polymorphism in the amino-terminal domain of GR results in an amino acid change (asparagine to serine at position 363). Because this polymorphism is located near the AF-1 region, it could affect transcriptional activation functions of GR. In a population study of this polymorphism, 6% of the subjects were heterozygous at this locus (38). Individuals with the polymorphism had a higher sensitivity to exogenously administered glucocorticoids, higher body mass index, and a marked trend toward lower bone mineral density. Because approximately 5% of patients appear to be at particular risk of developing side effects with glucocorticoid therapy, it is tempting to speculate that individuals with this polymorphism may represent a population at increased risk for glucocorticoid-induced side effects.

C. Glucocorticoid-Mediated Transcriptional Activation

Glucocorticoid receptors function primarily as ligand-activated transcription factors, and the classic concept of how glucocorticoids activate gene transcription is illustrated in Fig. 3 (reviewed in Ref. 39). Steroids are extremely lipophilic and enter the cell cytoplasm from the extracellular space primarily by passive diffusion. The GR is localized predominantly to the cytoplasm and enters the nucleus of the cell following activation by hormone. In the cytoplasm, the unliganded GR ($\sim$90 kDa) exists as a component of a large heteromeric complex ($\sim$330 kDa) that includes a dimer of heat shock protein 90 molecules, a subunit p23 protein, and any one of several immunophilin-related proteins (40,41). The heat shock proteins associated with GR appear to be important in maintaining GR in a conformation that is appropriate for ligand binding and for inhibition of GR translocation to the nucleus. Recent evidence suggests that unliganded, hsp-complexed GRs may exist in a dynamic equilibrium between nucleus and cytoplasm and shuttle continuously across the nuclear membrane in a manner similar to estrogen and progesterone receptors. Thus, factors in addition to heat shock protein binding may regulate GR nucleocytoplasmic trafficking (42).

Following ligand activation and nuclear localization, GR binds as a homodimer at GREs, which are specific palindromic DNA sequences found in and around genes that are transcriptionally activated GR. Initially, it was thought that the DNA sequence dictated only the position at which GR bound DNA. There is now evidence to suggest that the response element itself may affect the tran-

---

Figure 3 Glucocorticoid-mediated transcriptional activation. Prior to glucocorticoid binding, GR exists as a large multiunit complex in the cytoplasm, which includes two molecules of heat shock protein 90 (hsp90). Following activation by binding of glucocorticoid hormone (GC), GR undergoes an apparent conformational change, dissociates from the ''chaperone'' proteins, and translocates to the nucleus. In the nucleus, GR homodimers bind to a palindromic sequence termed a glucocorticoid response element (GRE) located in the regulatory regions of target gene. The bound GR homodimer interacts via coactivator proteins with the basal transcriptional machinery shown bound to the TATA box DNA sequence. The basal transcription complex includes TATA-binding protein (TBP), associated transcription factors (TAFs and TFIIs), and RNA polymerase II (pol II).

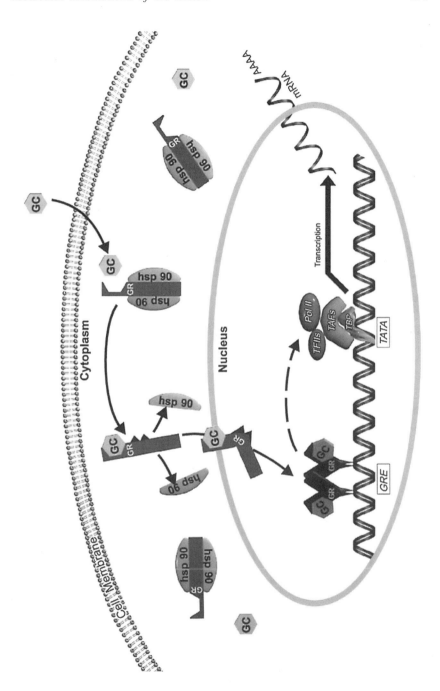

scription factor protein through allosteric effects, thus generating a pattern of regulation that is appropriate to the individual gene (43). Exactly how GR activates transcription has been somewhat unclear until recently. The accepted concept was that binding of the GR homodimer stabilized the basal transcription machinery through interacting proteins, but the identity of these proteins was unknown. Recently, several distinct groups of coactivator proteins have been identified that appear to participate in GR mediated transcriptional activation (44,45).

CBP (CREB-binding protein) is a ubiquitous nuclear coactivator that functions, at least in part, by uniting transcriptional activators, such as GR, with the basal transcription initiation complex. CBP was first discovered as a coactivator of CREB (46–48). A related protein, p300, shares extensive homology with CBP (49). The CBP and p300 make protein–protein interactions not only with CREB but also with steroid/nuclear receptors, including GR, and multiple other transcription factors (44). In addition, CBP/p300 have been shown to form protein–protein interactions with members of the basal transcription machinery, including RNA polymerase II (pol II), and the general transcription factors TFIIB and TATA-binding protein (TBP) (45).

Recently, other coactivator proteins that interact with GR have been identified (44,45,50). These coactivator proteins modulate GR activity and may play a role in the cell specificity of GR effects. Three distinct families of GR coactivators have been described. The first coactivator protein identified was the steroid receptor coactivator-1 (SRC-1), which interacts with the AF-2 region of the hormone binding domain of GR (27,28,51,52). This SRC family of 160-kDa proteins binds to the steroid/unclear receptor in a hormone-dependent manner via three leucine-rich motifs (LXXLL, where L denotes leucine and X is any amino acid) clustered in the central region of the SRC protein (53–55). Thus, the CBP/p300 and SRC family proteins that form interactions with both steroid/nuclear receptors and the basal transcription machinery may serve as a link between the DNA-bound GR and the general transcription factors in order to enhance transcription (Fig. 4). Other GR coactivators that have been identified include another p160 coactivator, termed glucocorticoid receptor interacting protein-1 (GRIP-1), and a 152-kDa protein, p/CIP (56–58).

Linking GR and the basal transcription machinery appears to be only one of the transcriptional activities of the coactivator proteins. In addition, the coactivators may play an even more intriguing role in gene transcription that involves modulation of chromatin structure. CBP/p300 and SRC-1 have histone acetyltransferase (HAT) activity that may influence promoter accessibility to transcription factors (59–61). Over 30 years ago, an association between histone acetylation and enhanced transcriptional activity was identified (62). Histones package all chromosomal DNA into chromatin, and the packaging of DNA into chromatin performs a critical role in regulating gene expression. The basic structural unit

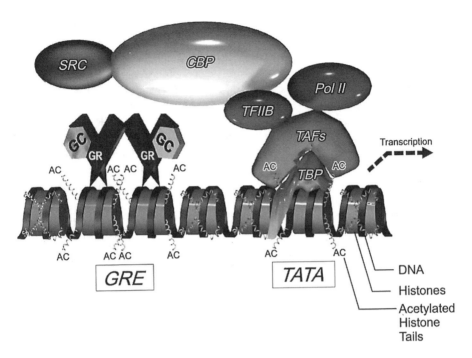

Figure 4 Interactions of GR with coactivators and chromatin. The basal transcription complex consisting of TBP, TAFs, TFIIB, and pol II is labeled as noted in the legend to Fig. 3. The interaction of GR with the basal transcription complex via coactivator proteins SRC (steroid receptor coactivator) and CBP is depicted. DNA is shown packaged into chromatin by histones. The repeating structural unit in chromatin is the nucleosome that consists of ~146 bp of DNA wrapped 1.75 superhelical turns around a core of histones. SRC and CBP, as well as some proteins in the basal transcription complex, have intrinsic histone acetyltransferase (HAT) activity and are able to acetylate histones. "Ac" indicates hyperacetylation of the histone tails. Acetylation of histone tails produces an allosteric change in the nucleosome conformation, destabilizes the interaction between the histone tails and DNA, and allows the nucleosomal DNA to become more accessible to transcription factors. The histone tails of the two nucleosomes at either end of the figure are hypoacetylated and interact tightly with the DNA, preventing transcription factor access to the DNA.

of chromatin is the nucleosome, which consists of ~146 bp of DNA wrapped more or less twice around an octamer of core histone proteins (see Fig. 4) (63,64). The functional consequence of chromatin packaging is to limit access of transcription factors to the DNA. Acetylation of histones occurs at lysine residues located on the amino-terminal tails of the histone, thereby neutralizing the positive charge of the histone tails and decreasing their affinity for the DNA. As a consequence of acetylation of the histone tails, the nucleosomal conformation is altered and the DNA becomes accessible to transcription factor (e.g., GR) binding at enhancer sites. In addition, to the intrinsic acetyltransferase activity of CBP/p300 and SRC family proteins, many other proteins with previously described functions in transcriptional regulation appear to be histone acetylases (59,61,65). Thus, in addition to providing a bridge between the DNA-bound GR and the basal transcription machinery, the coactivators may also supply the essential histone acetylation that alters the conformation of nucleosomes in the region and allows binding of factors necessary to enhance transcription. In addition to proteins with histone acetylation, a group of corepressor proteins with histone deacetylase (HDAC) activity has been identified (66–70).

The classic mechanism of GR-mediated transcriptional activation requires GR binding to DNA at a consensus GRE. Recently, transcriptional effects independent of DNA binding have been described for GR with the transcription factor STAT-5 (71,72). GR acts as a transcriptional coactivator for STAT-5 and enhances STAT-5-dependent transcription of the β-casein gene. The STAT-5/GR complex binds DNA independently of the GRE. Synergistic activation of transcription by GR without directly binding to DNA is not limited to interaction with STAT-5. In particular, IL-6-activated STAT-3 associates with ligand-bound GR to form a signaling complex that functions through an IL-6-responsive element in a synergistic manner (73). In addition, interactions of GR with CCAAT/enhancer binding protein and Oct transcription factors have been characterized (74–78).

Cross talk between β-adrenergic agonist and glucocorticoid signaling pathways may be an important interaction. In clinical studies of asthma patients, the addition of a long-acting β-agonist to inhaled steroid therapy provided superior asthma control when compared with increasing the dose of inhaled steroid (79,80). Eickelberg and coworkers have provided a possible molecular mechanism to explain this interaction between β-agonists and glucocorticoids (81). In experiments with cultured lung fibroblasts and vascular smooth muscle cells, β-agonists activated both GR translocation to the nucleus and DNA binding by GR. Although the mechanism through which activation of GR by β-agonists occurs is unclear at present, this interaction may be important in the apparent enhanced anti-inflammatory effects achieved by adding a long-acting β-agonist to inhaled steroid therapy.

III. Glucocorticoid Targets in Asthma

Glucocorticoids produce antiasthma effects by controlling expression of specific target genes. The exact target genes that are critical for glucocorticoid action in asthma are unknown, but the anti-inflammatory action of glucocorticoids probably involves the regulation of a number of genes. Glucocorticoids enhance transcription of several genes that may have significant inhibitory effects on the inflammatory process in asthma. An early proposal for the inhibitory mechanism of glucocorticoids was an increase in lipocortin-1 synthesis (82). Lipocortins are specific inhibitors of phospholipase A2, a presumed regulator in the production of prostaglandins, leukotrienes, and platelet activating factor. Although glucocorticoids can induce lipocortin-1 in several cell types relevant in asthma, the importance of the anti-inflammatory effects of lipocortin is uncertain. Glucocorticoids induce the expression of the type II IL-1 receptor, a decoy molecule for IL-1 (83). Increased levels of this IL-1 decoy receptor could produce anti-inflammatory activity by blocking the effects of IL-1. Because glucocorticoids increase expression of only a limited number of genes that appear to play a role in asthmatic inflammation, enhanced gene expression by glucocorticoids does not appear to the dominant mechanism for GR-mediated anti-inflammatory effects.

There is evidence that glucocorticoids activate transcription at the promoter for the β_2-adrenergic receptor and increase expression of these receptors in lung (84,85). Although not a direct anti-inflammatory mechanism, this effect of glucocorticoids could prevent downregulation of β-receptors during chronic β-agonist therapy. In asthmatic patients, prednisolone therapy has been shown to reverse β_2-adrenergic receptor downregulation induced by β_2-adrenergic agonist exposure (86). Also, because of the recent evidence suggesting a synergistic anti-inflammatory effect of glucocorticoids and β-agonists in asthma (79,80), the upregulation of β_2-adrenergic receptors by glucocorticoids may be important clinically.

Compared to gene activation, inhibition of gene expression may be particularly important in producing the anti-inflammatory effects of glucocorticoids. A variety of cytokines appear to play a major role in generating the inflammatory response in the lung. There is evidence that glucocorticoids limit expression of multiple inflammatory cytokines including IL-1 through IL-6, IL-11, IL-13, IL-16, GM-CSF, tumor necrosis factor-α (TNF-α), and the chemokines IL-8, RANTES, eotaxin, macrophage inflammatory protein-1a, and monocyte chemoattractant protein-1 (reviewed in Ref. 87). Another mechanism by which glucocorticoids may produce anti-inflammatory effects is inhibition of adhesion molecule expression in the lung. Glucocorticoids regulate expression of ICAM-1 and VCAM-1 (88–90), and this effect could decrease inflammatory cell migration into the airways. In addition, anti-inflammatory effects of glucocorticoids may be mediated by inhibiting expression of various enzymes. Nitric oxide synthase (NOS) can be induced by cytokines released during inflammation, leading to increased nitric oxide (NO) production. Although it is unclear whether NO plays a role in asthma, it is possible that NO may increase bronchial blood flow and inflammatory plasma exudation (91). Studies in mice lacking iNOS suggest that this enzyme may play an important role in the inflammatory process (92). The inducible form of NOS is potently inhibited by glucocorticoids, resulting in diminished NO generation. Glucocorticoids also inhibit induction of the inducible isoform of cyclo-oxygenase (COX-2) in airway epithelial cells, thus possibly decreasing the formation of prostaglandins in the airways (93).

IV. Repression of Gene Expression by Glucocorticoids

Most evidence suggests that glucocorticoid regulation of target genes occurs at the level of gene transcription, but there is evidence that regulation of gene expression for some cytokine genes is, at least partially, posttranscriptional (94,95). Repression of the IL-11, GM-CSF, and COX-2 genes in lung epithelial cells and fibroblasts is mediated by both transcriptional and posttranscriptional mechanisms (96–99), and the mechanisms may be cell type specific. For COX-2, the posttranscriptional mechanism for glucocorticoid-dependent repression requires GR-mediated transcription and involves shortening of COX-2 poly(A) tails (98). Nevertheless, the primary mechanism of glucocorticoid-mediated gene repression appears to be an effect on gene transcription.

At the transcriptional level, the molecular basis of glucocorticoid action is due to either GR-mediated induction of specific target genes as a result of sequence-specific DNA binding (Fig. 3) or GR-dependent repression of expression (reviewed in Refs. 2,100–102). Many of the antiasthma effects of glucocorticoids in asthma appear to be the result of downregulation or repression of target gene expression. Repression of target gene expression by glucocorticoids may occur by transcriptional interference, that is, when a transcription factor is prevented from successfully interacting with the transcription initiation complex by direct or indirect interactions with another transcription factor. Interference may occur through competition for a common cis-response element, by the formation of inactive complexes, or by competition for a common coactivator (49,103). There is evidence that expression of multiple cytokine genes is mediated, at least in part, by the transcription factors nuclear factor κB (NFκB) and activator protein 1 (AP-1). NFκB and AP-1 may be important targets for glucocorticoid-mediated repression cytokine gene expression in asthma (102,104,105). Several mechanisms for GR-mediated repression of gene transcription through transcriptional interference or crosstalk have been described.

A. Repression Through Direct Binding of GR to DNA

The model of a "negative GRE" (nGRE) has been proposed to explain glucocorticoid repression of prolactin, pro-opiomelanocortin, and osteocalcin gene expression (106–109). The ligand-activated GR binds to the nGRE sequences in the promoters of these genes and represses gene transcription, either through a direct destabilizing effect on the basal transcription complex or by exclusion of an activator factor. In the osteocalcin gene promoter, it has been shown that the location of GR binding to DNA overlaps with the TATA box (109). When glucocorticoid-activated GR binds at this site, it is able to displace the TATA-binding protein (TBP) and block transcription. Another example of GR-mediated repression, that is the result of DNA binding by GR, is inhibition at the proliferin gene promoter (110). A "composite GRE" sequence is present in the proliferin gene that consists of a GR binding site that overlaps with a binding site for AP-1. AP-1 is a dimeric transcription factor generally composed of the two proteins Fos and Jun, and repression of proliferin expression appears to be the result of GR blocking the transcriptional activation by AP-1. A composite GRE has also been identified in the c-*fos* gene promoter consisting of overlapping GR and serum response factor binding sites. In this case, it is not clear whether GR represses c-fos expression by excluding SRF binding or quenching the activity of bound serum response factor.

B. Repression Through Interaction with Activator Protein 1

Analyses of the promoters for many of the genes involved in inflammation have not demonstrated GRE or nGRE sequences essential for binding of activated GR. Thus, examples of transcriptional repression that require GR binding to the DNA may be the exception rather than the rule. A protein–protein interaction model of repression has been developed from data derived from multiple studies. An example is GR-mediated repression of AP-1 induction of the collagenase gene (110–112). Studies have clearly demonstrated that GR represses collagenase gene transcription but does not bind directly to the collagenase gene promoter. AP-1 functions as a transcriptional activator of the collagenase gene. DNA-independent protein–protein interactions between GR and the AP-1 components Jun and Fos are responsible for the GR inhibition of AP-1 regulated target genes (Fig. 5). Conversely, functional antagonism can also affect GR action, thus supporting the AP-1/GR protein–protein interaction model. Stimulation of AP-1 activity represses glucocorticoid-induced transcriptional activation at GRE-containing reporter genes, without AP-1 binding to DNA. The AP-1 family of transcription factors forms dimers by interaction at a bZip DNA-binding dimerization motif, termed a "leucine zipper." The results of deletion mapping studies are consistent with the possibility that the leucine zipper of Jun or Fos and the zinc finger of GR interact to form a heterodimer that prevents either from binding to DNA (110–112). Thus, these protein–protein interactions between GR and AP-1 add an additional aspect to the combinatorial control of gene expression and provide one mechanism for GR-mediated repression of gene expression.

Recently, the model of GR-mediated transcriptional repression independent of DNA binding has recently been corroborated by in vivo studies in mice.

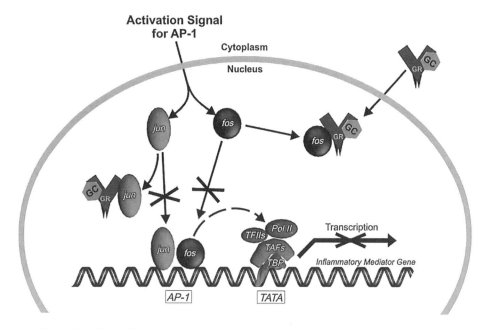

Figure 5   GR-mediated repression of AP-1 activity. Activation of Fos and Jun by signals from the cell surface induces Fos–Jun binding at the AP-1 DNA response element and target gene activation. Ligand-activated GR may interact with either Jun or Fos, and the resulting formation of inactive complexes between GR and Fos or Jun interferes with AP-1 target gene activation.

Reichardt and coworkers "knocked-in" a point mutation in the GR gene DNA-binding domain, leading to substitution of alanine by threonine at amino acid 458 in the second "zinc finger" (113). This mutation results in a dimerization-defective GR that is unable to bind cooperatively as a homodimer to GREs (114). In these mice (termed GR$^{dim/dim}$, for "dimerization defective") DNA-binding-dependent transcriptional activation of genes is defective (113). In addition to the defect in GRE-mediated gene induction, the mice are deficient in repression of genes that are regulated through nGREs, the prolactin and pro-opiomelanocortin genes. In contrast, transcriptional repression through protein–protein interactions is clearly intact in GR$^{dim/dim}$ mice. Interference with and repression of AP-1-regulated genes by GR are intact in cells isolated from GR$^{dim/dim}$ mice. Additional studies in the GR$^{dim/dim}$ mice will be helpful for addressing questions regarding crosstalk between GR and NFκB as well as other transcription factors. The issue of whether glucocorticoid-induced adverse effects are primarily the result of transcriptional activation or transcriptional repression functions of GR can also be addressed in the GR$^{dim/dim}$ mice. This is a particularly important question because of the availability of unique glucocorticoids that are more effective in activation of GR blockade of AP-1 and NFκB signaling than GR-mediated transcriptional activation (115,116). If the glucocorticoid-induced adverse effects are mediated by the transcriptional activation function of GR, these novel glucocorticoids would be effective anti-inflammatory agents with fewer side effects.

C. Inhibition of NFκB Signaling by Glucocorticoids

GR can inhibit AP-1 activity by the protein–protein interaction as described above, but it appears that AP-1 may regulate only a portion of the cytokine genes that are important in inflammation. The transcription factor NFκB is ubiquitous and is associated with the induction of multiple genes, including cytokines and other important inflammatory genes (105,117). The transcription factor NFκB activates genes encoding cytokines, chemokines, and adhesion molecules such as TNF-α, IL-1β, IL-6, IL-8, RANTES, GM-CSF, ICAM-1, and VCAM-1 (118).

NFκB is a member of the NFκB/Rel multigene family of transcription factors, whose activity is regulated by subcellular localization. Members of the NFκB/Rel family are characterized by a conserved stretch of 300 amino acids termed the "Rel homology domain." NFκB is a dimer most frequently composed of two subunits, p65 (RelA) and p50 (119). NFκB transcriptional activity occurs when the p65/p50 dimer binds DNA at specific decameric DNA sequences termed "κB sites" (Fig. 6). NFκB resides in the cytoplasm of unstimulated cells, and DNA binding and transcriptional activities of NFκB are tightly controlled by accessory proteins termed "inhibitory-κB (IκB) subunits." The IκB family of inhibitory molecules consists of several proteins including IκBα, IκBβ, IκBε, and IκBγ, but IκBα appears to play the central role in regulation of NFκB in most cells (120). IκB proteins bind to NFκB in the cytoplasm and block translocation to the nucleus and DNA binding by NFκB. NFκB is activated by various signals including TNF-α, IL-1β, stress, UV irradiation, oxidants, lipopolysaccharide, and viral agents. Activation signals lead to phosphorylation and degradation of IκB with subsequent activation of NFκB. IκBα synthesis is transcriptionally regulated by NFκB such that following NFκB activation, IκBα is resynthesized quickly and inactivates NFκB in the cytoplasm, thus terminating NFκB activity.

Chemical cross-linking and overexpression studies have shown that GR can interact directly with the p65 subunit of NFκB (121–123), thus blocking NFκB binding to DNA and transcriptional activity (Fig. 6). These data suggest a mechanism of NFκB inhibition by GR through a protein–protein interaction that is similar to the mechanism of GR interference with AP-1 activity. Recently, De Bosscher and coworkers have demonstrated that the GR/NFκB protein–protein interaction may interfere with the link between NFκB and the basal transcription machinery (124).

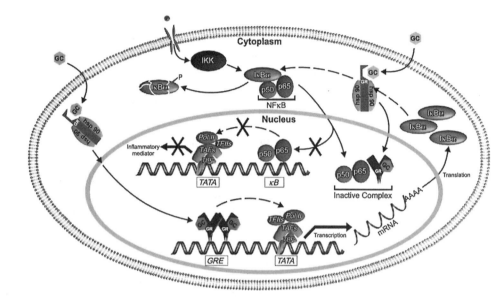

Figure 6   GR-mediated repression of NFκB activity. In the inactive state, NFκB (hetero-dimer of p65 and p50) is anchored in the cytoplasm by IκBα. Activation signals through cell surface receptors activate IκB kinase (IKK), which phosphorylates IκBα. Following phosphorylation, IκBα undergoes proteolytic degradation, and the NFκB heterodimer (p65/p50) is free to pass into the nucleus, where it binds to κB sites in the regulatory regions of inflammatory mediator genes and enhances transcription. GR may block NFκB activity by either of two mechanisms. Inhibition may occur through protein–protein inter-actions between ligand-activated GR and NFκB (inactive complex). This interaction either may prevent the p65/p50 NFκB heterodimer from binding at the κB response element or may interfere with the interaction of NFκB with the basal transcription machinery. A second proposed mechanism for GR-mediated inhibition of NFκB is enhanced transcrip-tion of the IκBα gene by GR. The enhanced synthesis of IκBα replaces the degraded IκBα and neutralizes the free NFκB, thus inhibiting NFκB activation.

Although considerable data support a protein–protein interaction between GR and NFκB as a mechanism of GR blockade of NFκB signaling, two groups of investigators (125,126) have reported that glucocorticoids are able to inhibit NFκB activity by transcriptional activation of the IκBα gene (Fig. 6). As de-scribed above, the activation of NFκB involves the targeted degradation of cyto-plasmic IκB inhibitor and translocation of NFκB to the nucleus, where it binds to κB-response elements of inducible genes. Induction of the IκBα gene by gluco-corticoids leads to an increased rate of IκBα protein synthesis. It is proposed that the increased expression of IκBα by glucocorticoids could block translocation of

NFκB to the nucleus (Fig. 6) (125,126). Furthermore, it was suggested that IκBα could actively remove NFκB from its promoter element in the nucleus. In several cell types, it was demonstrated that following stimulation by tumor necrosis factor in the presence of glucocorticoid, NFκB quickly reassociates with newly synthesized IκBα, thus markedly decreasing the amount of NFκB that translocates to the nucleus (125,126). This mechanism of inhibition of NFκB has not been supported by other studies in different cell types (127–131). Whether induction of IκBα by glucocorticoids is an important anti-inflammatory mechanism in asthma is a significant research question.

D. CREB-Binding Protein (CBP)/GR Interactions

As described above, a large number of coactivator proteins have been identified recently, primarily by two-hybrid screening. The CBP/p300 transcription factors appear to play an important role as coactivators for GR transcriptional activity. The CBP/p300 proteins are not only important coactivators for GR and other members of the steroid/nuclear receptor family but also for the transcription factors AP-1, NFκB, and STAT (49,50,132). The AP-1, NFκB, and STAT transcription factors perform an important role in transcriptional activation and expression of genes for inflammatory mediators.

Loss of one CBP gene allele, resulting in lower cellular CBP levels, appears to cause the Rubenstein–Taybi syndrome, which is associated with severe developmental defects (133,134). Although it is not entirely clear why p300 cannot compensate for the CBP deficiency, the Rubenstein–Taybi syndrome suggests that CBP is physiologically maintained at a limiting component in the cell and that competition for CBP may produce cross talk between different signaling pathways. Because CBP/p300 functions as a coactivator for both AP-1 as well as GR, it was proposed that mutual repression between GR and AP-1 or NFκB could result from competition for limiting amounts of CBP/p300. Indeed, the GR inhibition of AP-1 and NFκB activity can be abolished by overexpression of CBP or p300 (103,135–138). Thus, different transcription factors may interfere with one another by competing for limiting amounts of common cofactors such as CBP and p300, and this mechanism may be important in cross-signaling. This model has been challenged recently. De Bosscher and colleagues found that although extra CBP did stimulate NFκB-mediated transcriptional activation, it did not affect the relative levels of transcriptional repression mediated by GR (124).

As described above, CBP/p300 and other coactivators for GR have intrinsic histone acetyltransferase activity that may be essential for the alteration of chromatin structure that allows transcription factor binding and gene transcription (139). In addition to histone acetyltransferases, transcription factors with histone deacetylase activity have been identified recently and appear to be associated with repression of gene transcription (140–144). Although recruitment of histone deacetylases (HDACs) by the thyroid and retinoic acid nuclear receptors has been demonstrated as a mechanism of transcriptional repression, this has not been demonstrated for GR until recently. Ito and coworkers investigated the mechanism by which glucocorticoids repress of IL-1β-stimulated GM-CSF expression in epithelial cells (145). For GR-mediated repression of GM-CSF, the site of cross talk between GR and NFκB occurred at the level of regulation of histone H4 acetylation. IL-1β stimulated CBP-associated histone acetylation at the GM-CSF promoter, and activated GR inhibited the acetylation through direct inhibition of CBP-associated HAT activity and by recruitment of the corepressor, histone deacetylase 2 (HDAC2) (145).

V. Summary and Perspectives

Glucocorticoids are clearly the most effective anti-inflammatory agents in the management of asthma, and a better understanding of the molecular mechanisms of glucocorticoid action is an essential step in the development of more efficacious therapeutic agents. It will be critical to identify the specific GR-regulated target genes most important in asthma and to understand how GR interacts with other transcription factors in the combinatorial control of these genes. A feature that distinguishes glucocorticoid action from other types of steroid-regulated pathways is that most cell types express substantial levels of GR. Therefore, the molecular basis of cell-specific glucocorticoid responsiveness is not the result of cell-specific GR expression, as is the case for estrogen, progesterone, and androgen effects. Nevertheless, there are multiple examples of cell/tissue-specific effects of glucocorticoids on gene regulation (146–149). A possible explanation is the tissue-specific expression of coactivator and corepressor proteins that interact with GR, other transcription factors, and the basal transcription machinery. As outlined in this chapter, multiple coactivator proteins have been identified that interact with GR and modulate glucocorticoid activity. In addition, the recent report by Ito and coworkers demonstrating the recruitment of the HDAC2 to the transcription complex by GR activation is the first description of a corepressor protein interacting with GR (145). Further investigation in this area should lead to an enhanced understanding of GR-mediated transcriptional repression.

　　A clear understanding of whether side effects associated with glucocorticoid therapy are the result of GR transcriptional activation or transcriptional repression functions will be essential in the development of safer glucocorticoids. Analysis of GR mutant mice defective in GR dimerization and GR binding to DNA should allow assessment in vivo of the specific contribution of GR-mediated transcriptional activation and transcriptional repression in the development of glucocorticoid-induced side effects (113). If glucocorticoid-induced adverse effects are primarily the result of transcriptional activation by GR, agents that selectively activate GR transcriptional repression would theoretically be devoid of side effects. "Dissociated" glucocorticoids have been developed that dissociate GR-mediated transcriptional activation from repression of AP-1 (115). Recently, studies have demonstrated that synthetic glucocorticoids such as RU24782, RU24858, and RU40066 that lack transcriptional activating function are able to repress efficiently NFκB-dependent gene activation (116). Selective agents of the retinoic acid and estrogen receptors have been developed and have demonstrated clinical benefit (150,151). Thus, dissociated glucocorticoids may have great potential as safer and more efficacious antiasthma agents.

References

1. Barnes PJ, Pedersen S, Busse WW. Efficacy and safety of inhaled corticosteroids. New developments. Am J Respir Crit Care Med 1998; 157(3 Pt 2):S1–53.
2. Mangelsdorf DJ, Thummel C, Beato M, Herrlich P, Schutz G, Umesono K, Blumberg B, Kastner P, Mark M, Chambon P, et al. The nuclear receptor superfamily: the second decade. Cell 1995; 83(6):835–839.
3. Blumberg B, Evans RM. Orphan nuclear receptors—new ligands and new possibilities. Genes Dev 1998; 12(20):3149–3155.
4. Burnstein KL, Cidlowski JA. The down side of glucocorticoid receptor regulation. Mol Cell Endocrinol 1992; 83(1):C1–C8.
5. Okret S, Dong Y, Bronnegard M, Gustafsson JA. Regulation of glucocorticoid receptor expression. Biochimie 1991; 73(1):51–59.
6. Pepin MC, Pothier F, Barden N. Impaired type II glucocorticoid-receptor function in mice bearing antisense RNA transgene. Nature 1992; 355(6362):725–728.
7. Theriault A, Boyd E, Harrap SB, Hollenberg SM, Connor JM. Regional chromosomal assignment of the human glucocorticoid receptor gene to 5q31. Hum Genet 1989; 83(3):289–291.
8. Francke U, Foellmer BE. The glucocorticoid receptor gene is in 5q31–q32. Genomics 1989; 4(4):610–612.
9. Encio IJ, Detera-Wadleigh SD. The genomic structure of the human glucocorticoid receptor. J Biol Chem 1991; 266(11):7182–7188.
10. Strahle U, Schmidt A, Kelsey G, Stewart AF, Cole TJ, Schmid W, Schutz G. At least three promoters direct expression of the mouse glucocorticoid receptor gene. Proc Natl Acad Sci USA 1992; 89(15):6731–6735.
11. Nobukuni Y, Smith CL, Hager GL, Detera-Wadleigh SD. Characterization of the human glucocorticoid receptor promoter. Biochemistry 1995; 34(25):8207–8214.
12. Penuelas I, Encio IJ, Lopez-Moratalla N, Santiago E. cAMP activates transcription of the human glucocorticoid receptor gene promoter. J Steroid Biochem Mol Biol 1998; 67(2):89–94.
13. Bamberger CM, Bamberger AM, de Castro M, Chrousos GP. Glucocorticoid receptor beta, a potential endogenous inhibitor of glucocorticoid action in humans. J Clin Invest 1995; 95(6):2435–2441.

14. Oakley RH, Sar M, Cidlowski JA. The human glucocorticoid receptor beta isoform: expression, biochemical properties, and putative function. J Biol Chem 1996; 271(16):9550–9559.

15. de Castro M, Elliot S, Kino T, Bamberger C, Karl M, Webster E, Chrousos GP. The non-ligand binding beta-isoform of the human glucocorticoid receptor (hGR beta): tissue levels, mechanism of action, and potential physiologic role. Mol Med 1996; 2(5):597–607.

16. Oakley RH, Webster JC, Sar M, Parker CR Jr., Cidlowski JA. Expression and subcellular distribution of the beta-isoform of the human glucocorticoid receptor. Endocrinology 1997; 138(11):5028–5038.

17. Vottero A, Chrousos GP. Glucocorticoid receptor beta: view I. Trends Endocrinol Metab 1999; 10(8):333–338.

18. Leung DYM, Hamid Q, Vottero A, Szefler SJ, Surs W, Minshall E, Chrousos GP, Klemm DJ. Association of glucocorticoid insensitivity with increased expression of glucocorticoid receptor beta. J Exp Med 1997; 186(9):1567–1574.

19. Leung DY, Szefler SJ. New insights into steroid resistant asthma. Pediatr Allergy Immunol 1998; 9(1):3–12.

20. Hamid QA, Wenzel SE, Hauk PJ, Tsicopoulos A, Wallaert B, Lafitte JJ, Chrousos GP, Szefler SJ, Leung DY. Increased glucocorticoid receptor beta in airway cells of glucocorticoid-insensitive asthma. Am J Respir Crit Care Med 1999; 159(5Pt1): 1600–1604.

21. Miesfeld RL, Bloom JW. Glucocorticoid receptor structure and function. In: Schleimer RP, Busse WW, O'Byrne PM, eds. Inhaled Glucocorticoids in Asthma. New York: Marcel Dekker, 1996:3–27.

22. Bloom JW, Miesfeld RL. Molecular Mechanisms of Glucocorticoid Action. In: Szefler SJ, Leung DYM, eds. Severe Asthma: Pathogenesis and Clinical Management. New York: Marcel Dekker, 1996:255–284.

23. Tsai MJ, O'Malley BW. Molecular mechanisms of action of steroid/thyroid receptor superfamily members. Annu Rev Biochem 1994; 63:451–486.

24. Cavailles V, Dauvois S, L'Horset F, Lopez G, Hoare S, Kushner PJ, Parker MG. Nuclear factor RIP140 modulates transcriptional activation by the estrogen receptor. EMBO J 1995; 14(15):3741–3751.

25. Espinas ML, Roux J, Pictet R, Grange T. Glucocorticoids and protein kinase A coordinately modulate transcription factor recruitment at a glucocorticoid-responsive unit. Mol Cell Biol 1995; 15(10):5346–5354.

26. Wessely O, Deiner EM, Beug H, von Lindern M. The glucocorticoid receptor is a key regulator of the decision between self-renewal and differentiation in erythroid progenitors. EMBO J 1997; 16(2):267–280.

27. Torchia J, Glass C, Rosenfeld MG. Co-activators and co-repressors in the integration of transcriptional responses. Curr Opin Cell Biol 1998; 10(3):373–383.

28. Shibata H, Spencer TE, Onate SA, Jenster G, Tsai SY, Tsai MJ, O'Malley BW. Role of co-activators and co-repressors in the mechanism of steroid/thyroid receptor action. Recent Prog Horm Res 1997; 52:141–164.

29. Darimont BD, Wagner RL, Apriletti JW, Stallcup MR, Kushner PJ, Baxter JD, Fletterick RJ, Yamamoto KR. Structure and specificity of nuclear receptor–coactivator interactions. Genes Dev 1998; 12(21):3343–3356.

30. Freedman LP. Anatomy of the steroid receptor zinc finger region. Endocr Rev 1992; 13(2):129–145.

31. Dahlman-Wright K, Wright A, Carlstedt-Duke J, Gustafsson JA. DNA-binding by the glucocorticoid receptor: a structural and functional analysis. J Steroid Biochem Mol Biol 1992; 41(3–8):249–272.

32. Luisi BF, Xu WX, Otwinowski Z, Freedman LP, Yamamoto KR, Sigler PB. Crystallographic analysis of the interaction of the glucocorticoid receptor with DNA. Nature 1991; 352(6335):497–505.

33. Godowski PJ, Picard D, Yamamoto KR. Signal transduction and transcriptional regulation by glucocorticoid receptor–LexA fusion proteins. Science 1988; 241(4867):812–816.

34. Hollenberg SM, Evans RM. Multiple and cooperative trans-activation domains of the human glucocorticoid receptor. Cell 1988; 55(5):899–906.

35. Dahlman-Wright K, Almlof T, McEwan IJ, Gustafsson JA, Wright AP. Delineation of a small region within the major transactivation domain of the human glucocorticoid receptor that mediates transactivation of gene expression. Proc Natl Acad Sci USA 1994; 91(5):1619–1623.

36. Bodwell JE, Webster JC, Jewell CM, Cidlowski JA, Hu JM, Munck A. Glucocorticoid receptor phosphorylation: overview, function and cell cycle-dependence. J Steroid Biochem Mol Biol 1998; 65(1–6):91–99.

37. Rogatsky I, Trowbridge JM, Garabedian MJ. Potentiation of human estrogen receptor alpha transcriptional activation through phosphorylation of serines 104 and 106 by the cyclin A-CDK2 complex. J Biol Chem 1999; 274(32):22296–22302.

38. Huizenga NA, Koper JW, De Lange P, Pols HA, Stolk RP, Burger H, Grobbee DE, Brinkmann AO, De Jong FH, Lamberts SW. A polymorphism in the glucocorticoid receptor gene may be associated with and increased sensitivity to glucocorticoids in vivo. J Clin Endocrinol Metab 1998; 83(1):144–151.

39. Bloom JW. Molecular pharmacology of glucocorticoids. Clin Asthma Rev 1997; 1:99–107.

40. Smith DF, Toft DO. Steroid receptors and their associated proteins. Mol Endocrinol 1993; 7(1):4–11.

41. Cheung J, Smith DF. Molecular chaperone interactions with steroid receptors: an update [In Process Citation]. Mol Endocrinol 2000; 14(7):939–946.

42. Hache RJ, Tse R, Reich T, Savory JG, Lefebvre YA. Nucleocytoplasmic trafficking of steroid-free glucocorticoid receptor. J Biol Chem 1999; 274(3):1432–1439.

43. Lefstin JA, Yamamoto KR. Allosteric effects of DNA on transcriptional regulators. Nature 1998; 392(6679):885–888.

44. Collingwood TN, Urnov FD, Wolffe AP. Nuclear receptors: coactivators, corepressors and chromatin remodeling in the control of transcription. J Mol Endocrinol 1999; 23(3):255–275.

45. Robyr D, Wolffe AP, Wahli W. Nuclear hormone receptor coregulators in action: diversity for shared tasks. Mol Endocrinol 2000; 14(3):329–347.

46. Shikama N, Lyon J, La Thangue NB. The p300/CBP family: integrating signals with transcription factors and chromatin. Trends Cell Biol 1997; 7:230–236.

47. Goldman PS, Tran VK, Goodman RH. The multifunctional role of the co-activator CBP in transcriptional regulation. Recent Prog Horm Res 1997; 52:103–119.

48. Jenster G. Coactivators and corepressors as mediators of nuclear receptor function: an update. Mol Cell Endocrinol 1998; 143(1–2):1–7.

49. Janknecht R, Hunter T. Transcription: a growing coactivator network. Nature 1996; 383(6595):22–23.

50. Horwitz KB, Jackson TA, Bain DL, Richer JK, Takimoto GS, Tung L. Nuclear receptor coactivators and corepressors. Mol Endocrinol 1996; 10(10):1167–1177.

51. Onate SA, Tsai SY, Tsai MJ, O'Malley BW. Sequence and characterization of a coactivator for the steroid hormone receptor superfamily. Science 1995; 270(5240): 1354–1357.

52. Hong H, Darimont BD, Ma H, Yang L, Yamamoto KR, Stallcup MR. An additional region of coactivator GRIP1 required for interaction with the hormone-binding domains of a subset of nuclear receptors. J Biol Chem 1999; 274(6):3496–3502.

53. Torchia J, Rose DW, Inostroza J, Kamei Y, Westin S, Glass CK, Rosenfeld MG. The transcriptional co-activator p/CIP binds CBP and mediates nuclear-receptor function. Nature 1997; 387(6634):677–684.

54. Le Douarin B, Nielsen AL, Garnier JM, Ichinose H, Jeanmougin F, Losson R, Chambon P. A possible involvement of TIF1 alpha and TIF1 beta in the epigenetic control of transcription by nuclear receptors. EMBO J 1996; 15(23):6701–6715.

55. Heery DM, Kalkhoven E, Hoare S, Parker MG. A signature motif in transcriptional co-activators mediates binding to nuclear receptors. Nature 1997; 387(6634):733–736.

56. Hong H, Kohli K, Trivedi A, Johnson DL, Stallcup MR. GRIP1, a novel mouse protein that serves as a transcriptional coactivator in yeast for the hormone binding domains of steroid receptors. Proc Natl Acad Sci USA 1996; 93(10):4948–4952.

57. Hong H, Kohli K, Garabedian MJ, Stallcup MR. GRIP1, a transcriptional coactivator for the AF-2 transactivation domain of steroid, thyroid, retinoid, and vitamin D receptors. Mol Cell Biol 1997; 17(5):2735–2744.

58. Torchia J, Rose DW, Inostroza J, Kamei Y, Westin S, Glass CK, Rosenfeld MG. The transcriptional co-activator p/CIP binds CBP and mediates nuclear-receptor function. Nature 1997; 387(6634):677–684.

59. Struhl K. Histone acetylation and transcriptional regulatory mechanisms. Genes Dev 1998; 12(5):599–606.

60. Wolffe AP, Pruss D. Targeting chromatin disruption: Transcription regulators that acetylate histones. Cell 1996; 84(6):817–819.

61. Pazin MJ, Kadonaga JT. What's up and down with histone deacetylation and transcription? Cell 1997; 89(3):325–328.

62. Allfrey V, Faulkner RM, Mirsky AE. Acetylation and methylation of histones and their possible role in the regulation of RNA synthesis. Proc Natl Acad Sci USA 1964; 51:786–794.

63. Luger K, Mader AW, Richmond RK, Sargent DF, Richmond TJ. Crystal structure of the nucleosome core particle at 2.8 A resolution. Nature 1997; 389(6648):251–260.

64. Kornberg RD, Lorch Y. Twenty-five years of the nucleosome, fundamental particle of the eukaryote chromosome. Cell 1999; 98(3):285–294.

65. Struhl K, Moqtaderi Z. The TAFs in the HAT. Cell 1998; 94(1):1–4.

66. Tyler JK, Kadonaga JT. The "dark side" of chromatin remodeling: repressive effects on transcription. Cell 1999; 99(5):443–446.

67. Knoepfler PS, Eisenman RN. Sin meets NuRD and other tails of repression. Cell 1999; 99(5):447–450.

68. Maldonado E, Hampsey M, Reinberg D. Repression: targeting the heart of the matter. Cell 1999; 99(5):455–458.

69. Agarwal S, Viola JP, Rao A. Chromatin-based regulatory mechanisms governing cytokine gene transcription. J Allergy Clin Immunol 1999; 103(6):990–999.

70. Felsenfeld G. Chromatin unfolds. Cell 1996; 86(1):13–19.

71. Stocklin E, Wissler M, Gouilleux F, Groner B. Functional interactions between Stat5 and the glucocorticoid receptor. Nature 1996; 383(6602):726–728.

72. Stoecklin E, Wissler M, Moriggl R, Groner B. Specific DNA binding of Stat5, but not of glucocorticoid receptor, is required for their functional cooperation in the regulation of gene transcription. Mol Cell Biol 1997; 17(11):6708–6716.

73. Zhang Z, Jones S, Hagood JS, Fuentes NL, Fuller GM. STAT3 acts as a co-activator of glucocorticoid receptor signaling. J Biol Chem 1997; 272(49):30607–30610.

74. Chandran UR, Warren BS, Baumann CT, Hager GL, DeFranco DB. The glucocorticoid receptor is tethered to DNA-bound Oct-1 at the mouse gonadotropin-releasing hormone distal negative glucocorticoid response element. J Biol Chem 1999; 274(4):2372–2378.

75. Prefontaine GG, Lemieux ME, Giffin W, Schild-Poulter C, Pope L, LaCasse E, Walker P, Hache RJ. Recruitment of octamer transcription factors to DNA by glucocorticoid receptor. Mol Cell Biol 1998; 18(6):3416–3430.

76. Prefontaine GG, Walther R, Giffin W, Lemieux ME, Pope L, Hache RJ. Selective binding of steroid hormone receptors to octamer transcription factors determines transcriptional synergism at the mouse mammary tumor virus promoter. J Biol Chem 1999; 274(38):26713–2679.

77. Cram EJ, Ramos RA, Wang EC, Cha HH, Nishio Y, Firestone GL. Role of the CCAAT/enhancer binding protein-alpha transcription factor in the glucocorticoid stimulation of p21waf1/cip1 gene promoter activity in growth-arrested rat hepatoma cells. J Biol Chem 1998; 273(4):2008–2014.

78. Gottlicher M, Heck S, Herrlich P. Transcriptional cross-talk, the second mode of steroid hormone receptor action [see comments]. J Mol Med 1998; 76(7):480–489.

79. Greening AP, Ind PW, Northfield M, Shaw G. Added salmeterol versus higher-dose corticosteroid in asthma patients with symptoms on existing inhaled corticosteroid. Allen & Hanburys Limited UK Study Group. Lancet 1994; 344(8917):219–224.

80. Woolcock A, Lundback B, Ringdal N, Jacques LA. Comparison of addition of salmeterol to inhaled steroids with doubling of the dose of inhaled steroids. Am J Respir Crit Care Med 1996; 153(5):1481–1488.

81. Eickelberg O, Roth M, Lorx R, Bruce V, Rudiger J, Johnson M, Block LH. Ligand-independent activation of the glucocorticoid receptor by beta2-adrenergic receptor agonists in primary human lung fibroblasts and vascular smooth muscle cells. J Biol Chem 1999; 274(2):1005–1010.

82. Flower RJ. Lipocortin and the mechanism of action of the glucocorticoids. Br J Pharmacol 1988; 94(4):987–1015.

83. Re F, Muzio M, De Rossi M, Polentarutti N, Giri JG, Mantovani A, Colotta F. The type II "receptor" as a decoy target for interleukin 1 in polymorphonuclear leukocytes: characterization of induction by dexamethasone and ligand binding properties of the released decoy receptor. J Exp Med 1994; 179(2):739–743.

84. Collins S, Caron MG, Lefkowitz RJ. Beta-adrenergic receptors in hamster smooth muscle cells are transcriptionally regulated by glucocorticoids. J Biol Chem 1988; 263(19):9067–9070.

85. Mak JC, Nishikawa M, Shirasaki H, Miyayasu K, Barnes PJ. Protective effects of a glucocorticoid on downregulation of pulmonary beta 2-adrenergic receptors in vivo. J Clin Invest 1995; 96(1):99–106.

86. Brodde OE, Howe U, Egerszegi S, Konietzko N, Michel MC. Effect of predniso-lone and ketotifen on beta 2-adrenoceptors in asthmatic patients receiving beta 2-bronchodilators. Eur J Clin Pharmacol 1988; 34(2):145–150.

87. Barnes PJ. Anti-inflammatory actions of glucocorticoids: molecular mechanisms. Clin Sci (Colch) 1998; 94(6):557–572.

88. van de Stolpe A, Caldenhoven E, Raaijmakers JA, van der Saag PT, Koenderman L. Glucocorticoid-mediated repression of intercellular adhesion molecule-1 expres-sion in human monocytic and bronchial epithelial cell lines. Am J Respir Cell Mol Biol 1993; 8(3):340–347.

89. Tessier PA, Cattaruzzi P, McColl SR. Inhibition of lymphocyte adhesion to cyto-kine-activated synovial fibroblasts by glucocorticoids involves the attenuation of vascular cell adhesion molecule 1 and intercellular adhesion molecule 1 gene ex-pression. Arthr Rheum 1996; 39(2):226–234.

90. Atsuta J, Plitt J, Bochner BS, Schleimer RP. Inhibition of VCAM-1 Expression in Human Bronchial Epithelial Cells by Glucocorticoids. Am J Respir Cell Mol Biol 1999; 20(4):643–650.

91. Barnes PJ. NO or no NO in asthma? Thorax 1996; 51(2):218–220.

92. Wei XQ, Charles IG, Smith A, Ure J, Feng GJ, Huang FP, Xu D, Muller W, Mon-cada S, Liew FY. Altered immune responses in mice lacking inducible nitric oxide synthase. Nature 1995; 375(6530):408–411.

93. Mitchell JA, Belvisi MG, Akarasereenont P, Robbins RA, Kwon OJ, Croxtall J, Barnes PJ, Vane JR. Induction of cyclo-oxygenase-2 by cytokines in human pulmo-nary epithelial cells: regulation by dexamethasone. Br J Pharmacol 1994; 113(3): 1008–1014.

94. Bickel M, Iwai Y, Pluznik DH, Cohen RB. Binding of sequence-specific proteins to the adenosine- plus uridine- rich sequences of the murine granulocyte/macrophage colony-stimulating factor mRNA. Proc Natl Acad Sci USA 1992; 89(21):10001–10005.

95. Ristimaki A, Narko K, Hla T. Down-regulation of cytokine-induced cyclo-oxy-genase-2 transcript isoforms by dexamethasone: evidence for post-transcriptional regulation. Biochem J 1996; 318(Pt 1):325–331.

96. Wang J, Zhu Z, Nolfo R, Elias JA. Dexamethasone regulation of lung epithelial cell and fibroblast interleukin-11 production. Am J Physiol 1999; 276(1Pt1):L175–L185.

97. Zitnik RJ, Whiting NL, Elias JA. Glucocorticoid inhibition of interleukin-1-induced interleukin-6 production by human lung fibroblasts: evidence for transcriptional

and post-transcriptional regulatory mechanisms. Am J Respir Cell Mol Biol 1994; 10(6):643–650.

98. Newton R, Seybold J, Kuitert LM, Bergmann M, Barnes PJ. Repression of cyclo-oxygenase-2 and prostaglandin E2 release by dexamethasone occurs by transcriptional and post-transcriptional mechanisms involving loss of polyadenylated mRNA. J Biol Chem 1998; 273(48):32312–32321.

99. Adkins KK, Levan TD, Miesfeld RL, Bloom JW. Glucocorticoid regulation of GM-CSF: evidence for transcriptional mechanisms in airway epithelial cells. Am J Physiol 1998; 275(2Pt1):L372–L378.

100. Beato M, Herrlich P, Schutz G. Steroid hormone receptors: many actors in search of a plot. Cell 1995; 83(6):851–857.

101. De Bosscher K, Vanden Berghe W, Haegeman G. Mechanisms of anti-inflammatory action and of immunosuppression by glucocorticoids: negative interference of activated glucocorticoid receptor with transcription factors. J Neuroimmunol 2000; 109(1):16–22.

102. Adcock IM. Molecular mechanisms of glucocorticosteroid actions. Pulm Pharmacol Ther 2000; 13(3):115–126.

103. Kamei Y, Xu L, Heinzel T, Torchia J, Kurokawa R, Gloss B, Lin SC, Heyman RA, Rose DW, Glass CK, Rosenfeld MG. A CBP integrator complex mediates transcriptional activation and AP-1 inhibition by nuclear receptors. Cell 1996; 85(3):403–414.

104. Barnes PJ, Adcock I. Anti-inflammatory actions of steroids: molecular mechanisms. Trends Pharmacol Sci 1993; 14(12):436–441.

105. Barnes PJ, Karin M. Nuclear factor-kappaB: a pivotal transcription factor in chronic inflammatory diseases. N Engl J Med 1997; 336(15):1066–1071.

106. Sakai DD, Helms S, Carlstedt-Duke J, Gustafsson JA, Rottman FM, Yamamoto KR. Hormone-mediated repression: a negative glucocorticoid response element from the bovine prolactin gene. Genes Dev 1988; 2(9):1144–1154.

107. Drouin J, Sun YL, Chamberland M, Gauthier Y, De Lean A, Nemer M, Schmidt TJ. Novel glucocorticoid receptor complex with DNA element of the hormone-repressed POMC gene. EMBO J 1993; 12(1):145–156.

108. Stromstedt PE, Poellinger L, Gustafsson JA, Carlstedt-Duke J. The glucocorticoid receptor binds to a sequence overlapping the TATA box of the human osteocalcin promoter: a potential mechanism for negative regulation. Mol Cell Biol 1991; 11(6):3379–3383.

109. Meyer T, Carlstedt-Duke J, Starr DB. A weak TATA box is a prerequisite for glucocorticoid-dependent repression of the osteocalcin gene. J Biol Chem 1997; 272(49):30709–30714.

110. Miner JN, Yamamoto KR. The basic region of AP-1 specifies glucocorticoid receptor activity at a composite response element. Genes Dev 1992; 6(12B):2491–2501.

111. Yang-Yen HF, Chambard JC, Sun YL, Smeal T, Schmidt TJ, Drouin J, Karin M. Transcriptional interference between c-Jun and the glucocorticoid receptor: mutual inhibition of DNA binding due to direct protein–protein interaction. Cell 1990; 62(6):1205–1215.

112. Schule R, Rangarajan P, Kliewer S, Ransone LJ, Bolado J, Yang N, Verma IM,

Evans RM. Functional antagonism between oncoprotein c-Jun and the glucocorticoid receptor. Cell 1990; 62(6):1217–1226.

113. Reichardt HM, Kaestner KH, Tuckermann J, Kretz O, Wessely O, Bock R, Gass P, Schmid W, Herrlich P, Angel P, Schutz G. DNA binding of the glucocorticoid receptor is not essential for survival. Cell 1998; 93(4):531–541.

114. Heck S, Kullmann M, Gast A, Ponta H, Rahmsdorf HJ, Herrlich P, Cato AC. A distinct modulating domain in glucocorticoid receptor monomers in the repression of activity of the transcription factor AP-1. EMBO J 1994; 13(17):4087–4095.

115. Vayssiere BM, Dupont S, Choquart A, Petit F, Garcia T, Marchandeau C, Gronemeyer H, Resche-Region M. Synthetic glucocorticoids that dissociate transactivation and AP-1 transrepression exhibit antiinflammatory activity in vivo. Mol Endocrinol 1997; 11(9):1245–1255.

116. Vanden Berghe W, Francesconi E, De Bosscher K, Resche-Rigon M, Haegeman G. Dissociated glucocorticoids with anti-inflammatory potential repress interleukin-6 gene expression by a nuclear factor-kappaB-dependent mechanism. Mol Pharmacol 1999; 56(4):797–806.

117. Baeuerle PA, Baltimore D. NF-kappa B: ten years after. Cell 1996; 87(1):13–20.

118. Barnes PJ. Nuclear factor-kappa B. Int J Biochem Cell Biol 1997; 29(6):867–70.

119. Siebenlist U, Franzoso G, Brown K. Structure, regulation and function of NF-kappa B. Annu Rev Cell Biol 1994; 10:405–455.

120. Baldwin AS, Jr. The NF-kappa B and I kappa B proteins: new discoveries and insights. Annu Rev Immunol 1996; 14:649–683.

121. Ray A, Prefontaine KE. Physical association and functional antagonism between the p65 subunit of transcription factor NF-kappa B and the glucocorticoid receptor. Proc Natl Acad Sci USA 1994; 91(2):752–756.

122. Caldenhoven E, Liden J, Wissink S, Van de Stolpe A, Raaijmakers J, Koenderman L, Okret S, Gustafsson JA, Van der Saag PT. Negative cross-talk between RelA and the glucocorticoid receptor: a possible mechanism for the antiinflammatory action of glucocorticoids. Mol Endocrinol 1995; 9(4):401–412.

123. Mukaida N, Morita M, Ishikawa Y, Rice N, Okamoto S, Kasahara T, Matsushima K. Novel mechanism of glucocorticoid-mediated gene repression. Nuclear factor-kappa B is target for glucocorticoid-mediated interleukin 8 gene repression. J Biol Chem 1994; 269(18):13289–13295.

124. De Bosscher K, Vanden Berghe W, Vermeulen L, Plaisance S, Boone E, Haegeman G. Glucocorticoids repress NF-kappaB-driven genes by disturbing the interaction of p65 with the basal transcription machinery, irrespective of coactivator levels in the cell. Proc Natl Acad Sci USA 2000; 97(8):3919–3924.

125. Auphan N, DiDonato JA, Rosette C, Helmberg A, Karin M. Immunosuppression by glucocorticoids: inhibition of NF-kappa B activity through induction of I kappa B synthesis. Science 1995; 270(5234):286–290.

126. Scheinman RI, Cogswell PC, Lofquist AK, Baldwin AS, Jr. Role of transcriptional activation of I kappa B alpha in mediation of immunosuppression by glucocorticoids. Science 1995; 270(5234):283–286.

127. Adcock IM, Nasuhara Y, Stevens DA, Barnes PJ. Ligand-induced differentiation

of glucocorticoid receptor (GR) trans-repression and transactivation: preferential targetting of NF-kappaB and lack of I-kappaB involvement. Br J Pharmacol 1999; 127(4):1003–1011.

128. Brostjan C, Anrather J, Csizmadia V, Stroka D, Soares M, Bach FH, Winkler H. Glucocorticoid-mediated repression of NFkappaB activity in endothelial cells does not involve induction of IkappaBalpha synthesis. J Biol Chem 1996; 271(32): 19612–19616.

129. De Bosscher K, Schmitz ML, Vanden Berghe W, Plaisance S, Fiers W, Haegeman G. Glucocorticoid-mediated repression of nuclear factor-kappaB-dependent transcription involves direct interference with transactivation. Proc Natl Acad Sci USA 1997; 94(25):13504–13509.

130. Heck S, Bender K, Kullmann M, Gottlicher M, Herrlich P, Cato AC. I kappaB alpha-independent downregulation of NF-kappaB activity by glucocorticoid receptor. EMBO J 1997; 16(15):4698–4707.

131. Wissink S, van Heerde EC, vand der Burg B, van der Saag PT. A dual mechanism mediates repression of NF-kappaB activity by glucocorticoids. Mol Endocrinol 1998; 12(3):355–363.

132. Glass CK, Rose DW, Rosenfeld MG. Nuclear receptor coactivators. Curr Opin Cell Biol 1997; 9(2):222–232.

133. Hennekam RC, Tilanus M, Hamel BC, Voshart-van Heeren H, Mariman EC, van Beersum SE, van den Boogaard MJ, Breuning MH. Deletion at chromosome 16p13.3 as a cause of Rubinstein–Taybi syndrome: clinical aspects. Am J Hum Genet 1993; 52(2):255–262.

134. Petrij F, Giles RH, Dauwerse HG, Saris JJ, Hennekam RC, Masuno M, Tommerup N, van Ommen GJ, Goodman RH, Peters DJ, et al. Rubinstein–Taybi syndrome caused by mutations in the transcriptional co-activator CBP. Nature 1995; 376(6538):348–351.

135. Hanstein B, Eckner R, DiRenzo J, Halachmi S, Liu H, Searcy B, Kurokawa R, Brown M. p300 is a component of an estrogen receptor coactivator complex. Proc Natl Acad Sci USA 1996; 93(21):11540–11545.

136. Chakravarti D, LaMorte VJ, Nelson MC, Nakajima T, Schulman IG, Juguilon H, Montminy M, Evans RM. Role of CBP/P300 in nuclear receptor signalling. Nature 1996; 383(6595):99–103.

137. Sheppard KA, Phelps KM, Williams AJ, Thanos D, Glass CK, Rosenfeld MG, Gerritsen ME, Collins T. Nuclear integration of glucocorticoid receptor and nuclear factor-kappaB signaling by CREB-binding protein and steroid receptor coactivator-1. J Biol Chem 1998; 273(45):29291–29294.

138. Wadgaonkar R, Phelps KM, Haque Z, Williams AJ, Silverman ES, Collins T. CREB-binding protein is a nuclear integrator of nuclear factor-kappaB and p53 signaling. J Biol Chem 1999; 274(4):1879–1882.

139. Montminy M. Transcriptional activation. Something new to hang your HAT on. Nature 1997; 387(6634):654–655.

140. Alland L, Muhle R, Hou H, Jr., Potes J, Chin L, Schreiber-Agus N, DePinho RA. Role for N-CoR and histone deacetylase in Sin3-mediated transcriptional repression. Nature 1997; 387(6628):49–55.

141. Laherty CD, Yang WM, Sun JM, Davie JR, Seto E, Eisenman RN. Histone deacety-

lases associated with the mSin3 corepressor mediate mad transcriptional repression. Cell 1997; 89(3):349–356.

142. Hassig CA, Schreiber SL. Nuclear histone acetylases and deacetylases and transcriptional regulation: HATs off to HDACs. Curr Opin Chem Biol 1997; 1(3):300–308.

143. Nagy L, Kao HY, Chakravarti D, Lin RJ, Hassig CA, Ayer DE, Schreiber SL, Evans RM. Nuclear receptor repression mediated by a complex containing SMRT, mSin3A, and histone deacetylase. Cell 1997; 89(3):373–380.

144. Heinzel T, Lavinsky RM, Mullen TM, Soderstrom M, Laherty CD, Torchia J, Yang WM, Brard G, Ngo SD, Davie JR, Seto E, Eisenman RN, Rose DW, Glass CK, Rosenfeld MG. A complex containing N-CoR, mSin3 and histone deacetylase mediates transcriptional repression. Nature 1997; 387(6628):43–48.

145. Ito K, Barnes PJ, Adcock IM. Glucocorticoid receptor recruitment of histone deacetylase 2 inhibits interleukin-1beta-induced histone H4 acetylation on lysines 8 and 12. Mol Cell Biol 2000; 20(18):6891–6903.

146. Nechushtan H, Benvenisty N, Brandeis R, Reshef L. Glucocorticoids control phosphoenolpyruvate carboxykinase gene expression in a tissue specific manner. Nucleic Acids Res 1987; 15(16):6405–6417.

147. Eisenberger CL, Nechushtan H, Cohen H, Shani M, Reshef L. Differential regulation of the rat phosphoenolpyruvate carboxykinase gene expression in several tissues of transgenic mice. Mol Cell Biol 1992; 12(3):1396–1403.

148. Grange T, Roux J, Rigaud G, Pictet R. Two remote glucocorticoid responsive units interact cooperatively to promote glucocorticoid induction of rat tyrosine aminotransferase gene expression. Nucleic Acids Res 1989; 17(21):8695–8709.

149. Ivarie RD, Schacter BS, O'Farrell PH. The level of expression of the rat growth hormone gene in liver tumor cells is at least eight orders of magnitude less than that in anterior pituitary cells. Mol Cell Biol 1983; 3(8):1460–1467.

150. Gustafsson JA. Therapeutic potential of selective estrogen receptor modulators. Curr Opin Chem Biol 1998; 2(4):508–511.

151. Resche-Rigon M, Gronemeyer H. Therapeutic potential of selective modulators of nuclear receptor action. Curr Opin Chem Biol 1998; 2(4):501–517.

9

Nocturnal Asthma as a Component of Severe Asthma

E. RAND SUTHERLAND

National Jewish Medical and Research
Center
Denver, Colorado

RICHARD J. MARTIN

National Jewish Medical and Research
Center
University of Colorado
Denver, Colorado

I. Introduction

Nocturnal worsening of airflow limitation is an important part of the asthma clinical syndrome and must be considered an important factor in the diagnosis and management of asthma. As awareness of nocturnal asthma has increased, so too has its importance in defining severe asthma—nocturnal asthma symptoms are now an important component of current guidelines for grading asthma severity and determining appropriate asthma therapy (1). Nocturnal asthma presents special therapeutic considerations and is associated with significant morbidity and mortality. This chapter reviews relevant pathophysiologic, epidemiologic, and therapeutic concepts in nocturnal asthma and explores their relevance to severe asthma.

II. What Is Nocturnal Asthma?

Nocturnal symptoms are a common part of the asthma clinical syndrome. Studies of outpatients with asthma have indicated that approximately 40% of individuals with asthma experience nocturnal symptoms on a nightly basis and that up to

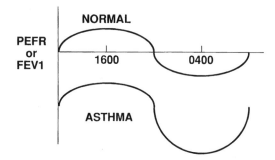

Figure 1 Both normal subjects (top) and asthmatic patients (bottom) have circadian alterations in lung function, with nadirs occurring at approximately 4 A.M. The circadian variation in lung function is increased in patients with asthma compared to that in nonasthmatic patients. (Reprinted from Ref. 83.)

75% of patients are awakened by asthma symptoms at least once per week (2). In many asthmatic patients, circadian variations in lung function are seen, with peak lung function occurring at approximately 4 P.M. and with a nadir in lung function seen at approximately 4 A.M. (see Fig. 1). The drop in lung function between these two time points may exceed 50% (3).

Nocturnal asthma may be defined as a drop in the forced expiratory volume in 1 sec (FEV_1) of $\geq 15\%$ from 4 P.M. to 4 A.M. in a subject who carries a diagnosis of asthma. This overnight decrement in lung function has been shown to correlate not only with increased symptoms of airway obstruction (4), but is also associated with increased airway responsiveness (5) and increased airway inflammation (6,7). Circadian variations in lung function are also seen in subjects without asthma, but the variation is only 5 to 8% (8). Up to 70% of sudden deaths and 80% of respiratory arrests in asthmatic patients occur during sleep (9). These clinical aspects of nocturnal asthma may be explained by unique inflammatory and physiologic perturbations and require special therapeutic considerations, as described below.

III. Pathophysiology of Nocturnal Asthma

Airway inflammation is the *sine qua non* of asthma, and circadian changes in cellular, humoral, and neurogenic inflammation have been shown to contribute directly to the pathogenesis of nocturnal asthma. The relatively recent addition of bronchoscopic sampling of the lower airways (including bronchoalveolar lavage and endo- and transbronchial biopsies) to the evaluation of subjects with

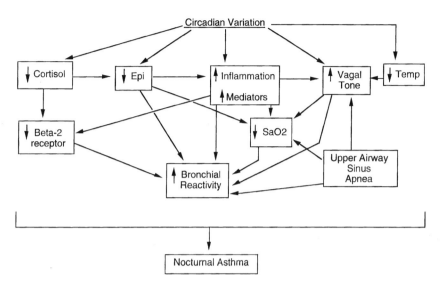

Figure 2 Mechanisms contributing to worsening of nocturnal asthma. Abbreviations: Epi, epinephrine; SaO₂, oxygen saturation. (Reprinted from Ref. 83.)

nocturnal asthma has yielded new insights into circadian changes in airway and alveolar inflammation. Circadian changes in airway inflammation are accompanied by other physiologic changes including downregulation of β2-adrenergic receptors (10), increased vagal tone (11), and circadian alterations in circulating epinephrine (12) and other endogenous bronchodilators, all of which combine to worsen airflow obstruction at night (Fig. 2).

IV. Inflammatory Mechanisms in Nocturnal Asthma

A. Eosinophils

Eosinophils are important effector cells in the pathogenesis of nocturnal asthma (13). Many investigators have demonstrated circadian variations in the number of eosinophils found in both the peripheral blood and airways of subjects with nocturnal asthma.

In 1995, Ulrik reported the results of a study designed to study the relationship between the number of peripheral blood eosinophils and markers of asthma disease activity (14). He studied 70 pediatric and young adult patients with asthma, 46 of whom had allergic asthma. The number of peripheral blood eosinophils was found to be closely correlated with asthma symptom scores [correlation coefficient (r) of 0.69, $P < 0.001$, in children and $r = 0.58$ in young adults] and inversely correlated with percentage FEV_1 predicted ($r = -0.75$, $P < 0.001$, in children and $r = -0.80$, $P < 0.001$, in young adults). In both children and young adults, the number of peripheral eosinophils was also closely correlated with diurnal variations in peak expiratory flow rates. As the number of peripheral blood eosinophils increased, so too did the percentage of diurnal variation in peak flow ($r = 0.81$, $P < 0.001$), ranging from variations of approximately 5% to variations as high as 70% (14).

Characteristics of circulating eosinophils also appear to influence circadian variations in asthma. Calhoun and colleagues studied 15 patients with asthma, 5 of whom had nocturnal asthma (15). The authors demonstrated that subjects with nocturnal asthma had a significantly greater number of circulating eosinophils and that the absolute number of peripheral blood eosinophils in these subjects at 4 A.M. was closely correlated with the degree of morning-to-evening variability in FEV_1 ($r = 0.7$, $P = 0.0007$). The percentage of low-density eosinophils, which have greater proinflammatory potential (16), was significantly greater in nocturnal asthmatics at 4 A.M. compared to that at 4 P.M. (41.5 vs. 16.6% of total eosinophils, $P = 0.03$). Additionally, the percentage of low-density eosinophils at 4 A.M. was significantly greater in nocturnal asthmatics compared to that in nonnocturnal asthmatics and normals (41.5 vs. 13.1%, $P = 0.004$, and 41.5 vs. 6.8%, $P < 0.02$, respectively). The percentage of low-density eosinophils in nocturnal asthmatics at 4 A.M. was closely correlated with evening-to-morning changes in FEV_1 ($r = 0.66$, $P = 0.002$). However, the proportion of low-density eosinophils and pulmonary function at 4 P.M. were similar in nocturnal asthmatics and nonnocturnal asthmatics. Finally, eosinophils in subjects with nocturnal asthma demonstrated longer survival in in vitro culture, also a feature of eosinophils with greater proinflammatory activity (15).

In a study which examined the relationship between circadian variations in plasma epinephrine and plasma cortisol and circulating eosinophils, Bates and colleagues studied 10 young adults with asthma, 6 of whom experienced at least one nocturnal decline in FEV_1 of $\geq 15\%$ during the course of the study (17). Circulating eosinophil counts were greater in subjects with nocturnal asthma and correlated with the frequency of nocturnal asthma ($r = 0.732$, $P = 0.02$) and average percentage decrease in FEV_1 ($r = 0.667$, $P = 0.035$). Plasma epinephrine levels varied in a circadian fashion and the concentration at 10 P.M. was significantly lower in subjects with nocturnal asthma compared to that in nonnocturnal asthmatics ($P = 0.039$). The authors concluded that patients with indicators of more severe inflammation (as manifested by higher circulating eosinophil counts) are at greater risk for nocturnal asthma, that the plasma epinephrine level and the time of its nadir determine whether nocturnal asthma develops, and that these effects of the variation in epinephrine levels are to some extent independent of epinephrine's regulation of airway tone (17). This additional effect of reduced plasma epinephrine levels may be due to its role as an endogenous bronchodilator.

B. Alveolar Tissue Inflammation

Prompted in part by evidence from autopsy studies (18) that the pathologic changes of asthma occur not only in large and small airways, but also in alveoli, Kraft and colleagues hypothesized in 1993 that significant alveolar tissue inflammation was present in patients with chronic, stable asthma. They studied 21 patients, 11 of whom had nocturnal asthma and 10 of whom had nonnocturnal asthma. Each subject underwent bronchoscopy with endobronchial and transbronchial biopsy at both 4 A.M. and 4 P.M. and morphometric analysis was utilized to determine the number and type of inflammatory cells per unit volume. The authors showed that there was a significant difference in the number of eosinophils per unit volume in nocturnal asthmatics compared to that of nonnocturnal asthmatics in alveolar tissue biopsies obtained at 4 A.M. [median-40.2 $\times$ 10^3 and interquartile range (IQ)-26.4–57.1 $\times$ 10^3 versus median-15.7 $\times$ 10^3 and IQ-2.1–35.2 $\times$ 10^3; $P = 0.05$ for the comparison]. No similar differences were demonstrated in the airway biopsies (see Fig. 3).

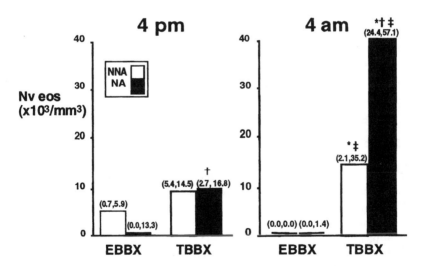

Figure 3 The number per unit volume (Nv) of eosinophils in endobronchial (airway, EBBX) and transbronchial (alveolar, TBBX) biopsies at 4 A.M. and 4 P.M. in subjects with nocturnal asthma (NA, solid bars) and nonnocturnal asthma (NNA, open bars). Values are expressed as medians with the 25–75 interquartile range in parentheses above each bar. *‡†, $P \leq 0.05$. (Reprinted from Ref. 7.)

Additionally, in subjects with nocturnal asthma, there was a circadian variation in the number of eosinophils seen in alveolar tissue, with a significantly greater number of eosinophils present at 4 A.M. (41.4 ± 8.6 × 10³ vs. 12.9 ± 4.3 × 10³; $P = 0.005$). The number of macrophages was also greater in nocturnal asthmatic alveolar tissue at 4 A.M. than at 4 P.M. No circadian differences in the number of airway inflammatory cells were demonstrated. In nonnocturnal asthmatics, no circadian differences in alveolar inflammatory cell numbers could be demonstrated. Increases in alveolar eosinophils in nocturnal asthmatics correlated with nocturnal decrements in FEV_1 ($r = -0.54$, $P = 0.03$); this relationship was not seen in airway tissue (7). The authors concluded that alveolar tissue inflammation was an important component of the inflammatory response in asthmatics and that circadian variations in alveolar tissue inflammation may play an important role in the pathogenesis of nocturnal asthma.

T-lymphocytes are also thought to play a central role in asthma pathogenesis (19). Inflammatory cytokines such as tumor necrosis factor-α (TNF-α), interleukin (IL) 4, IL-5, and IL-13 are produced by T-lymphocytes and facilitate eosinophil migration into tissues through vascular endothelium. In 1999, Kraft and colleagues (20) studied whether lymphocytes were responsible for recruitment of eosinophils into alveolar tissue in patients with nocturnal asthma. They demonstrated that nocturnal asthmatics had significantly greater numbers of CD4+ lymphocytes in alveolar tissue at 4 A.M. than did nonnocturnal asthmatics (median-9.8/mm² and IQ-5.6–30.8 vs. median-1.5/mm² and IQ-0–6.3; $P = 0.04$ for the comparison). Alveolar CD4+ cells correlated positively with the number of EG2+ eosinophils ($r = 0.66$, $P = 0.01$) and inversely with FEV_1 ($r = -0.68$, $P = 0.0018$) at 4 A.M. (20).

C. Exhaled Nitric Oxide

Levels of nitric oxide (NO) in exhaled air have been hypothesized to reflect airway inflammation (21). In a study designed to evaluate circadian variations in exhaled NO in nocturnal asthmatics, ten Hacken and colleagues showed that mean exhaled NO concentrations were significantly higher at all circadian time points in subjects with nocturnal asthma than in subjects with nonnocturnal asthma or in control subjects (22). Mean exhaled NO levels correlated with variations in peak expiratory flow rates of >15% between 4 A.M. and 4 P.M. ($r = 0.61$, $P < 0.01$) but not with FEV_1. Although mean exhaled NO levels were higher at 4 A.M. than at 4 P.M., the authors were unable to demonstrate a true circadian rhythm in exhaled NO levels in nocturnal asthmatics (22). The authors concluded that subjects with nocturnal asthma exhale greater amounts of NO during both the day and night and that this may reflect circadian variations in airway inflammation.

A subsequent study by Georges and colleagues (23) did find a circadian variation in exhaled nitric oxide in subjects with nocturnal asthma, although levels were shown (unexpectedly) to fall at 4 A.M. compared to those at 4 P.M. The authors studied five nocturnal asthmatics and five nonnocturnal asthmatics. The circadian pattern of exhaled NO was shown to be different between nocturnal and nonnocturnal asthmatics, and nocturnal asthmatics demonstrated a significant circadian decrease in exhaled NO levels, which were 77.2 ± 8.2 ppb at 4 P.M., 68.4 ± 8.7 ppb at 10 P.M. ($P < 0.003$), and 66.0 ± 8.5 ppb ($P < 0.001$) at 4 A.M. (23). Previous studies had demonstrated that exhaled NO could decrease in the setting of bronchoconstriction (24), but when the authors adjusted for changes in FEV_1 in a mixed-model analysis, only a portion of the decrease in exhaled NO could be attributed to bronchoconstriction. Therefore, the authors concluded that there is a nighttime drop in exhaled NO in subjects with nocturnal asthma and speculated that decreased levels of exhaled NO at night may in fact be pathogenic in nocturnal asthma due to either a loss of nitric oxide's endogenous bronchodilatory effect (23) or the proinflammatory activities of the conversion product peroxynitrite.

D. Neuroendocrine Variations in Nocturnal Asthma

Changes in both lung function and airway responsiveness have been documented in nocturnal asthma, and these changes have been related to normal circadian variations in several neurohormones. Peak serum cortisol levels occur upon awakening and decrease during the nocturnal hours; levels trough in the late evening (12). This variation in cortisol levels is seen in both normal and asthmatic subjects. In the setting of nocturnal asthma, this decrease in serum cortisol levels is important because of cortisol's anti-inflammatory effect on the chronically inflamed airways of asthmatic patients. In addition, cortisol is an important upregulator of β-adrenergic receptor numbers (25) and affinity, increasing the proportion of β-adrenergic receptors in the high-affinity state (26). Therefore, the nocturnal decrement in serum cortisol levels may lead to downregulation of β-adrenergic receptor numbers and affinity, thereby affecting response to both endogenous and exogenous bronchodilators and potentiating airflow limitation in nocturnal asthma (10).

Circulating serum levels of epinephrine also decrease at night. Nocturnal asthma symptoms occur at the time of night when the effect of this endogenous bronchodilator is most needed. In addition, vagal tone is increased at night, which further promotes bronchoconstriction (27).

Both the number and physiologic function of β2-adrenergic receptors are significantly decreased in asthmatic patients with nocturnal worsening compared to those of nonnocturnal asthmatics from 4 P.M. to 4 A.M. (10). Szefler and colleagues measured levels of plasma histamine, cortisol, epinephrine, cyclic adenosine monophosphate (cAMP), and leukocyte β-adrenergic receptors in 7 subjects with nocturnal asthma, 10 subjects with nonnocturnal asthma, and 10 normal controls. Plasma histamine, cortisol, epinephrine, and cAMP levels all fell at night, but no significant variations were found between the three groups, demonstrating that circadian decreases in neurohormone levels are not unique to nocturnal asthma. Significant differences in leukocyte β-adrenergic receptor density and function were demonstrated between nocturnal asthmatics and both nonnocturnal asthmatic and control subjects, however. Nocturnal asthmatic subjects demonstrated a 33% decrease in leukocyte β-adrenergic receptor density between 4 P.M. (294 ± 65 receptors/cell) and 4 A.M. (182 ± 46 receptors/cell; $P < 0.05$ for the comparison). Contrary to other reports (28), the authors were unable to demonstrate circadian alterations in leukocyte β-adrenergic receptor binding affinity, but there was significantly lower cAMP production in response to stimulation with the adrenergic agonist isoproterenol, with a 17 ± 7.3% increase in cellular cAMP in nocturnal asthmatic leukocytes at 4 A.M. versus an 80.2 ± 21.3% increase in normal subjects and a 69.4 ± 13.7% increase in nonnocturnal asthmatics ($P < 0.05$). The authors concluded that this diminished response to isoproterenol was due to either the change in leukocyte β-adrenergic receptor density or a postreceptor abnormality (10).

A number of genetic polymorphisms in the coding region of the β2-adrenergic receptor have been described, three of which (mutations at amino acids 16, 27, and 164) impart specific alterations in the biochemical and pharmacologic properties of the receptor (29–31). In 1995 Turki and colleagues (32) hypothesized that the mutation which substituted glycine (Gly16) for arginine (Arg16) at position 16 led to accelerated β-agonist-promoted downregulation of the β-agonist receptor and that Gly16 might be overrepresented in nocturnal asthma. In a study which compared the genotypes of 23 nocturnal asthmatic patients and 22 nonnocturnal asthmatic patients, the authors demonstrated that the frequency of the Gly16 allele was 80.4% in nocturnal asthmatics compared to 52.2% in the nonnocturnal asthmatics ($P = 0.007$). The presence of the Gly16 allele conferred an odds ratio of 3.8 for nocturnal asthma. There were no differences in the polymorphisms at positions 27 and 164 between the two groups (32). The authors concluded that the prevalence of the Gly16 allele appeared to be an important factor in determining the nocturnal asthma phenotype.

E. Alterations in Steroid Responsiveness in Nocturnal Asthma

In 1999, Kraft and colleagues presented the results of a study designed to determine glucocorticoid receptor (GR) binding characteristics and steroid responsiveness in subjects with nocturnal asthma (33). They showed that subjects with nocturnal asthma demonstrated a significantly lower GR binding affinity at 4

A.M. versus 4 P.M., as measured by an elevated dissociation constant (K_d) at 4 A.M. (22.2 ± 1.6 nmol/L) when compared with 4 P.M. (10.9 ± 0.7 nmol/L; $P = 0.0001$ for the comparison). Glucocorticoid receptor K_d, which is inversely related to receptor binding, did not change over the 24-h period in either nonnocturnal asthmatic or normal subjects. With the group of nocturnal asthmatic subjects there was a significant inverse correlation ($r = -0.65$, $P = 0.04$) between the GR K_d and FEV_1 at 4 A.M. This decreased affinity of the glucocorticoid receptor for corticosteroids may form the basis for nocturnal airway inflammation by decreasing the anti-inflammatory effects of both endogenous and therapeutic exogenous corticosteroids (33).

Alternative splicing of the GR pre-mRNA generates a second (β-) isoform of the GR (GR-β), which does not bind glucocorticoids and antagonizes the transactivating activity of the classic GR (34). Kraft and colleagues, in work complimentary to that described in the preceding paragraph, hypothesized that GR-β expression was increased at night in the lung macrophages of nocturnal asthmatics (35). They showed that in nocturnal asthmatics, the expression of GR-β was significantly increased in lung macrophages ($P = 0.001$) compared to that of nonnocturnal asthmatic subjects. The authors concluded that increased expression of GR-β in lung macrophages of nocturnal asthmatic patients may play a role in the decreased steroid responsiveness seen at night in nocturnal asthma (35).

V. Physiologic Variations in Nocturnal Asthma

A. Airways Resistance and Responsiveness in Nocturnal Asthma

In subjects with nocturnal asthma, there is a slow but progressive increase in lower airway resistance at night. This phenomenon is seen overnight both during sleep and wakefulness (Fig. 4), indicating that there is a circadian rhythm in lung function independent of sleep. Airway resistance is at its greatest in asthmatic patients during sleep, however, so one must conclude that unidentified factors associated with sleep are also important in determining levels of airflow limitation (36).

One physiologic indication of nocturnal increases in lower airways resistance is fall in peak expiratory flow rates (PEFR) at night. In nocturnal asthmatics who suffer recurrent symptoms and awakenings, there is a close correlation (r = 0.85, $P < 0.001$) between nocturnal symptoms and overnight fall in PEFR (5). In this study Martin and colleagues also showed that changes in PEFR were also correlated with the percentage predicted FEV_1 at 4 P.M. ($r = 0.73$, $P < 0.001$), the percentage predicted FEV_1 at 4 A.M. ($r = 0.84$, $P < 0.001$), and the percentage change in FEV_1 between 4 P.M. and 4 A.M ($r = 0.75$, $P < 0.001$) (5).

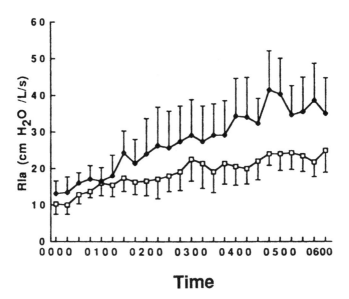

Time

Figure 4   Lower airway resistance (Rla) in asthmatic subjects between midnight and 6 A.M., both when awake (open square) and asleep (solid diamond). (Reprinted from Ref. 36.)

In this study, the authors also showed that there was a significant difference in airway responsiveness at 4 P.M. versus 4 A.M., with a PC_{20} (the concentration of methacholine required to provoke a 20% fall in FEV_1) of 1.80 ± 0.75 mg/ml at 4 P.M. versus 0.474 ± 0.16 mg/ml at 4 A.M. Using logarithmic transformation, there was a significant difference between the PC_{20} values at the two different time points, with $P < 0.002$. There was also a significant correlation between the overnight change in PEFR and the fall in FEV_1 in response to inhaled saline at 4 A.M., with an $r = 0.86$ and $P < 0.001$. The authors concluded that asthmatics with prominent nocturnal symptoms have a greater overnight decrement in their PEFR and that this drop in PEFR appears to be related to the level of methacholine and saline-induced airway responsiveness (5).

As noted above, peripheral airways and alveolar tissue changes are also important in the pathogenesis of nocturnal asthma. Involvement of these areas by inflammation results in increased resistance at the level of the peripheral airways as well. In 1990, Wagner and colleagues published the results of a study in which they utilized a wedged bronchoscopic technique to determine peripheral airway resistance at different flow rates in individuals with and without asthma (37). Although asthmatic and nonasthmatic subjects had similar baseline FEV_1, functional residual capacity (FVC), and specific airway conductance, asthmatic subjects had significantly increased peripheral airway resistance, confirming the physiologic import of inflammatory changes seen in peripheral airways (37).

B. Lung Volume Changes in Nocturnal Asthma

Circadian changes in lung volumes are seen in patients with and without nocturnal asthma. In normal volunteers, FRC falls between wakefulness and sleep, with the lowest values seen during rapid eye movement (REM) sleep (38). Asthmatic patients, who during daytime typically exhibit thoracic hyperinflation compared with normal subjects, have marked reductions in FRC during REM sleep such that during REM sleep asthmatic patients have FRC values nearly identical to those seen in normal volunteers (Fig. 5). This paradoxical response of an absence of thoracic hyperinflation despite significant decreases in FEV_1 defies the well-accepted hyperbolic relationship between airway resistance and lung volume (39)

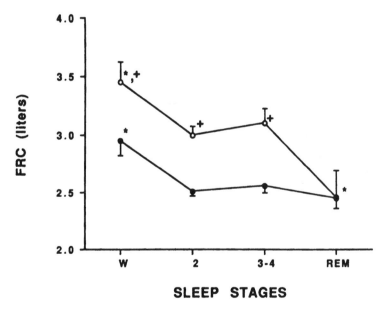

SLEEP STAGES

Figure 5 Changes in FRC during various sleep stages in subjects with nocturnal asthma (open circle) and normal controls (solid circle). $^+ P < 0.05$ for comparison between subjects with nocturnal asthma and normal controls; $*P < 0.05$ for comparisons between wakefulness and REM sleep versus all sleep stages in subjects with nocturnal asthma and for comparisons between wakefulness and all sleep stages in normal subjects. (Reprinted from Ref. 38.)

and may indicate that the normal relationship between volume and resistance is lost during sleep in subjects with nocturnal asthma.

C. Loss of Normal Airway–Parenchymal Interaction in Nocturnal Asthma

In 2000, Irvin and colleague published the results of a study of the interdependence of airways and lung parenchyma in the patient with nocturnal asthma (40). They studied five subjects with nocturnal asthma using whole-body plethysmography to evaluate the degree of interdependence of the parenchyma and airways during both sleep and wakefulness as assessed with volume–resistance relationships. They were able to demonstrate that lower pulmonary resistance (Rlp) increased during sleep in subjects with nocturnal asthma, from 16.2 ± 2.8 to 29.8 ± 9.6 cmH$_2$O/L/sec ($P < 0.001$). When continuous negative pressure (CNP) was applied to the thorax using a poncho cuirass to produce a thoracic gas volume (TGV) which approximated the subjects' awake TGV, airway resistance failed to fall significantly, with an Rlp at TGV of 29.8 ± 9.6 cmH$_2$O/L/sec versus an Rlp at TGV $+ 0.8$ L of 26.6 ± 7.4 cmH$_2$O/L/sec (see Fig. 6). In two subjects, airway resistance increased with this procedure.

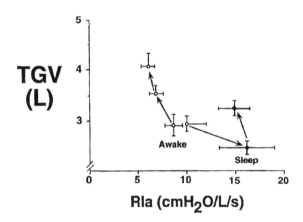

Figure 6   The effect of sleep on volume–resistance relationships in nocturnal asthma. During wakefulness (open circles) the volume–resistance relationship is intact as increasing lung volume produces a fall in lower airway resistance (Rla). During sleep (closed circles) Rla increases. If the lung is inflated with continuous negative pressure applied to the thorax, Rla does not fall appropriately. This indicates that "uncoupling" of the lung parenchyma and airways has occurred, indicating loss of the normal volume–resistance relationship. Data points are mean $\pm$ SEM for the five subjects. (Reprinted from Ref. 40.)

Over the course of the night, the amount of CNP required to increase TGV progressively increased. Respiratory system compliance was derived from the relationship between changes in CNP and resultant changes in thoracic gas volume. From early sleep to late sleep, respiratory system compliance fell from 0.079 ± 0.02 to 0.035 ± 0.002 cmH_2O/L, indicating that nocturnal asthma may be associated with up to a 50% fall in respiratory system compliance (40).

VI. Epidemiology of Nocturnal Asthma

The most comprehensive evaluation of the epidemiology of nocturnal asthma was published in 1988 by Turner-Warwick (2). She reported the results of a questionnaire designed to determine the prevalence of nocturnal symptoms in asthmatic patients. This questionnaire was distributed to approximately 26,000 primary care physicians in the United Kingdom.

A total of 7729 patients responded, and 74% reported awakening at least once per week with asthma symptoms; 64% reported nocturnal asthma symptoms at least three times per week (Table 1). The author noted that this overall frequency of nocturnal symptoms (74%) was identical to that found in a survey published in 1971. Furthermore, the introduction of inhaled corticosteroid preparations, which occurred in the time interval between the two surveys, appeared to have no impact on the prevalence of nocturnal symptoms among patients with asthma.

Among those 3015 patients who rated their asthma severity as "mild," 26% reported being awakened by symptoms nightly, indicating that patients and possibly their physicians did not view nocturnal symptoms as important in determining disease severity. When looking at this association across all severity

Table 1 Frequency of Nocturnal
Awakening in a Cohort of 7729
Asthmatics[a]

Frequency	Percentage of cohort
At least 1 night/month	94
At least 1 night/week	74
At least 3 nights/week	64
Every night	39

[a] Adapted from Ref. 2.

ratings, however, the author reported a "good correlation" between asthma severity as perceived by patients and the frequency of nocturnal awakening, with $P < 0.001$.

VII. Morbidity and Mortality in Nocturnal Asthma

As described above, nocturnal symptoms are an important part of the asthma clinical syndrome in some patients. Symptoms of dyspnea may occur throughout the hours of sleep, but they increase over the course of the night and tend to peak in the early morning hours. In a large pharmacologic study of nocturnal asthma 1525 of 1631 dyspneic episodes in 3129 patients occurred between the hours of 10 P.M. and 7 A.M., with the peak symptom frequency at 4 A.M. (see Fig. 7) (41). Also, patients with nocturnal asthma, even when clinically stable, have worse cognitive performance and worse objective and subjective sleep quality compared to normal volunteers (42).

Respiratory arrest due to airflow limitation is also more likely to happen at night. In their survey of 1169 consecutive hospital admissions for asthma exacerbation, Hetzel and colleagues reported 10 successful resuscitations for respiratory arrest in nine patients (9). Eight of the 10 respiratory arrests occurred between the hours of midnight and 6 A.M. A feature common to all these patients was the presence of large circadian variations in peak expiratory flow rates, with a fall seen in the early morning hours. Interestingly, although this phenomenon was seen in the majority of patients with respiratory arrest, it was also a feature common to approximately 30% of all patients admitted with acute asthma (9).

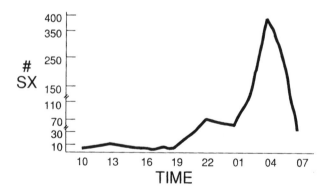

Figure 7   Frequency (# SX) and clock-hour distribution of nocturnal symptoms in 3129 patients with asthma. (Reprinted from Ref. 83 and redrawn from data in Ref. 41.)

The mechanisms that cause the nocturnal declines in airflow can, if uncompensated for by the patient or untreated by the physician, lead not only to respiratory arrest but to death, and in fact most deaths from asthma occur at night (43). In analysis of 38 asthma deaths that occurred in a group of patients between 35 and 64 years of age, Cochrane and Clark showed that of the 19 deaths that occurred following admission to acute care hospitalization, 13 (68%) occurred between the hours of midnight and 8 A.M. (44). The remainder of deaths occurred intermittently throughout the nonsleep portion of the 24-h circadian cycle. The authors also showed that 11 of the 19 patients who died had received sedative medications within 12 h of death. Although there did not appear to be significant differences in the use of sedatives when prescribing practices were compared between the 19 deaths and 19 surviving patients with asthma (44), this observation may indicate that there is a subset of patients with severe asthma who have blunted arousal to the stimulus of dyspnea. This blunted arousal mechanism may prevent patients from initiating compensatory physiologic mechanisms for the hypoventilation associated with nocturnal worsening of airflow limitation, thus increasing the likelihood of death from progressive airway obstruction. This would explain the observation of Hetzel and colleagues (9) that only a portion of the 30% of their cohort with significant circadian variations in airflow sustained respiratory arrest.

VIII. Therapeutic Considerations in Nocturnal Asthma

Also, as described above, circadian rhythms play an important role in the clinical manifestations of nocturnal asthma, but they may also play an important role in determining the efficacy of certain medications. For example, matching drug levels to biological need during the 24-h period may improve control of symptoms (45). This relatively new concept, called chronotherapy, is described in further detail below.

Treatment of nocturnal asthma is composed of pharmacologic interventions directed at inflammatory and other processes that cause airflow obstruction as well as adjunctive therapies to treat concurrent conditions which may worsen nocturnal asthma severity. Pharmacologic approaches to the treatment of nocturnal asthma are outlined in Table 2.

A. Pharmacologic Interventions in Nocturnal Asthma

Theophylline

Theophylline is an effective treatment for nocturnal asthma. Barnes and colleagues (46) conducted a study in 12 nocturnal asthmatic subjects to determine whether theophylline, administered as a single nighttime dose, could achieve ther-

Table 2 Pharmacologic Approach to the Treatment of Nocturnal Asthma[a]

Mild disease (10–20% overnight fall in PEFR)
    Inhaled corticosteroids
    If no improvement, add theophylline (sustained-release preparation) and/or
        inhaled long-acting β2-agonist
Moderate to severe disease (>20% fall in overnight PEFR)
    Inhaled corticosteroids plus theophylline (sustained-release preparation) or
        inhaled long-acting β2-agonist
    If no improvement, consider oral corticosteroids once daily (at 3 P.M.) or twice
        daily (at 8 A.M. and 3 P.M.) depending on relative severity of daytime and
        nocturnal symptoms
    Once symptoms and lung function have improved, add or continue sustained-
        release theophylline or inhaled long-acting β2-agonist and taper oral
        corticosteroids
Treatment of nocturnal awakenings
    Short-acting inhaled β2-agonist
    Consider inhaled anticholinergic agent

Note: PEFR, peak expiratory flow rate.
Adapted from Ref. 73.

apeutic drug levels and ameliorate nocturnal symptoms. They utilized a slow-release preparation of theophylline and targeted therapeutic levels of 8 to 15 mg/L (M = 10.9 mg/L) 10 h after administration. With this dosing strategy, they showed significant improvements in morning PEFR, with PEFR of 332 ± 31 L/min during treatment versus 283 ± 32 L/min during placebo ($P < 0.001$). There was also a significant decrease in rescue salbutamol (albuterol) use during treatment with theophylline (46). Many other studies (47–49) of sustained-release theophylline in nocturnal asthma have shown similar results, with improved morning peak flows, decreased awakenings, decreased use of rescue inhalers and subjective improvement in symptoms.

Control of spirometric indices and morning symptoms in nocturnal asthma depends on the type and dosing schedule of sustained-release theophylline preparations (48). Theophylline may be dosed according to a chronopharmacologic strategy, timing the dose to achieve therapeutic efficacy at the nadir of lung function in nocturnal asthma. Martin and colleagues compared twice-daily theophylline (Theo-Dur) versus once-daily theophylline (Uniphyll) in subjects with nocturnal asthma. Administration of the once-daily preparation at 7 P.M. resulted in a higher serum theophylline concentration at night than did an equivalent dose of the twice-daily preparation given at 7 P.M. and 7 A.M. The 7 A.M. FEV_1 was higher in subjects who received the once-daily preparation. These findings suggest that nocturnal asthmatics derive benefit from a therapeutic regimen designed to achieve peak serum theophylline concentrations at the time of night when airflow limitation is greatest, i.e., approximately 4 A.M. (48).

β2-Adrenergic Agonists

β2-Adrenergic agonists can be administered in either oral or inhaled forms. It was shown by Postma and colleagues in 1984 (50) and in subsequent studies (51) that an unequal morning and evening schedule of sustained-release oral terbutaline (Bricany) was advantageous in the treatment of nocturnal asthma. In patients with asthma and early morning dyspnea, this chronopharmacologic treatment schedule, which consisted of one-third of the dose (5 mg) at 8 A.M. and two-thirds (10 mg) at 8 P.M., designed to yield peak serum levels of terbutaline between midnight and 8 A.M., resulted in improvements in both lung function as manifested by elimination of the "morning dip" in PEFR and by a reduction in symptoms of dyspnea, cough, and nocturnal awakening (50). A 1985 study of the same regimen by Postma demonstrated prevention of the nocturnal fall in FEV_1, PaO_2 (arterial partial pressure of oxygen), and SaO_2 (arterial oxygen percent saturation) in eight patients with nocturnal asthma (52).

A subsequent study by Stewart and colleagues utilized the same sustained-release formulation of terbutaline and showed that an oral regimen of an identical dose of 7.5 mg twice daily significantly improved morning PEFR (259 L/min with treatment versus 213 L/min with placebo, $P < 0.02$), decreased nocturnal rescue inhaler use (1.3 vs. 1.9 puffs/night, $P < 0.02$), and did not appear to alter sleep quality (53).

Other oral bronchodilators have been evaluated in nocturnal asthma. Bogin and Ballard utilized a pulsed-release form of albuterol (Proventil Repetabs) in a randomized, double-blind, placebo-controlled crossover study to test its effects on lung function and awakenings in nocturnal asthma (54). All patients were concurrently receiving theophylline in addition to albuterol, with mean levels of 12.9 ± 0.8 µg/dl. In their cohort, the overnight drop in FEV_1 was significantly smaller when subjects received pulsed-release albuterol versus placebo ($P < 0.005$). Significant subjective improvement was also noted when patients were taking albuterol, and patients reported awakening from sleep less frequently during the albuterol-treatment phase of the study. No significant differences were noted with regard to rescue inhaler use or sleep-stage characteristics (other than awakening episodes) (54).

Salmeterol, a long-acting inhaled β-agonist has recently assumed prominence in the treatment of nocturnal asthma. A 1992 study by Fitzpatrick and colleagues (55) evaluated two different twice-daily doses of inhaled salmeterol, 50 µg and 100 µg b.i.d., in a crossover trial in 20 clinically stable patients with nocturnal asthma. Both doses of salmeterol produced significant improvements in both nocturnal awakenings and morning and daytime asthma symptoms. Peak expiratory flow readings were also significantly improved with both doses of salmeterol as was the overnight drop in PEFR. A significant decrease in the frequency of rescue salbutamol (albuterol) use was seen in patients during the high-dose salmeterol (100 µg b.i.d.) arm of the study. Minimal toxicity was seen from the drug, and the authors concluded that salmeterol at 50 mcg b.i.d. was a safe and effective treatment for nocturnal asthma (55).

In 1999, Lockey and colleagues (56) evaluated salmeterol's effects on spirometric indices and asthma-specific quality of life in 474 patients with significant nocturnal asthma. Patients were allowed to continue the use of theophylline if previously prescribed and were stratified based on serum theophylline level. As-needed albuterol was continued, and patients received either 42 µg b.i.d. of salmeterol or placebo in a double-blind, placebo-controlled fashion. Throughout the study there was a significant improvement in asthma-specific quality of life ($P \leq 0.005$) in the salmeterol group compared with baseline. Morning PEFR and mean FEV_1 were both significantly improved in the treatment group ($P \leq 0.002$ and $P \leq 0.004$, respectively). The effect on morning PEFR was seen independent of subjects' theophylline use. Salmeterol significantly increased the percentage of nights uninterrupted by awakenings due to asthma symptoms from 28 to 77% by the end of the treatment periods compared to 28 to 49% in those subjects receiving placebo ($P < 0.001$). Rescue albuterol use was also significantly decreased in the salmeterol treatment group (56).

When compared in a multicenter, double-blind, double-dummy, randomized crossover trial, both extended-release albuterol tablets (Volmax) and inhaled salmeterol compared favorable and resulted in similar degrees of bronchodilation and asthma symptom control (57). As in the studies cited previously, albuterol was administered in an unequal dosing schedule, with 5 mg in the morning and 10 mg in the evening, and salmeterol was dosed as 42 µg (two puffs) b.i.d. From information collected during an open-label phase of the study, the authors demonstrated that more patients preferred the inhaled agonists because patients noted fewer side effects, greater relief of symptoms, and decreased use of rescue albuterol (57).

The effect of salmeterol in nocturnal asthma does not appear to extend beyond mere bronchodilatory effects. In 1997, Kraft and colleagues published the results of a crossover trial of salmeterol, 100 µg b.i.d., versus placebo, using pathologic grade of lower airway inflammation (as assessed by bronchoalveolar lavage (BAL and biopsy) as an outcome. Although similar improvements in sleep quality and physiology as described in other studies (see above) were noted, there were no changes in airway responsiveness or indices of airway inflammation, including BAL cell count and differential, eosinophil cationic protein, Charcot–Leyden crystal protein, leukotriene B4, and thromboxane B2 (58).

Corticosteroids

Oral Corticosteroids

As with other forms of asthma, nocturnal asthma responds favorably to treatment with corticosteroids. Chronotherapy with oral corticosteroids is of particular importance in the treatment of nocturnal asthma. Studies by Reinberg and colleagues (59,60) have demonstrated that 3 P.M. is the optimal time for administration of corticosteroids. Beam and colleagues (61) utilized a double-blind, placebo-controlled, crossover design to evaluate the impact of a variably timed 50-mg oral dose of prednisone given at 8 A.M., 3 P.M., or 8 P.M. on overnight spirometry, blood eosinophil counts, and bronchoalveolar lavage cytology in seven subjects with nocturnal asthma. Compared to placebo, a single prednisone dose at 3 P.M. resulted in a reduction in the overnight percentage fall in FEV_1 (28.2 $\pm$ 7.3% fall vs. 10.4 $\pm$ 4.5% fall; $P = 0.04$) and improvement in the 4 A.M. FEV_1 (2.53 $\pm$ 0.38 L vs. 3.43 $\pm$ 0.38 L. $P = 0.03$). In contrast, neither the 8 A.M. nor the 8 P.M. prednisone dose resulted in overnight spirometric improvement compared to placebo. With the 3 P.M. prednisone dose, peripheral blood eosinophil counts were significantly reduced at both 8 P.M. and 4 A.M. The 3 P.M. dose also resulted in a pancellular reduction in bronchoalveolar lavage cytology ($P \leq$ to 0.05 for all cell lines compared to placebo). The authors concluded that a chronopharmacologic strategy for prednisone dosing could alter the inflammatory milieu and spirometric decline associated with nocturnal worsening of asthma (61).

Inhaled Corticosteroids

Once-daily inhaled corticosteroid preparations are also effective in the treatment of nocturnal asthma. Wempe and colleagues studied the effect of once-daily budesonide in subjects with nocturnal asthma and showed improvements in mean FEV1, reduction in airway responsiveness as measured by methacholine PC_{20}, and improved 4 A.M. FEV_1. Treatment with budesonide also improved asthma symptoms and reduced the number of awakenings compared to placebo (62). Other studies of budesonide (63,64) and beclomethasone (65) have shown similar results.

Chronotherapeutic dosing is important with inhaled corticosteroids as well. Pincus and colleagues compared the efficacy of chronotherapeutic dosing of inhaled triamcinolone, 800 µg once daily at 3 P.M., versus traditional 200 µg q.i.d. dosing in a cohort of 30 asthmatics, 17 of whom (8 in the once-daily group and 9 in the q.i.d. group) had nocturnal asthma (66). The authors showed that once-daily dosing at 3 P.M. was equally efficacious and did not increase side effects (66). When these authors compared the effects of more convenient once-daily dosing schedules (8 A.M. or 5:30 P.M.) to traditional q.i.d. dosing, they showed that early evening (5:30 P.M.) dosing was preferable to morning (8 A.M.) dosing, which did not produce comparable effects to q.i.d. dosing with regard to morning or evening PEFR (67).

Combination and Other Pharmacologic Interventions in Nocturnal Asthma

Inhaled corticosteroids and inhaled long-acting bronchodilators may be used in combination in the treatment of nocturnal asthma. Weersink and colleagues showed that the combination of fluticasone propionate and salmeterol xinafoate appeared to provide greater protection against airway responsiveness to adenosine monophosphate than did salmeterol alone, but that either drug alone or their combination provided comparable therapeutic effects with regard to circadian variation of spirometric indices (68).

The role of sodium cromoglycate and nedocromil are limited in patients with nocturnal asthma (69–72). The effects of these agents, particularly nedocromil, are best seen after 4 to 12 weeks of therapy, which suggests that the effect is most likely due to properties other than these drugs' reduction of mast cell degranulation (73).

Inhaled anticholinergic medications have little effect on the overnight fall in pulmonary function seen in patients with nocturnal asthma. Much of this lack of effect is due to the short half-life of currently available inhaled anticholinergic drugs. Coe and Barnes (74) studied the effect of the quarternary anticholinergic oxitropium bromide in a low-dose regimen (0.2 mg) administered at bedtime. They were able to identify a group of subjects with improvements in overnight lung function but could not identify features that differentiated responders from nonresponders (74).

B. Nonpulmonary and Nonpharmacologic Therapy for Nocturnal Asthma

Nasal Continuous Positive Airway Pressure

A concurrent diagnosis of obstructive sleep apnea should always be considered in the patient with nocturnal asthma. Nasal continuous positive airway pressure (CPAP), a well-accepted therapeutic intervention for patients with sleep apnea, also has a role in this subset of patients with nocturnal asthma. Chan and colleagues showed that nasal CPAP resulted in significant improvements in both morning and evening PEFR, symptoms, and medication use in patients with nocturnal asthma and obstructive sleep apnea (75). Nasal CPAP does not improve the overnight drop in FEV_1 in patients with nocturnal asthma in the absence of obstructive sleep apnea, however (76). A full polysomnographic evaluation along with spirometry pre- and postsleep should be obtained in patients in whom concurrent nocturnal asthma and obstructive sleep apnea are considered so that nasal CPAP may be employed if necessary.

Treatment of Gastroesophageal Reflux

The relationship between nocturnal asthma and gastroesophageal reflux remains controversial. It has been hypothesized that gastroesophageal reflux of gastric acid, which can occur during sleep due to a combination of increased gastric acid secretion and supine posture, may result in reflex bronchospasm from increased vagal tone (73). Tan and colleagues (77) measured airway resistance and esophageal pH in nocturnal asthmatic subjects with and without reflux esophagitis. The increase in lower airway resistance was not affected by the presence or absence of esophageal acid. Furthermore, the overnight fall in FEV_1 stayed constant in the presence or absence of acid in nocturnal asthmatics with or without reflux esophagitis (77). This study did not examine concurrent aspiration, so although reflux of gastric acid did not appear to be a direct trigger of bronchoconstriction, aspiration as a potential trigger was not excluded. Treatment of gastroesophageal reflux in asthma should be based primarily on symptoms of reflux and should not be employed empirically in the treatment of nocturnal asthma.

Treatment of Rhinitis and Sinusitis

Chronic rhinitis and sinusitis are common in patients with asthma, and although the mechanisms by which these states worsen asthma is not clear, both daytime and nocturnal asthma symptoms will improve as the sinuses clear (73). Airway resistance has been shown to increase due to aspiration of inflammatory sinus secretions in animal models (78). Reflex bronchoconstriction and mouth- breathing may also be important factors in the worsening of bronchoconstriction in asthmatic patients with rhinosinusitis (79). Therapy with nasal corticosteroids, oral decongestants, and nasal saline irrigation are beneficial in the majority of patients.

Other Nonpharmacologic Interventions

Airway cooling at night may play an important role in the triggering of nocturnal asthma (80). Chen and Chai explored this potential mechanism of bronchospasm and showed that breathing air at 37°C and 100% relative humidity reduced bronchospasm compared with breathing room air (81). Patients often find this therapy uncomfortable, however, and for that reason it has little practical value.

Weiner and colleagues studied inspiratory muscle training in nocturnal asthmatics, hypothesizing that inspiratory muscle training would result in increased strength and endurance, thereby improving asthma symptoms (82). The authors demonstrated that inspiratory muscle training, when used for 6 months, improves inspiratory muscle strength and endurance and results in improvement in asthma symptoms, hospitalizations for asthma, emergency department contact, absence from school or work, and medication consumption in patients with asthma (82). Inspiratory muscle training, although not commonly used, may serve as a potential nonpharmacologic strategy in nocturnal asthma.

IX. Conclusion

Nocturnal asthma is an important phenotype within the asthma clinical syndrome that, if not treated appropriately, can result in significant morbidity and mortality. Unique physiologic and inflammatory characteristics exist which form the substrate for this phenotype. Knowledge of these characteristics, along with an understanding of the specific therapies directed at the circadian nature of this disease can result in significant improvements in lung function, sleep quality, and asthma-specific quality of life.

References

1. National Heart, Lung and Blood Institute. Guidelines for the Diagnosis and Management of Asthma. Washington, DC: Expert Panel Report 2, 1997.
2. Turner-Warwick M. Epidemiology of nocturnal asthma. Am J Med 1988; 85:6–8.
3. Martin RJ. Location of airway inflammation in asthma and the relationship to circadian change in lung function. Chronobiol Int 1999; 16:623–630.
4. Van Keimpema AR, Ariaansz M, Tamminga JJ, Nauta JJ, Postmus PE. Nocturnal waking and morning dip of peak expiratory flow in clinically stable asthma patients during treatment: occurrence and patient characteristics. Respiration 1997; 64:29–34.
5. Martin RJ, Cicutto LC, Ballard RD. Factors related to the nocturnal worsening of asthma. Am Rev Respir Dis 1990; 141:33–38.
6. Jarjour NN, Busse WW. Cytokines in bronchoalveolar lavage fluid of patients with nocturnal asthma. Am J Respir Crit Care Med 1995; 152:1474–1477.
7. Kraft M, Djukanovic R, Wilson S, Holgate ST, Martin RJ. Alveolar tissue inflammation in asthma. Am J Respir Crit Care Med 1996; 154:1505–1510.
8. Hetzel MR, Clark TJ. Comparison of normal and asthmatic circadian rhythms in peak expiratory flow rate. Thorax 1980; 35:732–738.
9. Hetzel MR, Clark TJ, Branthwaite MA. Asthma: analysis of sudden deaths and ventilatory arrests in hospital. Br Med J 1977; 1:808–811.
10. Szefler SJ, Ando R, Cicutto LC, Surs W, Hill MR, Martin RJ. Plasma histamine, epinephrine, cortisol, and leukocyte beta-adrenergic receptors in nocturnal asthma. Clin Pharmacol Ther 1991; 49:59–68.
11. Morrison JF, Pearson SB, Dean HG. Parasympathetic nervous system in nocturnal asthma. Br Med J (Clin Res Ed) 1988; 296:1427–1429.
12. Barnes P, Fitzgerald G, Brown M, Dollery C. Nocturnal asthma and changes in circulating epinephrine, histamine, and cortisol. N Engl J Med 1980; 303:263–267.
13. Gleich GJ. The eosinophil and bronchial asthma: current understanding. J Allergy Clin Immunol 1990; 85:422–436.

14. Ulrik CS. Peripheral eosinophil counts as a marker of disease activity in intrinsic and extrinsic asthma. Clin Exp Allergy 1995; 25:820–827.

15. Calhoun WJ, Bates ME, Schrader L, Sedgwick JB, Busse WW. Characteristics of peripheral blood eosinophils in patients with nocturnal asthma. Am Rev Respir Dis 1992; 145:577–581.

16. Frick WE, Sedgwick JB, Busse WW. The appearance of hypodense eosinophils in antigen-dependent late phase asthma. Am Rev Respir Dis 1989; 139:1401–1406.

17. Bates ME, Clayton M, Calhoun W, Jarjour N, Schrader L, Geiger K, Schultz T, Sedgwick J, Swenson C, Busse W. Relationship of plasma epinephrine and circulating eosinophils to nocturnal asthma. Am J Respir Crit Care Med 1994; 149:667–672.

18. Carroll N, Elliot J, Morton A, James A. The structure of large and small airways in nonfatal and fatal asthma. Am Rev Respir Dis 1993; 147:405–410.

19. Djukanovic R, Roche WR, Wilson JW, Beasley CR, Twentyman OP, Howarth RH, Holgate ST. Mucosal inflammation in asthma. Am Rev Respir Dis 1990; 142:434–457.

20. Kraft M, Martin RJ, Wilson S, Djukanovic R, Holgate ST. Lymphocyte and eosinophil influx into alveolar tissue in nocturnal asthma. Am J Respir Crit Care Med 1999; 159:228–234.

21. Kharitonov SA, Yates D, Robbins RA, Logan-Sinclair R, Shinebourne EA, Barnes PJ. Increased nitric oxide in exhaled air of asthmatic patients. Lancet 1994; 343:133–135.

22. ten Hacken NH, van der Vaart H, van der Mark TW, Koeter GH, Postma DS. Exhaled nitric oxide is higher both at day and night in subjects with nocturnal asthma. Am J Respir Crit Care Med 1998; 158:902–907.

23. Georges G, Bartelson BB, Martin RJ, Silkoff PE. Circadian variation in exhaled nitric oxide in nocturnal asthma. J Asthma 1999; 36:467–473.

24. Silkoff PE, McClean PA, Slutsky AS, Caramori M, Chapman KR, Gutierrez C, Zamel N. Exhaled nitric oxide and bronchial reactivity during and after inhaled beclomethasone in mild asthma. J Asthma 1998; 35:473–479.

25. Fraser CM, Venter JC. The synthesis of beta-adrenergic receptors in cultured human lung cells: induction by glucocorticoids. Biochem Biophys Res Commun 1980; 94:390–397.

26. Davies AO, Lefkowitz RJ. In vitro desensitization of beta adrenergic receptors in human neutrophils: attenuation by corticosteroids. J Clin Invest 1983; 71:565–571.

27. Martin RJ. Small airway and alveolar tissue changes in nocturnal asthma. Am J Respir Crit Care Med 1998; 157:S188–S190.

28. Titinchi S, Al Shamma M, Patel KR, Kerr JW, Clark B. Circadian variation in number and affinity of beta 2-adrenoceptors in lymphocytes of asthmatic patients. Clin Sci 1984; 66:323–328.

29. Reihsaus E, Innis M, MacIntyre N, Liggett SB. Mutations in the gene encoding for the beta 2-adrenergic receptor in normal and asthmatic subjects. Am J Respir Cell Mol Biol 1993; 8:334–339.

30. Green SA, Cole G, Jacinto M, Innis M, Liggett SB. A polymorphism of the human beta 2-adrenergic receptor within the fourth transmembrane domain alters ligand binding and functional properties of the receptor. J Biol Chem 1993; 268:23116–23121.

31. Green SA, Turki J, Innis M, Liggett SB. Amino-terminal polymorphisms of the human beta 2-adrenergic receptor impart distinct agonist-promoted regulatory properties. Biochemistry 1994; 33:9414–9419.

32. Turki J, Pak J, Green SA, Martin RJ, Liggett SB. Genetic polymorphisms of the beta 2-adrenergic receptor in nocturnal and nonnocturnal asthma. Evidence that Gly16 correlates with the nocturnal phenotype. J Clin Invest 1995; 95:1635–1641.

33. Kraft M, Vianna E, Martin RJ, Leung DYM. Nocturnal asthma is associated with reduced glucocorticoid receptor binding affinity and decreased steroid responsiveness at night. J Allergy Clin Immunol 1999; 103:66–71.

34. Hamid QA, Wenzel SE, Hauk PJ, Tsicopoulos A, Wallaert B, Lafitte JJ, Chrousos GP, Szefler SJ, Leung DY. Increased glucocorticoid receptor beta in airway cells of glucocorticoid-insensitive asthma. Am J Respir Crit Care Med 1999; 159:1600–1604.

35. Kraft M, Leung DYM, Martin RJ, Hamid QA. Reduced steroid responsiveness at night in asthma is due to increased glucocorticoid receptor beta expression in lung macrophages. Am J Respir Crit Care Med 1999; 159:A632.

36. Ballard RD, Tan WC, Kelly PL, Pak J, Pandey R, Martin RJ. Effect of sleep and sleep deprivation on ventilatory response to bronchoconstriction. J Appl Physiol 1990; 69:490–497.

37. Wagner EM, Liu MC, Weinmann GG, Permutt S, Bleecker ER. Peripheral lung resistance in normal and asthmatic subjects. Am Rev Respir Dis 1990; 141:584–588.

38. Ballard RD, Irvin CG, Martin RJ, Pak J, Pandey R, White DP. Influence of sleep on lung volume in asthmatic patients and normal subjects. J Appl Physiol 1990; 68:2034–2041.

39. Briscoe WA, Dubois AB. The relationship between airways resistance, airways conductance and lung volume in subjects of different age and body size. J Clin Invest 1958; 37:1279–1285.

40. Irvin CG, Pak J, Martin RJ. Airway-parenchyma uncoupling in nocturnal asthma. Am J Respir Crit Care Med 2000; 161:50–56.

41. Dethlefsen U, Repgas R. Ein neues Therapieprinzip bei Nachtlichen Asthma. Klin Med 1985; 80:44–47.

42. Fitzpatrick MF, Engleman H, Whyte KF, Deary IJ, Shapiro CM, Douglas NJ. Morbidity in nocturnal asthma: sleep quality and daytime cognitive performance. Thorax 1991; 46:569–573.

43. Cochrane GM. Asthma deaths at night. In: Barnes PJ, Levy J, eds. Nocturnal Asthma. London: Royal Society of Medicine, 1984:11–15.

44. Cochrane GM, Clark JH. A survey of asthma mortality in patients between ages 35 and 64 in the Greater London hospitals in 1971. Thorax 1975; 30:300–305.

45. Smolensky MH, Reinberg AE, Martin RJ, Haus E. Clinical chronobiology and chronotherapeutics with applications to asthma. Chronobiol Int 1999; 16:539–563.

46. Barnes PJ, Greening AP, Neville L, Timmers J, Poole GW. Single-dose slow-release aminophylline at night prevents nocturnal asthma. Lancet 1982; 1:299–301.

47. Goldenheim PD, Conrad EA, Schein LK. Treatment of asthma by a controlled-release theophylline tablet formulation: a review of the North American experience with nocturnal dosing. Chronobiol Int 1987; 4:397–408.

48. Martin RJ, Cicutto LC, Ballard RD, Goldenheim PD, Cherniack RM. Circadian vari-

ations in theophylline concentrations and the treatment of nocturnal asthma. Am Rev Respir Dis 1989; 139:475–478.

49. Elias-Jones AC, Higenbottam TW, Barnes ND, Godden DJ. Sustained release theophylline in nocturnal asthma. Arch Dis Child 1984; 59:1159–1161.

50. Postma DS, Koeter GH, Meurs H, Keyzer JJ. Slow release terbutaline in nocturnal bronchial obstruction: relation of terbutaline dosage and blood levels with circadian changes in peak flow values. Annu Rev Chronopharmacol 1984; 1:101–104.

51. Koeter GH, Postma DS, Keyzer JJ, Meurs H. Effect of oral slow-release terbutaline on early morning dyspnoea. Eur J Clin Pharmacol 1985; 28:159–162.

52. Postma DS, Koeter GH, Mark TW, Reig RP, Sluiter HJ. The effects of oral slow-release terbutaline on the circadian variation in spirometry and arterial blood gas levels in patients with chronic airflow obstruction. Chest 1985; 87:653–657.

53. Stewart IC, Rhind GB, Power JT, Flenley DC, Douglas NJ. Effect of sustained release terbutaline on symptoms and sleep quality in patients with nocturnal asthma. Thorax 1987; 42:797–800.

54. Bogin RM, Ballard RD. Treatment of nocturnal asthma with pulsed-release albuterol. Chest 1992; 102:362–366.

55. Fitzpatrick MF, Mackay T, Driver H, Douglas NJ. Salmeterol in nocturnal asthma: a double blind, placebo controlled trial of a long acting inhaled beta 2 agonist. Br Med J 1990; 301:1365–1368.

56. Lockey RF, DuBuske LM, Friedman B, Petrocella V, Cox F, Rickard K. Nocturnal asthma: effect of salmeterol on quality of life and clinical outcomes. Chest 1999; 115:666–673.

57. Martin RJ, Kraft M, Beaucher WN, Kiechel F, Sublett JL, LaVallee N, Shilstone J. Comparative study of extended release albuterol sulfate and long-acting inhaled salmeterol xinafoate in the treatment of nocturnal asthma. Ann Allergy Asthma Immunol 1999; 83:121–126.

58. Kraft M, Wenzel SE, Bettinger CM, Martin RJ. The effect of salmeterol on nocturnal symptoms, airway function, and inflammation in asthma. Chest 1997; 111:1249–1254.

59. Reinberg A, Gervais P, Chaussade M, Fraboulet G, Duburque B. Circadian changes in effectiveness of corticosteroids in eight patients with allergic asthma. J Allergy Clin Immunol 1983; 71:425–433.

60. Reinberg A, Halberg F, Falliers CJ. Circadian timing of methylprednisolone effects in asthmatic boys. Chronobiologia 1974; 1:333–347.

61. Beam WR, Weiner DE, Martin RJ. Timing of prednisone and alterations of airways inflammation in nocturnal asthma. Am Rev Respir Dis 1992; 146:1524–1530.

62. Wempe JB, Tammeling EP, Postma DS, Auffarth B, Teengs JP, Koeter GH. Effects of budesonide and bambuterol on circadian variation of airway responsiveness and nocturnal symptoms of asthma. J Allergy Clin Immunol 1992; 90:349–357.

63. Toogood JH, Baskerville JC, Jennings B, Lefcoe NM, Johansson SA. Influence of dosing frequency and schedule on the response of chronic asthmatics to the aerosol steroid, budesonide. J Allergy Clin Immunol 1982; 70:288–298.

64. Malo JL, Cartier A, Merland N, Ghezzo H, Burek A, Morris J, Jennings BH. Four-times-a-day dosing frequency is better than a twice-a-day regimen in subjects requiring a high-dose inhaled steroid, budesonide, to control moderate to severe asthma. Am Rev Respir Dis 1989; 140:624–628.

65. Horn CR, Clark TJ, Cochrane GM. Inhaled therapy reduces morning dips in asthma. Lancet 1984; 1:1143–1145.

66. Pincus DJ, Szefler SJ, Ackerson LM, Martin RJ. Chronotherapy of asthma with inhaled steroids: the effect of dosage timing on drug efficacy. J Allergy Clin Immunol 1995; 95:1172–1178.

67. Pincus DJ, Humeston TR, Martin RJ. Further studies on the chronotherapy of asthma with inhaled steroids: the effect of dosage timing on drug efficacy. J Allergy Clin Immunol 1997; 100:771–774.

68. Weersink EJ, Douma RR, Postma DS, Koeter GH. Fluticasone propionate, salmeterol xinafoate, and their combination in the treatment of nocturnal asthma. Am J Respir Crit Care Med 1997; 155:1241–1246.

69. Ruffin R, Alpers JH, Kroemer DK, Rubinfeld AR, Pain MC, Czarny D, Bowes G. A 4-week Australian multicentre study of nedocromil sodium in asthmatic patients. Eur J Respir Dis Suppl 1986; 147:336–339.

70. Morgan AD, Connaughton JJ, Catterall JR, Shapiro CM, Douglas NJ, Flenley DC. Sodium cromoglycate in nocturnal asthma. Thorax 1986; 41:39–41.

71. Hetzel MR, Clarke JH, Gillam SJ, Isaac P, Perkins M. Is sodium cromoglycate effective in nocturnal asthma? Thorax 1985; 40:793–794.

72. Bernstein IL, Siegel SC, Brandon ML, Brown EB, Evans RR, Feinberg AR, Friedlaender S, Krumholz RA, Hadley RA, Handelman NI, Thurston D, Yamate M. A controlled study of cromolyn sodium sponsored by the Drug Committee of the American Academy of Allergy. J Allergy Clin Immunol 1972; 50:235–245.

73. Martin RJ, Kraft M. Nocturnal asthma: therapeutic considerations. Clin Immunother 1996; 6:443–453.

74. Coe CI, Barnes PJ. Reduction of nocturnal asthma by an inhaled anticholinergic drug. Chest 1986; 90:485–488.

75. Chan CS, Woolcock AJ, Sullivan CE. Nocturnal asthma: role of snoring and obstructive sleep apnea. Am Rev Respir Dis 1988; 137:1502–1504.

76. Martin RJ, Pak J. Nasal CPAP in nonapneic nocturnal asthma. Chest 1991; 100: 1024–1027.

77. Tan WC, Martin RJ, Pandey R, Ballard RD. Effects of spontaneous and simulated gastroesophageal reflux on sleeping asthmatics. Am Rev Respir Dis 1990; 141: 1394–1399.

78. Brugman SM, Larsen GL, Henson PM, Honor J, Irvin CG. Increased lower airways responsiveness associated with sinusitis in a rabbit model. Am Rev Respir Dis 1993; 147:314–320.

79. Shturman-Ellstein R, Zeballos RJ, Buckley JM, Souhrada JF. The beneficial effect of nasal breathing on exercise-induced bronchoconstriction. Am Rev Respir Dis 1978; 118:65–73.

80. Chen WY, Horton DJ, Weiser PC. Airway obstruction induced by body cooling in asthmatics. Physiology 1977; 20:16.

81. Chen WY, Chai H. Airway cooling and nocturnal asthma. Chest 1982; 81:675–680.

82. Weiner P, Azgad Y, Weiner M. Inspiratory muscle training during treatment with corticosteroids in humans. Chest 1995; 107:1041–1044.

83. Martin RJ. Nocturnal asthma: an overview. In: Martin RJ, ed. Nocturnal Asthma: Mechanisms and Treatment. Mount Kisco, NY: Futura, 1993:71–115.

10

Complementary and Alternative Therapies for Asthma

ESTHER L. LANGMACK

National Jewish Medical and Research Center
Denver Colorado

I. Introduction

Complementary and alternative medicine (CAM) encompasses therapies that are not traditionally taught in medical schools or employed in conventional Western medical practice. A therapy is complementary when used in addition to, or in conjunction with, conventional drugs or treatments, whereas an alternative therapy is used in place of conventional medical therapy. Many CAM therapies originate in diverse cultural healing practices dating back hundreds or thousands of years.

Use of CAM is increasing in the United States. Between 1990 and 1997, the percentage of individuals using CAM in the United States grew from 33.8 to 42.1% (1). During this 7-year period, the percentage of survey respondents using CAM for "lung problems" rose from 8.8 to 13.2% and the number using CAM for allergies nearly doubled from 8.7 to 16.6% (1). It is estimated that $27 billion was spent out-of-pocket on CAM therapies in 1997, an amount which approaches the $29.3 billion spent out-of-pocket for all U.S. physician services in the same year (1). Despite widespread and increasing use, 61.5% of those who used CAM did not discuss it with their medical doctor (1).

It has been hypothesized that patients use CAM because they are discontent with conventional medical care. In fact, dissatisfaction with conventional medicine does not appear to motivate most patients to use CAM. In a U.S. survey study, factors which predicted CAM use included poorer health status, higher level of education, and a holistic orientation to health, but not dissatisfaction with conventional medicine (2). In this study, only 4.4% of respondents reported that they relied primarily on alternative therapies; most used CAM in a complementary fashion. Most respondents felt that CAM was beneficial because it provided relief of symptoms or was more effective than standard medical treatment for their health problems. Concerns about the side effects and costs of conventional medications and a desire for a more active role in maintaining health may also motivate some patients to use CAM (3).

II. CAM for Asthma

How often asthmatics turn to CAM therapies, such as herbal remedies, homeopathy, acupuncture, yoga, hypnosis, or special diets, for relief has not been studied extensively. In one of the few studies to focus on asthmatics' use of CAM, 601 adult asthmatics from pulmonary and allergy specialty practices in Northern California were surveyed about their use of herbs, coffee, black tea, over-the-counter epinephrine or ephedrine for asthma (4). Eight percent of respondents used herbal remedies, 6% used epinephrine or ephedrine, and 6% used coffee or black tea. More women used herbal preparations, while more men used epinephrine- or ephedrine-containing products. Asthma-specific quality of life was worse among those using herbs, coffee, or black tea. Herbal product use was associated with an increased risk of hospitalization, while coffee or black tea use was associated with increased risk of both emergency department visits and hospitalization. Adherence to conventional medical therapy for asthma was not assessed in this study. Nonetheless, these findings suggest that CAM use may be a marker for severe or poorly controlled asthma.

Severe asthmatics may be more likely than those with milder disease to use CAM. Ernst and colleagues surveyed 17,000 members of the United Kingdom National Asthma Campaign about CAM use (5). Respondents who described their asthma as "severe" were roughly two to three times more likely than those with "mild" asthma to have tried CAM for asthma. Of 3837 respondents, the majority (59%) had used some form of CAM for asthma. The five most popular therapies were breathing techniques (30%), homeopathy (12%), herbalism (11%), yoga (9%), and acupuncture (7%). Most patients obtained information about CAM through friends and relatives (27%), the media (16%), or their general practitioner (13%). Twenty-three percent felt that CAM improved their asthma symptoms "to a great extent," while the majority (53%) felt that CAM had improved their asthma symptoms "to some extent" or "to a slight extent."

III. Botanicals

Crude plant materials and extracts, termed herbs or botanicals, have been used to treat asthma and other respiratory ailments for centuries. Some respiratory medications used today were derived from plants employed in traditional healing practices. These include guaifenesin (from guaiac wood), theophylline (from tea leaves), and cromolyn (from the Indian plant *Ammi visnaga*). In traditional practices, botanicals often complement other healing modalities. For example, in traditional Chinese medicine, herbs are integrated into a treatment program for asthma that includes acupuncture, diet, and behavioral prescriptions. In the Indian Ayurvedic tradition, herbal remedies may complement the practice of yoga.

Of all CAM therapies, use of herbal preparations is increasing the most rapidly. Between 1990 and 1997, use of herbal medicines rose from 2.5 to 12.1% of respondents in a U.S. survey, a greater increase than for any other CAM modality studied during this time period (1). In 1996, sales of herbal products in the United States totaled more than $1.5 billion and were estimated to be increasing at a rate of roughly 25% per year (6). Annual sales of herbal products are subtantially larger in European countries. As herbal product use has grown, so has the realization that these preparations are not always inert concoctions, but that they may contain one or more pharmacologically active ingredients with potential beneficial and adverse effects.

Dozens of botanicals have been used to treat asthma (Table 1) and the associated conditions of allergies and allergic rhinitis. Although many have been evaluated in animal models of asthma or in vitro, few have been evaluated in clinical trials. None have been rigorously tested for their efficacy or safety in treating human asthma. A detailed discussion of all of the botanicals used to treat asthma is beyond the scope of this chapter, but comprehensive reviews can be found in the literature (7–9).

Botanicals used to treat asthma may be selected for their potential to ameliorate asthma symptoms or their antibacterial or anti-inflammatory properties. Licorice, ginger, and *Pinellia*, for example, have antitussive effects (8), while mullein (10) and ginseng (7) are expectorants. *Datura stramonium* (jimson weed), which was smoked in cigarettes by asthmatics in the 19th and early 20th centuries, reduces sputum production through its anticholinergic action (9). Other botanicals, including cinnamon, peony, licorice, and *Gingko biloba* are valued for their antibacterial properties (8).

Of botanicals with bronchodilator activity, the Chinese plant *ma huang* (*Ephedra sinica*) is perhaps the most widely used. It is a central ingredient of Chinese and Japanese herbal preparations for asthma and allergic rhinitis. L-Ephedrine, the predominant active constituent of *ma huang*, is also found in Western products advocated for treatment of asthma, obesity, and fatigue and for producing euphoria (11). L-Ephedrine, an α- and β-adrenergic receptor agonist, was

Table 1 Herbal Products Used in the Treatment of Asthma by Culture[a]

Chinese

Aconite	Cuscutae (dodder)	*Ligusticum chuan xiong*	*Poria cocos* (hoelen)
Artemesia	*Dioscorae* (Chinese yam)	*Longdan jiechuan*	*Prunus armeniacae* (apricot/kernel)
Asarum	*Epimedium*	*Lumbricus spencer*	*Psoralae*
Aster	*Fritillaria*	*Ma huang* (*Ephedra sinica*)	*Rehmannia*
Astragalus	Gecko	Magnolia	*Schisandra*
Aurantii	*Ge ji* antiasthma pill	Minor Blue Dragon	*Scutellaria* (skullcap)
Bupleurum	*Ginkgo biloba*	Minor *Blupleurum* combination	*Sinomenum*
Cinnabar	Ginseng	*Morus* (mulberry)	*Trichosanthes*
Cinnamon	Gypsum	*Ophiopogum* (lily turf)	*Tussilago* (coltsfoot)
Cistanchis	*Juglandis*	Peony	*Wen yang* pill
Citrus reticulae	*Kan-lin* preparation	Perilla	*You gui* pill
Coptis (goldenthread)	Kidney reinforcing regimen	*Pinellia*	*Zingiber* (ginger)
Curculigo	Licorice		*Zizyphus* (Chinese date)
Cornus			

Japanese

Hange-koboku-to	*Sho-saiko-to*
Moku-boi-to	*Sho-seiryu-to*
Saiboku-to	
Shinpi-to	

Indian

Adhatoda vasica (Malabar nut)	*Croton tiglium*
Coleus forskholii	*Picrorrhiza kurroa*
Albizzia lebbek	*Tylophora indica/asthmatica* (Indian ipecac)

Latin American

Aloe barbadensis	*Desmodium* (*amor seco*)
	Galphimia glauca

Hawaiian

Allium cepa (cebolla/onion)	

Western

Sophora chryso phylla (mamane, mamani)	*Aleurites moluccana* (kukui, candlenut)	*Solanum americum* (popol, glossy nightshade)
	Piper methysticum (kawa, kava)	
Chinese skullcap	Goldenseal	*Ma huang*
Coltsfoot	Licorice	

[a] Adapted from Ref. 7.

once used to treat asthma in conventional Western medicine, before the advent of inhaled β2-agonists. Inhaled β2-agonists, however, have a much more favorable risk/benefit ratio compared to ephedrine (12), which has greater propensity for undesirable central nervous system and cardiac stimulation. Pseudoephedrine and phenylpropanolamine are other constituents of *ma huang*. *Pinellia*, a botanical found in many Asian herbal remedies, also contains ephedrine (7).

Some botanicals have been shown to attenuate various aspects of asthmatic airway inflammation in animal or in vitro studies. For example, in animal studies, gingkolide compound BN 52021 from *Gingko biloba* antagonized the bronchoconstrictor and eosinophil chemoattractant activities of platelet activating factor (7), a lipid-derived inflammatory mediator. Ginseng, licorice, *Scutellaria baicalensis*, and *Zizyphi fructusia* reduced serum IgE, as reflected by a decrease in passive cutaneous anaphylaxis in rats (13). *Shinpi-to* (TJ-85) inhibited release of leukotriene C4 (LTC_4) and LTB_4 from rat basophilic leukemia-2H3 cells in vitro (14). *Saiboku-to*, a Japanese preparation consisting of a mixture of botanicals, decreased histamine release from sensitized guinea pig lung tissue (15).

In human studies, pretreatment of eight atopic, mild asthmatics with oral gingkolide BN 52063 for 3 days attenuated early bronchoconstriction after inhaled allergen challenge (16). Hsieh studied 334 asthmatic children classified according to the principles of traditional Chinese medicine (17). Children were treated with one of three Chinese herbal combinations or placebo for 6 months. A placebo effect was observed: The herb and placebo groups all had improvements in asthma symptom scores, peak expiratory flow rates (PEFR), and conventional medication usage during the study. However, two of the three herbal groups had significantly greater PEFR (10–20 Lmin higher) at some, but not all, time points during treatment compared to the placebo group. In this same study, each of the three herbal preparations reduced eosinophils and LTC_4 in bronchoalveolar lavage fluid and increased airway conductance in a guinea pig model of allergen-induced asthma. However, the effects of botanicals upon airway inflammation in asthmatic humans have not been described in the medical literature.

The anti-inflammatory activity of some botanicals may be mediated by their effects on corticosteroid production or metabolism. In rats, ginseng saponin (18) and saikosaponin (19), a component of *bupleurum* (*saiko*), increased plasma ACTH and corticosterone levels. Other agents appear to increase circulating levels of both endogenous and exogenous corticosteroids by inhibiting 11β-dehydroxysteroid dehydrogenase, the enzyme that catalyzes the reversible conversion of cortisol to cortisone and prednisolone to prednisone. Inhibition of 11β-dehydroxysteroid dehydrogenase increases plasma levels of cortisol and prednisolone, which are metabolically active. In healthy human volunteers, glycyrrhetinic acid, the active metabolite of glycyrrhizin from *Glycyrrhiza glabra* (licorice), increased the ratio of plasma cortisol to cortisone (20). Licorice is found in several Asian herbal products, including Chinese Minor Blue Dragon and *saiboku-to*.

Saiboku-to has been shown to alter glucocorticoid pharmacokinetics, resulting in increased serum levels of prednisolone (21). In addition to licorice, several other *saiboku-to* ingredients, *Perilla frutescens*, *Zizyphus vulgaris*, *Magnolia offician-alis*, and *Scutellaria baicalensis*, have also been reported to inhibit 11β-dehydroxy-steroid dehydrogenase (22).

The corticosteroid-sparing effects of *saiboku-to* have been the focus of a few small studies of corticosteroid-dependent asthmatics. In one study, 64 steroid-dependent adult asthmatics treated with saiboku-to for 12 weeks had lower asthma symptom scores than the untreated group (23). Eleven patients were able to reduce their doses of oral corticosteroids by at least 50%, while two were able to withdraw from oral corticosteroids altogether. In a separate, uncontrolled study, 71% of 40 steroid-dependent asthmatics either stopped or decreased their oral corticosteroids during treatment with *saiboku-to* for 6 to 24 months (24). Unfortunately, neither of these clinical studies adequately described the protocol for reducing corticosteroids, *saiboku-to*'s impact on objective measures of lung function, or its side effects.

Although herb-containing remedies may be derived from natural sources, their use is not always safe. Adverse effects associated with use of these products are likely underrecognized and underreported (25). In the United States, herbal products are classified as dietary supplements and are therefore exempt from legislation requiring pre- and postmarket safety surveillance, unlike conventional pharmaceuticals. Consequently, manufacturers of herbal remedies need not demonstrate efficacy, purity, or potency of ingredients, and quality controls in manufacturing are not required. The amount of active ingredient in products may vary greatly (26). In addition, the U.S. Food and Drug Administration (FDA) does not regulate or routinely test herbal products imported from outside of the United States. In contrast, botanicals in many European countries are regulated in a manner similar to conventional pharmaceuticals and medical prescriptions are required for some preparations.

Adverse effects associated with botanicals may result from the pharmacologically active agents in the plant itself. For example, L-ephedrine, the active ingredient of *ma huang*, has been associated with adverse effects ranging in severity from nausea and vomiting to seizure, stroke, and fatal myocardial infarction (11). The U.S. FDA warns against taking more than 8 mg of *ma huang* every 6 h, or more than 24 mg per day, and it recommends against use for more than 7 consecutive days (10). As with any plant product, hypersensitivity reactions may occur, ranging in severity from dermatitis to anaphylaxis (25). *Saiboku-to* use has been associated with pneumonitis (27). Glycyrrhizin, one of the active agents in licorice, is well known for its mineralocorticoid side effects, including hypokalemia and sodium retention (20).

Adverse effects may also result from the presence of adulterants that have been intentionally or inadvertently added to the botanical preparation. Undeclared heavy metals (lead, mercury, cadmium, and arsenic), sedatives (diazepam and chlordiazepoxide), and stimulants (ephedrine and caffeine) have been found in some Chinese and Ayurvedic herbal remedies (25). Some preparations sold for pain relief have been shown to be adulterated with aspirin or ibuprofen (Kshirsagar, 1993), drugs which pose a danger to aspirin-sensitive asthmatics. Others products contain undeclared corticosteroids such as dexamethasone and triamcinolone (25).

Botanicals may interact significantly with other botanicals or prescription medications. Use of herbs by patients taking prescription drugs is common. In one study, of the 44% of respondents who regularly took prescription medications, nearly one in five (18.4%) reported concurrent use of at least one herbal remedy, high-dose vitamin, or both (1). Of the botanicals used for asthma, *ma huang* is contraindicated in patients taking monoamine oxidase (MAO) inhibitors, ephedrine, β-blockers, phenothiazines, pseudoephedrine, or theophylline (10). *Gingko biloba* and ginger both enhance the anticoagulant effects of aspirin and warfarin (10). Licorice interacts with corticosteroids, aldactone, diuretics, and digoxin (10). More information about side effects and interactions with prescription medications can be found elsewhere (7,10,28,29).

In summary, few data support the use of botanicals in the treatment of asthma at this time. Patients and physicians should nevertheless be familiar with the adverse effects of botanicals and their potential for interactions with other botanicals and prescription medications. Reports of hepatotoxicity associated with a few Chinese herbal remedies have prompted some authors to recommend periodic liver function testing for patients taking these preparations (30). Herbal remedies should be discontinued at least 2 weeks before surgery (10). In general, pregnant or nursing women should avoid botanicals because very little is known about their safety in these situations. Extreme vigilance is necessary when children, the elderly, or individuals with complex medical illness take herbal preparations. As with any other CAM therapy, conventional asthma medications should not be reduced except under medical supervision.

IV. Homeopathy

Homeopathy is an 18th-century practice based on the principle that "like cures like" when taken in extremely small doses. In classic homeopathy, a detailed history is taken about the patient's physical and psychological symptoms, a process that may itself have a salutary effect. A plant, animal, or mineral extract is then chosen, which, if given in a sufficiently high dose, would cause such symptoms. For example, if an allergic patient complains of watering eyes, *Allium cepa* (onion) might be selected. This extract is then diluted in an alcohol solution to such a great extent that there are often virtually no molecules of the extract present in the final dilution, which is administered orally to the patient. Succussion, the process of striking the tube at each stage of dilution, is believed to imprint the solvent with the desired therapeutic effect of the original extract. According to homeopathic principles, the more dilute the solution, the greater its alleged potency. Extracts used in the homeopathic treatment of asthma include bee and snake venoms, arsenicals, strychnine, lobelia, bittersweet, club moss, ambergris, charcoal, nitrates, bromine, and gold (9).

In the practice of homeopathic immunotherapy, or isopathy, a particular pollen or other allergen, such as dust mite, which is believed to precipitate asthma or allergic rhinitis, is administered in extremely dilute solutions. A few studies have reported positive effects of homeopathic immunotherapy on allergic rhinitis (31,32). In one randomized, double-blind, placebo-controlled study of 28 patients with moderately severe allergic asthma (33), treatment with a homeopathic preparation of diluted allergen for 4 weeks reduced the global severity of asthma symptoms, as measured with a 100 mm visual analog scale. Symptom severity improved by 7.2 mm in the treatment group, while it worsened by 7.8 mm in the placebo group, resulting in a significant difference between groups ($P = 0.003$). There was a trend ($P = 0.08$) toward a greater increase in forced expiratory volume in 1 sec (FEV_1) percentage predicted for the treatment group. In the treatment group, the median increase in FEV_1 percentage predicted was 3% compared to a 7% decline in the placebo group. There were no significant differences between groups in scores for severity of nocturnal asthma, morning chest tightness, daytime asthma, cough, nasal symptoms, medication usage, or PEFR.

Clinical trials of homeopathy have not been of high quality (34), in general, and evidence that homeopathy is effective for asthma (35) or any other clinical condition studied is lacking (36). Moreover, the biophysical mechanism of action of homeopathic preparations awaits plausible scientific explanation. Unlike herbal remedies, however, which may contain sufficient quantities of pharmacologically active substances to produce adverse reactions, properly manufactured homeopathic preparations are highly dilute and are therefore unlikely to cause adverse effects. However, as with herbal remedies and dietary supplements, homeopathic remedies are exempt from FDA regulation in the United States (37). In addition, solutions of some plant extracts prepared by practitioners of phytotherapy, a related discipline, may be more concentrated and could potentially have toxic effects.

V. Acupuncture

Acupuncture is a therapeutic modality in which fine needles are placed at various depths into specific points along the body surface. Originating in China thousands of years ago, acupuncture has become part of many healing traditions and is gaining acceptance worldwide. A survey in the United Kingdom revealed that 7% of 3837 asthmatic respondents had tried acupuncture, and the majority (71%) felt that acupuncture was at least slightly helpful (5). The physiological mechanisms through which acupuncture may improve asthma are unknown and have never been investigated systematically.

Several studies have reported acute improvement in pulmonary function after acupuncture. Yu and Lee demonstrated that needling the Din Chuan point, a location specific for asthma, during an acute asthma attack increased the mean FEV_1 by 58% and forced vital capacity (FVC) by 29%, whereas no significant improvement was observed with needling of control points (38). Virsik and colleagues reported a 24.5% increase in mean FEV_1 30 min after acupuncture in stable, moderate to severe asthmatics (39). Specific airway conductance (SGaw) increased by as much as 95% and PEFR by 23% after acupuncture. Significant improvements in SGaw and PEFR, but not FEV_1, lasted up to 2 h (39). Using the forced oscillation technique, Takishima and colleagues found that needling the Suitotsu point near the stellate ganglion in the neck decreased respiratory resistance by ≥20% in more subjects than stimulation of a sham point (40).

The ability of acupuncture to attenuate bronchospasm induced by histamine, methacholine, and exercise challenge has also been studied. In two studies (38,41) acupuncture had no effect on histamine-induced bronchoconstriction. In a well-designed and executed study, Tashkin and colleagues found that acupuncture attenuated acute bronchospasm induced by methacholine, as reflected by modest improvements in SGaw, FEV_1, and thoracic gas volume, compared to sham acupuncture, nebulized saline, or no intervention (42). Unlike isoproterenol, however, acupuncture did not effectively reverse methacholine-induced bronchoconstriction, and it had a slower onset of action. In children with exercise-induced bronchospasm, acupuncture 20 min before running on a treadmill reduced airflow obstruction by nearly 50% (43). However, in a separate study, acupuncture had no effect on exercise-induced bronchospasm (44).

Of studies examining the efficacy of acupuncture for treating chronic asthma, two studies (45,46) are particularly well designed. In Tashkin and colleagues' study, 25 moderate-to-severe asthmatic adults and children received 4 weeks of standardized, biweekly acupuncture or sham acupuncture in a double-blind crossover design (46). Acupuncture had no significant effect on symptoms, medication use, or pulmonary function during the treatment period or for 3 to 4 weeks after treatment ended. They concluded that acupuncture was not effective treatment for chronic asthma. In contrast, Christensen and colleagues reported positive results. Their study compared the effect of 5 weeks of biweekly, standardized, electroacupuncture therapy to sham electroacupuncture in 17 moderate-to-severe adult asthmatics (45). A significant increase in PEFR and a significant decrease in β2-agonist use were observed in the electroacupuncture group, compared to the sham group, after 2 weeks of treatment, but improvement was not sustained thereafter. The magnitude of the mean increase in PEFR was approximately 50 L/min. β2-Agonist use was reduced by 53% in the electroacupuncture group. In the electroacupuncture group, asthma symptoms improved over the course of the study, compared to baseline, but there was no significant difference compared to the sham electroacupuncture group. Christensen et al. concluded that acupuncture was a moderately effective treatment for chronic asthma. Other investigators have reported improvement in chronic asthma after acupuncture treatment in uncontrolled trials (47,48).

Acupuncture is generally considered safe, but certain adverse effects have been reported. The incidence of adverse effects has not been carefully studied. The most common adverse events are vasovagal reactions (dizziness, syncope, and nausea) and transient skin injury (bruising, dermatitis, or hematoma formation) (49,50). The actual incidence of life-threatening or fatal injuries related to acupuncture is estimated to be extremely low, but transmission of infectious diseases, such as hepatitis B, human immunodeficiency virus (HIV), nerve damage, pneumothorax, and other organ punctures have been reported (49,50). Serious adverse events are believed to be more common when acupuncture is practiced by inadequately trained individuals (50).

VI. Yoga and Hypnosis

Therapies that focus on the mind–body connection and emphasize relaxation or altered states of consciousness have been advocated for use in asthma. These techniques include biofeedback, transcendental meditation, mental imagery, yoga, and hypnosis. Of these, yoga and hypnosis have been the most extensively evaluated in clinical studies.

Yoga is an important component of Ayurvedic medicine, an ancient Indian healing tradition that is still practiced today. Traditional yoga practice includes breathing exercises, cleansing rituals, postures and stretching, and meditation (51). Nagarathna found that asthmatics who practiced yoga exercises, breath-slowing techniques, and meditation for 6 weeks had fewer episodes of asthma, greater PEFR, and decreased use of asthma medications compared to matched controls (52). Singh and colleagues examined the effect of pranayama breathing, one aspect of yogic practice, upon asthma (53). Subjects were trained in this breathing method using a device that imposes a 1:2 ratio between inspiration and expiration and slows breathing frequency. Compared to control subjects, those who used the device for 2 weeks had decreased bronchial reactivity to inhaled histamine, but no improvement in medication use, PEFR, or FEV_1. Vendanthan reported that practice of yoga breathing exercises, postures, and meditation resulted in a more positive attitude, greater relaxation, and a trend toward reduced medication usage in asthmatics (54). The results of some studies suggest that hypnosis may be an effective therapy for chronic asthma (55,56), exercise-induced asthma (57), and acute asthma exacerbations (58,59). Most studies, however, have reported positive effects of hypnosis on subjective parameters, such as asthma symptoms or medication use (60). The evidence that hypnosis produces enduring improvements in pulmonary function is mixed at best (60). Potential difficulties with hypnosis include the fact that only asthmatics who are sufficiently susceptible to hypnotic suggestion appear to benefit from this technique (55). Access to an experienced hypnotist and regular, long-term practice at home also appear to be necessary for benefits to be realized (60).

Yoga, hypnosis, and therapies that incorporate breathing techniques and relaxation are likely safe for most patients when used as an adjunct to conventional asthma therapy. Some authors, however, have raised the concern that these modalities may simply alter patient perception and promote tolerance to physiological warning signs of worsening asthma, such as wheezing, respiratory muscle fatigue, or carbon dioxide retention. This could delay institution of conventional treatment (61).

VII. Dietary Modifications

Special diets and vitamin and mineral supplements have proved popular with some patients with asthma (62). Dietary modifications include elimination diets and adherence to diets low in sodium (63). Dietary supplementation with magnesium (64), vitamin C (65), and selenium (66) have also been studied.

During elimination diets, foods such as seafood, milk, eggs, wheat, chocolate, cheeses, and nuts, which are believed to cause allergic reactions, are avoided (64). The efficacy of restricted diets for treatment of asthma has not been rigorously evaluated. In double-blind, placebo-controlled food challenges, however, the number of asthmatics who develop significant decrements in FEV_1 after ingesting particular foods is small, ranging from 2 to 7% (67–69). Immunoglobulin E-mediated responses to food appear to play a minor role in chronic adult asthma, although they may play a larger role in childhood asthma. Certain food additives, such as tartrazine, monosodium glutamate, and sodium metabisulfite may provoke bronchospasm and should be avoided by susceptible individuals. As long as adequate nutrition is maintained, elimination diets pose little health risk.

Magnesium has been shown in an in vitro study to relax rabbit bronchial smooth muscle (70). Intravenous magnesium infusion (1–3 g) had a modest, acute bronchodilator effect in emergency-department (71) and hospitalized (72) patients with asthma exacerbations: however, other investigators found no significant effects (73). Although some epidemiological evidence suggests that low dietary intake of magnesium is associated with a lower FEV_1 (74), asthmatics are not magnesium deficient, based on measurements of serum and blood cellular magnesium concentrations (75). Use of β2-agonists has been associated with reductions in skeletal muscle (76) and serum (77) magnesium concentrations; however, the clinical importance of these findings is uncertain. In chronic asthma, supplementation with 400 mg of magnesium per day for 3 weeks produced no significant improvement in FEV_1 or PD_{20} for methacholine, but it did reduce asthma symptom scores (78). Side effects of oral magnesium supplementation include dyspepsia and diarrhea (79). Patients with renal disease should not take magnesium supplements without medical supervision.

It has been proposed that asthmatic airways are subject to increased oxidative stress (80). Vitamin C (ascorbic acid) and selenium are antioxidants. Asthmatics have been reported to have lower plasma concentrations of vitamin C (81) and selenium (82) than controls, but it is not clear how these findings relate to airway inflammation or physiology (62). There is some evidence that short-term vitamin C supplementation (1–2 g/day) may decrease bronchospasm provoked by methacholine (83), exercise (84), and histamine (85), although negative results have also been reported (86). There is less evidence that either long-term vitamin C or selenium supplementation impacts chronic asthma. One 6-month study of vitamin C supplementation in 10 asthmatic children suggested that vitamin C may improve pulmonary function by reducing the frequency of upper respiratory tract infections or improving neutrophil chemotaxis (87). Selenium supplementation (100 μg/day for 14 days) in adult asthmatics was not associated with improvement in lung function or airway hyperresponsiveness to histamine (66). In large doses, vitamin C may cause dyspepsia, diarrhea, and nephrolithiasis. Vitamin C increases serum estrogen levels and reduces the anticoagulant effects of warfarin. Symptoms of selenium overdosage include nausea, vomiting, diarrhea, and fatigue (88).

Recognition of cysteinyl leukotrienes (LTC_4, LTD_4, and LTE_4) as mediators of bronchoconstriction and airway inflammation in asthma led to the hypothesis that a diet rich in fish oil will improve asthma. When ω-3 fatty acids found in fish oil are ingested, eicosapentaenoic acid and docosahexaenoic acid replace arachidonic acid in cell membranes. As a result, less arachidonic acid is available for synthesis of cysteinyl leukotrienes and LTB_4. Fish oil supplementation reduced cysteinyl leukotriene and LTB_4 production in stimulated peripheral blood mononuclear cells from normal subjects (89). In asthmatics, fish oil reduced peripheral blood neutrophil LTB_4 generation and chemotaxis (90), but it did not improve airway hyperresponsiveness to histamine or exercise, symptom severity, or bronchodilator use (90,91). Contrary to what might be expected, fish oil supplementation may have a deleterious effect in aspirin-sensitive asthma. In a study of 10 aspirin-intolerant asthmatics, fish oil supplementation was associated with a deterioration in asthma control, reflected by lower PEFR and greater broncho-dilator use (92). Side effects of fish oil include unpleasant taste, diarrhea, prolongation of bleeding time, and altered glucose metabolism (79).

VIII. Conclusions

The scientific evidence available to date does not support a role for CAM in the treatment of asthma. Although some CAM therapies appear to have positive effects in asthma, information about the potential risks, mechanisms of action, and benefits is limited. Significant methodological problems weaken conclusions that can be drawn from many studies. Subject groups, for example, are often small and poorly characterized with regard to asthma severity and use of conventional medications. Even in studies of better quality, the magnitude of effects reported is rarely equivalent to that obtained with conventional medications. Although some botanicals appear to have anti-inflammatory effects in vitro and in animal models, there is no convincing evidence that CAM therapies decrease airway inflammation in humans. All of these factors severely restrict application of results to contemporary clinical practice.

Despite limited information, it seems likely that some asthmatics, perhaps especially those with more severe disease, will continue to turn to CAM for relief. Some CAM therapies, such as yoga or relaxation, likely pose little harm to patients and may reduce the psychological stress of chronic asthma, which can be of significant value. Homeopathy, elimination diets, and vitamin and mineral supplements are relatively safe for most patients. Herbal remedies may pose a greater risk. However, discussing CAM openly with patients presents a unique opportunity to clarify the risks and benefits of both conventional and CAM therapies. Understanding the patient's cultural background and personal perspectives on chronic illness, which may motivate them to use CAM, can also strengthen the therapeutic alliance.

References

1. Eisenberg DM, Davis RB, Ettner SL, Appel S, Wilkey S, Van Rompay M, Kessler RC. Trends in alternative medicine use in the United States, 1990–1997: results of a follow-up national survey. J Am Med Assoc 1998; 280:1569–1575.

2. Astin JA. Why patients use alternative medicine: results of a national study. J Am Med Assoc 1998; 279:1548–1553.

3. Jonas WB. Alternative medicine—learning from the past, examining the present, advancing to the future. J Am Med Assoc 1998; 280:1616–1618.

4. Blanc PD, Kuschner WG, Katz PP, Smith S, Yelin EH. Use of herbal products, coffee or black tea, and over-the-counter medications as self-treatments among adults with asthma. J Allergy Clin Immunol 1997; 100:789–791.

5. Ernst E. Complementary therapies for asthma: what patients use. J Asthma 1998; 35:667–671.

6. Muller J, Clauson K. Pharmaceutical consideration of common herbal medicines. Am J Managed Care 1997; 3:1753–1770.

7. Bielory L, Lupoli K. Herbal interventions in asthma and allergy. J Asthma 1999; 36:1–65.

8. But P, Chang C. Chinese herbal medicine in the treatment of asthma and allergies. Clin Rev Allergy Immunol 1996; 14:253–269.

9. Ziment I. Unconventional therapy in asthma. Clin Rev Allergy Immunol 1996; 14: 289–320.

10. Fetrow C, Avila J. The Complete Guide to Herbal Medicines. Springhouse, PA: Springhouse Corporation, 1999.

11. Anonymous. Adverse events associated with ephedrine-containing products— Texas, December 1993–September 1995. J Am Med Assoc 1996; 276:1711–1712.

12. Popa VT. Clinical pharmacology of adrenergic drugs. J Asthma 1984; 21:183–207.

13. Koda A, Nishiyori T, Nagai H, Matsuura N, Tsuchiya H. [Anti-allergic actions of traditional oriental medicine—actions against types I and IV hypersensitivity reactions]. Nippon Yakurigaku Zasshi 1982; 80:31–41.

14. Hamasaki Y, Kobayashi I, Hayasaki R, Zaitu M, Muro E, Yamamoto S, Ichimaru T, Miyazaki S. The Chinese herbal medicine, shinpi-to, inhibits IgE-mediated leukotriene synthesis in rat basophilic leukemia-2H3 cells. J Ethnopharmacol 1997; 56: 123–131.

15. Nishiyori T, Tsuchiya H, Inagaki N. Effect of saiboku-to, a blended Chinese traditional medicine, on type I hypersensitivity reation, particularly on experimentally-caused asthma (Japanese, English abstract). Nippon Yakurigaku Zasshi-Folia Pharmacol Jpn 1983; 85:7–16.

16. Guinot P, Brambilla C, Duchier J, Braquet P, Bonvoisin B, Cournot A. Effect of BN 52063, a specific PAF-acether antagonist, on bronchial provocation test to allergens in asthmatic patients: a preliminary study. Prostaglandins 1987; 34:723–731.

17. Hsieh KH. Evaluation of efficacy of traditional Chinese medicines in the treatment of childhood bronchial asthma: clinical trial, immunological tests and animal study: Taiwan Asthma Study Group. Pediatr Allergy Immunol 1996; 7:130–140.

18. Hiai S, Yokoyama H, Oura H. Features of ginseng saponin-induced corticosterone secretion. Endocrinol Jpn 1979; 26:737–740.

19. Hiai S, Yokoyama H, Nagasawa T, Oura H. Stimulation of the pituitary–adrenocortical axis by saikosaponin of Bupleuri radix. Chem Pharm Bull (Tokyo) 1981; 29: 495–499.

20. MacKenzie MA, Hoefnagels WH, Jansen RW, Benraad TJ, Kloppenborg PW. The influence of glycyrrhetinic acid on plasma cortisol and cortisone in healthy young volunteers. J Clin Endocrinol Metab 1990; 70:1637–1643.

21. Homma M, Oka K, Ikeshima K, Takahashi N, Niitsuma T, Fukuda T, Itoh H. Different effects of traditional Chinese medicines containing similar herbal constituents on prednisolone pharmacokinetics. J Pharm Pharmacol 1995; 47:687–692.

22. Homma M, Oka K, Niitsuma T, Itoh H. A novel 11 beta-hydroxysteroid dehydrogenase inhibitor contained in saiboku-to, a herbal remedy for steroid-dependent bronchial asthma. J Pharm Pharmacol 1994; 46:305–309.

23. Egashira Y, Nagano H. A multicenter clinical trial of TJ-96 in patients with steroid-dependent bronchial asthma: a comparison of groups allocated by the envelope method. Ann NY Acad Sci 1993; 685:580–583.

24. Nakajima S, Tohda Y, Ohkawa K, Chihara J, Nagasaka Y. Effect of saiboku-to (TJ-96) on bronchial asthma: induction of glucocorticoid receptor, beta-adrenaline receptor, IgE-Fc epsilon receptor expression and its effect on experimental immediate and late asthmatic reaction. Ann NY Acad Sci 1993; 685:549–560.

25. Ernst E. Harmless herbs?: a review of the recent literature. Am J Med 1998; 104: 170–178.

26. Anonymous. Herbal roulette. Consumer Rep. 1995; November:698–705.

27. Temaru R, Yamashita N, Matsui S, Ohta T, Kawasaki A, Kobayashi M. [A case of drug induced pneumonitis caused by saiboku-To]. Nihon Kyobu Shikkan Gakkai Zasshi 1994; 32:485–490.

28. PDR. Physicians' Desk Reference for Herbal Medicines. Vol. 1. Montvale, NJ: Medical Economics Company, 1998:1244.

29. Blumenthal M, Goldberg A, Brinckmann J. Herbal Medicine. In: Blumenthal M, ed. Expanded Commission E. Monographs. Vol. 1. Newton: Integrative Medicine Communications, 2000:519.

30. Perharic L, Shaw D, Colbridge M, House I, Leon C, Murray V. Toxicological problems resulting from exposure to traditional remedies and food supplements. Drug Saf 1994; 11:284–294.

31. Reilly DT, Taylor MA, McSharry C, Aitchison T. Is homoeopathy a placebo response?: controlled trial of homoeopathic potency, with pollen in hayfever as model. Lancet 1986; 2:881–886.

32. Ludtke R, Wiesenauer M. [A meta-analysis of homeopathic treatment of pollinosis with Galphimia glauca]. Wien Med Wochenschr 1997; 147:323–327.

33. Reilly D, Taylor MA, Beattie NG, Campbell JH, McSharry C, Aitchison TC, Carter R, Stevenson RD. Is evidence for homoeopathy reproducible? Lancet 1994; 344: 1601–1606.

34. Kleijnen J, Knipschild P, ter Riet G. Clinical trials of homoeopathy [published erratum appears in Br Med J 1991; 302(6780):818]. Br Med J 1991; 302:316–323.

35. Linde K, Jobst KA. Homeopathy for chronic asthma. Cochrane Database Syst Rev 2000; 2.

36. Linde K, Clausius N, Ramirez G, Melchart D, Eitel F, Hedges LV, Jonas WB. Are the clinical effects of homeopathy placebo effects?: a meta-analysis of placebo-controlled trials [published erratum appears in Lancet 1998; 17;351(9097):220]. Lancet 1997; 350:834–843.

37. Wagner M. Is homeopathy 'new science' or 'new age'? Sci Rev Altern Med 1997; 1:7–12.

38. Yu DY, Lee SP. Effect of acupuncture on bronchial asthma. Clin Sci Mol Med 1976; 51:503–509.

39. Virsik K, Kristufek P, Bangha O, Urban S. The effect of acupuncture on pulmonary function in bronchial asthma. Prog Resp Res 1980; 14:271–275.

40. Takishima T, Mue S, Tamura G, Ishihara T, Watanabe K. The bronchodilating effect of acupuncture in patients with acute asthma. Ann Allergy 1982; 48:44–49.

41. Tandon MK, Soh PF. Comparison of real and placebo acupuncture in histamine-induced asthma: a double-blind crossover study. Chest 1989; 96:102–105.

42. Tashkin DP, Bresler DE, Kroening RJ, Kerschner H, Katz RL, Coulson A. Comparison of real and simulated acupuncture and isoproterenol in methacholine-induced asthma. Ann Allergy 1977; 39:379–387.

43. Fung KP, Chow OK, So SY. Attenuation of exercise-induced asthma by acupuncture. Lancet 1986; 2:1419–1422.

44. Chow OK, So SY, Lam WK, Yu DY, Yeung, CY. Effect of acupuncture on exercise-induced asthma. Lung 1983; 161:321–326.

45. Christensen PA, Laursen LC, Taudorf E, Sorensen SC, Weeke B. Acupuncture and bronchial asthma. Allergy 1984; 39:379–385.

46. Tashkin DP, Kroening RJ, Bresler DE, Simmons M, Coulson AH, Kerschnar H. A controlled trial of real and simulated acupuncture in the management of chronic asthma. J Allergy Clin Immunol 1985; 76:855–864.

47. Shao JM, Ding YD. Clinical observation on 111 cases of asthma treated by acupuncture and moxibustion. J Tradit Chin Med 1985; 5:23–25.

48. Choudhury KJ, FFoulkes-Crabbe DJO. Acupuncture for bronchial asthma. Altern Med 1989; 3:127–132.

49. MacPherson H. Fatal and adverse events from acupuncture: allegation, evidence, and the implications. J Altern Complement Med 1999; 5:47–56.

50. Lytle CD. Safety and regulation of acupuncture needles and other devices. Consensus Development Conference on Acupuncture, Bethesda, MD, Nov. 3–5, 1997.

51. Goyeche JR, Abo Y, Ikemi Y. Asthma: the yoga perspective. Part II: yoga therapy in the treatment of asthma. J Asthma 1982; 19:189–201.

52. Nagarathna R, Nagendra HR. Yoga for bronchial asthma: a controlled study. Br Med J (Clin Res Ed) 1985; 291:1077–1079.

53. Singh V, Wisniewski A, Britton J, Tattersfield A. Effect of yoga breathing exercises (pranayama) on airway reactivity in subjects with asthma. Lancet 1990; 335:1381–1383.

54. Vedanthan PK, Kesavalu LN, Murthy KC, Duvall K, Hall MJ, Baker S, Nagarathna S. Clinical study of yoga techniques in university students with asthma: a controlled study. Allergy Asthma Proc 1998; 19:3–9.

55. Ewer TC, Stewart DE. Improvement in bronchial hyper-responsiveness in patients with moderate asthma after treatment with a hypnotic technique: a randomised controlled trial. Br Med J (Clin Res Ed) 1986; 293:1129–1132.

56. Morrison JB. Chronic asthma and improvement with relaxation induced by hypnotherapy. J R Soc Med 1988; 81:701–704.

57. Ben-Zvi Z, Spohn WA, Young SH, Kattan M. Hypnosis for exercise-induced asthma. Am Rev Respir Dis 1982; 125:392–395.

58. Aronoff GM, Aronoff S, Peck LW. Hypnotherapy in the treatment of bronchial asthma. Ann Allergy 1975; 34:356–362.

59. Ferreiro O. Hypnosis—its use in acute attacks of bronchial asthma. Hypnosis 1993; 20:236.

60. Hackman RM, Stern JS, Gershwin ME. Hypnosis and asthma: a critical review. J Asthma 2000; 37:1–15.

61. Carlson CM, Sachs MI. Is alternative medicine an alternative for the treatment of asthma? [Editorial] J Asthma 1994; 31:149–151.
62. Monteleone CA, Sherman AR. Nutrition and asthma. Arch Intern Med 1997; 157: 23–34.
63. Burney PG, Neild JE, Twort CH, Chinn S, Jones TD, Mitchell WD, Bateman C, Cameron IR. Effect of changing dietary sodium on the airway response to histamine. Thorax 1989; 44:36–41.
64. Hackman RM, Stern JS, Gershwin ME. Complementary and alternative medicine and asthma. Clin Rev Allergy Immunol 1996; 14:321–336.
65. Bielory L, Gandhi R. Asthma and vitamin C. Ann Allergy 1994; 73:89–96.
66. Hasselmark L, Malmgren R, Zetterstrom O, Unge G. Selenium supplementation in intrinsic asthma. Allergy 1993; 48:30–36.
67. Onorato J, Merland N, Terral C, Michel FB, Bousquet J. Placebo-controlled double-blind food challenge in asthma. J Allergy Clin Immunol 1986; 78:1139–1146.
68. Novembre E, de Martino M, Vierucci A. Foods and respiratory allergy. J Allergy Clin Immunol 1988; 81:1059–1065.
69. Bock SA. Respiratory reactions induced by food challenges in children with pulmonary disease. Pediatr Allergy Immunol 1992; 3:188–194.
70. Spivey WH, Skobeloff EM, Levin RM. Effect of magnesium chloride on rabbit bronchial smooth muscle. Ann Emerg Med 1990; 19:1107–1112.
71. Skobeloff EM, Spivey WH, McNamara RM, Greenspon L. Intravenous magnesium sulfate for the treatment of acute asthma in the emergency department. J Am Med Assoc 1989; 262:1210–1213.
72. Noppen M, Vanmaele L, Impens N, Schandevyl W. Bronchodilating effect of intravenous magnesium sulfate in acute severe bronchial asthma. Chest 1990; 97:373–376.
73. Tiffany BR, Berk WA, Todd IK, White SR. Magnesium bolus or infusion fails to improve expiratory flow in acute asthma exacerbations. Chest 1993; 104:831–834.
74. Britton J, Pavord I, Richards K, Wisniewski A, Knox A, Lewis S, Tattersfield A, Weiss S. Dietary magnesium, lung function, wheezing, and airway hyperreactivity in a random adult population sample. Lancet 1994; 344:357–362.
75. de Valk HW, Kok PT, Struyvenberg A, van Rijn HJ, Haalboom JR, Kreukniet J, Lammers JW. Extracellular and intracellular magnesium concentrations in asthmatic patients. Eur Respir J 1993; 6:1122–1125.
76. Gustafson T, Boman K, Rosenhall L, Sandstrom T, Wester PO. Skeletal muscle magnesium and potassium in asthmatics treated with oral beta 2-agonists. Eur Respir J 1996; 9:237–240.
77. Bodenhamer J, Bergstrom R, Brown D, Gabow P, Marx JA, Lowenstein SR. Frequently nebulized beta-agonists for asthma: effects on serum electrolytes. Ann Emerg Med 1992; 21:1337–1342.
78. Hill J, Micklewright A, Lewis S, Britton J. Investigation of the effect of short-term change in dietary magnesium intake in asthma. Eur Respir J 1997; 10:2225–2229.
79. Drug Facts and Comparisons, 2000 Edition. St. Louis: Wolters Kluwer Company, 2000.
80. Greene LS. Asthma, oxidant stress, and diet. Nutrition 1999; 15:899–907.

81. Aderele WI, Ette SI, Oduwole O, Ikpeme SJ. Plasma vitamin C (ascorbic acid) levels in asthmatic children. Afr J Med Med Sci 1985; 14:115–120.

82. Stone J, Hinks LJ, Beasley R, Holgate ST, Clayton BA. Reduced selenium status of patients with asthma. Clin Sci 1989; 77:495–500.

83. Mohsenin V, Dubois AB, Douglas JS. Effect of ascorbic acid on response to methacholine challenge in asthmatic subjects. Am Rev Respir Dis 1983; 127:143–147.

84. Schachter EN, Schlesinger A. The attenuation of exercise-induced bronchospasm by ascorbic acid. Ann Allergy 1982; 49:146–151.

85. Bucca C, Rolla G, Oliva A, Farina JC. Effect of vitamin C on histamine bronchial responsiveness of patients with allergic rhinitis. Ann Allergy 1990; 65:311–314.

86. Malo JL, Cartier A, Pineau L, L'Archeveque J, Ghezzo H, Martin RR. Lack of acute effects of ascorbic acid on spirometry and airway responsiveness to histamine in subjects with asthma. J Allergy Clin Immunol 1986; 78:1153–1158.

87. Anderson R, Hay I, van Wyk H, Oosthuizen R, Theron A. The effect of ascorbate on cellular humoral immunity in asthmatic children. S Afr Med J 1980; 58:974–977.

88. Parfitt K, ed. Martindale, The Complete Drug Reference. London, UK: Pharmaceutical Press, 1999:1353–1354.

89. Lee TH, Hoover RL, Williams JD, Sperling RI, Ravalese JD, Spur BW, Robinson DR, Corey EJ, Lewis RA, Austen KF. Effect of dietary enrichment with eicosapentaenoic and docosahexaenoic acids on in vitro neutrophil and monocyte leukotriene generation and neutrophil function. J Engl J Med 1985; 312:1217–1224.

90. Arm JP, Horton CE, Mencia-Huerta JM, House F, Eiser NM, Clark TJ, Spur BW, Lee TH. Effect of dietary supplementation with fish oil lipids on mild asthma. Thorax 1988; 43:84–92.

91. Thien FC, Mencia-Huerta JM, Lee TH. Dietary fish oil effects on seasonal hay fever and asthma in pollen- sensitive subjects. Am Rev Respir Dis 1993; 147:1138–1143.

92. Picado C, Castillo JA, Schinca N, Pujades M, Ordinas A, Coronas A, Agusti-Vidal A. Effects of a fish oil enriched diet on aspirin intolerant asthmatic patients: a pilot study. Thorax 1988; 43:93–97.

11

Gastroesophageal Reflux in Severe Asthma

DONNA L. BRATTON

National Jewish Medical and Research Center
Denver, Colorado

PHILIP D. HANNA

Rocky Mountain Gastrointestinal Motility Center
Swedish Medical Center
Englewood, Colorado

I. Introduction

Retrograde movement of gastric contents into the esophagus is gastroesophageal reflux (GER). While both asthma and gastroesophageal reflux disease (GERD) are common in the general population, mounting data place GERD as a substantial contributor to asthma in many patients. There is a higher prevalence of GERD in patients with asthma than in the general population, and recent studies have begun to shed light on the mechanisms by which GERD alters airway function. Importantly, improvement in asthma with newer and more effective treatment of GERD underscores the importance of its identification and treatment. The fact that GERD can be silent in as many as 33% of adults with asthma (1,2) and 44% of infants with daily wheezing (3) necessitates a high index of suspicion, even in the absence of symptoms. Furthermore, evidence suggests that just as GERD can exacerbate asthma, asthma can exacerbate GERD, establishing a vicious cycle. As such, GERD must always be considered in the treatment of the patient with severe asthma. It should be noted, however, that most of our research on asthma and GERD that demonstrates their intimate association and interlocked mechanisms and treatment has been conducted in populations without regard to stratification for disease severity—for either asthma or GERD. Hence the discussion of GERD in severe asthma must at times be drawn from indirect and imperfect data.

II. GERD Prevalence in the Normal Population and in Asthma

Over 20% of the American population has symptomatic acid reflux at least once per month and 7% has daily heartburn (4,5). On the other hand, infrequent acid reflux is a normal, physiologic event. It is more frequent in the upright position than in the supine position (with ''normal'' reflux occurring between 4–6% of total upright time and less than 1.2% of total supine time).

Since some acid reflux is normal, the question is what constitutes ''abnormal'' acid reflux? The most widely used criteria are those developed by Johnson and Demeester (6) utilizing data from 24-h probe testing. A numerical score is derived that estimates the potential for the development of *histologic* esophagitis. This score does not directly reflect the amount of acid reflux that is present but numerically weights some reflux events (e.g., nocturnal or prolonged) greater than others since they are more likely to produce *esophageal* damage. Extrapolating the use of this score to other organ systems may not be appropriate. There is some evidence of a correlation between the degree of esophageal damage and asthma symptoms (see below), but studies utilizing esophageal acid perfusion before and after healing of esophagitis have not been done to verify this impression.

The prevalence of abnormal acid reflux in asthma patients is even less clear. Various studies have put the figure between 32–80% (1,7–10), but two representative recent series show a prevalence of GER in adults and children with asthma between 60–80% and 50–75%, respectively (11,12), which is much higher than that seen in the general population. This wide range is due to differences in how GERD is determined. Researchers have relied on patient reports of heartburn. Bernstein provocation studies, 24-h pH testing, and so on. The latter is by far the most reliable and ''silent'' (i.e., nonreported) reflux has been found consistently in one-quarter to one-third of asthma patients (2,13) and more recently in as many as 62% (14).

In a recent study by Field et al., 109 asthma patients referred to a university-based outpatient asthma clinic were questioned for symptoms of GER and asthma medication use (15). Their answers were compared to those of nonasthmatic subjects attending either a research or family practice clinic. Asthma patients, compared to control subjects, experienced significantly ($P < 0.05$) more heartburn (45% vs. 11%), regurgitation (21% vs. 10%), and dysphagia (24% vs. 10%) during the week prior to the clinic visit (15). Similar differences between asthma and control groups were seen if symptoms were scored for the previous 3 or 6 weeks. Of note, 41% of asthmatic subjects noted respiratory symptoms associated with GERD symptoms and 28% used rescue inhalers while experiencing GERD symptoms. Inhaler use was correlated with both severity of heartburn and regurgitation. A recent study by Harding et al. (1) has shown that 78% of respiratory symptoms (90% of coughs) were associated with esophageal acid events (as determined by 24-h pH testing). Studies of children with severe asthma have shown similarly high prevalence of GERD. In a recent outcome study, GERD was demonstrated in 57% of 98 consecutively evaluated children referred for severe asthma to the National Jewish Medical and Research Center (16). Similarly, Shapiro and Christie found a prevalence of 47% among children with steroid-dependent asthma (17). In infants with daily wheezing, 64% (54 of 84) evaluated by 24-h esophageal pH monitoring were found to have GERD (3). An important question, but one that has received little attention to date, is whether the use of increasingly effective asthma medications (including systemic corticosteroids), may modulate the symptoms of GERD or the inflammatory component (esophageal or airway—see below) such that the relationship of GER in severe asthma is obscured. The presence of possible atypical or extrapulmonary manifestations of GERD should further raise suspicion for this diagnosis (Table 1).

The prevalence and importance of GERD in nocturnal asthma is still debated. It is clear that nocturnal reflux is more damaging to the esophagus (i.e., causes greater histologic damage) than upright reflux because of more prolonged acid contact with the mucosa. In a small study of pediatric patients with severe nocturnal asthma (symptoms $\geq$ to 100 nights or mornings per year), 10 of 18 (56%) had a positive esophageal acid perfusion test (the "Bernstein test" has unclear significance in this setting) compared to 16% of patients with less severe asthma (18). In a study conducted in the early 1980s at National Jewish in Denver, 64% of 25 children with severe asthma with a nocturnal component were diagnosed with abnormal GERD (19). In a recent study, Cuttitta et al. (20) continuously and simultaneously monitored esophageal pH and airway resistances in 7 asthmatic subjects with moderate to severe GERD. They found a significant

Table 1 Extrapulmonary and Atypical Manifestations of GERD

Pharyngitis	Loss of dental enamel
Paroxysmal laryngospasm	Odynophagia
Vocal cord dysfunction	Dysphagia
Laryngitis	Breathlessnes
Dysphonia	Obstructive sleep apnea
Persistent cough	Noncardiac chest pain
Water brash	Growth failure (children)
Otalgia	Iron deficiency anemia
Sinusitis	

increase in lower respiratory resistance during both short- (<5 min) and long- (>5 min) duration reflux episodes. There was also a correlation between the area under the curve of lower airway resistance and the duration of the reflux episode. This is in contradistinction to the findings of Tan (21), possibly because that group studied only patients with mild GERD.

Concurrent with the many changes in the physiology of the airway (see Chapter 10) there are multiple changes involving the gastrointestinal system that occur during sleep (22,23). These include decreased gastric emptying (causing increased reflux), decreased esophageal motility (which may cause prolonged esophageal acid contact time), and decreased upper esophageal sphincter pressure (increased risk of aspiration). Just as in airway physiology, circadian rhythms may play a role as well. Plasma epinephrine levels are lower and parasympathetic tone increases at night (23). There may also be a circadian change in circulating hormones that modulate pulmonary lymphocyte release of proinflammatory cyto-kines (23). Such pervasive hormonal and inflammatory events may impact GI tract functioning and inflammation as well. In addition, as noted below, proton pump inhibitor (PPI) therapy is less effective at controlling acid production at night. All of these factors, and probably others, could contribute to worsening of both nocturnal asthma and GERD.

The degree of esophageal damage may be an important determinant in the possible relationship of GERD and asthma. GERD obviously can cause a wide spectrum of esophageal disease ranging from heartburn without macroscopic mu-cosal damage, to frank ulcerations, to Barrett's mucosa, with its associated in-creased risk of cancer. In a prospective study, Sontag (24) performed endoscopy on 186 consecutive asthma patients irrespective of their complaints of GERD. Thirty-nine percent were found to have esophageal mucosal erosions, ulcerations, or Barrett's mucosa. El-Serag (25) evaluated the records of 101,366 VA patients with a discharge diagnosis of erosive esophagitis or esophageal stricture. The odds-ratio for a concomitant diagnosis of asthma was 1.51 (CI 1.43–1.59).

Several studies have suggested that frank esophagitis increases the severity of asthma symptoms. Nakase (26) studied 72 adult asthmatics, all of whom under-went endoscopy. Group 1 ($n = 52$) had no mucosal breaks, Group 2 ($n = 15$) had mucosal erythema or erosions and Group 3 ($n = 5$) had frank ulcerations. Groups 2 and 3 all received treatment consisting of lansoprozole (30 mg q.d.) and cisapride (2.5 mg b.i.d.) for 8 weeks. Prior to treatment, the severity of asthma was graded 1–4 based on the scale outlined in the *Global Strategy for Asthma Management and Prevention* (27). Asthmatics with the worst mucosal disease (Group 3) had the most severe asthma at the initiation of therapy and this was the only group to show significant improvement in both morning and evening PEFR. Group 3 also was the only one to show a significant decrease in inhaled bronchodilator use compared to pretreatment. Anderson (28) performed esopha-geal acid infusions in three groups of patients: Group 1, esophagitis but no asthma

(n = 10); Group 2, asthma but no esophagitis (n = 21); and Group 3, asthma plus esophagitis (n = 8). Only Group 3 experienced a significant increase in pulmonary airway resistance (Raw) and a decrease in peak expiratory flow rate (PEF).

Why would the presence of esophagitis increase the severity of asthma? Mucosal breaks could increase the neurogenic afferent input to the brainstem and, therefore, bronchoconstrictive vagal efferent output to the airways (see discussion below). No studies have been done in asthma, but Ing et al. (29) showed that in cough patients whose cough was stimulated by esophageal acid perfusion, pretreatment of the esophagus with lignocaine blocked the precipitation of coughing. Presumably, the afferent limb of the autonomic reflex was blocked.

III. The Vicious Cycle of Asthma and GERD

As stated above, asthma, particularly severe asthma, can predispose to GERD just as GERD can contribute to asthma severity, thus establishing a vicious cycle. An understanding of the interlocked mechanisms by which these two disorders affect each other is important in our understanding of disease pathogenesis (Table 2).

Table 2 Factors That Contribute to the Vicious Cycle of Asthma and GERD

Factors Seen in Asthma that Promote GERD
    Transient LES relaxations—may be increased due to autonomic dysfunction in asthma
    LES hypotension—may be increased due to autonomic dysfunction in asthma
    Hiatal hernia
    Esophageal dysmotility
    Pulmonary hyperinflation
    Cough
    Obesity
    Upper airway resistance syndrome
    Obstructive apnea
    Steroid-induced myopathy (diaphragm)
    Asthma medications—particularly theophylline and oral β-agonists; corticosteroids?
Mechanisms by Which GERD Aggravates Asthma
    Reflex-mediated alterations of respiratory function—laryngo- and bronchoesophageal reflexes
    Airway hyperresponsiveness
    Neurogenic inflammation
    Microaspiration

A. Factors That Promote GERD in Patients with Asthma

Pathologic GERD is caused by two mechanisms. A hypotensive lower esophageal sphincter (LES) with a resting pressure of less than 10 mmHg can lead to reflux. (Surgeons would include a shortened LES or the displacement of the LES into the chest in the definition of a defective LES.) However, 65–75% of all patients with GERD have normal resting LES pressure and a normal anatomical LES. In these cases GERD is due to abnormal transient LES relaxations (TLESRs) (30). TLESRs are responsible for the belching reflex and are normal. In patients with GERD, they occur more frequently, are more prolonged, and are more likely to lead to reflux of gastric contents (30). Relaxation of the LES is mediated through the vagus nerve with nitric oxide as the postganglionic neurotransmitter. The crural diaphragm normally relaxes to admit food boluses to the stomach and also relaxes during TLESRs via a brainstem reflex and the phrenic nerve, but what mediates relaxation is not fully understood. Recent evidence indicates that γ-amino butyric acid is involved as a central inhibitory neurotransmitter (31).

Lower Esophageal Sphincter Hypotension

Lower esophageal sphincter (LES) hypotension is prevalent in asthma. Kjellen et al. (32) found that 27% of asthmatics had LES hypotension. Sontag et al. (11) found that of 104 consecutively studied asthma patients, LES pressures were significantly lower than those of controls, with asthmatics registering mean pressures of 12.6 vs 18.4 mmHg for normal controls. Low LES pressure alone, however, is not sufficient to cause GERD. Normally, the LES pressure rises when the valve is subjected to the stress of increased intragastric pressure (i.e., a normally responsive LES). This LES pressure rise should be higher than the rise in intragastric pressure, thus preventing acid reflux. However, in chronic GERD, esophageal damage can cause the LES to be less responsive, often allowing intragastric pressure to rise above LES pressure, which results in flow of material into the esophagus.

Other Factors That Alter LES Function

Other stresses on the LES also can lead to reflux. Studies have shown that acute bronchospasm (induced by histamine or methacholine inhalation) in asthma patients results in the generation of greater pleural negative pressure and increases the frequency of GER (33). During maximum inspiratory efforts, normal subjects can generate transdiaphragmatic pressures of 300 cmH_2O without causing GER (34). This huge pressure difference is mitigated by augmentation of LES pressure by crural diaphragm contraction, which compresses the LES as the diaphragm flattens during inspiration (Fig. 1). Several factors may alter this protective mechanism in patients with asthma. First, the presence of a hiatal hernia (whether

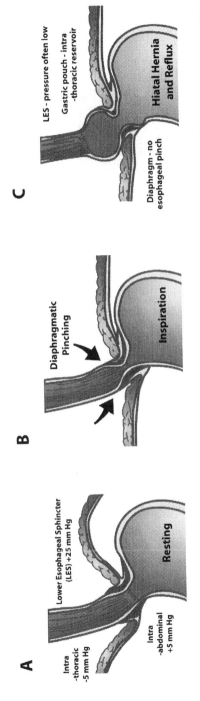

Figure 1 Diaphragmatic augmentation of LES pressure and hiatal hernia effect. (A) At end expiration, the diaphragm is relaxed and the transdiaphragmatic pressure difference of 10 mmHg is more than offset by the normal LES resting pressure of 25 mmHg and reflux is prevented. (B) At end inspiration, the diaphragm has contracted and "pinches" the gastroesophageal (GE) junction, which augments the LES pressure. This counters the increase in negative intrathoracic pressure, which accompanies inspiration, and reflux is prevented. (C) A hiatal hernia displaces the GE junction into the chest. When the diaphragm contracts with inspiration, the LES pressure is not augmented and the "pinch" occurs below the LES. This actually increases the likelihood of reflux since a reservoir is created just below the LES. When the LES opens (during normal swallowing or during TLESR's), gastric fluid is waiting just below and is more easily refluxed.

transient or fixed) displaces the LES into the chest and prevents this pressure augmentation. Hiatal hernias (HH) are more frequently found in asthmatics and contribute to the observed increase in GERD. Carmona-Sanchez found HH in 62% of asthmatics and in 34% of controls ($P = 0.02$) (35). Also, TLESRs are more frequent in patients with HH, thus leading to increased reflux (36). Acid reflux itself may be causal in the development of hiatal hernia. In animal models, esophageal acidification results in esophageal shortening through longitudinal smooth muscle fiber contraction, which can ultimately lead to submucosal fibrosis (37,38).

Second, hyperinflation of the lungs in severe airway obstruction flattens the diaphragm (which places the crural diaphragm at a functional disadvantage, therefore contributing to LES dysfunction) and increases abdominal pressure promoting GER (39–41). Additionally, crural diaphragm contraction is inhibited during TLESRs and thus the thoracoabdominal pressure difference that can increase during more forceful inspiration is not effectively neutralized and leads to reflux. Of importance, bronchodilator therapy alone in the absence of specific GERD therapy can improve GER (42).

Obesity also increases intraabdominal pressure and promotes GERD. In a recent study of 80 school-age children and adolescents admitted for evaluation of severe asthma at National Jewish, 50% were either morbidly obese [body mass index (BMI) >95th percentile] or at risk of morbid obesity (BMI >85th percentile). Increasing BMI was significantly associated with the diagnosis of GERD ($P < 0.01$) and correlated with oral corticosteroid dose and poor functional endurance (both $P < 0.0001$) (16). Additionally, the association of upper airway resistance syndrome and obstructive sleep apnea, more frequent in obese subjects, has been positively correlated with GERD (43). Data suggest that obstructive sleep apnea will increase negative intrathoracic pressures, which will aggravate GERD, and that GERD can contribute to obstructive sleep apnea perhaps by contributing to arousals that disturb sleep architecture (43–47). These factors—hyperinflation, lower and/or upper airway obstruction, coughing, and obesity—are frequently encountered in the patient with severe asthma, can exacerbate GERD, and must be specifically addressed in the treatment of severe asthma.

Esophageal Dysmotility

Since all people have some reflux, the esophagus is called upon to quickly remove the acid. Gravity helps when the body is held upright. But reflux also initiates esophageal contraction waves that push the acid back into the stomach ("secondary peristaltic contractions"). GERD patients frequently have ineffective esophageal peristalsis, which can lead to poor esophageal acid clearance. This is manifested primarily as low-amplitude contractions or nontransmitted contractions.

Kahrilas found that 25% of GERD patients with mild esophagitis and 48% with ulcerative esophagitis had peristaltic dysfunction (48). Fouad found that 53% of asthma patients had ineffective esophageal motility compared to only 19% of nonasthmatics with heartburn (49). Kjellen et al. (32) found that 38% of 97 consecutively studied asthmatics had evidence of dysmotility and Campo (28) demonstrated it in 68% of asthmatics in a smaller series. Esophageal acid contact time is greater in asthma patients than in healthy controls and has been demonstrated to be abnormal in 32–82% of asthmatic patients (1,11,49,50). Sontag et al. (11) found that 82% (85/104) of consecutive asthma patients (recruited regardless of the presence or absence of reflex symptoms) had elevated esophageal acid contact times. Prolonged esophageal acid contact time is often seen during supine positioning during sleep (50) and is thought to aggravate nocturnal asthma. Although some studies have not shown an association of nocturnal asthma and GERD (21,51,52), delayed clearance of esophageal acid in sleep has been associated with nocturnal asthma by others (19,53,54) (see above).

Autonomic Dysregulation of Esophageal Function

Since both LES pressure and TLESRs are autonomically regulated, and since autonomic dysregulation (with increased cholinergic activity; see Chapter 4) has been demonstrated in asthmatic subjects (53,55–57), the hypothesis of autonomic dysregulation of esophageal function in patients with asthma and GERD is obvious. Lodi et al. (58), using 73 autonomic function tests of the cardiovascular system, demonstrated that a hypervagal response was present in 51% (8/15), a hyperadrenergic response in 8%, and a mixed response in 14% of asthmatic subjects with GERD. Though the assessments were confined to effects of the vagus on the cardiovascular system, these findings corroborate others, suggesting generalized autonomic dysfunction in asthma. Whether autonomic dysfunction of the esophagus in patients with asthma (particularly severe asthma) and GERD will be identified remains to be seen.

Medications Used in the Treatment of Asthma

Medications used for the treatment of asthma have long been suspected of contributing to GERD. Slow-release theophylline has been shown to lower LES pressure and increase reflux by as much as 24% (17,59), although others have not found this association (1,60). Oral β-agonists may also decrease LES pressure (61); however, inhaled agents have been found to cause no significant change in GERD parameters, pH probe, or esophageal motility studies (11,62–65). Studies looking for association of GERD and asthma therapy in subjects undergoing treatment with various medications have found the association to be independent of drug therapy for asthma (11,15,18,66,67). In the patient with severe steroid-dependent asthma, it has been hypothesized that myopathy of the crural diaphragm may contribute significantly to LES dysfunction (68,69,70). No studies have been done to evaluate the effects of steroids on esophageal function, but reflux esophagitis, esophageal dysmotility, and LES hypotension have been found to be more common in patients with Cushing's syndrome (71).

B. Mechanisms by Which GERD Contributes to Asthma

Review of the literature shows that there is evidence from animal and human studies for (1) reflex-mediated changes in pulmonary functioning; (2) heightened nonspecific airway hyperreactivity and (3) neurogenic airway inflammation, all resulting from esophageal acidification/injury; and (4) bronchoconstriction and airway inflammation resulting from microaspiration of refluxed material.

Reflex-Mediated Changes in Pulmonary Functioning in GER

Changes in pulmonary functioning in animals and humans in response to either acid reflux or acid infusion into the esophagus have been demonstrated. These include changes in airway caliber and function as measured by increased pulmonary resistance and decreased compliance, peak expiratory flow rate, FEV_1, and arterial blood gas (72). Esophageal acid instillation or distention of the esophagus by an intraesophageal balloon in a dog model increased respiratory resistance, a response that was ablated by vagotomy (73). In humans, Wright et al. (74) found significant reductions in airflow and arterial oxygen saturation after esophageal acid infusion. Schan et al. (66) found that esophageal acid infusion caused a small but significant decrease in PEF in asthma patients with GERD, asthma patients without GERD, GERD patients without asthma, and normal controls. Asthma subjects were found to have more pronounced decrements in PEF that persisted past the time required for acid clearance (66). A second infusion of normal saline restored the PEF in all subjects except for the patients with asthma and GERD, whose PEF remained low. Similarly, acid infusions have shown continued increases in specific airway resistance 40 min after acid clearance form the esophagus (75). A small but significant drop in FEV_1 was documented in a study of moderate to severe asthmatics and this drop in function correlated with the level of bronchial hyperresponsiveness (52).

Of note, changes in airway function have shown dependence on the amount of acid instilled and may be delayed for up to 90 min or more (76), and thus some studies may not have assessed optimally for changes in pulmonary function. Another confounding factor is the presence of a positive Bernstein test (sensation of pain during an esophageal acid infusion test) as a measure of esophageal inflammation. Whereas some studies have shown altered pulmonary function regardless of Bernstein test positivity, other studies have demonstrated these changes only in patients exhibiting a positive Bernstein test (28,32,72,77,78).

This would suggest that a certain severity of GERD or esophageal inflammation may be required to see demonstrable effects on pulmonary function (see above). While the above studies describe significant changes in airway caliber/ function, the magnitude of such changes was generally near the threshold for statistical significance [reviewed in (79)]. Indeed, other studies have not demonstrated significant changes in airway caliber or function following esophageal acid infusion (21,80). More subtle, but probably more common, are changes in minute ventilation, respiratory rate, and the sensation of dyspnea [discussed in (81)]. To this end, Field et al. (82) showed in a group of nonasthmatic subjects with esophageal disease that esophageal acid infusion resulted in significant increases in respiratory rate (13.6 to 15.8 breaths/min) and minute ventilation (7.1 to 8.5 L/min) while not changing other respiratory parameters. Chest discomfort and sensation of respiratory effort were correlated with minute ventilation. Again, the changes in the latter were most pronounced in subjects reporting a positive Bernstein test. As these subjects did not have asthma, such studies should be conducted in asthmatic patients of varying severity and hyperresponsivity. Of note, changes in minute ventilation, respiratory rate, and the sensation of dyspnea may well result in increased use of bronchodilators (15,83), which in theory can contribute to β-agonist desensitization and worsening asthma (84). Certainly, dyspnea seemingly out of proportion with changes in pulmonary function should prompt investigation to rule out abnormal GERD rather than prompt an escalation of asthma medication (2,82,85,86).

Both the tracheobronchial tree and the esophagus originate embryonically from the foregut and as such share vagal innervation, which includes sensory afferents and noncholinergic, nonadrenergic efferents (NANC) (see Chapter 4), in addition to cholinergic innervation. For the most part, the changes in airway caliber/function from esophageal acid infusion have been ablated by anticholinergic agents (74,75,87), demonstrating that the cholinergic fibers running in the vagus nerve are largely responsible for the changes in airway caliber/function. The discovery of esophageal mechanochemoreceptors which affect bronchial tone (75,88), with similarities to receptors localized to other extrapulmonic sites (nasopharynx and sinuses) (89–91), establishes the afferent arm. As such, esophageal mechanical distention, irritation, or frank injury from acid and possibly other refluxed material (pepsin, bile salts, and activated pancreatic enzymes) (92,93) initiates a reflex arch that results in changes in airway functioning.

Airway Hyperresponsiveness in GERD

Several studies have shown that the finding of excessive GER or esophageal acid infusion is associated with enhanced bronchial reactivity to various nonspecific agents. Herve et al. (94) studied the effect of acid infusion on subsequent response to isocapnic hyperventilation and methacholine responsiveness. They found that following acid infusion the degree of bronchospasm exhibited was significantly increased (approximately doubled) to a given challenge with dry air. Additionally, the provocative dose of methacholine producing a 20% reduction in FEV_1 (PC_{20}) was significantly reduced. Similarly, an increase in reactivity to histamine following ingestion of a dilute acid drink (pH 3.1) was also found in 8 of 18 children with moderate to severe asthma, the majority of whom also exhibited abnormal nocturnal GER on pH probe monitoring (76). Of note, baseline pulmonary function was not altered by ingestion of acid except in two children given a 10-fold stronger solution. Similarly to the effects of acid infusion on changes in airway caliber/function described above, the hyperresponsiveness of the airway to esophageal acid is also blocked by atropine given prior to acid instillation (94).

Interesting work from Vincent et al. (7) showed that in 105 consecutive patients, methacholine PC_{20} correlated with the number of reflux episodes on 24-h pH testing. Similarly, Erkstrom and Tibbling (95) demonstrated that bronchial reactivity to histamine was correlated with subclinical bronchospasm in asthmatic patients with reflux-associated respiratory symptoms. Together these data suggest that GER primes the airways to be more hyperresponsive to a host of irritant and nonspecific stimuli. Though severe asthma has not been extensively studied, the implications of this work are that in patients with severe asthma and GERD, treatment of GERD may decrease their overall hyperresponsiveness and need for medication, though this has not been formally tested.

Neurogenic Inflammation in GER

Though it is known that inflammation in severe asthma is heterogeneous, no thorough assessment of airway inflammation has been made to date in patients with asthma with and without GERD or before and after effective GERD therapy in those patients with GERD. The possibility of neurogenic inflammation in GERD-induced airway disease comes from an evolving understanding of neurogenic inflammation induced in several rodent species but also in the skin (96), nose (97,98), and gut of humans (99).

As described above, unmyelinated sensory afferent nerves are localized in the airway and esophageal epithelium, where they are stimulated by a variety of noxious chemical and mechanical stimuli. Such stimulation leads to centrally integrated neurotransmission that results in the perception of pain and protective reflexes (e.g., cough and laryngo- or bronchospasm) as well as antidromic stimulation by local axon reflexes of nonadrenergic, noncholinergic nerve fibers running in the vagus nerve to the viscera (airways and esophagus). These local axon reflexes result in the release of the proinflammatory tachykinins (substance P and neurokinin A) that cause vasodilation, plasma extravasation, smooth muscle contraction (bronchospasm), modulation of airway parasympathetic activity, mucus secretion, and inflammatory cell recruitment (96,100,101–104). Interesting work by Hamamoto et al. (105), using a guinea pig model, has shown that acid instillation into the esophagus resulted in neurogenic airway edema. Mechanistically, it appeared that this involved local axon reflexes between the esophagus and airways, resulting in release of substance P into the airways. This response was inhibited by a substance P inhibitor and was enhanced by inhibition of neutral endopeptidase, an enzyme responsible for degradation of substance P. The animals had been atropinized to ablate effects of the cholinergic system and vagotomy only partially ablated the response. Aspiration of the infusate was not required for these responses, as the esophagus had been separated and surgically closed proximally.

No studies of neurogenic inflammation in GERD exacerbation of asthma have been explored in humans. However, there is some evolving evidence for abnormal NANC activity in humans with asthma (see Chapter 4). Tachykinin-containing nerves are generally sparse in human airways (101,106), but some investigators have reported increased density and altered morphology of substance P-containing nerve fibers in asthmatic airways compared to those of normal airways (107), though this has not been confirmed by others (108–110). The receptors for tachykinins NK_1 and NK_2 have been demonstrated on airway smooth muscle, blood vessels, glands, airway ganglion neurons, and on airway epithelium (102,111–113) and expression of NK_2 mRNA has been demonstrated to be greater in subjects with asthma than in normal subjects (114). Finally, the tachykinins have been shown to cause bronchospasm (106,115,116; and see Chapter 4), and increased levels of tachykinins have been identified in the bronchoalveolar lavage fluid and sputum of subjects with asthma and are associated with acute bronchospasm (117,118). However, to date, employment of tachykinin antagonists have been disappointing in the mediation of nonspecific bronchoconstrictory stimuli (hypertonic saline and exercise) (119,120). Ultimately, defining the role of tachykinins in mediating neurogenic airway inflammation and airway functional changes due to GERD awaits the use of specific and potent antagonists in trials of selected patients with asthma and GERD.

Microaspiration

Compared to the relatively small decrements in airway caliber/function following esophageal acid infusion discussed above, microaspiration of refluxed acid or application of acid directly to the tracheal mucosa in animals (to simulate microaspiration) leads to significant reductions in airway functioning in the absence of chemical pneumonitis (41,121). Tuchman et al. (121) showed in a feline model that 10 mL of acid instilled into the esophagus resulted in a 1.5-fold increase in total lung resistance, whereas 0.5 mL instilled into the trachea resulted in a 5-fold increase. Three methods have been used in the attempt to identify microaspiration in humans with GERD and asthma: pH probe testing, radioisotope scanning, and recovery of lipid-laden macrophages at bronchoscopy (75,122–125). Dual-channel 24-h pH testing has been used to differentiate between distal and proximal esophageal acid exposure: pH electrodes are placed 5 cm above the lower esophageal sphincter (LES) and just below the upper esophageal sphincter (UES). While distal esophageal acidification is much more common than proximal acidification–e.g., Gastall et al. found that abnormal distal acid reflux was twice as common as proximal acid reflux in 27 asthmatics over a 24-h period (126)—proximal reflux (PR) raises the possibility of microaspiration (75,126–128). When PR is associated with simultaneous symptoms, aspiration is assumed to have occurred. This assumption may not be correct since distal esophageal acidification has also occurred and the symptoms may be reflexive. Several studies have not demonstrated a reliable relationship between PR and symptoms in asthmatics (9,127,129) despite showing a relationship between symptoms and distal reflux. Furthermore, studies employing radioisotope techniques generally fail to demonstrate microaspiration (130,131), and the use of lipid-laden alveolar macrophages recovered at bronchoscopy to make the diagnosis is neither specific nor highly sensitive. However, aspiration does sometimes occur. Varkey (132) used dual-channel recording (one electrode in the proximal esophagus and one just above the upper esophageal sphincter in the pharynx) in 19 asthmatics and showed that proximal reflux occurred in 31% of distal esophageal reflux episodes. Five percent of these proximal reflux events were associated with pharyngeal reflux. Jack et al. (133) monitored esophageal and tracheal pH simultaneously in 4 patients with severe asthma. There were 37 episodes of prolonged (i.e., >5 min) proximal acid reflux and 5 of these were associated with tracheal acidification. Significant deterioration of pulmonary function was noted during these aspiration episodes. Overall, it is thought that microaspiration plays a role in a minority of adults with asthma, though it may be more common in young children, where it has been causally linked to chronic cough and recurrent pneumonias as well as asthma (particularly nocturnal asthma) (53,134). Further testing, possibly on selected subgroups of patients, is needed.

Mechanistically, in animal models the increase in total lung resistance induced by direct tracheal acidification can be abolished by bilateral cervical vagotomy, again demonstrating the role of the vagus nerve in this bronchoconstrictory (and bronchoprotective) response (135). Aspiration of acid (and other noxious components of refluxate) may also induce nonspecific bronchial hyperreactivity by altering airway afferent nerve excitability (100). Alternatively, cytokines and mediators produced at the site of airway epithelial injury may recruit inflammatory cells or generate tachykinin-mediated inflammation and bronchoconstriction via local axon reflexes (see above) (136). In the extreme, massive aspiration results in profound inflammation of the lungs and respiratory distress and injury (137–140).

IV. Diagnosis of GERD in the Patient with Severe Asthma

A. Diagnostic Tests

Barium Swallow

Reflux of barium is frequently seen on UGI studies and has been reported in 25% of patients without reflux symptoms undergoing these examinations (141). Although some studies have shown barium studies to be fairly sensitive and specific, especially when abdominal compression is utilized (142), more recent studies comparing barium studies and 24-h pH testing have questioned this (143). Since virtually all people have at least some reflux at some point during the day, the demonstration of barium reflux during this examination is of little value. The demonstration of esophageal ulcerations, strictures, and disordered motility are more specific findings for GERD.

Endoscopy

Endoscopy is a much more sensitive test for esophageal mucosal damage due to reflux than are barium studies. When esophagitis is seen, the diagnosis of GERD is clinched. However, with the recent availability of OTC H_2 receptor antagonists and the widespread prescribing of antisecretory medications for a variety of complaints, esophagitis is often not found at endoscopy in GERD patients because of prior treatment. In a study by Bell (144), patients with documented pathologic GERD (by 24-h pH testing) who were scheduled to undergo fundoplication were evaluated by endoscopy preoperatively. There was no correlation between the degree of esophageal inflammation and the magnitude of documented GERD, apparently because virtually all patients had been treated with antisecretory agents before evaluation.

Although endoscopy should not be an initial test in evaluating patients with suspected GERD associated asthma, it should be used in certain situations. If significant GERD symptoms have been present for more than 5 years, then the incidence of Barrett's esophagitis increases and endoscopy should be done to exclude this premalignant condition. Also, if bleeding, odynophagia, or dysphagia is present, then endoscopy is indicated.

Twenty-Four-Hour pH Testing

This tool has been shown to be the most sensitive method to demonstrate esophageal reflux (145,146). It has a reported sensitivity and specificity of >90% (145,146), though a recent study using two consecutive 24-h periods suggested less than optimal reproducibility of the test with a false negative rate of 19% for the first day (147). Also, false negative results may be seen in 20–50% of proximal 24-h pH testing (148). This test can document both pathologic reflux as well as correlate acid reflux with symptoms. Schnatz (9) reported that of 54 patients suspected of having cough or asthma related to GERD, only those patients with abnormal 24-h pH tests had symptom improvement with treatment (71%). In a recent study, Harding (1) evaluated 199 asthmatics with 24-h pH testing. One hundred sixty-four (82%) had typical reflux symptoms and, of these, 118 (72%) had abnormal 24-h pH studies. In the asthmatic group without complaints of heartburn or regurgitation, 29% still had pathologic reflux. In addition, 79% of all respiratory symptoms occurred simultaneously or within 5 min of a drop in esophageal pH to below 4.

Twenty-four-hour pH testing can also be used to confirm effectiveness of antisecretory therapy. Katzka (149) looked at 45 patients with GERD symptoms who remained symptomatic despite treatment with omeprazole (20 mg twice a day). Poor esophageal acid control (defined as distal esophageal acidification >1.6% of total time) was found in 31% of patients. Harding and Richter (150) showed that 30% of asthmatics treated with omeprazole (20 mg q.d.) continued to have pathologic GERD on subsequent 24-h pH testing. They advocate testing in all asthma patients suspected of having GERD-related symptoms who fail initial therapy to verify adequacy of acid suppression treatment.

New technology employing esophageal probes to detect liquid flow as impedance changes may offer the opportunity to investigate the role of nonacidic reflux in asthma in patients in whom acid suppressive therapy is successful. However, this technology is in its infancy and will require further study and validation.

V. Asthma Outcomes with Treatment of GERD

A. Outcomes of Medical Therapy

Multiple trials have been conducted to evaluate the effects of the treatment of GERD on asthma. Most of these can be criticized on many levels: small sample size, short duration of therapy, poor documentation of GER suppression and esophagitis healing, and so on. All early trials utilized H_2 receptor antagonists (occasionally with the addition of cisapride). More recently, PPI therapy has been studied—almost exclusively with omeprazole. Omeprazole is a much more potent inhibitor of gastric acid secretion than are H_2 receptor antagonists (151) and only studies which include PPI therapy should be seriously considered as utilizing effective therapy (152).

Field recently reviewed all medical trials to 1996 (82). At that time, there were only four studies in which PPI therapy was studied. Two studies (153,154) treated asthmatic patients for only 4 weeks and one study (155) treated for 6 weeks. In the study by Meier et al., 29% (4/15) of patients demonstrated improved pulmonary function (20% or more change in FEV_1) in response to omeprazole (155). Of note, however, of the 11 patients labeled omeprazole nonresponders, 5 (45%) had evidence of incomplete healing of esophagitis on endoscopy. Since up to 12 weeks of treatment is needed to see a maximal response to therapy (150), results from these studies are suspect. Only one study (150) was of 3 months' duration and verified adequacy of antisecretory therapy with 24-h pH testing with subsequent dosage adjustments. Seventy-three percent of patients with both asthma and GERD demonstrated improvement in PEF (20% or more) or a decrease in asthma symptoms. However, this series was small (only 30 patients) and had no control or placebo arm. Acknowledging these shortcomings, Field found that when taken together, these four studies showed medical reflux therapy improved asthma symptoms and asthma medication use but did not improve pulmonary function.

Since Field's review, three more studies have been published (13,156–157). Levin et al. studied nine asthmatics treated with either omeprazole (20 mg daily) or placebo for 8 weeks in a double-blind, randomized, crossover fashion (156). They found that after omeprazole therapy patients had a higher morning and evening PEFR ($P = 0.025$). They also showed statistically improved activity limitation ($P = 0.039$), asthma symptoms ($P = 0.049$), and emotions ($P = 0.040$), as scored on the Asthma Quality of Life Questionnaire (158), compared to placebo.

Boeree et al. looked at 36 allergic and nonallergic subjects who had either asthma or COPD with severe airway hyperresponsiveness despite treatment with inhaled corticosteroids (157). All patients had GERD documented by 24-h testing but only 14 of 36 patients (39%) had reflux symptoms (dysphagia, heartburn, or regurgitation). Treatment was with omeprazole (40 mg b.i.d.) or placebo for 3 months in a randomized, double blind non-cross-over fashion. Reversibility of airway obstruction (defined as the absolute increase in FEV_1 as percentage predicted after inhaled ipratropium), FEV_1, vital capacity, and PEF measurements showed no improvement with treatment. Except for nocturnal cough, respiratory symptoms did not improve. Criticisms of this study include small sample size with low power, the inclusion of COPD patients (who might be expected to respond differently (159), and a high rate of drug noncompliance (13 of 36 took less than 75% of pills). Twenty-four-hour pH testing was done at the end of the study and a significant improvement in esophageal acid contact time was noted. However, it is not stated whether the treatment failures had adequate esophageal acid suppression compared to the responders.

Kijljander et al. looked at 107 unselected asthmatic patients who subsequently underwent 24-h pH testing (13). Fifty-seven (53%) patients were found to have GERD and were randomized to treatment with omeprazole (40 mg q.d.) or placebo for 8 weeks. After a 2-week wash-out period they were crossed over. Thirty-five percent of patients had no reflux symptoms. No improvement in daytime symptoms was seen ($P = 0.14$), but a significant improvement in nocturnal symptoms ($P = 0.04$) was noted primarily in patients with more severe reflux ($P = 0.002$). FEV_1 improved only in patients with intrinsic asthma ($P = 0.049$).

B. Outcomes of Surgical Therapy

The surgical literature on the treatment outcomes in asthma is even less clear. Field (81) reviewed all published reports (English) from 1966 to 1998. Twenty-four articles were identified and 19 separated asthma patients from other subjects. Only 2 studies were controlled, 10 had 10 or fewer patients, and 2 were in abstract form only. When all asthma patients were combined for evaluation, 417 patients were identified. Antireflux surgery improved GERD symptoms in 90%, asthma symptoms in 79%, asthma medication use in 88%, and pulmonary function in 27%. Essentially all studies could be criticized for multiple reasons, including small sample size, lack of a control group, nonrandomization, poor definition and documentation of asthma and GERD, lack of objective criteria and documentation of response to therapy, and insufficient follow-up. Of note, few studies have been conducted to directly compare surgical and medical therapy (160) and none to date compare the superior therapy utilizing PPIs to surgery.

C. Approach to GERD Therapy in the Patient with Severe Asthma

Since GERD is very common in asthma (the best studies suggest the figure is between 69 and 82%) (10), an empiric trial of antireflux therapy is reasonable in any patient with significant asthma. Also, since silent reflux is present in a third or more of asthmatics (see above), neither a history of symptoms nor diagnostic testing (e.g., 24-h pH monitoring and endoscopy) is mandatory before trial institution because of the high prevalence of GERD in asthma and the additional expense.

O'Connor (161) studied 11 empiric treatment strategies and found that omeprazole 20 mg/day for 3 months followed by pH testing in nonresponders was the most cost-effective. However, Harding et al. have shown that 30% of asthmatics needed at least 20 mg b.i.d. to control acid reflux (150). Additionally, Peghini et al. have recently shown that the nocturnal gastric pH rises above 4 for significant periods of time in up to 70% of subjects on omeprazole therapy, even in patients taking 20 mg b.i.d. (162). Finally, several investigators have suggested that other noxious agents (such as pepsin and bile) in gastric refluxate could damage the esophageal mucosa (163–168) and lead to reflexive airway restriction. (It is well known that significant reflux esophagitis can occur in patients after total gastrectomy!) These noxious agents also are damaging to the airways in the minority of patients felt to have microaspiration-related asthma symptoms.

Thus, a stepwise approach to an empiric trial utilizing the strategy suggested by O'Connor (161) could take 6–9 months. Such a strategy is often not

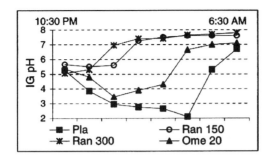

Figure 2 Summary pH profile. Median hourly intragastric (IG) pH in 12 subjects receiving four treatments given at bedtime in addition to 20 mg omeprazole twice daily. Pla: placebo; Ran 150: 150 mg ranitidine; Ran 300: 300 mg ranitidine; Ome 20: 20 mg omeprazole. (From Ref. 162.)

appropriate in severe, steroid—dependent asthma. For all the above reasons, an aggressive, and often empiric, trial of therapy consisting of a combination of proton pump inhibitor, H_2 receptor antagonist, and prokinetic agent [e.g., omeprazole (0.7–3.3 mg/kg for children up to the adult dose of 20-mg b.i.d.), ranitidine (4–6 mg/kg for children up to the adult dose of 150 mg h.s.), and metaclopramide (0.1–0.2 mg/kg for children up to the adult dose of 10–20 mg h.s.)] is the best approach in the patient with severe asthma. Adding an H_2 receptor antagonist at night has been shown to abolish the breakthrough gastric acid secretion (169) that is often seen with PPI use (see above) (Fig. 2). Prokinetic agents (metaclopramide and cisapride) have been shown to be primarily effective in preventing supine reflux (170). Use of these agents at night diminishes reflux of nonacid material and may increase the chance of success of the trial (170,171). It appears that all PPI medications are equally effective (at equivalent dosages) and any substitution is acceptable. The same is true of the H_2 receptor antagonists. The duration of the therapeutic trial should be at least 3 months in order to see the maximum effect (150).

If a significant response to therapy is seen, then long-term treatment is needed. GERD is a chronic disease that rarely spontaneously resolves. At a minimum, daily treatment with a PPI will usually be needed. If symptoms recur while the patient is on daily A.M. PPI treatment [PPI's are more effective if taken in the morning (172,173)], then addition of an H_2 receptor antagonist at h.s. is the most cost-effective next step. If no response to an empiric trial is seen, then a 24-h pH study should be performed to verify adequate acid suppression. If this shows acid suppression, then acid reflux is probably not contributing to the patient's asthma symptoms (10).

Surgery is also a viable option for long-term therapy. It should only be considered in patients who have a clear-cut response to an empiric trial of medical therapy or in patients with life-threatening episodes of nocturnal asthma in whom medical management is deemed inadequate or impractical. Open fundoplication has been shown to prevent significant reflux in 75–90% of patients (174–177). Currently, laparoscopic fundoplication surgery is being used almost exclusively in appropriate patients, but the long-term success of these procedures is yet to be determined. Short and mid-term follow-up studies demonstrate that the laparoscopic approach is equivalent to the open approach (178,179). Laparoscopic fundoplication may be preferable to the traditional approach in patients with severe asthma and poor healing due to corticosteroid use, though further studies in these patients will be needed.

VI. Conclusions

Compelling data support a role for GERD in the exacerbation of asthma in many patients. Mechanistic studies establish reflex-mediated changes in pulmonary function, inflammation, airway hyperresponsiveness, and microaspiration as the pathophysiologic basis of its contribution to asthma. Studies demonstrating improvements in asthma accompanying increasingly effective GERD treatment will further strengthen the hypothesis of causality, and such studies are beginning to establish appropriate therapeutic guidelines. That GERD is prevalent in asthma and frequently ''silent'' makes it an appropriate consideration in the treatment of any patient with severe or escalating asthma.

References

1. Harding SM, Guzzo MR, Richter JE. 24-h esophageal pH testing in asthmatics: respiratory symptom correlation with esophageal acid events. Chest 1999; 115(3): 654–659.
2. Irwin RS, Curley FJ, French CL. Difficult-to-control asthma. Contributing factors and outcome of a systematic management protocol. Chest 1993; 103:1662–1669.
3. Sheikh S, Stephen T, Howell L, Eid N. Gastroesophageal reflux in infants with wheezing. Pediatr Pulmonol 1999; 28(3):181–186.
4. Locke GR, 3rd, Talley NJ, Fett SL, Zinsmeister AR, Melton LJ, 3rd. Prevalence and clinical spectrum of gastroesophageal reflux: a population-based study in Olmsted County, Minnesota. Gastroenterology 1997; 112(5):1448–1456.
5. Nebel OT, Fornes MF, Castell DO. Symptomatic gastroesophageal reflux: incidence and precipitating factors. Am J Dig Dis 1976; 21(11):953–956.
6. Johnson LF, Demeester TR. Twenty-four-hour pH monitoring of the distal esophagus. A quantitative measure of gastroesophageal reflux. Am J Gastroenterol 1974; 62(4):325–332.

7. Vincent D, Cohen-Jonathan AM, Leport J, Merrouche M, Geronimi A, Pradalier A, Soule JC. Gastro-oesophageal reflux prevalence and relationship with bronchial reactivity in asthma. Eur Respir J 1997; 10(10):2255–2259.

8. Dal Negro R, Pomari C, Micheletto C, Turco P, Tognella S. Prevalence of gastro-oesophageal reflux in asthmatics: an Italian study. Ital J Gastroenterol Hepatol 1999; 31(5):371–375.

9. Schnatz PF, Castell JA, Castell DO. Pulmonary symptoms associated with gastro-esophageal reflux: use of ambulatory pH monitoring to diagnose and to direct therapy. Am J Gastroenterol 1996; 91(9):1715–1718.

10. Harding SM, Sontag SJ. Asthma and gastroesophageal reflux. Am J Gastroenterol 2000; 95(suppl 8):23–32.

11. Sontag S, O'Connell S, Khandelwal S, Miller T, Nemchausky B, Serlovsky R. Most asthmatics have GER with or without bronchodilator therapy. Gastroenterology 1990; 99:613–620.

12. Tucci F, Resti M, Fontana R, Novembre E, Lami CA, Vierucci A. Gastroesophageal reflux and bronchial asthma: prevalence and effect of cisapride therapy. J Pediatr Gastroenterol Nutr 1993; 17(3):265–270.

13. Kiljander TO, Salomaa ER, Hietanen EK, Terho EO. Gastroesophageal reflux in asthmatics: A double-blind, placebo-controlled crossover study with omeprazole [In Process Citation]. Chest 1999; 116(5):1257–1264.

14. Harding SM, Guzzo MR, Richter JE. The prevalence of gastroesophageal reflux in asthma patients without reflux symptoms [In Process Citation]. Am J Respir Crit Care Med 2000; 162(1):34–39.

15. Field SK, Underwood M, Brant R, Cowie RL. Prevalence of gastroesophageal reflux symptoms in asthma. Chest 1996; 109:316–322.

16. Bratton D, Price M, Gavin L, Glenn K, Brenner M, Gelfand E, Klinnert M. Impact of a multidisciplinary day program on disease and health care costs in children and adolescents with severe asthma: a two year follow-up study. Ped Pulmonol 2001; 31(3):177–189.

17. Shapiro GG, Christie DL. Gastroesophageal reflux in steroid-dependent asthmatic youths. Pediatrics 1979; 63:207–212.

18. Gustafsson PM, Kjellman NI, Tibbling L. Oesophageal function and symptoms in moderate and severe asthma. Acta Paediatr Scand 1986; 75(5):729–736.

19. Martin ME, Grunstein MM, Larsen GL. The relationship of gastroesophageal reflux to nocturnal wheezing in children with asthma. Ann Allergy 1982; 49(6):318–322.

20. Cuttitta G, Cibella F, Visconti A, Scichilone N, Bellia V, Bonsignore G. Spontaneous gastroesophageal reflux and airway patency during the night in adult asthmatics. Am J Respir Crit Care Med 2000; 161(1):177–181.

21. Tan WC, Martin RJ, Pandey MR, Ballard RD. Effects of spontaneous and simulated gastroesophageal reflux on sleeping asthmatics. Am Rev Respir Dis 1990; 141:1394–1399.

22. Harding SM. Nocturnal asthma: role of nocturnal gastroesophageal reflux. Chronobiol Int 1999; 16(5):641–662.

23. D'Alonzo GE, Ciccolella DE. Nocturnal asthma: physiologic determinants and current therapeutic approaches. Curr Opin Pulm Med 1996; 2(1):48–59.

24. Bou-Abboud CF, Wayland H, Paulsen G, Guth PH. Microcirculatory stasis pre-

cedes tissue necrosis in ethanol-induced gastric mucosal injury in the rat. Dig Dis Sci 1988; 33(7):872–877.

25. el-Serag HB, Sonnenberg A. Comorbid occurrence of laryngeal or pulmonary disease with esophagitis in United States military veterans. Gastroenterology 1997; 113(3):755–760.

26. Nakase H, Itani T, Mimura J, Kawasaki T, Komori H, Tomioka H, Chiba T. Relationship between asthma and gastro-oesophageal reflux: significance of endoscopic grade of reflux oesophagitis in adult asthmatics. J Gastroenterol Hepatol 1999; 14(7):715–722.

27. NHLBI. World Health Organization Workshop Report. Geneva: World Health Organization, 1993.

28. Andersen LI, Schmidt A, Bundgaard A. Pulmonary function and acid application in the esophagus. Chest 1986; 90(3):358–363.

29. Ing AJ, Ngu MC, Breslin AB. Pathogenesis of chronic persistent cough associated with gastroesophageal reflux. Am J Respir Crit Care Med 1994; 149(1):160–167.

30. Mittal RK, Holloway R, Dent J. Effect of atropine on the frequency of reflux and transient lower esophageal sphincter relaxation in normal subjects. Gastroenterology 1995; 109(5):1547–1554.

31. Lidums I, Lehmann A, Checklin H, Dent J, Holloway RH. Control of transient lower esophageal sphincter relaxations and reflux by the GABA(B) agonist baclofen in normal subjects. Gastroenterology 2000; 118(1):7–13.

32. Kjellen G, Brundin A, Tibbling L, Wranne B. Oesophageal function in asthmatics. Eur J Respir Dis 1981; 62(2):87–94.

33. Moote DW, Lloyd DA, McCourtie DR, Wells GA. Increase in gastroesophageal reflux during methacholine-induced bronchospasm. J Allergy Clin Immunol 1986; 78:619–623.

34. Goldman JM, Bennett JR. Gastro-oesophageal reflux and asthma: a common association, but of what clinical importance? Gut 1990; 31(1):1–3.

35. Carmona-Sanchez R, Valdovinos-Diaz MA, Facha MT, Aguilar L, Cachafeiro M, Solana S, Carrillo G, Chapela R, Mejia M, Perez-Chavira R, Salas J. [Hiatal hernia in asthmatic patients: prevalence and its association with gastroesophageal reflux]. Rev Invest Clin 1999; 51(4):215–220.

36. Kahrilas PJ, Shi G, Manka M, Joehl RJ. Increased frequency of transient lower esophageal sphincter relaxation induced by gastric distention in reflux patients with hiatal hernia. Gastroenterology 2000; 118(4):688–695.

37. Paterson WG, Kolyn DM. Esophageal shortening induced by short-term intraluminal acid perfusion in opossum: a cause for hiatus hernia? Gastroenterology 1994; 107(6):1736–1740.

38. Jones MP, Schubert ML. Initiation and perpetuation of gastroesophageal reflux disease. Gastroenterology 1998; 115(5):1296–1298.

39. Holmes PW, Campbell AH, Barter CE. Acute changes of lung volumes and lung mechanics in asthma and in normal subjects. Thorax 1978; 33(3):394–400.

40. Roussos C, Macklem PT. The respiratory muscles. N Engl J Med 1982; 307(13):786–797.

41. Boyle JT, Tuchman DN, Altschuler SM, Nixon TE, Pack AI, Cohen S. Mechanisms

for the association of gastroesophageal reflux and bronchospasm. Am Rev Respir Dis 1985; 131(5):S16–S20.

42. Singh V, Jain NK. Asthma as a cause for, rather than a result of, gastroesophageal reflux. J Asthma 1983; 20(4):241–243.

43. Ing AJ, Ngu MC, Breslin AB. Obstructive sleep apnea and gastroesophageal reflux. Am J Med 2000; 108(suppl 4a):120–125.

44. Zaragoza RH, Szefler SJ, Bratton DL. Therapeutic manipulations in severe nocturnal asthma: a non-conventional approach in a severe high risk asthmatic. J Asthma 1992; 29:281–287.

45. Kerr P, Shoenut JP, Millar T, Buckle P, Kryger MH. Nasal CPAP reduces gastroesophageal reflux in obstructive sleep apnea syndrome. Chest 1992; 101(6):1539–1544.

46. Kerr P, Shoenut JP, Steens RD, Millar T, Micflickier AB, Kryger MH. Nasal continuous positive airway pressure: a new treatment for nocturnal gastroesophageal reflux? J Clin Gastroenterol 1993; 17(4):276–280.

47. Teramoto S, Ohga E, Matsui H, Ishii T, Matsuse T, Ouchi Y. Obstructive sleep apnea syndrome may be a significant cause of gastroesophageal reflux disease in older people [letter; comment]. J Am Geriatr Soc 1999; 47(10):1273–1274.

48. Kahrilas PJ, Dodds WJ, Hogan WJ, Kern M, Arndorfer RC, Reece A. Esophageal peristaltic dysfunction in peptic esophagitis. Gastroenterology 1986; 91(4):897–904.

49. Fouad YM, Katz PO, Hatlebakk JG, Castell DO. Ineffective esophageal motility: the most common motility abnormality in patients with GERD-associated respiratory symptoms. Am J Gastroenterol 1999; 94(6):1464–1467.

50. Campo S, Morini S, Re MA, Monno D, Lorenzetti R, Moscatelli B, Bologna E. Esophageal dysmotility and gastroesophageal reflux in intrinsic asthma. Dig Dis Sci 1997; 42(6):1184–1188.

51. Hughes DM, Spier S, Rivlin J, Levison H. Gastroesophageal reflux during sleep in asthmatic patients. J Pediatr 1983; 102(5):666–672.

52. Ekstrom T, Tibbling L. Gastro-oesophageal reflux and triggering of bronchial asthma: a negative report. Eur J Respir Dis 1987; 71(3):177–180.

53. Jolley SG, Herbst JJ, Johnson DG. Eosphageal pH monitoring during sleep identifies children with respiratory symptoms from gastroesphageal reflux. Gastroenterology 1981; 80:1501–1506.

54. Mattox HE, Richter JE. Prolonged ambulatory esophageal pH monitoring in the evaluation of gastroesophageal reflux disease. Am J Med 1990; 89(3):345–356.

55. Kaliner M. The cholinergic nervous system and immediate hypersensitivity. 1. Eccrine sweat responses in allergic patients. J Allergy Clin Immunol 1976; 58(2):308–315.

56. Kaliner M, Shelhamer JH, Davis PB, Smith LJ, Venter JC. Autonomic nervous system abnormalities and allergy [clinical conference]. Ann Intern Med 1982; 96(3):349–357.

57. Kallenbach JM, Webster T, Dowdeswell R, Reinach SG, Millar RN, Zwi S. Reflex heart rate control in asthma: evidence of parasympathetic overactivity. Chest 1985; 87(5):644–648.

58. Lodi U, Harding SM, Coghlan HC, Guzzo MR, Walker LH. Autonomic regulation in asthmatics with gastroesophageal reflux. Chest 1997; 111(1):65–70.

59. Ekström T, Tibbling L. Gastro-oesophageal reflux and nocturnal asthma. Eur Respir J 1988; 1:636–638.

60. Hubert D, Gaudric M, Guerre J, Lockhart A, Marsac J. Effect of theophylline on gastroesophageal reflux in patients with asthma. J Allergy Clin Immunol 1988; 81(6):1168–1174.

61. DiMarino AJ, Jr., Cohen S. Effect of an oral beta2-adrenergic agonist on lower esophageal sphincter pressure in normals and in patients with achalasia. Dig Dis Sci 1982; 27(12):1063–1066.

62. Michoud MC, Leduc T, Proulx F, Perreault S, Du Souich P, Duranceau A, Amyot R. Effect of salbutamol on gastroesophageal reflux in healthy volunteers and patients with asthma [published erratum appears in J Allergy Clin Immunol 1992; 89(3):778]. J Allergy Clin Immunol 1991; 87(4):762–767.

63. Schindlbeck NE, Heinrich C, Huber RM, Muller-Lissner SA. Effects of albuterol (salbutamol) on esophageal motility and gastroesophageal reflux in healthy volunteers. J Am Med Assoc 1988; 260(21):3156–3158.

64. Sontag SJ, O'Connell S, Khandelwal S, Miller T, Nemchausky B, Schnell TG, Serlovsky R. Effect of positions, eating, and bronchodilators on gastroesophageal reflux in asthmatics. Dig Dis Sci 1990; 35(7):849–856.

65. Sontag SJ, Schnell TG, Miller TQ, Khandelwal S, O'Connell S, Chejfec G, Greenlee H, Seidel UJ, Brand L. Prevalence of oesophagitis in asthmatics. Gut 1992; 33:872–876.

66. Schan CA, Harding SM, Haile JM, Bradley LA, Richter JE. Gastroesophageal reflux-induced bronchoconstriction. Chest 1994; 106:731–737.

67. Theodoropoulos DS, Lockey RF, Boyce HW, Jr., Bukantz SC. Gastroesophageal reflux and asthma: a review of pathogenesis, diagnosis, and therapy. Allergy 1999; 54(7):651–661.

68. Decramer M, Lacquet LM, Fagard R, Rogiers P. Corticosteroids contribute to muscle weakness in chronic airflow obstruction. Am J Respir Crit Care Med 1994; 150(1):11–16.

69. Dekhuijzen PN, Decramer M. Steroid-induced myopathy and its significance to respiratory disease: a known disease rediscovered. Eur Respir J 1992; 5(8):997–1003.

70. Gallagher CG. Respiratory steroid myopathy [editorial; comment]. Am J Respir Crit Care Med 1994; 150(1):4–6.

71. German SV, Marova EI, Razlivakhin Iu A, Petrova EA. [Esophageal lesions in Cushing's syndrome and corticosteroma]. Probl Endokrinol (Mosk) 1988; 34(1): 18–22.

72. Mansfield LE, Stein MR. Gastroesophageal reflux and asthma: a possible reflex mechanism. Ann Allergy 1978; 41:224–226.

73. Mansfield LE, Hameister HH, Spaulding HS, Smith NJ, Glab N. The role of the vague nerve in airway narrowing caused by intraesophageal hydrochloric acid provocation and esophageal distention. Ann Allergy 1981; 47(6):431–434.

74. Wright RA, Miller SA, Corsello BF. Acid-induced esophagobronchial-cardiac reflexes in humans. Gastroenterology 1990; 99(1):71–73.

75. Harding SM, Schan CA, Guzzo MR, Alexander RW, Bradley LA, Richter JE. Gastroesophageal reflux-induced bronchoconstriction. Chest 1995; 108:1220–1227.
76. Wilson NM, Charette L, Thomson AH, Silverman M. Gastro-oesophageal reflux and childhood asthma: the acid test. Thorax 1985; 40:592–597.
77. Spaulding HS, Mansfield LE, Stein MR. Further investigation of the association between gastroesophageal reflux and bronchoconstriction. J Allergy Clin Immunol 1982; 69:516–521.
78. Davis RS, Larsen GL, Grunstein MM. Respiratory response to intraesophageal acid infusion in asthmatic children during sleep. J Allergy Clin Immunol 1983; 72:393–398.
79. Field SK. A critical review of the studies of the effects of simulated or real gastro-esophageal reflux on pulmonary function in asthmatic adults. Chest 1999; 115(3):848–856.
80. Wesseling G, Brummer RJ, Wouters EF, ten Velde GP. Gastric asthma? No change in respiratory impedance during intraesophageal acidification in adult asthmatics. Chest 1993; 104(6):1733–1736.
81. Field SK, Gelfand GA, McFadden SD. The effects of antireflux surgery on asthmatics with gastroesophageal reflux. Chest 1999; 116(3):766–774.
82. Field SK, Sutherland LR. Does medical antireflux therapy improve asthma in asthmatics with gastroesophageal reflux?: a critical review of the literature. Chest 1998; 114(1):275–283.
83. Ekström T, Lindgren BR, Tibbling L. Effects of ranitidine treatment on patients with asthma and a history of gastro-oesophageal reflux: a double blind crossover study. Thorax 1989; 44:19–23.
84. Sears MR. Is the routine use of inhaled beta-adrenergic agonists appropriate in asthma treatment? No. Am J Respir Crit Care Med 1995; 151(3/1):600–601.
85. Pratter MR, Curley FJ, Dubois J, Irwin RS. Cause and evaluation of chronic dyspnea in a pulmonary disease clinic. Arch Intern Med 1989; 149(10):2277–2282.
86. DePaso WJ, Winterbauer RH, Lusk JA, Dreis DF, Springmeyer SC. Chronic dyspnea unexplained by history, physical examination, chest roentgenogram, and spirometry: analysis of a seven-year experience. Chest 1991; 100(5):1293–1299.
87. Ing AJ, Ngu MC, Breslin AB. Chronic persistent cough and clearance of esophageal acid. Chest 1992; 102(6):1668–1671.
88. Fisher AB, DuBois AB, Hyde RW. Evaluation of the forced oscillation technique for the determination of resistance to breathing. J Clin Invest 1968; 47(9):2045–2057.
89. Tomori Z, Widdicombe JG. Muscular, bronchomotor and cardiovascular reflexes elicited by mechanical stimulation of the respiratory tract. J Physiol (Lond) 1969; 200(1):25–49.
90. Kaufman J, Wright GW. The effect of nasal and nasopharyngeal irritation on airway resistance in man. Am Rev Respir Dis 1969; 100(5):626–630.
91. Slavin RG. Sinusitis in adults and its relation to allergic rhinitis, asthma, and nasal polyps. J Allergy Clin Immunol 1988; 82(5/2):950–956.
92. Lin KM, Ueda RK, Hinder RA, Stein HJ, DeMeester TR. Etiology and importance of alkaline esophageal reflux. Am J Surg 1991; 162(6):553–557.
93. Stein HJ, Feussner H, Kauer W, DeMeester TR, Siewert JR. Alkaline gastroesopha-

geal reflux: assessment by ambulatory esophageal aspiration and pH monitoring. Am J Surg 1994; 167(1):163–168.

94. Herve P, Denjean A, Jian R, Simonneau G, Duroux P. Intraesophageal perfusion of acid increases the bronchomotor response to methacholine and to isocapnic hyperventilation in asthmatic subjects. Am Rev Respir Dis 1986; 134:986–989.

95. Ekstrom T, Tibbling L. Esophageal acid perfusion, airway function, and symptoms in asthmatic patients with marked bronchial hyperreactivity. Chest 1989; 96(5): 995–998.

96. Otsuka M, Yoshioka K. Neurotransmitter functions of mammalian tachykinins. Physiol Rev 1993; 73(2):229–308.

97. Braunstein G, Fajac I, Lacronique J, Frossard N. Clinical and inflammatory responses to exogenous tachykinins in allergic rhinitis [published erratum appears in Am Rev Respir Dis 1993; 148(6/1):following 1700]. Am Rev Respir Dis 1991; 144(3/1):630–635.

98. Philip G, Sanico AM, Togias A. Inflammatory cellular influx follows capsaicin nasal challenge. Am J Respir Crit Care Med 1996; 153(4/1):1222–1229.

99. Arakawa T, Uno H, Fukuda T, Higuchi K, Kobayashi K, Kuroki T. New aspects of gastric adaptive relaxation, reflex after food intake for more food: involvement of capsaicin-sensitive sensory nerves and nitric oxide. J Smooth Muscle Res 1997; 33(3):81–88.

100. Canning B. Inflammation in asthma. The role of nerves and the potential influence of gastroesophageal reflux disease. In: Stein MR, ed. Gastroesophageal Reflux Disease and Airway Disease. New York: Marcel Dekker, 1999:19–54.

101. Lundberg JM, Hokfelt T, Martling CR, Saria A, Cuello C. Substance P-immunoreactive sensory nerves in the lower respiratory tract of various mammals including man. Cell Tissue Res 1984; 235(2):251–261.

102. Ellis JL, Undem BJ, Kays JS, Ghanekar SV, Barthlow HG, Buckner CK. Pharmacological examination of receptors mediating contractile responses to tachykinins in airways isolated from human, guinea pig and hamster. J Pharmacol Exp Ther 1993; 267(1):95–101.

103. Ellis JL, Undem BJ. Pharmacology of non-adrenergic, non-cholinergic nerves in airway smooth muscle. Pulm Pharmacol 1994; 7(4):205–223.

104. Holzer P. Local effector functions of capsaicin-sensitive sensory nerve endings: involvement of tachykinins, calcitonin gene-related peptide and other neuropeptides. Neuroscience 1988; 24(3):739–768.

105. Hamamoto J, Kohrogi H, Kawano O, Iwagoe H, Fujii K, Hirata N, Ando M. Esophageal stimulation by hydrochloric acid causes neurogenic inflammation in the airways in guinea pigs. J Appl Physiol 1997; 82(3):738–745.

106. Fuller RW. Pharmacology of inhaled capsaicin in humans. Respir Med 1991; 85(suppl A):31–34.

107. Ollerenshaw SL, Jarvis D, Sullivan CE, Woolcock AJ. Substance P immunoreactive nerves in airways from asthmatics and nonasthmatics. Eur Respir J 1991; 4(6): 673–682.

108. Howarth PH, Djukanovic R, Wilson JW, Holgate ST, Springall DR, Polak JM. Mucosal nerves in endobronchial biopsies in asthma and non-asthma. Int Arch Allergy Appl Immunol 1991; 94(1–4):330–333.

109. Lilly CM, Bai TR, Shore SA, Hall AE, Drazen JM. Neuropeptide content of lungs from asthmatic and nonasthmatic patients. Am J Respir Crit Care Med 1995; 151 (2/1):548–553.

110. Chanez P, Springall D, Vignola AM, Moradoghi-Hattvani A, Polak JM, Godard P, Bousquet J. Bronchial mucosal immunoreactivity of sensory neuropeptides in severe airway diseases. Am J Respir Crit Care Med 1998; 158(3):985–990.

111. Naline E, Molimard M, Regoli D, Emonds-Alt X, Bellamy JF, Advenier C. Evidence for functional tachykinin NK1 receptors on human isolated small bronchi. Am J Physiol 1996; 271(5/1):L1763–1767.

112. Castairs JR, Barnes PJ. Autoradiographic mapping of substance P receptors in lung. Eur J Pharmacol 1986; 127(3):295–296.

113. Yu XY, Undem BJ, Spannhake EW. Protective effect of substance P on permeability of airway epithelial cells in culture. Am J Physiol 1996; 271(6 Pt 1):L889–895.

114. Bai TR, Zhou D, Weir T, Walker B, Hegele R, Hayashi S, McKay K, Bondy GP, Fong T. Substance P (NK1)- and neurokinin A (NK2)-receptor gene expression in inflammatory airway diseases. Am J Physiol 1995; 269(3 Pt 1):L309–317.

115. Barnes PJ, Baraniuk JN, Belvisi MG. Neuropeptides in the respiratory tract. Part I. Am Rev Respir Dis 1991; 144(5):1187–1198.

116. Barnes PJ, Baraniuk JN, Belvisi MG. Neuropeptides in the respiratory tract. Part II. Am Rev Respir Dis 1991; 144(6):1391–1399.

117. Nieber K, Baumgarten CR, Rathsack R, Furkert J, Oehme P, Kunkel G. Substance P and beta-endorphin-like immunoreactivity in lavage fluids of subjects with and without allergic asthma. J Allergy Clin Immunol 1992; 90(4 Pt 1):646–652.

118. Tomaki M, Ichinose M, Miura M, Hirayama Y, Yamauchi H, Nakajima N, Shirato K. Elevated substance P content in induced sputum from patients with asthma and patients with chronic bronchitis. Am J Respir Crit Care Med 1995; 151(3 Pt 1): 613–617.

119. Fahy JV, Wong HH, Geppetti P, Reis JM, Harris SC, Maclean DB, Nadel JA, Boushey HA. Effect of an NK1 receptor antagonist (CP-99,994) on hypertonic saline-induced bronchoconstriction and cough in male asthmatic subjects. Am J Respir Crit Care Med 1995; 152(3):879–884.

120. Ichinose M, Miura M, Yamauchi H, Kageyama N, Tomaki M, Oyake T, Ohuchi Y, Hida W, Miki H, Tamura G, Shirato K. A neurokinin 1-receptor antagonist improves exercise-induced airway narrowing in asthmatic patients. Am J Respir Crit Care Med 1996; 153(3):936–941.

121. Tuchman DN, Boyle JT, Pack AI, Scwartz J, Kokonos M, Spitzer AR, Cohen S. Comparison of airway responses following tracheal or esophageal acidification in the cat. Gastroenterology 1984; 87(4):872–881.

122. Heyman S, Kirkpatrick JA, Winter HS, Treves S. An improved radionuclide method for the diagnosis of gastroesophageal reflux and aspiration in children (milk scan). Radiology 1979; 131(2):479–482.

123. Chernow B, Johnson LF, Janowitz WR, Castell DO. Pulmonary aspiration as a consequence of gastroesophageal reflux: a diagnostic approach. Dig Dis Sci 1979; 24(11):839–844.

124. Colombo JL, Hallberg TK. Pulmonary aspiration and lipid-laden macrophages: in search of gold (standards). Pediatr Pulmonol 1999; 28(2):79–82.

125. Colombo JL, Hallberg TK. Recurrent aspiration in children: lipid-laden alveolar macrophage quantitation. Pediatr Pulmonol 1987; 3(2):86–89.

126. Gastal OL, Castell JA, Castell DO. Frequency and site of gastroesophageal reflux in patients with chest symptoms. Studies using proximal and distal pH monitoring. Chest 1994; 106(6):1793–1796.

127. Cucchiara S, Santamaria F, Minella R, Alfieri E, Scoppa A, Calabrese F, Franco MT, Rea B, Salvia G. Simultaneous prolonged recordings of proximal and distal intraesophageal pH in children with gastroesophageal reflux disease and respiratory symptoms. Am J Gastroenterol 1995; 90(10):1791–1796.

128. Dobhan R, Castell DO. Normal and abnormal proximal esophageal acid exposure: results of ambulatory dual-probe pH monitoring. Am J Gastroenterol 1993; 88:25–29.

129. Wo JM, Hunter JG, Waring JP. Dual-channel ambulatory esophageal pH monitoring. A useful diagnostic tool? Dig Dis Sci 1997; 42(11):2222–2226.

130. Castell DO. Asthma and gastroesophageal reflux. Chest 1989; 96:2–3.

131. Ghaed N, Stein MR. Assessment of a technique for scintigraphic monitoring of pulmonary aspiration of gastric contents in asthmatics with gastroesophageal reflux. Ann Allergy 1979; 42(5):306–308.

132. Varkey B. Abstract. Chest 1992; 102:152S.

133. Jack CIA, Calverley PMA, Donnelly RJ, Tran J, Russell G, Hind CRK, Evans CC. Simultaneous tracheal and oesophageal pH measurements in asthmatic patients with gastro-oesophageal reflux. Thorax 1995; 50:201–204.

134. Berquist WE, Rachelefsky GS, Kadden M. Gastroesophageal reflux-associated recurrent pneumonia and chronic asthma in children. Pediatrics 1981; 68:29–35.

135. Harding S. GERD, airway disease, and the mechanisms of interaction. In: Stein MR, ed. Gastroesophageal Reflux and Airway Disease. New York: Marcel Dekker, 1999:139–178.

136. Martling CR, Lundberg JM. Capsaicin sensitive afferents contribute to acute airway edema following tracheal instillation of hydrochloric acid or gastric juice in the rat. Anesthesiology 1988; 68(3):350–356.

137. Folkesson HG, Matthay MA, Hebert CA, Broaddus VC. Acid aspiration-induced lung injury in rabbits is mediated by interleukin-8-dependent mechanisms. J Clin Invest 1995; 96(1):107–116.

138. Schwartz DJ, Wynne JW, Gibbs CP, Hood CI, Kuck EJ. The pulmonary consequences of aspiration of gastric contents at pH values greater than 2.5. Am Rev Respir Dis 1980; 121(1):119–126.

139. Wynne JW, Modell JH. Respiratory aspiration of stomach contents. Ann Intern Med 1977; 87(4):466–474.

140. Mays EE, Dubois JJ, Hamilton GB. Pulmonary fibrosis associated with tracheobronchial aspiration: a study of the frequency of hiatal hernia and gastroesophageal reflux in interstitial pulmonary fibrosis of obscure etiology. Chest 1976; 69(4):512–515.

141. Lemire S. Assessment of clinical severity and investigation of uncomplicated gastroesophageal reflux disease and noncardiac angina-like chest pain. Can J Gastroenterol 1997; 11(suppl B):37B–40B.

142. Sellar RJ, De Caestecker JS, Heading RC. Barium radiology: a sensitive test for gastro-oesophageal reflux. Clin Radiol 1987; 38(3):303–307.

143. Johnston BT, Troshinsky MB, Castell JA, Castell DO. Comparison of barium radiology with esophageal pH monitoring in the diagnosis of gastroesophageal reflux disease. Am J Gastroenterol 1996; 91(6):1181–1185.

144. Bell RC, Hanna P, Mills MR, Bowrey D. Patterns of success and failure with laparoscopic Toupet fundoplication. Surg Endosc 1999; 13(12):1189–1194.

145. DeVault KR, Castell DO. Guidelines for the diagnosis and treatment of gastroesophageal reflux disease: Practice Parameters Committee of the American College of Gastroenterology. Arch Intern Med 1995; 155(20):2165–2173.

146. Kahrilas PJ, Quigley EM. Clinical esophageal pH recording: a technical review for practice guideline development. Gastroenterology 1996; 110(6):1982–1996.

147. Mahajan L, Wyllie R, Oliva L, Balsells F, Steffen R, Kay M. Reproducibility of 24-hour intraesophageal pH monitoring in pediatric patients. Pediatrics 1998; 101(2):260–263.

148. Vaezi MF, Schroeder PL, Richter JE. Reproducibility of proximal probe pH parameters in 24-hour ambulatory esophageal pH monitoring. Am J Gastroenterol 1997; 92(5):825–829.

149. Katzka DA, Paoletti V, Leite L, Castell DO. Prolonged ambulatory pH monitoring in patients with persistent gastroesophageal reflux disease symptoms: testing while on therapy identifies the need for more aggressive anti-reflux therapy [see comments]. Am J Gastroenterol 1996; 91(10):2110–2113.

150. Harding SM, Richter JE, Guzzo MR, Schan CA, Alexander RW, Bradley LA. Asthma and gastroesophageal reflux: acid suppressive therapy improves asthma outcome. Am J Med 1996; 100(4):395–405.

151. Maton PN. Omeprazole. N Engl J Med 1991; 324(14):965–975.

152. Chiba N. Proton pump inhibitors in acute healing and maintenance of erosive or worse esophagitis: a systematic overview. Can J Gastroenterol 1997; 11(suppl B): 66B–73B.

153. Ford GA, Oliver PS, Prior JS, Butland RJ, Wilkinson SP. Omeprazole in the treatment of asthmatics with nocturnal symptoms and gastro-oesophageal reflux: a placebo-controlled cross-over study. Postgrad Med J 1994; 70(823):350–354.

154. Teichtahl H, Kronborg IJ, Yeomans ND, Robinson P. Adult asthma and gastro-oesophageal reflux: the effects of omeprazole therapy on asthma. Aust N Z J Med 1996; 26(5):671–676.

155. Meier JH, McNally PR, Punja M, Freeman SR, Sudduth RH, Stocker N, Perry M, Spaulding HS. Does omeprazole (prilosec) improve respiratory function in asthmatics with gastroesophageal reflux?: a double-blind, placebo-controlled crossover study. Dig Dis Sci 1994; 39(10):2127–2133.

156. Levin TR, Sperling RM, McQuaid KR. Omeprazole improves peak expiratory flow rate and quality of life in asthmatics with gastroesophageal reflux. Am J Gastroenterol 1998; 93(7):1060–1063.

157. Boeree MJ, Peters FT, Postma DS, Kleibeuker JH. No effects of high-dose omeprazole in patients with severe airway hyperresponsiveness and (a)symptomatic gastro-oesophageal reflux. Eur Respir J 1998; 11(5):1070–1074.

158. Juniper EF, Guyatt GH, Epstein RS, Ferrie PJ, Jaeschke R, Hiller TK. Evaluation of impairment of health related quality of life in asthma: development of a questionnaire for use in clinical trials. Thorax 1992; 47(2):76–83.

159. Ducoloné A, Vandevenne A, Jouin H, Grob J-C, Coumaros D, Meyer C, Burghard G, Methlin G, Hollender L. Gastroesophageal reflux in patients with asthma and chronic bronchitis. Am Rev Respir Dis 1987; 135:327–332.

160. Larrain A, Carrasco E, Galleguillos F, Sepulveda R, Pope CE, II. Medical and surgical treatment of nonallergic asthma associated with gastroesophageal reflux. Chest 1991; 99:1330–1335.

161. O'Connor JF, Singer ME, Richter JE. The cost-effectiveness of strategies to assess gastroesophageal reflux as an exacerbating factor in asthma. Am J Gastroenterol 1999; 94(6):1472–1480.

162. Peghini PL, Katz PO, Bracy NA, Castell DO. Nocturnal recovery of gastric acid secretion with twice-daily dosing of proton pump inhibitors. Am J Gastroenterol 1998; 93(5):763–767.

163. McCallum RW. Pharmacologic modulation of motility. Yale J Biol Med 1999; 72(2–3):173–180.

164. Richter J. Do we know the cause of reflux disease? Eur J Gastroenterol Hepatol 1999; 11(suppl 1):3–9.

165. Morris GP, Feldman MJ, Barclay RL, Paterson WG. Esophagitis as the outcome of progressive failures of the defensive repertoire. Can J Gastroenterol 1997; 11(suppl B):28B–36B.

166. Kauer WK, Peters JH, DeMeester TR, Ireland AP, Bremner CG, Hagen JA. Mixed reflux of gastric and duodenal juices is more harmful to the esophagus than gastric juice alone: the need for surgical therapy re-emphasized. Ann Surg 1995; 222(4): 525–531.

167. Bremner CG, Mason RJ. 'Bile' in the oesophagus. Br J Surg 1993; 80(11):1374–1376.

168. Stoker DL, Williams JG. Alkaline reflux oesophagitis. Gut 1991; 32(10):1090–1092.

169. Peghini PL, Katz PO, Castell DO. Ranitidine controls nocturnal gastric acid break-through on omeprazole: a controlled study in normal subjects. Gastroenterology 1998; 115(6):1335–1339.

170. Inauen W, Emde C, Weber B, Armstrong D, Bettschen HU, Huber T, Scheurer U, Blum AL, Halter F, Merki HS. Effects of ranitidine and cisapride on acid reflux and oesophageal motility in patients with reflux oesophagitis: a 24 hour ambulatory combined pH and manometry study. Gut 1993; 34(8):1025–1031.

171. Lieberman DA, Keeffe EB. Treatment of severe reflux esophagitis with cimetidine and metoclopramide. Ann Intern Med 1986; 104(1):21–26.

172. Fraser AG, Sawyerr AM, Hudson M, Smith MS, Pounder RE. Morning versus evening dosing of lansoprazole 30 mg daily on twenty-four-hour intragastric acidity in healthy subjects. Aliment Pharmacol Ther 1996; 10(4):523–527.

173. Chiverton SG, Howden CW, Burget DW, Hunt RH. Omeprazole (20 mg) daily given in the morning or evening: a comparison of effects on gastric acidity, and plasma gastrin and omeprazole concentration. Aliment Pharmacol Ther 1992; 6(1): 103–111.

174. Rantanen TK, Halme TV, Luostarinen ME, Karhumaki LM, Kononen EO, Isolauri JO. The long term results of open antireflux surgery in a community-based health care center. Am J Gastroenterol 1999; 94(7):1777–1781.

175. Luostarinen M. Nissen fundoplication for gastro-oesophageal reflux disease: long-term results. Ann Chir Gynaecol 1995; 84(2):115–120.

176. Luostarinen M. Nissen fundoplication for reflux esophagitis: long-term clinical and endoscopic results in 109 of 127 consecutive patients. Ann Surg 1993; 217(4):329–337.

177. Martinez de Haro LF, Ortiz A, Parrilla P, Garcia Marcilla JA, Aguayo JL, Morales G. Long-term results of Nissen fundoplication in reflux esophagitis without strictures: clinical, endoscopic, and pH-metric evaluation. Dig Dis Sci 1992; 37:523–527.

178. Rantanen TK, Salo JA, Salminen JT, Kellokumpu IH. Functional outcome after laparoscopic or open Nissen fundoplication: a follow-up study. Arch Surg 1999; 134(3):240–244.

179. Eshraghi N, Farahmand M, Soot SJ, Rand-Luby L, Deveney CW, Sheppard BC. Comparison of outcomes of open versus laparoscopic Nissen fundoplication performed in a single practice. Am J Surg 1998; 175(5):371–374.

12

Application of Imaging Procedures in the Diagnosis and Management of Severe Asthma

STEVEN P. JENSEN, DAVID A. LYNCH, and JOHN D. NEWELL, Jr.

University of Colorado Health Sciences Center
Denver, Colorado

I. Introduction

Medical imaging techniques play an important role in the diagnosis and management of severe asthma. Properly applied, medical imaging may enhance the clinician's understanding of the anatomic and physiologic perturbations that are at the root of the patient's disease. Medical imaging may also allow for timely detection of complications or important superimposed conditions that may affect the clinical course of the severe asthmatic. Furthermore, medical imaging may assist in the differentiation of severe asthma from other disease processes with which it may be confused. This is vitally important, as the therapies for these various conditions may differ significantly (1,2).

II. Medical Imaging Tools in the Assessment of Severe Asthma

The armamentarium of medical imaging tools that find utility in the diagnosis and management of patients with severe asthma include plain film radiography, digital radiography, fluoroscopy, conventional and helical computed tomography

(CT), high resolution computed tomography (HRCT), and nuclear medicine radionuclide imaging.

A. Plain Film Radiography

The chest radiograph retains its position as the primary mode of investigation of diseases of the thorax. Standard posteroanterior (PA) and lateral projections are vital in the investigation of chest abnormalities, whereas specialized projections, such as oblique, lordotic, and lateral decubitus projections, play a role in further investigation and clarification of particular findings or abnormalities. The antero-posterior (AP) projection can be used rather than the PA projection in patients who are less mobile or who are unable to cooperate. Although the highest quality radiographs are obtained with fixed equipment, properly selected film and screen combinations, and high-kilovoltage techniques (115–160 kVp), portable radiography may also be of value in imaging those unable to fully cooperate or those to whom the imaging department is inaccessible. Portable radiographs have the disadvantages of lower peak kilovoltage technique, longer exposures, and shorter X-ray source to film distances, resulting in greater distortion of images due to geometric and magnification factors (3).

Although expiratory chest radiographs can help detect focal air trapping, their sensitivity for pneumothorax is similar to that of inspiratory radiographs (4). Therefore, their routine use adds no information to that obtained from the inspiratory chest radiograph.

B. Digital Radiography

While plain film radiography produces an image by exposure of a sheet of radiographic film, its newer cousin, digital radiography, depends on exposure of either a reusable photostimulable phosphor plate or a selenium-based drum or plate detector. In either case, the X-ray energy from the exposure is stored in the receptor until it is extracted from the detector as digital data corresponding to a two-dimensional matrix. The digital data may than be used to produce an image on an electronic monitor or on film. Digital radiography has wider exposure latitude than plain film radiography. In other words, diagnostically useful images may be produced from a broader range of X-ray exposures than is allowable with conventionally produced radiographs. Thus, an exposure that might result in an unusable, underexposed, or overexposed conventional plain film may, in many cases, still result in a diagnostically useful image using digital radiography. An additional advantage of digital radiography is the ability to transmit digital data electronically in such a manner that images may be viewed on monitors in locations remote from the site of image acquisition. Conventionally produced radiographs may also be converted to digital data by a film digitizer. The digital data may then be stored or electronically transmitted to be viewed on a monitor or photographed on film elsewhere (3).

C. Fluoroscopy

Fluoroscopy may be utilized in dynamic assessment of diaphragmatic function and lung expansion and in the analysis of suspected nodules or other radiographically detected findings. Perhaps more importantly in the setting of severe asthma, fluoroscopy is routinely used in conjunction with radiographic contrast materials in the study of the alimentary tract. Alimentary tract abnormalities that may play a role in the exacerbation of asthma or simulation of asthma, such as laryngeal penetration/aspiration and gastroesophageal reflux disease, may be detected with properly performed fluoroscopic studies (3).

D. Computed Tomography and High-Resolution Computed Tomography

A full discussion of the physics of computed tomography (CT) is beyond the scope of this text. However, in simplified terms, CT produces medical images by collecting data from multiple X-ray exposures passing through a plane through a subject. These exposures are usually made as an X-ray tube and detector rotate around the subject within a gantry. This process is described as an axial scan acquisition. The data collected in this process is then mathematically processed, and an image is formed by assigning a particular density or attenuation value to each pixel within a matrix representing the plane that was scanned. In this manner, a two-dimensional cross-sectional image is created. Helical or spiral CT is a more advanced variation of this technique, in which the X-ray source and detector rotate around the subject in the x–y plane as there is simultaneous translation of the subject in the z axis. This results in a spiral or helical path of the X rays through the subject. A continuous data set is produced, representing that spiral or helical path. The continuous data set is then mathematically reconstructed into two-dimensional cross-sectional images by interpolation of data both above and below the assigned image plane (3).

Several variables affect the spatial resolution and detail available in images from both axially and helically (spirally) acquired CT scans. One of the chief variables is the thickness of the scan slice. This is determined by the degree of collimation of the X-ray beam at it passes through the subject. Narrower collimation produces a narrower X-ray beam, resulting in a thinner slice of imaged tissue. This, in turn, results in less volume averaging artifact and greater detail within the image. Modern CT scanners are capable of collimation of the X-ray beam to thicknesses between 1 and 10 mm. High-resolution computed tomography (HRCT) employs the narrower end of the collimation spectrum (generally 1.0 or 1.5 mm) and high-detail reconstruction algorithms to produce images with very high spatial resolution. HRCT has found extensive utility in pulmonary imaging because of the exquisite detail that is produced and the enhanced potential for correlation of images with anatomy, histology, and pathology (3).

E. Nuclear Medicine

Nuclear medicine lung ventilation and perfusion scanning has a limited role in the evaluation of patients with asthma. Scintigraphic imaging of the lungs after inhalation or intravenous injection of various radiotracers allows assessment of pulmonary ventilation or perfusion, respectively. Ventilation and perfusion scanning may be performed either alone or in conjunction with one another, depending on the nature of the clinical question (3).

F. Sinus Radiography and Computed Tomography

Paranasal sinus disease, which may be associated with asthma in some cases, may be imaged with plain film or digital radiography as well as computed tomography.

G. Procedures of Historical Interest

Planar tomography of the thorax and bronchography are now primarily of historical interest. CT and HRCT have largely supplanted both of these techniques. Planar tomography employs the inverse movement of the X-ray source and the film during exposure, resulting in blurring of the image from all but a slab of tissue of variable thickness (thickness is dependent on magnitude of the motion of the X-ray source and film). Bronchography, now rarely performed, utilized instillation of contrast material into the bronchial tree, followed by radiography. Bronchography had been used primarily in the evaluation of bronchiectasis, a role that is now filled by HRCT (3).

III. Indications for Imaging in Severe Asthma

The clinician is frequently faced with the question "Is an imaging study indicated in the diagnosis and/or management of my patient?" This question is as appropriate for severe asthma as it is for any other medical condition. The question is also particularly important in this era of attempted health cost containment. Every procedure, laboratory test, or imaging study should add value to the patient's medical care and management. Additional studies or procedures that will not affect the patient's care or management do not add such value.

A number of investigators have evaluated the efficacy of chest radiographs in patients with asthma. Patient populations and clinical circumstances have varied somewhat in these studies, and a wide range of recommendations has resulted from these investigations. A brief review of some of these studies and the resulting recommendations follows.

Zieverink et al. (5) reviewed 528 adult and 464 pediatric chest radiographs, obtained in the emergency room or pediatric walk-in clinic. Patients included in the study were considered to have uncomplicated asthma, as defined by the American Thoracic Society. Only 2.2% of the adult chest radiographs demonstrated abnormalities, and the investigators concluded that chest radiographs are unnecessary in adult asthmatics unless the patient is unresponsive to bronchodilator therapy or is being admitted to the hospital. Approximately 13% of asthmatic children had abnormal radiographs. Chest radiographs were felt to be appropriate and potentially helpful in children with rales, rhonchi, and wheezing.

Findley and Sohn (6) reviewed 90 episodes of acute asthma in adults seen in an emergency room. One patient had a new infiltrate due to allergic aspergillosis, while 6 patients had minimal, stable interstitial abnormalities. The remainder of the radiographs were either normal (50 cases) or demonstrated hyperinflation (33 cases). The investigators concluded that chest radiographs are probably indicated only when pneumonia, a complication of asthma, or a condition mimicking asthma is suspected.

Heckerling (7) found a low incidence of chest radiograph abnormalities in 106 patients with acute asthma (2% with pneumonia and 5% with other abnormalities). He concluded that chest radiographs are not routinely needed in patients with acute asthma because they rarely have pneumonia.

Blair et al. (8) reported a retrospective review of 563 adult asthma patients seen in an emergency room setting. Of the 197 patients in whom chest radiographs were obtained, 42% had abnormal radiographic findings (hyperinflation and bronchial wall thickening were regarded as abnormalities in this series). Only 9% of the radiographed patients had complicated asthma, manifested by infiltrates or atelectasis on the chest radiographs. Therefore, only 3% of the entire group of asthma patients had radiographic abnormalities that would change medical management. Blair also indicated that within their institution, chest radiographs are obtained in adult patients if it is the initial episode of asthma in a patient older than 50 years of age, there is a poor response to bronchodilator therapy, or the patient exhibits fever or purulent sputum production.

Similarly, Sherman et al. (9) reported radiographic abnormalities resulting in clinically significant management changes in 4.5% of 242 patients hospitalized for exacerbation of COPD. Fifty-six percent of these patients had asthma, while the remainder had emphysema or chronic bronchitis. They proposed that chest radiographs be obtained in such patients when the white blood cell count exceeds 15 billion/L, the PMN leukocyte count exceeds 8 billion/L, there is a history of congestive heart failure or coronary artery disease, or the patient presents with chest pain or edema.

White and colleagues (10) reported a series of 54 adult asthmatics admitted to a hospital after failure of a 12-h course of bronchodilator therapy. Major radiographic abnormalities were found in 34% of the patients, while minor abnormalities were found in 41% of patients. They concluded that chest radiographs should be obtained in all adult patients admitted to the hospital for acute asthma.

Rossi et al. (11) reviewed a series of adult asthmatic patients that were admitted to the hospital. Chest radiographic abnormalities were detected in 50%, leading to management changes in only 5% of patients. Paranasal sinus radiographs, on the other hand, were abnormal 85% of the time and resulted in alteration of treatment in 29% of cases. While they felt that obtaining chest radiographs in severe cases of asthma may be advisable, they also recommended consideration of sinus radiographs in this population of patients, given the high incidence of sinus abnormalities and the frequency with which therapy was altered in such patients.

Tsai and colleagues (12) studied a series of patients admitted to the hospital with obstructive airway disease, dividing the patients into two groups, complicated and uncomplicated. Patients were classified as complicated if they met any of the following conditions: COPD, fever, or temperature greater than 37.8° C, heart disease, drug abuse, seizures, immunosuppression, other pulmonary disease, or a history of thoracic surgery. In the group of complicated patients, chest radiographic abnormalities resulted in alteration of clinical management in 26 of 84 (31%) admissions. Within the group of uncomplicated patients, chest radiographic findings altered the course of clinical management in only 1 of 44 (2%) patients. By limiting admission chest radiographs to those patients determined to be complicated, based on the clinical criteria noted above, these investigators believed that the need for admission chest radiographs could be reduced by about 34%.

In summary, a variety of recommendations regarding the utility of the chest radiograph have been suggested in the literature. Many of the studies described above included a much broader spectrum of patients than the severe asthmatic patients we are considering in this text. It would seem logical that, given the greater severity of disease and the increased importance in identifying complications early in the clinical course, one should be more liberal in obtaining chest radiographs in the group of patients with severe asthma than in the asthma population as a whole. On the other hand, careful consideration of each patient's clinical course and current condition may allow one to reduce the need for chest radiographs, even in the severe asthma population, thereby decreasing medical costs and radiation exposure to the patient.

Chest CT scanning, a technically more demanding and higher cost study, should be utilized in even fewer patients than chest radiography. However, chest CT plays a vital role in identifying complications of asthma, particularly allergic bronchopulmonary aspergillosis (ABPA). CT may also be very useful in identifying other conditions that may mimic severe asthma. Prime examples of such conditions are hypersensitivity pneumonitis, emphysema, interstitial lung diseases, and certain forms of bronchiolitis (13). In addition, HRCT is useful in assessing concomitant emphysema in smokers with severe asthma (14). Therefore, CT of the chest is indicated in patients with severe asthma in whom the clinical features or physiology suggest ABPA, emphysema, interstitial lung disease, or small airways disease.

IV. Key Imaging Findings in Severe Asthma

In this section, the chest radiographic and CT/HRCT findings of severe asthma are reviewed. Alimentary tract and sinus findings are also discussed. The key features of asthma on chest radiographs and chest CT include bronchial wall thickening, bronchial luminal narrowing, bronchial dilatation, and air trapping. Other features, such as mucous plugging, pulmonary consolidation, atelectasis, pneumomediastinum, and pneumothorax, are also occasionally seen in asthmatics.

A. Chest Radiographic Findings in Severe Asthma

Paganin et al. (15) reviewed the chest radiographs of 57 adult patients with chronic asthma of varying severity. Bronchial wall thickening was the most common abnormality identified, present in between 22 and 46% of patients, depending on the graded severity of the asthma (Fig. 1). Consolidation and/or infiltrates were seen in a few patients with moderate (10%) and severe (23%) asthma. Emphysema was present in 2 (15%) of the patients with severe asthma. Pneumomediastinum was observed in 1 patient with milder asthma. It is notable that Paganin did not consider hyperinflation to be a radiographic abnormality because

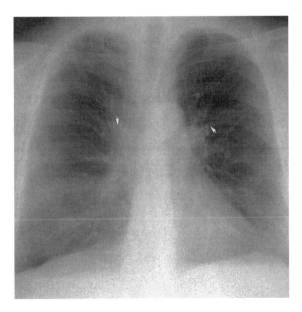

Figure 1 Chest radiograph of 54-year-old male with asthma reveals hyperinflation and bronchial wall thickening (arrows).

of its common occurrence in asthmatics as well as its poor specificity. Similarly, some other investigators have ignored hyperinflation when considering the chest radiographic abnormalities of asthma (5,7,16).

Eggleston et al. (16) reviewed 515 pediatric asthma admissions, of which 479 had chest films. Approximately 22% of radiographs demonstrated abnormalities other than hyperinflation. Perihilar infiltrates were most common (18%), followed by atelectasis (most commonly in the right middle lobe). Infiltrates occurred most commonly in the younger age group, those less than 6 years old. Pneumomediastinum was also relatively common, especially in older children (15.5% of patients over 10 years old demonstrated pneumomediastinum), and it was more commonly seen in more severe asthma.

Hodson and colleagues (17) described the radiologic abnormalities in 117 adult patients (over 15 years of age) admitted to Brompton Hospital with uncomplicated asthma. Those with pneumonia or ABPA were excluded from this study. They described two patterns of overinflation (hyperinflation) of the thorax, with one pattern consisting of simple pulmonary overinflation and the second pattern also showing enlargement of the pulmonary hilar vessels when compared to the intrapulmonary vessels. Hodson utilized a number of radiographic criteria in diagnosing overinflation, including depression of hemidiaphragms to the level of the anterior seventh ribs or below, lung length the same as or greater than lung width, heart diameter less than 11.5 cm, and retrosternal transradiancy greater than 3.5 cm in anteroposterior dimension. Overinflation was observed in 22 of the 117 patients, constant in 14, and reversible with resolution of the acute asthma attack in 8. Interestingly, the overinflation was seen in patients with an earlier onset of asthma symptoms (31% of patients with onset of asthma occurring between birth and age 15 and 0% of patients with onset of asthma after 30 years of age). This overinflation described by Hodson almost certainly reflects air trapping in these patients (Fig. 2).

In the article by Blair et al. (8), a number of radiographic findings of asthma were described. In uncomplicated asthma, hyperaeration, bronchial wall thickening, and transient pulmonary arterial hypertension were reported. Subjective assessment of hyperaeration, on the basis of increased retrosternal lucency, anterior bowing of the sternum, bulging of the intercostal spaces, and flattening of the hemidiaphragms, was thought to be as valuable as any objective methods used for evaluating hyperaeration. Pneumonitis, segmental or lobar atelectasis, pneumomediastinum, and pneumothorax were findings associated with complicated asthma. Consequences of long-term corticosteroid use were also noted, including mediastinal fat deposition, osteoporosis, avascular necrosis, and increased incidence of infections. Some of these consequences may be radiographically evident.

Rothstein et al. (18) evaluated total lung capacity in acute asthma by measuring radiographic lung volumes. Measurements were performed during acute

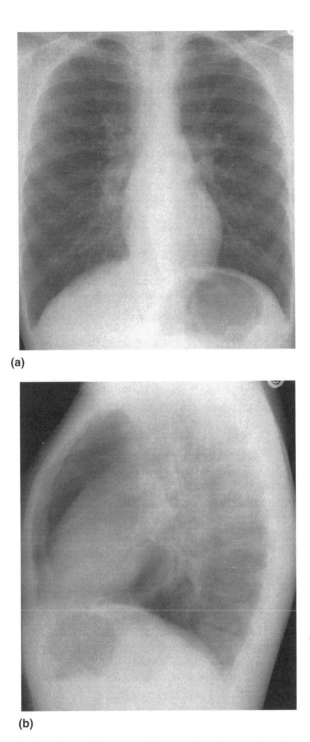

(a)

(b)

Figure 2 PA (a) and lateral (b) chest radiographs in a 14-year-old male asthmatic demonstrate hyperinflation and bronchial wall thickening.

asthma attacks as well as following improvement due to therapy. This study generally demonstrated a small decrease in total lung capacity as asthma improved, although some of the individual patients actually demonstrated slight increases in total lung capacity with improvement in their asthma symptoms.

Asthma usually involves the lungs symmetrically. However, an interesting case of reversible unilateral (left-sided) airway obstruction in a 32-year-old woman has been reported. Air trapping was observed radiographically in the left lung. Bronchoscopy demonstrated patency of the visible airways, with no evidence of obstructive tumor, mucous plug, or foreign body. Left-lung hyperinflation resolved with bronchodilator treatment. The reason for this unusual unilateral airway obstruction was not clear (19).

B. CT and HRCT Findings in Severe Asthma

A number of investigators have analyzed the HRCT features of asthma. The focus has been on several key features: air trapping, bronchial wall thickening and luminal narrowing, bronchial dilatation, and bronchial hyperreactivity.

Park et al. (20) compared HRCT findings in 39 asthmatics and 14 healthy controls. Although they found air trapping involving areas greater than one pulmonary segment to be more frequent in the asthmatic group (50%) than in the control group (14%), they found no significant difference in the prevalence of milder degrees of air trapping between the two groups.

Newman et al. (21) utilized quantitative techniques and density mask software in assessing expiratory and inspiratory air trapping in asthmatics compared to normal controls. CT pixels with an attenuation value of less than -900 Hounsfield units were considered to be indicative of air trapping. On expiratory HRCT and expiratory standard CT studies, a significantly higher proportion of these lower attenuation pixels were identified within the lungs of asthmatics compared to the normal controls, allowing for differentiation of the two groups. HRCT with 1.5-mm collimation was superior to standard CT with 10-mm collimation in identifying the areas of air trapping. Inspiratory CT scans revealed more overlap between the two groups and were less useful in distinguishing the two groups. The use of density mask software and quantitative techniques, though effective in identifying air trapping associated with asthma, may be too time consuming to gain widespread clinical usage.

Webb et al. (22) studied the changes in lung attenuation in 10 healthy, young male subjects on inspiratory and expiratory HRCT scans. Although lung attenuation usually decreased homogeneously with expiration, 4 of the 10 subjects demonstrated regional inhomogeneity of lung attenuation with rapid exhalation, indicating air trapping. Thus, one must realize that air trapping visible by HRCT expiratory images may not be an uncommon finding, even in normal individuals.

Lucidarme et al. (23) correlated findings on HRCT expiratory scans with PFT data. They analyzed air trapping on the basis of the lack of appropriate increase in lung attenuation with expiration (Fig. 3). The extent of air trapping was scored as a percentage by comparing the cross-sectional area of the lung affected by air trapping to the total cross-sectional area of lung. They also analyzed the change in cross-sectional area of the lungs between inspiratory and expiratory scans and calculated a "reduction score." These investigators found air trapping in subjects with chronic airways disease both with and without evidence of airway obstruction on PFTs. However, no air trapping was identified in the control group of 10 healthy subjects.

Bronchial wall thickening in asthma has also been the focus of a number of investigators. Paganin et al. (15) compared HRCT findings in those with asthma of varying severity with those of normal controls and found that the prevalence of bronchial wall thickening increased with increasingly severe asthma. For example, bronchial wall thickening was evident on the CT scans of

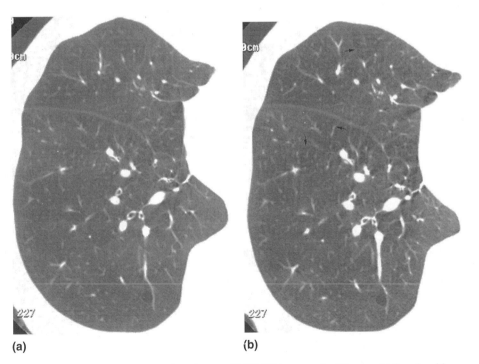

(a)   **(b)**

Figure 3 Inspiratory (a) and expiratory (b) HRCT images of a 63-year-old female with severe asthma. Patchy lucent zones (arrows) on expiratory image indicate expiratory air trapping. There is a small cyst in the right lower lobe.

15% of patients with mild asthma and of 23% of patients with more severe asthma. Furthermore, the prevalence of bronchial wall thickening was similar prior to and following treatment in a subgroup of patients treated with corticosteroids, suggesting some degree of irreversibility of the wall thickening (Figs. 4 and 5).

Okazawa et al. (24) used projection-magnification techniques to make detailed assessments of airway wall thickness, wall cross-sectional area, and luminal caliber on HRCT studies of asthmatics and healthy controls. Measurements were made both prior to and following bronchostimulation with methacholine chloride. Following methacholine challenge, for similar reductions in FEV_1, similar magnitudes of reduction in luminal area were seen in the two groups. Within the smaller airways, walls were significantly thickened in the asthmatic group compared to those of controls. Furthermore, in asthmatics, airway wall area did not decrease with bronchoconstriction, as it did in the normal control group. This fact may contribute to airway hyperresponsiveness in asthmatics.

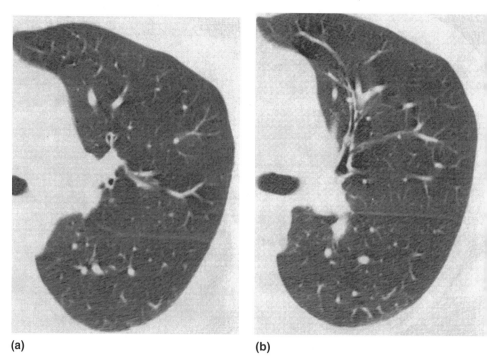

(a)   (b)

Figure 4 HRCT images of a 37-year-old female with severe asthma reveal bronchial wall thickening with luminal narrowing. Left upper lobe bronchi are shown both in cross section (a) and parallel to the scan plane (b).

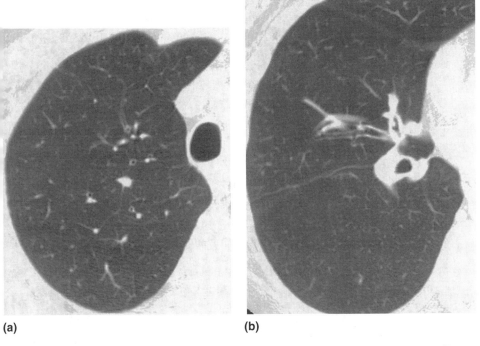

(a) **(b)**

Figure 5 HRCT images of a 48-year-old female with severe asthma demonstrate wall thickening and luminal narrowing involving medium-sized (a) and larger (b) airways.

Awadh et al. (25) conducted a study of airway wall thickness in asthma of varying severity (mild to near fatal) compared to that of normal controls. Precise measurements were made, using a projection-magnification technique. All of the asthma groups had thickened airway wall compared to normal subjects. Subjects with more severe asthma demonstrated a greater degree of wall thickening than those with milder asthma.

Park et al. (20) demonstrated that bronchial wall thickening on HRCT was more prevalent among asthmatics (44%) than among healthy subjects (4%). Additionally, the prevalence of bronchial wall thickening was found to be greater in asthmatics with severe airflow obstruction than in those with mild or no airflow obstruction.

Several published reports have indicated that bronchiectasis is commonly seen in asthma. Park et al. (20) reported bronchial dilatation in 24% of HRCT readings of patients with asthma of varying severity. Paganin and colleagues (15,26) reported relatively high frequencies of bronchiectasis, from 20 to 80%, depending on the severity of the asthma. Lynch et al. (27) analyzed individual bronchi and found that bronchial luminal caliber exceeded the caliber of the accompanying pulmonary artery quite frequently (36% of the bronchi of asthmatics and 26% of bronchi of normal subjects). At least one dilated bronchus was seen in 77% of asthmatic patients and in 59% of control subjects. Ward et al. (28) found that bronchiectasis was present on CT in 11 (29%) of 38 asthmatic patients. The differing prevalence of bronchiectasis or bronchial dilatation found in these studies is probably related to differing patient populations and differing definitions of bronchiectasis.

Brown, Herold, and colleagues (29,30) reported changes in airway caliber and airway pressure in anesthetized dogs after a challenge of histamine. Okazawa et al. (24) studied the reactivity of the airways in response to inhaled methacholine in asthmatics and healthy subjects.

We recently conducted a study (31) reviewing HRCT scans of 30 patients with severe asthma. The most frequent HRCT features were bronchial wall thickening in 30 (100%), expiratory air trapping in 19 of 22 examinations that included expiratory images (87%), inspiratory air trapping in 18 (60%), and bronchial luminal narrowing in 12 (40%). Minimal ground-glass opacity was found in 10 (33%) and evidence of pulmonary arterial hypertension was found in 8 (27%) of the severe asthma patients. Other HRCT features were found with less frequency (0–17%) in the severe asthma patients in this study. Of note, central bronchiectasis was found in 4 (13%) and peripheral bronchiectasis was found in 2 (7%) of these 30 severe asthmatics.

C. Alimentary Tract and Paranasal Sinus Findings in Severe Asthma

High incidences of gastroesophageal reflux (GER), hiatal hernia, and heartburn symptoms have been described in asthmatic patients by a number of investigators (32–34). Spontaneous GER and infusion of acid into the distal esophagus, simulating GER, have resulted in physiologic evidence of bronchoconstriction (35–37). Vagal nerve reflexes are thought to play a key role in this bronchoconstrictive response to GER or acid stimulation (34,38). Furthermore, medical and surgical treatment of GER disease has been shown to result in improvement in asthma symptoms and pulmonary function testing (39,40).

Medical imaging of GER disease is limited primarily to upper gastrointestinal tract studies (esophagram or upper GI series). The examiner should note any occurrence of spontaneous or provoked GER during the performance of these examinations. GER can be provoked by maneuvers that increase intraabdominal pressure, such as coughing, straight leg raising, Valsalva maneuver, or having a patient roll from a supine position with barium suspension in the gastric fundus. GER may also be induced by having a patient swallow water while lying in a right posterior oblique position with barium suspension in the gastric fundus.

This very sensitive provocative maneuver is termed the ''water siphon test.'' Hiatal hernias and reflux-induced changes of the distal esophagus, such as longitudinal fold thickening and ulcers or erosions, may also be observed on such contrast studies. Esophageal strictures may be present in those with chronic GER disease. These studies, usually performed fluoroscopically, also permit evaluation of esophageal function or dysfunction, which may contribute to GER disease.

Chest radiographs effectively demonstrate some of the larger hiatal hernias, which often contain an air–fluid level. Chest CT scans allow identification of smaller hiatal hernias when careful attention is paid to the gastroesophageal junction and the diaphragmatic hiatus. Esophageal wall thickening due to reflux esophagitis may also be recognized on CT scans of the chest or abdomen.

Scintigraphic studies have been used to monitor GER over time after oral administration of radiotracer-labeled liquids or solids. The frequency and magnitude of episodes of GER can be estimated from such examinations (41).

An association between inflammatory disease of the paranasal sinuses and asthma has also become apparent. Schwartz et al. (42) found that 47% of patients with acute exacerbations of asthma had abnormal sinus radiographs. Plain film sinus abnormalities included mucosal membrane thickening, cysts or rounded densities, opacified sinuses, and air–fluid levels. Since maxillary sinus abnormalities were most frequent, the most useful radiographic projection was thought to be the Waters' view. In this series, clinical history was found to be a poor predictor of whether sinus radiographs would be abnormal.

As mentioned earlier, Rossi et al. (11) found that radiographic abnormalities of the sinuses were more frequently found than chest radiographic abnormalities in acute asthma. Furthermore, sinus radiographs are more likely than chest radiographs to alter clinical management of the acute asthma patient.

Newman et al. (43) studied the relationship between chronic sinusitis and asthma as well as allergy and eosinophilia. Sinus CT scans were scored according to the degree of nasal passage and ostiomeatal complex obstruction and the extent of mucosal thickening within the sinuses. The association between chronic sinusitis and asthma was found to be strong only in those patients with extensive sinus disease. This study employed high-resolution, direct coronal CT scanning of the sinuses. Phillips and Platts-Mills (44) have emphasized the importance of proper preparation for sinus CT scans, including pretreatment with antibiotics and decongestants.

In the era of functional endoscopic sinus surgery (FESS), direct coronal CT scanning of the sinuses has become the study of choice, largely replacing sinus plain films (45,46) (Fig. 6). Coronal scans serve as a roadmap to the surgeon performing FESS. Limited axial scanning of the sinuses has been used in screening for sinusitis (47).

MRI has also found limited application in evaluation of the paranasal sinuses and surrounding structures. MRI may be useful in the analysis of develop-

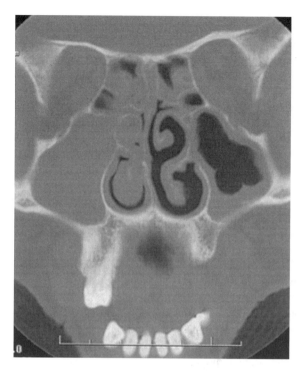

Figure 6 Extensive sinusitis in a 56-year-old female with asthma. Coronal CT scan demonstrates extensive mucosal thickening and opacification of maxillary antra and ethmoid air cells.

ment of the sinuses (48). It may also be of value in the analysis of complicated sinusitis, intraorbital and intracranial abnormalities associated with sinusitis, and neoplasm involving the sinuses and nasal cavity (45).

V. Imaging the Complications of Asthma

A. Pneumonia

Superimposed or concurrent pneumonia is sometimes suspected in the patient with an acute asthma attack. Bacteria, Mycoplasma, and viral agents are all possible sources of infection. As discussed in a preceding section, a broad range of results have been reported regarding the utility of a chest radiograph in the patient with severe asthma (5–12). In general, the incidence of pneumonia in patients with acute asthma has been found to be relatively low. However, since the presence of pneumonia would certainly affect the treatment of the asthmatic patient, one should strongly consider obtaining a chest radiograph in the asthmatic patient who is unresponsive to bronchodilator therapy, is febrile, or has an elevated WBC count or in whom concurrent pneumonia is suspected. Chest radiographs should be reviewed carefully for areas of consolidation or interstitial abnormalities that could represent pneumonia.

B. Pneumomediastinum

Pneumomediastinum is a surprisingly frequent finding in acute asthma, especially in the pediatric population. Eggleston et al. (16) identified pneumomediastinum in 5.4% of admission chest radiographs of children and adolescents with acute asthma. Dattwyler et al. (49) reported a series of 11 asthmatic patients, ranging in age from 13 to 31 years, in whom pneumomediastinum was discovered. Most of these patients presented with cough, chest pain, and dyspnea. None of these patients required specific therapy for the pneumomediastinum. Macklin (50) theorized that overinflation of the lungs can cause rupture of alveoli that are adjacent to the vascular sheaths, leading to air tracking along the vascular sheaths into the mediastinum. From the mediastinum, air may escape into the neck and chest wall soft tissues. Radiographic findings of pneumomediastinum include air within the mediastinum, air surrounding the pulmonary arteries, and neck and chest wall soft tissue emphysema.

C. Pneumothorax

Pneumothorax is a less common complication of asthma than pneumomediastinum. It may occur in conjunction with pneumomediastinum. It is most frequently seen in the asthmatic being treated with intermittent positive pressure ventilation, but may also occur spontaneously. It may be a fatal complication, so recognition is vital (8,16,51–54). PA and lateral chest radiographs are effective in demonstrating pneumothoraces. Expiratory PA films may increase the visibility of a pneumothorax by increasing the proportion of the volume of the pneumothorax to the total volume of the hemithorax as well as the difference in density of the lung compared to the surrounding pleural air (8). However, a more recent article by Seow et al. (4) showed that inspiratory and expiratory films are equally sensitive for pneumothorax detection.

D. Allergic Bronchopulmonary Aspergillosis

Allergic bronchopulmonary aspergillosis (ABPA) may affect 1–2% of patients with chronic asthma (55). It is usually caused by inhalation of spores of *Aspergillus fumigatus*, but it may also be caused by *Aspergillus glaucus*, *Aspergillus niger*, *Aspergillus terreus*, *Aspergillus flavus*, *Aspergillus oryzae*, or *Aspergillus ochraceus*. Fungi other than *Aspergillus* species may also cause illness, in which case it is termed allergic bronchopulmonary fungosis (ABPF) (56–59). The classic features of ABPA are asthma, immediate skin reactivity to *A. fumigatus*, serum precipitins to *A. fumigatus*, recurrent pulmonary infiltrates, peripheral blood eosinophilia, elevated serum IgE, central bronchiectasis, and elevated IgE and IgA antibodies to *A. fumigatus*. Although central bronchiectasis is classic, some patients with ABPA do not demonstrate this finding (55,60,61).

Early diagnosis and treatment of patients with ABPA is critical, since damage to the airways from the chronic inflammation can be limited by appropriate treatment, usually with corticosteroids, sometimes complemented by antifungal agents (55,60,61).

Medical imaging is crucial in the detection of the recurrent pulmonary infiltrates and central bronchiectasis that are characteristic of ABPA (Fig. 7). Chest radiography may identify these features, but the key imaging role is now filled by HRCT (62,63). Bronchography, once the gold standard in the diagnosis of bronchiectasis, carries with it the risks of impaired ventilation and diffusion, bronchospasm, and toxic effects of local anesthetic applied to respiratory epithelium. Hence, bronchography should not be performed in asthmatics, further emphasizing the need for HRCT in the evaluation of possible bronchiectasis in asthmatics (62). An HRCT–pathology correlation study demonstrated 87% sensitivity for HRCT in the identification of bronchiectasis proven on pathologic specimens (64).

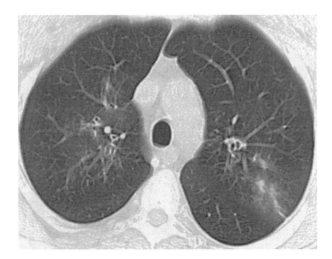

Figure 7 Thirty-seven-year-old asthmatic with ABPA. HRCT demonstrates cylindric bronchiectasis in the left upper lobe segmental bronchi and focal consolidation posteriorly, presumed due to eosinophilic infiltration.

Bronchiectasis consists of irreversible dilatation of bronchi, usually accompanied by bronchial wall thickening. The CT findings of bronchiectasis include circular shadows exceeding the caliber of the adjacent pulmonary artery ("signet ring" sign) and "tramlines," or parallel bronchial walls, extending for a distance within the sectional plane (65). The loss of normal tapering of bronchi, evident within bronchi that are parallel to the plane of a CT scan section, has been described as the best early sign of bronchiectasis (13,66). Bronchiectasis seen in the outer third of the lung is considered peripheral, while all other bronchiectasis is considered central (65). HRCT studies at different altitudes (sea level versus 1600 m above sea level) have suggested that hypoxic bronchodilatation and vasoconstriction may alter the typical caliber proportions of these structures. Therefore, some caution should be exercised in diagnosing bronchiectasis where such physiologic conditions may exist (67).

In comparing HRCT findings of patients with ABPA to those with non-ABPA asthma, Neeld and associates (62) found bronchial dilatation in 41% of lung lobes in those with ABPA compared to 15% in the non-ABPA asthmatic group. All of the bronchiectasis in the control group was cylindrical, whereas the ABPA group demonstrated cylindrical, varicose, and cystic forms of bronchiectasis (Fig. 8). Bronchial wall thickening and upper lobe involvement by bronchial dilatation were commonly seen in both groups. The relative insensitivity of chest radiography was highlighted by the fact that

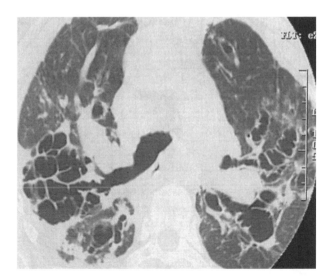

Figure 8 Fifty-year-old asthmatic with ABPA. HRCT demonstrates severe cystic bronchiectasis.

only 5 of 9 patients with bronchiectasis identified by HRCT had plain film abnormalities.

Similarly, Angus et al. (63) found a much higher incidence of bronchial dilatation in ABPA patients (43 of 102 examined pulmonary lobes) than in non-ABPA asthmatics (3 of 66 examined pulmonary lobes). Again, bronchial wall thickening was commonly seen in both groups of patients. Pleural thickening was commonly seen in patients with ABPA but seen in only a few instances in the non-ABPA group.

In yet another report, Ward et al. (28) found bronchiectasis in 42 (95%) of 44 patients with ABPA and in 11 (29%) of 38 asthmatics without ABPA. In addition, the bronchiectasis of ABPA was more often varicose or cystic compared to the cylindrical bronchiectasis typically seen in asthmatics without ABPA. These investigators suggested that bronchiectasis involving three or more lobes, centrilobular nodules, and mucoid impaction are strongly suggestive of ABPA.

Certainly, there are many other causes of bronchiectasis. Reiff et al. (68) reviewed a series of patients with idiopathic bronchiectasis, ABPA, hypogammaglobulinemia, impaired mucociliary clearance, or cystic fibrosis. In general, the bronchiectasis of ABPA and cystic fibrosis was more widespread than the bronchiectasis of other causes. Central bronchiectasis was more common in ABPA. Cylindrical bronchiectasis was the most common form seen in all causes of bronchiectasis, but the ABPA patients had a higher incidence of varicose and cystic bronchiectasis than the other groups. Despite these generalizations, making a specific diagnosis based on HRCT findings alone is hazardous. Clinical correlation should be sought when the HRCT demonstration of central bronchiectasis raises the possibility of ABPA.

Mucoid impaction within dilated or nondilated bronchi may also be observed in ABPA as well as in other conditions such as cystic fibrosis, bronchial atresia, intrapulmonary sequestration, and proximal bronchial obstruction (65). High attenuation of the material constituting mucous plugs has been reported in association with ABPA (69,70).

E. Churg–Strauss Syndrome

Churg–Strauss syndrome is seen almost exclusively in patients with asthma. This syndrome consists of a systemic necrotizing vasculitis, sometimes associated with eosinophilia and/or extravascular granuloma formation. The vasculitis may affect the lungs, skin, kidneys, and peripheral nerves. Patchy, migratory consolidations or ground-glass opacities, which may be peripheral or random in distribution, are the most common findings on radiographs or CT scans. The findings are nonspecific (1,71). Extrapulmonary findings may be very helpful in arriving at the proper diagnosis. For example, sinus radiographs or CT scans may detect the commonly detected sinus disease. Physical examination of the patient may reveal an associated skin rash (72) (Fig. 9).

F. Eosinophilic Pneumonia

Eosinophilic pneumonia may also occur in patients with asthma. Mayo et al. (73) reported CT findings in six patients with chronic eosinophilic pneumonia, four of whom had histories of asthma. The key radiologic and CT finding of eosinophilic pneumonia is predominantly peripheral air space consolidation. The peripheral nature of the consolidation is more readily apparent on CT studies than on chest radiographs. The presence of blood eosinophilia may help secure the diagnosis of eosinophilic pneumonia when the peripheral consolidation pattern is recognized.

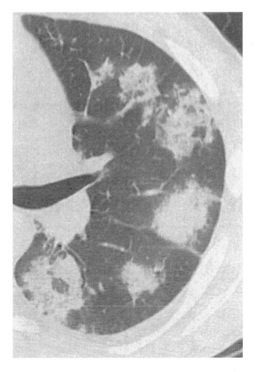

Figure 9 Churg–Strauss syndrome in a 37-year-old with severe asthma, treated with leukotriene antagonists. Chest radiograph (a) and HRCT images (b and c) revealed multifocal bilateral pulmonary consolidation.

VI. Detection of Conditions Which May Mimic Severe Asthma

A. Bronchiolitis Obliterans

Bronchiolitis obliterans, also known as obliterative bronchiolitis or constrictive bronchiolitis, is a small airways disease that is histologically characterized by proliferation of fibrous tissue in the bronchiolar walls (74,75). While many cases of bronchiolitis obliterans are cryptogenic, the condition also occurs in the setting of connective tissue diseases such as rheumatoid arthritis, toxic fume inhalation, antecedent lower respiratory tract infection, chronic rejection of lung or heart–lung transplantation, graft versus host disease associated with bone marrow transplantation, chronic hypersensitivity pneumonitis, Swyer–James syndrome, and use of drugs such as penicillamine and cocaine (74–81).

Bronchiolitis obliterans is characterized clinically by irreversible airway obstruction. Clinical diagnosis requires exclusion of emphysema, chronic bronchitis, asthma, and other causes of airway obstruction (77). The clinical differentiation of bronchiolitis obliterans from severe asthma may be difficult, especially when the latter exhibits irreversible or only partially reversible airway obstruction.

We studied the HRCT findings in 30 severe asthma and 14 bronchiolitis obliterans patients. We discovered that broad overlap exists in the HRCT findings of these two conditions. Specifically, inspiratory and expiratory air trapping, bronchial wall thickening, and bronchial luminal narrowing are commonly seen in both conditions. However, inspiratory and expiratory air trapping tend to be more extensive in bronchiolitis obliterans than in severe asthma. In addition, a mosaic pattern of lung attenuation, presumably due to a combination of air trapping and hypoxic vasoconstriction, is commonly seen in bronchiolitis obliterans (50% in our series) but is uncommonly seen in severe asthma (3% in our series). Identification of the mosaic pattern of lung attenuation on HRCT is therefore suggestive of bronchiolitis obliterans when considering a patient with obstructive airways disease. In the absence of this mosaic pattern, differentiation of bronchiolitis obliterans and severe asthma by HRCT remains difficult (31) (Fig. 10).

B. Chronic Bronchitis

Chronic bronchitis is a clinical diagnosis characterized by a chronic productive cough for 3 months or longer in each of 2 consecutive years. Other causes of chronic cough should be excluded before this diagnosis is made. Radiographic findings of chronic bronchitis primarily consist of bronchial wall thickening and normal lung volumes. Pulmonary hyperinflation is thought to be rare in chronic bronchitis. As the radiographic findings are nonspecific, the greatest utility of the chest radiograph is in the exclusion of other processes that might mimic chronic

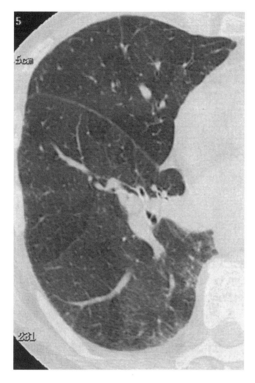

Figure 10 Mosaic pattern of lung attenuation is apparent on this inspiratory HRCT image in an 82-year-old female with bronchiolitis obliterans.

bronchitis (13,82). Differentiation of severe asthma from chronic bronchitis is usually possible by analysis of history and clinical features rather than by dependence on imaging findings.

C. Emphysema

Pulmonary emphysema, the permanent enlargement of air spaces distal to the terminal bronchioles and associated wall destruction, is usually easier to detect on HRCT than on chest radiographs, depending on the severity of the emphysema. The classic radiographic findings of emphysema are increased pulmonary radiolucency and vascular attenuation, which is manifest by a decreased number of vessels, fewer vascular branches, increased branching angles, and straightening of vessels. Increased peribronchovascular interstitial opacities may also be seen in some patients, particularly those with cor pulmonale (83). HRCT can readily identify macroscopic areas of lung destruction, which may be panlobular, centrilobular, distal acinar (paraseptal), or irregular in morphology (83,84). Panlobular emphysema, which may be seen in α1-antitrypsin deficiency, often has a lower lobe predominance. Centrilobular emphysema, the most common variety and strongly associated with cigarette smoking, generally has an upper lung zone predominance. Distal acinar emphysema is subpleural and may lead to large bulla formation. Irregular (paracicatricial) emphysema occurs in areas of fibrosis and scarring (84). Quantitative techniques, in which areas of lung attenuation below a certain Hounsfield unit threshold are identified, have been used for the identification of not only macroscopic emphysema, but also microscopic areas of emphysema (83–85). Obviously, asthma and emphysema may be concurrent conditions, especially in cigarette smokers. CT can be helpful in identifying emphysema in such patients (14) (Fig. 11).

D. Bronchiectasis

Bronchial dilatation or bronchiectasis may occur in uncomplicated asthma as well as in asthma associated with ABPA (15,20,26,27). A host of other causes of bronchiectasis exist, including cystic fibrosis, ciliary dyskinesia, immunodeficiency disorders, tracheobronchomegaly, toxic gas inhalation, α1-antitrypsin deficiency, rheumatoid arthritis, childhood infections, mycobacterial infection (particularly with *Mycobaterium avium* complex), bacterial pneumonia, and chronic aspiration. Many cases of bronchiectasis are also idiopathic (13). HRCT is very useful in identifying the presence, extent, and distribution of bronchiectasis.

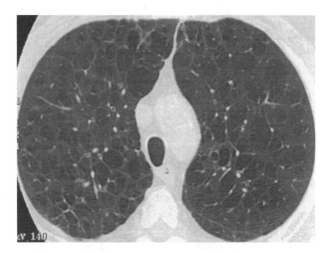

Figure 11 Extensive centrilobular emphysema is well demonstrated by HRCT in this 70-year-old male.

E. Hypersensitivity Pneumonitis

Hypersensitivity pneumonitis, or extrinsic allergic alveolitis, in its acute, sub-acute, and chronic phases, may in some cases cause diagnostic confusion with severe asthma, especially when an obvious inhaled organic antigen is not identified. Although chest radiographs may demonstrate abnormalities such as ground-glass opacity, peribronchial thickening, or a diffuse granular pattern (86), HRCT has been found to be more sensitive in the detection of hypersensitivity pneumonitis (86,87). HRCT findings in acute and subacute hypersensitivity pneumonitis include poorly defined centrilobular nodules, ground-glass opacities, and patchy air space consolidation (87–89) (Fig. 12). In more chronic cases of hypersensitivity pneumonitis, focal decreased attenuation and mosaic perfusion, ground-glass opacities, small nodules, focal air trapping or emphysema, and fibrosis have been described (86,90–92). Thus, identification of such radiographic or HRCT features in a patient with acute or chronic respiratory symptoms may prompt further investigation into exposure history, and a cause of hypersensitivity pneumonitis may eventually be identified.

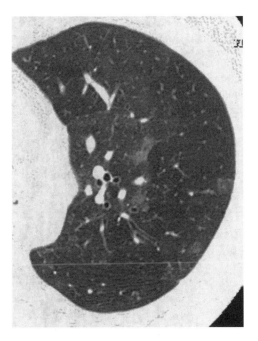

Figure 12 Hypersensitivity pneumonitis in this 45-year-old female is manifest on HRCT as patchy ground-glass opacity with a large area of decreased lung attenuation in the lateral lung.

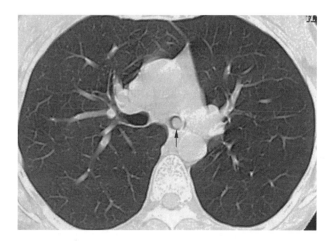

Figure 13   This 44-year-old female presented with shortness of breath. Pulmonary function testing revealed irreversible airway obstruction. CT scan demonstrates a mass nearly completely occluding the left mainstem bronchus. The mass was a bronchial carcinoid.

F. Large Airway Obstruction

Finally, large airway obstruction may occasionally cause confusion with asthma. Vocal cord dysfunction (VCD), the paradoxical closure of the vocal cords with inspiration, may simulate asthma or may coexist with asthma (93–97). The diagnosis of VCD is dependent on laryngoscopic observation of the vocal cords. Imaging studies of the thorax in VCD are usually normal. Stenosis or mass involving the trachea or bronchi may also present with symptoms mimicking asthma. Careful attention to the large airways on chest radiographs and chest CT scans may allow diagnosis of such obstructive lesions. Helicor CT section through suspicious areas may elucidate the nature of the lesions (Fig. 13).

VII. Conclusion

Medical imaging tools and their application in the diagnosis and management of severe asthma have been reviewed. Properly applied, medical imaging may reflect the anatomic and physiological abnormalities responsible for signs and symptoms in the severe asthmatic. Imaging may allow identification of important complications of severe asthma. Finally, a number of conditions that mimic or may be confused with asthma may be recognized through imaging procedures. Future research in the imaging of severe asthma will focus on quantitating the amount of large and small airway disease using quantitative spiral and high-resolution

CT techniques. Future research will try to identify imaging patterns to distinguish severe asthma from less severe forms and bronchiolitis.

References

1. Lynch DA. Imaging of asthma and its complications. Thoracic Imaging 1999 (Syllabus). Amelia Island, FL: Society of Thoracic Radiologists, Mar 21–25, 1999.
2. Snider GL. Distinguishing among asthma, chronic bronchitis, and emphysema. Chest 1985; 87(suppl):35–39.
3. Fraser RS, Müller NL, Colman N, Paré PD, eds. Methods of radiologic investigation. Diagnosis of Diseases of the Chest. 4th ed. Philadelphia: W. B. Saunders, 1999: 299–338.
4. Seow A, Kazerooni EA, Cascade PN, Pernicano PG, Neary M. Comparison of upright inspiratory and expiratory chest radiographs for detecting pneumothoraces. AJR 1996; 166:313–316.
5. Zieverink SE, Harper AP, Holden RW, Klatte EC, Brittain H. Emergency room radiography of asthma: an efficacy study. Radiology 1982; 145:27–29.
6. Findley LJ, Sahn SA. The value of chest roentgenograms in acute asthma in adults. Chest 1981; 80:535–536.
7. Heckerling PS. The need for chest roentgenograms in adults with acute respiratory illness. Arch Intern Med 1986; 146:1321–1324.
8. Blair DN, Coppage L, Shaw C. Medical imaging in asthma. J Thorac Imag 1986; 1(2):23–35.
9. Sherman S, Skoney JA, Ravikrishnan KP. Routine chest radiographs in exacerbations of chronic obstructive pulmonary disease. Arch Intern Med 1989; 149:2493–2496.
10. White CS, Cole RP, Lubetsky HW, Austin JHM. Acute asthma: admission chest radiography in hospitalized adult patients. Chest 1991; 100:14–16.
11. Rossi OVJ, Lahde S, Laitinen J, Huhti E. Contribution of chest and paranasal sinus radiographs to the management of acute asthma. Int Arch Allergy Immunol 1994; 105:96–100.
12. Tsai TW, Gallagher EJ, Lombardi G, Gennis P, Carter W. Guidelines for the selective ordering of admission chest radiography in adult obstructive airway disease. Ann Emerg Med 1993; 22:1854–1858.
13. Newell JD, Chan ED, Martin RJ. Imaging of airway disease. In: Lynch DA, Newell JD, Lee JS, eds. Imaging of Diffuse Lung Disease. Hamilton: B. C. Decker, 2000: 171–197.
14. Kondoh Y, Taniguchi H, Yokoyama S, Taki F, Takagi K, Satake T. Emphysematous change in chronic asthma in relation to cigarette smoking: assessment by computed tomography. Chest 1990; 97:845–849.
15. Paganin F, Trussard V, Seneterre E, Chanez P, Giron J, Godard P, Senac JP, Michel FB, Bousquet J. Chest radiography and high resolution computed tomography of the lungs in asthma. Am Rev Respir Dis 1992; 146:1084–1087.
16. Eggleston PA, Ward BH, Pierson WE, Bierman, CW. Radiographic abnormalities in acute asthma in children. Pediatrics 1974; 54:442–449.

17. Hodson ME, Simon G, Batten JC. Radiology of uncomplicated asthma. Thorax 1974; 29:296–303.
18. Rothstein MS, Zelefsky MN, Eichacker PQ, Rudolph DJ, Williams MH. Radiographic measurement of total lung capacity in acute asthma. Thorax 1989; 44:510–512.
19. DiFrancia M, Barbier D, Orehek J. Left lung asthma. Chest 1993; 104:1919–1920.
20. Park CS, Müller NL, Worthy SA, Kim JS, Awadh N, Fitzgerald M. Airway obstruction in asthmatic and healthy individuals: inspiratory and expiratory thin-section CT findings. Radiology 1997; 203:361–367.
21. Newman KB, Lynch DA, Newman LS, Ellegood D, Newell JD. Quantitative computed tomography detects air trapping due to asthma. Chest 1994; 106:105–109.
22. Webb WR, Stern EJ, Kanth N, Gamsu G. Dynamic pulmonary CT: findings in healthy adult men. Radiology 1993; 186:117–124.
23. Lucidarme O, Coche E, Cluzel P, Mourey-Gerosa I, Howarth N, Grenier P. Expiratory CT scans for chronic airway disease: correlation with pulmonary function test results. AJR 1998; 170:301–307.
24. Okazawa M, Müller NL, McNamara AE, Child S, Verburgt L, Pare PD. Human airway narrowing measured using high resolution computed tomography. Am J Respir Crit Care Med 1996; 154:1557–1562.
25. Awadh N, Müller NL, Park CS, Abboud RT, Fitzgerald JM. Airway wall thickness in patients with near fatal asthma and control groups: assessment with high resolution computed tomographic scanning. Thorax 1998; 53:248–253.
26. Paganin F, Seneterre E, Chanez P, Daures JP, Bruel JM, Michel FB, Bousquet J. Computed tomography of the lungs in asthma: influence of disease severity and etiology. Am J Respir Crit Care Med 1996; 153:110–114.
27. Lynch DA, Newell JD, Tschomper BA, Cink TM, Newman LS, Bethel R. Uncomplicated asthma in adults: comparison of CT appearance of the lungs in asthmatic and healthy subjects. Radiology 1993; 188:829–833.
28. Ward S, Heyneman L, Lee MJ, Leung AN, Hansell, DM, Müller NL. Accuracy of CT in the diagnosis of allergic bronchopulmonary aspergillosis in asthmatic patients. AJR 1999; 173:937–942.
29. Brown RH, Herold CJ, Hirshman CA, Zerhouni EA, Mitzner W. In vivo measurements of airway reactivity using high-resolution computed tomography. Am Rev Respir Dis 1991; 144:208–212.
30. Herold CJ, Brown RH, Mitzner W, Links JM, Hirshman CA, Zerhouni EA. Assessment of pulmonary airway reactivity with high-resolution CT. Radiology 1991; 181:369–374.
31. Jensen SP, Lynch DA, Brown KK, Wenzel SE, Newell JD. High resolution CT features of severe asthma and bronchiolitis obliterans. Chicago, IL: Annual Meeting of the Radiological Society of North America, Nov 26–Dec 1, 2000.
32. Mays EE. Intrinsic asthma in adults: association with gastroesophageal reflux. J Am Med Assoc 1976; 236:2626–2628.
33. Sontag SJ. Gut feelings about asthma: the burp and the wheeze. Chest 1991; 99:1321–1324.
34. Cunningham ET, Ravich WJ, Jones B, Donner MW. Vagal reflexes referred from

the upper aerodigestive tract: an infrequently recognized cause of common cardiore-spiratory responses. Ann Intern Med 1992; 116:575–582.

35. Tan WC, Martin RJ, Pandey R, Ballard RD. Effects of spontaneous and simulated gastroesophageal reflux on sleeping asthmatics. Am Rev Respir Dis 1990; 141: 1394–1399.

36. Ekström T, Tibbling L. Esophageal acid perfusion, airway function, and symptoms in asthmatic patients with marked bronchial hyperreactivity. Chest 1989; 95:995–998.

37. Schan CA, Harding SM, Haile JM, Bradley LA, Richter JE. Gastroesophageal reflux-induced bronchoconstriction: an intraesophageal acid infusion study using state-of-the-art technology. Chest 1994; 106:731–737.

38. Mansfield LE, Hameister HH, Spaulding HS, Smith NJ, Glab N. The role of the vagus nerve in airway narrowing caused by intraesophageal hydrochloric acid provocation and esophageal distention. Ann Allergy 1981; 47:431–434.

39. Larrain A, Carrasco E, Galleguillos F, Sepulveda R, Pope CE. Medical and surgical treatment of nonallergic asthma associated with gastroesophageal reflux. Chest 1991; 99:1330–1335.

40. Harper PC, Bergner A, Kaye MD. Antireflux treatment for asthma: improvement in patients with associated gastroesophageal reflux. Arch Intern Med 1987; 147:56–60.

41. Roy CC, Silverman A, Alagille D. Pediatric Clinical Gastroenterology. 4th ed. St. Louis: Mosby-Year Book, 1995:163–166.

42. Schwartz HJ, Thompson JS, Sher TH, Ross RJ. Occult sinus abnormalities in the asthmatic patient. Arch Intern Med 1987; 147:2194–2196.

43. Newman LJ, Platts-Mills TAE, Phillips CD, Hazen KC, Gross CW. Chronic sinusitis: relationship of computed tomographic findings to allergy, asthma, and eosinophilia. J Am Med Assoc 1994; 271:363–367.

44. Phillips CD, Platts-Mills TAE. Chronic sinusitis: relationship between CT findings and clinical history of asthma, allergy, eosinophilia, and infection. AJR 1995; 164: 185–187.

45. Yousem DM. Imaging of sinonasal inflammatory disease. Radiology 1993; 188: 303–314.

46. Laine FJ, Smoker WRK. The ostiomeatal unit and endoscopic surgery: anatomy, variations, and imaging findings in inflammatory diseases. AJR 1992; 159:849–857.

47. Witte RJ, Heurter JV, Orton DF, Hahn FJ. Limited axial CT of the paranasal sinuses in screening for sinusitis. AJR 1996; 167:1313–1315.

48. Scuderi AJ, Harnsberger HR, Boyer RS. Pneumatization of the paranasal sinuses: normal features of importance to the accurate interpretation of CT scans and MR images. AJR 1993; 160:1101–1104.

49. Dattwyler RJ, Goldman MA, Bloch KJ. Pneumomediastinum as a complication of asthma in teenage and young adult patients. J Allergy Clin Immunol 1979; 63:412–416.

50. Macklin CC. Transport of air along sheaths of pulmonic blood vessels from alveoli to mediastinum: clinical implications. Arch Intern Med 1939; 64:913.

51. Burke GJ. Pneumothorax complicating acute asthma. S Afr Med J 1979; 55:508–510.

52. Legge DA, Tiede JJ, Peters GA et al. Death from tension pneumothorax and chlor-
     promazine cardiorespiratory collapse as separate complications of asthma. Ann Al-
     lergy 1969; 27:23–29.
53. Karetzky MS. Asthma mortality associated with pneumothorax and intermittent pos-
     itive pressure breathing. Lancet 1975; 1:828–829.
54. Bierman CW. Pneumomediastinum and pneumothorax complicating asthma in chil-
     dren. Am J Dis Child 1967; 114:42.
55. Greenberger PA, Miller TP, Roberts M, Smith LL. Allergic bronchopulmonary as-
     pergillosis in patients with and without evidence of bronchiectasis. Ann Allergy
     1993; 70:333–338.
56. Backman K, Roberts M, Patterson R. Allergic bronchopulmonary mycosis caused
     by Fusarium vasinfectum. Am J Respir Crit Care Med 1995; 152:1379–1381.
57. Kamei K, Unno H, Nagao K, Kuriyama T, Nishimura K. Allergic bronchopulmonary
     mycosis caused by the basidiomycetous fungus Schizophyllum commune. Clin In-
     fect Dis 1994; 18:305–309.
58. Lee TM, Greenberger PA, Oh S, Patterson R, Roberts M, Liotta JL. Allergic bron-
     chopulmonary candidiasis: case report and suggested diagnostic criteria. J Allergy
     Clin Immunol 1987; 80:816–820.
59. Miller MA, Greenberger PA, Amerian R et al. Allergic bronchopulmonary mycosis
     caused by Pseudallescheria boydii. Am Rev Respir Dis 1993; 148:810–812.
60. Greenberger PA. Diagnosis and management of allergic bronchopulmonary aspergil-
     losis. Allergy Proc 1994; 15:335–339.
61. Denning DW, Van Wye JE, Lewiston NJ, Stevens DA. Adjunctive therapy of al-
     lergic bronchopulmonary aspergillosis with itraconozole. Chest 1991; 100:813–
     819.
62. Neeld DA, Goodman LR, Gurney JW, Greenberger PA, Fink JN. Computerized
     tomography in the evaluation of allergic bronchopulmonary aspergillosis. Am Rev
     Respir Dis 1990; 142:1200–1205.
63. Angus RM, Davies M-L, Cowan MD, McSharry C, Thomson NC. Computed tomo-
     graphic scanning of the lung in patients with allergic bronchopulmonary aspergillosis
     and in asthmatic patients with a positive skin test to Aspergillus fumigatus. Thorax
     1994; 49:586–589.
64. Kang EY, Müller RR, Müller NL. Bronchiectasis: comparison of preoperative thin-
     section CT and pathologic findings in resected specimens. Radiology 1995; 195:
     649–654.
65. McGuiness G, Naidich DP, Leitman BS, McCauley DI. Bronchiectasis: CT evalua-
     tion. AJR 1993; 160:253–259.
66. Lynch DA. Imaging of asthma and allergic bronchopulmonary mycosis. Radiol Clin
     North Am 1998; 36(1):129–142.
67. Kim JS, Müller NL, Park CS, Lynch DA, Newman LS, Grenier P, Herold CJ. Bron-
     choarterial ratio on thin section CT: comparison between high altitude and sea level.
     J Comput Assist Tomogr 1997; 21(2):306–311.
68. Reiff DB, Wells AU, Carr DH, Cole PJ, Hansell DM. CT findings in bronchiectasis:
     limited value in distinguishing between idiopathic and specific types. AJR 1995;
     165:261–267.
69. Goyal R, White CS, Templeton PA, Britt EJ, Rubin LJ. High attenuation mucous

plugs in allergic bronchopulmonary aspergillosis: CT appearance. J Comput Assist Tomogr 1992; 16:649–650.

70. Logan PM, Müller NL. High-attenuation mucous plugging in allergic bronchopulmonary aspergillosis. Can Assoc Radiol J 1996; 47:374–377.

71. Worthy SA, Müller NL, Hansell DM, Flower CDR. Churg–Strauss syndrome: the spectrum of pulmonary CT findings in 17 patients. AJR 1998; 170:297–300.

72. Li GW, Dickey BF, Green LK, Manian P. Recurrent asthma, sinusitis, and rash in a 63-year-old man. Chest 1995; 108:1451–1453.

73. Mayo JR, Müller NL, Road J, Sisler J, Lillington G. Chronic eosinophilic pneumonia: CT findings in six cases. AJR 1989; 153:727–730.

74. Fraser RS, Müller NL, Colman N, Paré PD, eds. Bronchiolitis. Diagnosis of Diseases of the Chest. 4th ed. Philadelphia: W. B. Saunders, 1999:2321–2357.

75. King TE. Bronchiolitis obliterans. Lung 1989; 167:69–93.

76. Garg K, Lynch DA, Newell JD, King TE. Proliferative and constrictive bronchiolitis: classification and radiologic features. AJR 1994; 162:803–808.

77. Hansell DM, Rubens MB, Padley SPG, Wells AU. Obliterative bronchiolitis: individual CT signs of small airways disease and functional correlation. Radiology 1997; 203:721–726.

78. Lau DM, Siegel MJ, Hildebolt CF, Cohen AH. Bronchiolitis obliterans syndrome: thin-section CT diagnosis of obstructive changes in infants and young children after lung transplantation. Radiology 1998; 208:783–788.

79. Lentz D, Bergin CJ, Berry GJ, Stoehr C, Theodore J. Diagnosis of bronchiolitis obliterans in heart-lung transplantation patients: importance of bronchial dilatation on CT. AJR 1992; 159:463–467.

80. Worthy SA, Park CS, Kim JS, Müller NL. Bronchiolitis obliterans after lung transplantation: high resolution CT findings in 15 patients. AJR 1997; 169:673–677.

81. Skeens JL, Fuhrman CR, Yousem SA. Bronchiolitis obliterans in heart-lung transplantation patients: radiologic findings in 11 patients. AJR 1989; 153:253–256.

82. Takasugi JE, Godwin JD. Radiology of chronic obstructive pulmonary disease. Radiol Clin N Am 1998; 36:29–55.

83. Thurlbeck WM, Müller NL. Emphysema: definition, imaging, and quantification. AJR 1994; 163:1017–1025.

84. Stern EJ, Frank MS. CT of the lung in patients with pulmonary emphysema: diagnosis, quantification, and correlation with pathologic and physiologic findings. AJR 1994; 162:791–798.

85. Genevois PA, De Vuyst P, Sy M, Scillia P, Chaminade L, de Maertelaer V, Zanen J, Yernault JC. Pulmonary emphysema: quantitative CT during expiration. Radiology 1996; 199:825–829.

86. Buschman DL, Gamsu G, Waldron JA, Klein JS, King TE. Chronic hypersensitivity pneumonitis: use of CT in diagnosis. AJR 1992; 159:957–960.

87. Lynch DA, Rose CS, Way D, King TE. Hypersensitivity pneumonitis: sensitivity of high-resolution CT in a population-based study. AJR 1992; 159:469–472.

88. Silver SF, Müller NL, Miller RR, Lefcoe MS. Hypersensitivity pneumonitis: evaluation with CT. Radiology 1989; 173:441–445.

89. Akira M, Kita N, Higashihara T, Sakatani M, Kozuka T. Summer-type hypersensitiv-

ity pneumonitis: comparison of high-resolution CT and plain radiographic findings. AJR 1992; 158:1223–1228.

90. Hansell DM, Wells AU, Padley SPG, Müller NL. Hypersensitivity pneumonitis: correlation of individual CT patterns with functional abnormalities. Radiology 1996; 199:123–128.

91. Remy-Jardin M, Remy J, Wallaert B, Müller NL. Subacute and chronic bird breeder hypersensitivity pneumonitis: sequential evaluation with CT and correlation with lung function tests and bronchoalveolar lavage. Radiology 1993; 189:111–118.

92. Adler BD, Padley SPG, Müller NL, Remy-Jardin M, Remy J. Chronic hypersensitivity pneumonitis: high-resolution CT and radiographic features in 16 patients. Radiology 1992; 185:91–95.

93. Martin RJ, Blager FB, Gay ML, Wood RP. Paradoxic vocal cord motion in presumed asthmatics. Semin Respir Med 1987; 8:332–337.

94. Brugman SM, Newman K. Vocal cord dysfunction. Med/Sci Update 1993; 11:1–5.

95. Corren J, Newman KB. Vocal cord dysfunction mimicking bronchial asthma. Postgrad Med 1992; 92:153–156.

96. Christopher KL, Wood RP, Eckert RC, Blager FB, Raney RA, Souhrada JF. Vocal-cord dysfunction presenting as asthma. N Engl J Med 1983; 308:1566–1570.

97. Newman KB, Dubester SN. Vocal cord dysfunction: masquerader of asthma. Semin Respir Crit Care Med 1994; 15:161–167.

13

Chronic Infection and Severe Asthma

DAVID N. PHAM and MONICA KRAFT

National Jewish Medical and Research Center
Denver, Colorado

I. Introduction

Asthma affects an estimated 4 to 5 million children and up to 8% of the general population in the United States, which results in health care costs of approximately 4.6 billion annually (1–3). It is a chronic inflammatory disease whose etiologic mechanism is poorly understood. In the 1960s to 1970s it was suggested that viral and bacterial agents played an important causative role in wheezing in allergic individuals and its recurrence in asthmatic children (4–5). Documentation of this causal relationship, however, was poor and proved inconclusive.

It has been characterized and generally recognized that viral infections inducing upper respiratory infections often exacerbate established asthma (6–7). In contrast, information on nonviral infectious inducers or promoters of asthma remains scarce. There are data that bacterial organisms, specifically *Chlamydia pneumoniae* and *Mycoplasma pneumoniae*, may be associated with asthma exacerbation, possibly as factors in its pathogenesis (8–9). As the data regarding the role of bacterial infection in severe asthma are scant, in this chapter we discuss the role of these organisms in the exacerbation and pathogenesis of asthma in general.

II. *Chlamydia pneumoniae*

Chlamydia pneumoniae is a common respiratory pathogen and has been implicated in endemic and epidemic cases of community acquired pneumonia (9). The organism is characterized as an obligate intracellular organism with extraordinarily high seroprevalence, as 30–50% of adults worldwide are seropositive for *C. pneumoniae* (10–11). The seroepidemiologic data indicate that virtually all persons are infected with the organism at least once during their lives and it is believed that many *C. pneumoniae* infections are asymptomatic (11–13). Infections with chlamydia have been documented to persist up to 11 months in adults (14). *Chlamydia pneumoniae* has also been associated with disease states such as coronary heart disease and asthma (15–16).

Grayston et al. were the first to document wheezing after an acute lower respiratory tract infection caused by *Chlamydia psittaci* in a patient (17). Grayston and colleagues reported a case of 35-year-old male who presented to clinic complaining of a sore throat. On chest radiograph, he was found to have a left lower lobe infiltrate, and erythromycin (1 g/day for 5 days) therapy was initiated. Throat-swab culture revealed *C. psittaci*, TWAR strain. Despite antibiotic therapy, the patient never completely returned to baseline. He presented again and was found to have expiratory wheezing on auscultation. A repeat throat-swab culture for chlamydia was negative. Since the TWAR strain had been isolated, the patient was initiated on tetracycline (2 g/day for 7 days), which resulted in complete resolution of his symptoms. This longer term therapy was efficacious and resulted in resolution of wheezing.

Subsequently, the first association between *C. pneumoniae* and asthma was described by Hahn et al. (16), who evaluated 365 consecutive patients who presented with symptoms of lower respiratory tract illness to four primary clinics surrounding Madison, Wisconsin. At time of enrollment, pharyngeal culture and serum samples were obtained and patients were asked to return in 4 weeks during the convalescent phase for serologic testing. Seventy-one exposed patients were matched to unexposed patients by age, sex, smoking status, and month of illness. The criteria for serodiagnosis exposure to *C. pneumoniae* antibody titer utilized both complement fixation (CF) and microimmunofluorescence (MIF) testing. Acute infection was characterized by (1) a fourfold titer rise in IgG between two serum samples 4 weeks apart, (2) a single specimen with an IgM titer of at least 1:16, or (3) an IgG titer of at least 1:512. A preexisting *C. pneumoniae* antibody was defined as an IgM titer less than 1:16 and an IgG titer greater than 1:16 and less than 1:512.

Based on these criteria, 19 patients were diagnosed with acute *C. pneumoniae* infection including pharyngitis, sinusitis, and laryngitis. Fifteen (74%) of 19 demonstrated acute *C. pneumoniae* antibody (IgM), 14 (74%) had IgM titers less than 1:16, and 13 (68%) had *C. pneumoniae* CF titers of less than 1:32. Of the

19 patients with increased IgM antibody, 3 (16%) were wheezing at the time of enrollment and 6 (32%) developed evidence of bronchospasm (4 with wheezing and 2 with decreased peak expiratory flow rates) later in the course of their illness. Due to the high rate of wheezing, Hahn et al. evaluated the magnitude of *C. pneumoniae* titer and found a dose–response relationship between the antibody titer level and the prevalence of wheezing (Table 1). This interpretation must be taken cautiously in light of the high seroprevalence of *C. pneumoniae*. A further change is likely not to be sufficient to state a dose–response relationship. The high seroprevalence of *C. pneumoniae* (10–11) and the ability of *C. pneumoniae* to persist (14) may suggest false positivity in these studies.

Additionally, the 6-month follow-up, Hahn et al. showed that 21 of the 71 exposed patients (29.6) and 5 (7%) of the unexposed matched control patients were diagnosed with asthmatic bronchitis or developed asthma following respiratory illness. The additional history of atopy increased the association of *C. pneumoniae* exposure (OR, 4.6; 95% CI, 1.2–17.6) and asthmatic bronchitis (OR, 8.0; 95% CI, 2.2–28.7). A dose–response relationship was observed such that the higher the *C. pneumoniae* titer, the higher the incidence of patients diagnosed with asthma following respiratory illness (Table 2).

Hahn et al. then showed that *C. pneumoniae* was associated with acute wheezing episode (18) and can lead to the development of chronic asthma (19). In one series of patients, they showed that 12 of 131 patients (9.2%) at the 6-month follow-up had a prior history of respiratory illness prior to the diagnosis of asthma (18). Five of the 12 (41.7%) were newly diagnosed asthmatics and had moderate to severe obstructive lung disease and 7 (58.3%) showed exacerbation of previously diagnosed asthma. Of the 5 newly diagnosed asthmatics, 2 had serologic evidence for acute *C. pneumoniae* infection. In another consecutive series of 163 primary-care outpatient adolescents and adults with reactive airways

Table 1 Wheezing and *Chlamydia pneumoniae* Antibody Titer

Antibody titer	No. (%) with wheeze[a]	Odds ratios		95% CI[b]
		Crude	Adjusted[b]	
<1:16	17/149 (11.4)	1.0 (Referent)	1.0 (Referent)	—
1:16	11/70 (15.7)	1.4	1.2	0.51–2.9
1:32	13/73 (17.8)	1.7	1.4	0.60–3.2
1:64	10/44 (22.7)	2.3	1.9	0.73–5.0
≥1:128	10/29 (34.5)	4.1	3.5	1–9.7

Note. Adapted from Ref. 16.

[a] Patients with wheezing at time of enrollment in study.

[b] Derived from logistic regression, controlled for age, sex, smoking, duration of illness prior to enrollment, season of illness, and sampling: test for trend, $P = 0.01$. CI, confidence interval.

Table 2   Diagnosis of Asthmatic Bronchitis Before and After Illness

| Titer category | Before illness* ($n = 142$) | After illness* | | Odds ratios (95% CI)+ |
		Total group ($n = 142$)	Nonatopic patients ($n = 115$)	
Seronegative	2/71 (3)	5/71 (7)	1/60 (2)	1.0 (Referent)
Nondiagnostic (1:64)	1/40 (3)	8/40 (20)	6/32 (19)	4.6 (1.2–17.6)
Nondiagnostic (≥1:128)	1/15 (7)	7/15 (47)	4/10 (40)	12.5 (2.5–62.6)
Acute antibody	0/16 (0)	6/16 (38)	6/13 (46)	12.0 (2.2–65)

Note. Adapted from Ref. 16.

[a] Number of patients with bronchospasm per total patients. Numbers in parentheses indicate percentages.

[b] Odds ratios for the total group after illness, derived from logistic regression controlled for age, sex, season of illness; test for trend in the odds ratios, $P = 0.0006$. CI, confidence interval.

disease, first-ever wheezing episode or chronic asthma first encountered between 1988 and 1994 were followed prospectively (19). Twenty patients (12%) were diagnosed with *C. pneumoniae* infection by serology (15 patients), culture isolation (3 patients), or both (2 patients). Of the 20 patients, 10 wheezed for the first time and 6 subsequently developed chronic asthma.

Several other studies have also shown a similar serologic association between *C. pneumoniae* and acute, chronic, and nonatopic asthma as well as exacerbation of asthma (20–22). Allegra et al. evaluated 74 adult outpatients diagnosed with acute exacerbation of asthma who were recruited through an allergy clinic (20). Fifty-seven subjects tested positive via skin prick for at least one common antigen, whereas 17 suffered from intrinsic asthma. The 74 patients were evaluated by means of MIF testing for acute and convalescent (≥3 weeks) IgG antibodies to several infectious agents. Of the 74 patients, 15 (20%) presented with seroconversion (a fourfold rise in IgG antibody at least 3 weeks after enrollment) to either viral or bacterial pathogens. Six patients (8%) were considered infected with *C. pneumoniae*, 1 with *M. pneumoniae*, and 1 with both *C. pneumoniae* and *M. pneumoniae* by the following serologic criteria: Acute infection was defined as a fourfold rise in IgG titer ≥ 1:16, a fourfold rise in IgM titer ≥1:16, IgM titer ≥1:16, or IgG ≥1:512; and a preexisting infection was defined as IgG ≥1: 512. Treatment with antibiotics resulted in resolution of the asthma exacerbation in 5 of the 8 seroconverters and the other 3 showed improved symptoms. However, the serologic data for seroconversion presented by Allegra and colleagues did not appear to correlate with culture data. Of the patients considered to be infected with *C. pneumoniae*, one patient, who demonstrated pharyngeal swab culture positivity, demonstrated only a twofold increase in IgG titers, from 1:

Table 3 IgG Titers and Serological Classifications of Acute Asthma, Chronic Asthma, and Control Groups

	Acute asthma ($n = 123$)	Chronic asthma ($n = 46$)	Controls ($n = 1518$)
IgG Titers			
Range	0–512	0–256	0–512
Median	0	16	0
Mean	24.3	33.7	19.6
Acute infection	7 (5.7%)	2 (4.3%)	87 (5.7%)
Unadjusted odds ratio (95% CI)	1.02 (0.46–2.25)	1.02 (0.24–4.34)	1.00
Adjusted odds ratio (95% CI)	0.81 (0.32–2.05)	1.07 (0.13–8.65)	1.00
Previous infection	18 (14.6%)	16 (34.8%)	193 (12.7%)
Unadjusted odds ratio (95% CI)	1.18 (0.70–1.99)	3.66 (1.95–6.90)	1.00
Adjusted odds ratio (95% CI)	0.92 90.49–1.70)	3.99 (1.60–9.97)	1.00
No infection	98 (79.7%)	28 (60.9%)	1238 (81.6%)

Note. Adapted from Ref. 21.

128 at enrollment to 1:256 at convalescence. Furthermore, there was significant variability in IgG titers at baseline and subsequent convalescent titers with baseline titers ranging from negative to 1:128 and convalescent titers ranging from 1:64 to 1:1024. Thus, consistency in criteria regarding infection is necessary in order to determine a link to asthma.

Cook et al. evaluated patients with acute asthma and control subjects and followed 1687 patients prospectively over a 24-month period (21). Patients with acute asthma defined on the basis of episodes of wheezing requiring immediate treatment with nebulized bronchodilators showed rapid clinical improvement. Patients who showed a history of chronic sputum production or emphysema, known or suspected immunodeficiency, hypergammaglobulinemia, connective tissue disease, or other autoimmune diseases were excluded in order to avoid false-positive and negative states. Acute infection or reinfection was defined by titers of IgG $\geq 1:512$ or IgM $\geq 1:8$ or convalescent samples revealing a fourfold increase in IgG. Titers indicating previous infection without recrudescence were presumed to be IgG levels from 1:64 to 1:256, undetectable IgM titers, and/or no significant rise in IgG.

Utilizing the above criteria, they found a significant association between the presence of *C. pneumoniae* antibody titers in the chronic asthma group (16 in 46, or 34.8%) compared to those in the nonasthma control group (193 in 1518, or 12.7%) (Table 3). However, they were unable to show any significant difference in acute reinfection (5.7%), previous infection (14.6%), and no infection (79.7%) in the acute asthma and control groups 5.7, 12.7, and 81.6%, respectively. This study by Cook et al. (21) differs from other studies (18–20) in that acute infection was defined by an arbitrary value for IgG of 1:512, whereas others have used a fourfold rise in titer and/or IgG of 1:512. Another difference may be due to the lack of follow-up with both the acute asthma group (29 of 123) and the control group (282 of 1518) in order to obtain convalescent titers. Therefore, Cook and colleagues were unable to show any significant difference in acute reinfection, previous infection, and no infection in the acute asthma and control groups.

Von Hertzen et al., utilizing different serologic criteria for positivity (IgG ≥ 1:128, IgM ≥ 1:20, and IgA ≥1:32), showed a significant association between the presence of *C. pneumoniae* antibody and female patients with longstanding nonatopic asthma (22). They enrolled 435 consecutive patients with symptoms suggestive of asthma, rhinitis, and allergy. Asthma was diagnosed utilizing the following three criteria: (1) a history of characteristic symptoms, (2) a response to 200 μg salbutamol of ≥ 15% increase in forced expiratory volume in 1 sec (FEV$_1$) or in peak flow value (PEF) or diurnal variation ≥20% in PEF during a 1-week follow-up, and (3) an increase in bronchial responsiveness to histamine challenge testing, defined as a provocative dose of histamine causing a reduction of 15% in FEV$_1$. Increased bronchial responsiveness was further graded arbitrarily as mild (from >0.4 to 1.6 mg), moderate (from >0.1 to 0.4 mg), or severe (from ≤0.1 mg) (23). These patients were divided into groups of recent-onset asthma (*n* = 224), established within 7 years of the study; and chronic asthma (*n* = 108), established more than 7 years before the study; and controls (*n* = 98). Patients with concomitant chronic obstructive pulmonary disease or chronic cough were excluded.

In female patients, elevated serum IgG antibody levels to *C. pneumoniae* were observed to occur in 11% of controls, 28% of recent-onset asthmatics, and 43% of asthmatics with nonatopic longstanding disease, whereas for men the respective values were 33, 50, and 64% (Fig. 1). When controlling for age, sex, and smoking, there was significant association between IgG titer levels and longstanding asthma [odds ratio (OR) of 3.3, 95% confidence interval (CI) of 1.6–6.8] and recent asthma (OR 2.3, 95% CI 1.2–4.4). A stronger association was observed among women with longstanding asthma (OR 4.2, 95% CI 1.6–10.9) and for recent asthma (OR 3.0, 95% CI 1.3–7.2). Men showed higher prevalence but no statistical difference between the control and asthma groups. Furthermore, when the analysis was performed in atopics and nonatopic asthmatics regardless of gender, nonatopic longstanding asthma was significantly associated with elevated IgG antibody levels to *C. pneumoniae* (OR 6.0, 95% CI 2.1–17.1).

Emre et al. evaluated 118 children with acute episodes of wheezing; *C. pneumoniae* was cultured from the nasopharynx swab of 13 (11%) children with wheezing, whereas it was found in only 2 (5%) sex-matched healthy controls (24). Three of the 13 culture-positive children with wheezing had serologic evidence

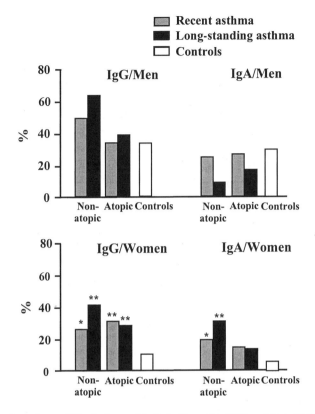

Figure 1 Prevalence (%) of elevated IgG (a titer of ≥128) and IgA (>32) antibody levels according to group structure and sex. *$P < 0.05$; ** $P < 0.01$. (Adapted from Ref. 22.)

(fourfold rise in IgG, IgG ≥ 1:512, or IgM ≥ 1:16) of acute infection. Several other studies have only shown 1–13% of culture isolation of *C. pneumoniae* (20,25,30) in association with patients with asthma or community acquired pneumonia (CAP).

IgE and IgA have also been shown to be associated with *C. pneumoniae* and asthma (26–27). Emre et al. examined the sera of 45 children in the following four groups: 14 children with chronic asthma who presented with acute episodes of wheezing, 11 children with community acquired pneumonia associated with culture-proven *C. pneumoniae* infection, 11 asthmatic children with acute exacerbation but cultures negative for *C. pneumoniae*, and 9 asymptomatic patients with cultures negative for *C. pneumoniae*. By immunoblot assay utilizing *C. pneumoniae* proteins, he showed 12 of the 14 culture-positive asthmatics (85.7%) with acute exacerbation, whereas only 1 of 11 culture-positive patients (9.1%) with CAP demonstrated an IgE antibody against *C. pneumoniae*. Additionally, Emre et al. showed no correlation between culture data to the standard serologic criteria used by others as a measure of *C. pneumoniae* positivity (fourfold rise in IgG, single IgG $\geq 1:512$, or IgM titer of $\geq 1:16$). Only 1 of the 14 culture-positive asthmatic and none of the 11 culture-positive CAP children had serologic evidence of chlamydia infection by these criteria. IgE was present in 2 of 11 culture-negative asthmatics and 2 of 9 culture-negative asymptomatic patients. Although it did not demonstrate cause and effect, this study suggests that *C. pneumoniae* can elicit an IgE response. Given the strong relationship between IgE, atopy, and asthma, this may be a mechanism by which infectious organisms contribute to asthma pathogenesis.

Serum IgA has also been proposed to be a useful marker in diagnosing chronic infections, since it has a short half-life (28) and its continuous presence is indicative of persistent immune stimulation (29). Hahn et al. showed that 18 of 25 patients (72%) with recent-onset mild asthma and 20 of 45 sex- and age-matched controls demonstrated positivity of at least 1:10 (27). In a different 13-month longitudinal study, 108 asthmatic children were asked to keep a daily diary of respiratory symptoms and peak flow rates (30). When respiratory symptoms were reported, nasal aspirates were obtained to measure secretory IgA (sIgA) directed against *C. pneumoniae*. As the frequency of respiratory symptoms increased, a sevenfold increase in sIgA directed against *C. pneumoniae* was observed. These preliminary studies suggest IgA is produced in response to *C. pneumoniae* infection, but its relationship to asthma requires further study.

In contrast, the development of polymerase chain reaction (PCR) has provided an alternative diagnostic tool to show the association between chlamydia and asthma. Utilizing primers against the major outer membrane proteins (MOMP) gene sequence, Cunningham et al. evaluated *C. pneumoniae* by PCR from nasal aspirates (30). Children recruited from this study were asked to maintain diary cards of upper and lower respiratory symptoms and PEF. The investigator was notified and nasal aspirates were obtained when PEF fell ≥ 50 L/min or when respiratory symptoms occurred.

Surprisingly, similar numbers of patients demonstrated PCR positivity whether or not they were symptomatic (68 of 292, or 23%) or asymptomatic (18 of 65, or 28%). Interestingly, subjects found to be PCR positive with one reported episode were likely to remain PCR positive after subsequent reported respiratory episodes. Recurrent acute infection increased the likelihood of PCR positivity to 35%, whereas 18% of patients were PCR negative initially and then became PCR positive with reported symptoms.

With regard to PCR positivity in asthma, Miyashita et al., however, showed lower frequency of PCR positivity in both asthmatics (9 of 168, or 5.4%) and normal controls (1 in 108, or 0.9%) experiencing acute exacerbations (31). The difference in isolation techniques between Cunningham and colleagues, who employed nasal aspirates, and Miyashita et al., who employed nasal swab with isolation culture, may not fully explain the prevalence difference observed in both the asthmatic and nonasthmatic control groups. Another possible explanation for the difference between the frequency of PCR positivity for the two groups may be related to the age of the study groups. Cunningham's study group was composed of children between 9 and 10 years of age, whereas the mean age of Miyashita's study group was 49 years. The prevalence of infection with *C. pneumoniae* is greater in children than in adults (32–34). Both groups used different probe sequences to a high conserved region of the MOMP gene for the *Chlamydia* genus, making this an unlikely reason for the differences (35).

Culture isolates of *C. pneumoniae* have been associated with acute wheezing episodes in children with asthma. *Chlamydia pneumoniae* has been considered a fastidious organism and is difficult to recover in initial culture (36). Culture is considered the least sensitive method used in the identification of these organisms. An initial study by Hahn et al. demonstrated culture positivity in only 1 of 365 subjects (16). With the discovery of the HEp-2, an immortalized human tracheal cell line (37) which allows chlamydia to propagate after infection, follow-up studies by Hahn et al. showed slight improvement in isolation and culture of *C. pneumoniae* in 3 of 163 patients (19). The very small incremental improvement in culture technique is probably not sufficient to use this technique to identify chlamydial infection in large population-based studies.

III. *Mycoplasma pneumoniae*

Mycoplasma pneumoniae is another common upper respiratory tract pathogen that affects children and adults worldwide (38). The exact cause-and-effect relationship between *M. pneumoniae* and asthma remains to be determined. In 1970, Berkovich et al. evaluated 84 asthmatic patients ages 6 months to 16 years who presented through the winter of 1967 to 1968 with acute episodes of wheezing (5). Throat and rectal swabs, blood cultures, and serum were obtained at the initial visit and at follow-up visits 2 to 4 weeks later. Utilizing microtiter techniques from 84 paired serum samples, 27 of the 84 patients demonstrated a fourfold change in IgG antibodies, consistent with acute infection. Specifically, they demonstrated serologic evidence of infection to influenza types A and B, respiratory syncytial virus, parainfluenza virus, adenovirus, and *M. pneumoniae* infections in 27 of 84 patients (32.1%) associated with acute wheezing episodes. Of the 27 patients, 7 demonstrated *M. pneumoniae*-positive antibody titers at baseline and 5 of these individuals' titers increased by at least four-fold at 2- to 4-week follow-up. Two of these 7 patients had fourfold or greater decrease in antibody titers, suggestive of resolution of acute infection. Similarly, Huhti et al.

found that 27 of 63 patients (42.8%) hospitalized with severe asthma had viral or mycoplasma infections (39). Of these 27 patients, 5 had positive serologic evidence of mycoplasma infections. A fourfold change in antibody levels from paired blood sera, obtained 14 to 18 days apart, was taken as positive evidence of infection.

Subsequently, respiratory tract infection with *M. pneumoniae* was shown to predispose the individual to developing airway hyperresponsiveness. Mok et al. followed 50 children with prior history of *M. pneumoniae* respiratory tract infection over a period of 1.5 to 9.5 years (40). These 50 children were chosen from 103 cases of *M. pneumoniae* infection at the Royal Hospital in Edinburgh from January 1968 to 1975 through review of case records at the Regional Virus Laboratory in Edinburgh, Scotland. Chest radiographs of the 50 children at the time of acute illness revealed pneumonic consolidation (19 children), patchy infiltrate (19 children), or hyperinflation (2 children) or were normal (10 children). Five of the 50 children developed persistent cough or wheeze for the first time after mycoplasma illness and all five children had increase bronchial reactivity after exercise challenge.

Sabato et al. evaluated 108 children presenting with *M. pneumoniae* infection, defined as having serologic titers of greater than 1:160, and 48 of these children were followed for 3 years after their acute illness (41). During the acute infectious period, the incidence of wheezing was found to be 40% in some patients and for others was their first (number of patients not stated). Of the patients wheezing for the first time, five wheezed subsequently, although the specific time was not reported. They also showed that after 1 week of antibiotic therapy with erythromycin, nonasthmatic mycoplasma-infected subjects had significantly greater bronchodilator response (9.4 ± 4.9%) compared to healthy nonasthmatic, uninfected children (3.6 ± 3.8%) at 1 month after the infection, $P < 0.01$. Although this bronchodilator response does not meet American Thoracic Society criteria (42) as a significant bronchodilator response consistent with asthma, these data suggest that *M. pneumoniae* infection may affect airway function beyond the period of acute infection.

PCR has also been applied to detect *M. pneumoniae* from patients with chronic stable asthma. Kraft et al. evaluated 18 chronic stable asthmatic and 11 healthy nonasthmatic control subjects from the surrounding Denver, Colorado, metropolitan area from June 1994 to April 1996 (43). Both asthmatics and control subjects underwent bronchoscopy with endobronchial biopsy (EBBX) from the fourth- or fifth-generation airways, protected brushing of the large airways, and bronchoalveolar lavage (BAL). The location of the biopsies was randomized to the right or left lower lobe, followed by brushing and BAL of the right middle lobe or lingula of the opposite lung. Throat swabs and nasal specimens were also obtained. The specimens were inoculated directly into mycoplasma-specific media for evaluation by culture and PCR. One biopsy specimen was embedded into paraffin for mycoplasma PCR only. *Mycoplasma pneumoniae* PCR utilized the primer sequence to the P1 adhesion gene and the 16S ribosomal RNA (rRNA) gene (44–45). Our laboratory utilized a stringent conservative approach, which demands positivity from two primers from samples obtained from one site or positivity from two different sites, and we were able to detect 10 of 18 (55%) subjects with chronic, stable asthma and 1 of 11 control subjects with *M. pneumoniae* from BAL fluid and endobronchial biopsy specimens from the lower airways. When a more liberal approach was taken, where a patient was considered positive if one or more sites demonstrated PCR positivity, the number of positive patients increased to 11 of 18 asthmatics and 2 of 11 control subjects. The distribution of the PCR-positive patients is shown in Fig. 2. All cultures for *M. pneumoniae* were negative. Both asthmatics and control subjects were antibody negative for IgG and IgM directed against *M. pneumoniae*, as determined by enzyme-linked immunosorbent assay.

According to these results, our chronic stable asthmatics appear to be chronically infected or colonized with *M. pneumoniae* despite culture and serologic negativity (41). One possibility is that PCR positivity persisted after an upper respiratory infection, as shown in a guinea pig model (46). However, the subjects had not experienced a recent upper respiratory infection at least 3 months prior to entry into the study. Therefore, it is possible that *M. pneumoniae* is allowed to remain in an abnormal airway and contribute to ongoing inflammation or is

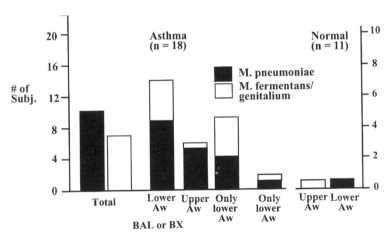

Figure 2 The number of asthmatic subjects positive for *M. pneumoniae, M. fermentans,* and *M. genitalium* by PCR in the lower airway (Lower AW) and upper airway only (Only Upper Aw). Solid bars represent the number of subjects who were PCR positive for *M. pneumoniae*; open bars represent the number of subjects positive for *M. fermentans* and *M. genitalium* BAL, bronchoalveolar lavage; BX, biopsy. (Adapted from Ref. 43.)

a marker of disease. Further study is required to better understand the mechanism of *M. pneumoniae* in chronic asthma.

IV. Serologic, Culture, and Polymerase Chain Reaction Testing

The majority of the studies reviewed thus far have utilized either serologic testing alone or in combination with PCR and/or cultures to describe the association with *C. pneumoniae* and *M. pneumoniae* in asthma. Interpretation of this association is difficult, especially when using serologic testing, in light of its highly nonspecific and nonsensitive nature. First, *C. pneumoniae* has been described to infect at least once during an individual's life and it is believed that many are asymptomatic carriers (11–14). As such, many of the studies show healthy asymptomatic individuals with high IgG titers (16,21,22,43). Additionally, the serologic criteria are fairly arbitrary, as they were proposed without being correlated with culture results. This correlation with culture results, however, is suspect because these organisms are isolated in only 13% of patients with radiographically confirmed community acquired pneumonia (25). It is also necessary to keep in mind that culture positivity may not always correlate with serologic evidence (30,47). Second, tests such as MIF utilize monoclonal and polyclonal antibodies that cross-react with other *Chlamydia* lipopolysaccharide antigens. Similar cross-reactivity can also occur within *Mycoplasma*. A number of studies state that this cross-reactivity can be differentiated by fluorescence pattern when compared to other species-specific major outer membrane proteins (MOMP). However, the MOMP gene appears to be highly conserved in the chlamydial species (35). This nucleotide homology can be as high as 75%. Hammerschlag and colleagues have reported that patients evaluated for *C. pneumoniae* infections produce MIF antibodies to *Chlamydia trachomatis* in similar titers (47). Third, there is a significant association between smoking and *C. pneumoniae* seropositivity. Smoking increases the incidence of upper respiratory tract infection and as such increases the relative risk of seropositivity. Karvonen et al. estimated relative risk of *C. pneumoniae* seropositivity at 1.5 times greater than that of those who have never smoked, and there was no significant difference when gender differences were compared (49). The majority of the studies evaluating IgG as a reflection of *C. pneumoniae* infection may misclassify and overestimate the incidence, since smoking was not taken into account. Last, in evaluating elderly adult patients, rheumatoid arthritis and other autoimmune diseases, specifically those with rheumatoid factor (RF) positivity, can cause false-positive *C. pneumoniae* IgG and IgM antibody measurements. Verkooyen et al. evaluated 25 patients with active rheumatoid arthritis but without respiratory illness; 14 were also *C. pneumoniae*

IgG and IgM positive (50). Absorption of IgG from these RF-containing sera invariably resulted in disappearance of reactivity in the MIF IgM assay.

Recently, Routes et al. showed no significant difference in *C. pneumoniae* antibody titers between adult onset asthmatics and control subjects (51). In this retrospective, parallel-group study, serum samples from inpatients, outpatients, and hospital workers were obtained from the clinical laboratory at the National Jewish Medical and Research Center. Forty-six patients met the American Thoracic Society criteria (42) for the diagnosis of asthma and had onset of asthma symptoms after the age of 40 years. Titers of IgG and IgM antibodies to *C. pneumoniae* were measured by MIF in the adult-onset asthmatics and age- and sex-matched controls. There was no significant difference in the proportion of adult-onset asthmatic or control subjects with IgG titers against *C. pneumoniae* criteria that would signify acute infection (IgG $\geq 1:512$), indeterminate exposure ($1:16 \geq$ IgG $< 1:512$), or seronegativity (IgG $< 1:16$) (Fig. 3).

The same difficulties associated with MIF testing can also occur with PCR. Since the majority of PCR primers utilize the species-specific MOMP gene (35),

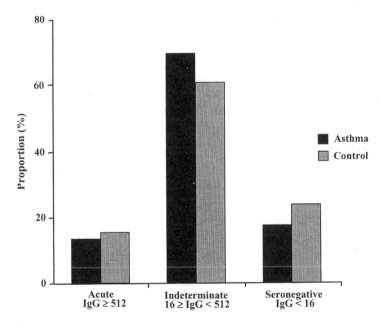

Figure 3 IgG antibody titers in asthmatics and control subjects. Levels of IgG *C. pneumoniae* antibody titers in asthmatics and control subjects indicating acute infection, prior exposure (indeterminate), or no prior exposure. (Adapted from Ref. 16.)

it is possible to have species cross-reactivity occur and result in falsely high positivity. A PCR primer for *C. pneumoniae*, the MOMP-omp1 gene sequence published as IOL207, was utilized by Cunningham et al. (30) and has been shown to cross-react with other chlamydia species, due to high homologies within the variable sequence domain IV of the MOMP gene (52). This shared homology between *C. pneumoniae* and *Chlamydia trachomatis* can be as high as 30% (53). However, Cunningham et al. stated that this primer sequence does not cross-react with other chlamydia species (30). Since his symptomatic (23%) and asymptomatic (28%) subjects exhibited high PCR positivity for *C. pneumoniae*, the question arises as to whether this primer pair was tested against the different serovars of *C. trachomatis* or *Chlamydia psittaci*. In addition, different primer pairs directed against different gene products for *C. pneumoniae* have been utilized. Kraft et al. utilized a PCR primer specific for the 16S rRNA gene and were unable to detect *C. pneumoniae* in any of the 18 chronic stable asthmatics and 11 healthy control subjects (43). This 16S rRNA primer sequence has been shown to be highly specific and sensitive to *C. pneumoniae* and does not cross-react with *C. trachomatis* (54). Similarly, PCR primers against the P1 adhesion gene, the 16S rRNA gene, and *M. pneumoniae* do not appear to cross-react with other mycoplasma isolates from humans (44–45).

The least sensitive method uses culture isolates of *Chlamydia* and *M. pneumoniae*. Culture positivity varies between 1 and 20% (16,19,20,25). The reasons behind the low yield may be related to suboptimal site localization for sampling and that the site of colonization has not yet been identified. Another possibility may be related to the clinical specimen, which may contain a small number of organisms such that optimal existing culture conditions are unable to detect growth.

V. Role of Antibiotic Testing

Since the link between chronic bacterial infection and asthma has been investigated and not yet established, a number of investigators, including Allegra et al. (20), Hahn et al. (55–56), Emre et al. (35), and Kraft et al. (57), have treated their *C. pneumoniae* and *M. pneumoniae*-positive asthmatic patients with antibiotics. The majority of the studies used macrolides to show complete remission or at least significant improvement in asthma symptoms and/or physiology and/or discontinuation of oral steroids. These investigators speculated that the mechanism for the observed improvement may be related to the antimicrobial activity against chlamydia and mycoplasma. However, it is also possible that macrolides also have nonmicrobial activities. They can delay steroid clearance (58), alter inflammation (59–61), and decrease bronchial hyperresponsiveness (62). Hahn et al., however, argued that these effects are less likely since improvement persisted >10 weeks after cessation of antibiotics (55). Wildfeuer et al. showed that within polymorphonuclear leukocytes the half-life was 210 ± 69 h after administration of a 3-day regimen of 500 mg of azithromycin once daily (63). As such, it is possible that the anti-inflammatory effects of the dosing regimen used by Hahn et al., composed of 1000 mg of azithromycin weekly for 3 to 6 weeks, may still persist.

Three other studies described the use of doxycycline or levofloxacin, instead of the use of macrolides, to treat *C. pneumoniae* infection detected via culture, PCR, and/or serology positivity. Hahn et al. enrolled 46 patients with moderate to moderately severe stable chronic asthma in an open-label study (55). Thirty patients were treated with a macrolide (29 were treated with azithromycin and 1 with erythromycin) and 16 were treated with doxycycline. Hahn et al. found that 54% appeared to benefit from antibiotic treatment. Subgroup analysis separating the effects of macrolide treatment and those of doxycycline on *C. pneumoniae* was not performed. In a smaller study by Allegra et al. (20), 7 patients with acute exacerbation of asthma demonstrated serologic evidence of acute *C. pneumoniae* infection. Two of the 7 patients were treated with 2-week course of doxycycline, resulting in cure of their asthma. Four patients with acute exacerbation of asthma and PCR positivity of a nasopharyngeal specimen for *C. pneumoniae* underwent treatment with levofloxacin for 14 to 21 days. Remission of their asthma symptoms occurred within 90 days after treatment and nasopharyngeal specimens became PCR negative for *C. pneumoniae*.

In one recently submitted study, we treated 31 of 55 chronic stable asthmatics who demonstrated PCR positivity for *M. pneumoniae* (57). These patients underwent a double-blind, placebo-controlled trial of 500 mg of clarithromycin twice daily or placebo for 6 weeks. During the randomization of 52/55 subjects, 26 individuals received clarithromycin, of which 16 were PCR positive for mycoplasma, and 26 received placebo, of which 13 were PCR positive for mycoplasma. The PCR-positive patients demonstrated improvement when they received treatment with clarithromycin. Improvement in the FEV_1 (13.2%, $P <$ 0.01) was demonstrated for the PCR-positive patients who received clarithromycin compared to the PCR-positive group who received placebo. These data suggest that macrolides appear to benefit those asthmatic patients who demonstrate PCR positivity for *M. pneumoniae*. The mechanism is not clear, as macrolides have both antimicrobial and anti-inflammatory effects (58–62,64,65). As the current PCR technique is qualitative, we are assuming we are reducing organism burden, but we cannot say this conclusively, as some patients were still PCR positive after therapy. Current investigation with an animal model of *M. pneumoniae* will hopefully clarify this issue (66).

Treatment of asthmatic patients with antibiotics is not recommended until further studies can validate the infectious cause of asthma. If such studies are to occur, a bactericidal agent against *C. pneumoniae* and *M. pneumoniae* should be used. Macrolide studies should be designed to control for all the nonmicrobial activities if possible. The tetracyclines or quinolones may serve as alternatives.

VI. Conclusion

A growing body of evidence suggests that *C. pneumoniae* and *M. pneumoniae* may play important roles in inducing and promoting asthma. The evidence for *C. pneumoniae* thus far shows only an association. Stringent studies correlating serologic markers with culture positivity and using specific PCR primers that can detect different *C. pneumoniae* and yet not cross-react with all serovars against *C. psittaci* and *C. trachomatis* (67) must be performed. With regard to *M. pneumoniae*, the body of literature is less problematic. Cross-reactivity associated with serologic and PCR data is not observed. The population studies, however, remain few in number. Larger population studies need to be performed. Thus, the current data are intriguing, as they suggest a relationship between specific bacterial organisms and asthma. Further studies, possibly employing animal models, are needed to demonstrate cause and effect.

References

1. Buist AS. Asthma mortality: what have we learned? J Allergy Clin Immunol 1989; 84:275–283.
2. Weiss KB, Wagener DK. Changing pattern of asthma mortality: identify target populations at high risk. J Am Med Assoc 1990; 264:683–685.
3. National Institutes of Health, National Heart, Lung, and Blood Institute Data Fact Sheet. Bethesda, MD: National Institutes of Health, 1995.
4. Freeman GL. Wheezing associated with respiratory tract infections in children: the role of specific infectious agents in allergic respiratory manifestations. Clin Pediatr 1966; 5:586–592.
5. Berkovich S, Millian SJ, Snyder RD. The association of viral and mycoplasma infections with recurrence in the asthmatic child. Ann Allergy 1970; 28:43–49.
6. Pattemore PK, Johnston SL, Bardin PG. Viruses as precipitants of asthma symptoms. I. Epidemiology. Clin Exp Allergy 1992; 22:325–336.
7. Johnston SL, Pattermore PK, Sanderson G, Smith S, Lampe F, Josephs LK, Symington P, O'Toole S, Myint SH, Tyrrell DAJ, Holgate ST. Community study of role of virus infections in exacerbations of asthma in 9-11 year old children. Br Med J 1995; 310:1225–1228.
8. Leaver R, Weinberg EG. Is Mycoplasma pneumoniae a preciprocating factor in acute severe asthma in children? S Afr Med J 1985; 68:78–79.
9. Grayston JT, Campbell LA, Kuo CC, Mordhorst C, Saikku P, Thom D, Wang SP. A new respiratory tract pathogen: Chlamydia pneumoniae, strain TWAR. J Infect Dis 1990; 161:618–625.

10. Grayston JT, Wang SP, Kuo CC, Campbell LA. Current knowledge on Chlamydia pneumoniae, strain TWAR, an important cause of pneumonia and other acute respiratory diseases. Eur J Microbiol Infect Dis 1989; 8:191–202.

11. Saikku P. The epidemiology and significance of Chlamydia pneumoniae. J Infect 1992; 25:27–34.

12. Gnarpe, J, Gnarpe H, Sundelof B. Epidemic prevalence of Chlamydia pneumoniae in subjectively healthy persons. Scand J Infect Dis 1991; 23:387–388.

13. Hyman CL, Augenbraun MH, Roblin PM, Schachter J, Hammerschlag MR. Asymptomatic respiratory-tract infection with Chlamydia pneumoniae TWAR. J Clin Microbiol 1992; 29:2082–2083.

14. Hammerschlag MR, Chirgwin K, Roblin PM, Gelling M, Dumornay W, Mandel L, Smith P, Schachter J. Persistent infection with Chlamydia pneumoniae following acute respiratory illness. Clin Infect Dis 1992; 14:178–82.

15. Saikku P, Leinonen M, Mattila K, Ekman MR; Nieminen MS, Makela PH, Huttunen JK, Valtonen V. Serological evidence of an association of a novel Chlamydia, TWAR, with chronic coronary heart disease and acute myocardial-infarction. Lancet 1988; 2:983–986.

16. Hahn DL, Dodge RW, Golubjatnikov R. Association of Chlamydia pneumoniae (Strain TWAR) infection with wheezing, asthmatic bronchitis, and adult-onset asthma. J Am Med Assoc 1991; 266:225–230.

17. Grayston TJ, Kuo CC, Wang SP, Altman J. A new Chlamydia psittaci, TWAR, isolated in acute respiratory tract infections. N Engl J Med 1986; 315:161–168.

18. Hahn DL, Golubjatnikov R. Asthma and Chlamydia infection: A case series. J Fam Pract 1994; 38:589–595.

19. Hahn DL, McDonald R. Can acute Chlamydia pneumoniae respiratory tract infection initiate chronic asthma? Ann Allergy Asthma Immunol 1998; 81:339–344.

20. Allegra L, Blasi F, Centanii S, Cosentini R, Denti F, Raccanelli R, Tarsia P, Valenti V. Acute exacerbation of Chlamydia pneumoniae infection. Eur Respir J 1994; 7: 2165–2168.

21. Cook PJ, Davies P, Tunnicliffe W, Ayres JG, Honeybourne D, Wise R. Chlamydia pneumoniae and asthma. Thorax 1998; 53:254–259.

22. von Hertzen L, Toyrola M, Gimishanov A, Bloigu A, Leinonen M, Saikku P, Haahtela T. Asthma, atopy, and Chlamydia pneumoniae antibodies in adults. Clin Exp Allergy 1999; 29:522–528.

23. Sovijärvi A, Malmberg P, Reinikainen K, Rytilä P, Poppius H. A rapid dosimetric method with controlled tidal breathing for histamine challenge. Chest 1993; 104: 164–170.

24. Emre U, Robbin PM, Gelling M, Dumornay W, Rao M, Hammerschlag MR, Schachter J. 1994. The association of Chlamydia pneumoniae infection and reactive airway disease in Children. Arch Pediatr Adolesc Med 1994; 148:727–732.

25. Block S, Hedrick HJ, Hammerschlag MR, Cassell GH, Craft JC. Mycoplasma pneumoniae and Chlamydia pneumoniae in pediatric community-acquired pneumonia: comparative efficacy and safety of clarithromycin vs. erythromycin ethylsuccinate. Pediatr Infect Dis 1995; 14:471–477.

26. Emre U, Sokolovskaya N, Roblin PM, Schachter J, Hammerschlag MR. Detection

of anti-Chlamydia pneumoniae IgE in children with reactive airway disease. J Infect Dis 1995; 172:265–267.

27. Hahn DL, Anttila T, Saikku P. Association of Chlamydia pneumoniae IgA antibodies with recently symptomatic asthma. Epidemiol Infect 1996; 117:513–517.

28. Carayannapoulos L, Capra JD. Immunoglobulins: structure and function. In: Fundamental Immunology. 3rd ed. New York: Raven Press, 1993.

29. Samra Z, Soffer Y. IgA anti-Chlamydia antibodies as a diagnostic tool for monitoring of active chlamydial infection. Eur J Epidemiol 1993; 8:882–884.

30. Cunningham AF, Johnston SL, Julious SA, Lampe FC, Ward ME. Chronic Chlamydia pneumoniae infection and asthma exacerbations in children. Eur Respir J 1998; 11:345–349.

31. Miyashita N, Kubota Y, Nakajima M, Niki Y, Kawane H, Matsushima T. Chlamydia pneumoniae and exacerbation in adults. Ann Allergy Asthma Immunol 1998; 80: 405–409.

32. Normann E, Gnarpe J, Gnarpe H, Wettergren B. Chlamydia pneumoniae in children with acute respiratory tract infection. Acta Pediat 1998; 8:23–27.

33. Marrie TJ, Grayston JT, Wang SP, Kuo CC. Pneumonia associated with the T WAR strain of Chlamydia. Ann Intern Med 1987; 106:507–511.

34. Grayston JT, Diwan VK, Cooney M, Wang SP. Community- and hospital-acquired pneumonia associated with Chlamydia TWAR infection demonstrated serologically. Arch Intern Med 1989; 149:169–173.

35. Carter MW, Al-Mahdawi SAH, Giles IG, Treharne JD, Ward ME, Clarke IN. Nucleotide sequence and taxonomic values of the major outer membrane protein gene of Chlamydia pneumoniae IOL-207. J Gen Microbiol 1991; 137:465–475.

36. Thom DH, Grayston JT. Infections with Chlamydia pneumoniae strain TWAR. Clin Chest Med 1991; 12:245–256.

37. Roblin PM, Dumornay W, Hammerschlag MR. Use of Hep-2 cells for improved isolation and passage of Chlamydia pneumoniae. J Clin Microbiol 1992; 30:1968–1971.

38. Clyde WA. Mycoplasma pneumoniae respiratory disease symposium: summation and significance. Yale J Biol Med 1983; 56:523–527.

39. Huhti E, Mokka T, Nikoskelainen J, Halonen P. Association of viral and mycoplasma infections with exacerbations of asthma. Ann Allergy 1974; 33:145–149.

40. Mok JYQ, Waugh PR, Simpson H. Mycoplasma infection: a follow-up study of 50 children with respiratory illness. Arch Dis Child 1979; 54:506–511.

41. Sabato AR, Martin AJ, Marmion BP, Kok TW, Cooper DM. Mycoplasma pneumoniae: acute illness, antibiotics, and subsequent pulmonary function. Arch Dis Child 1984; 59:1034–1037.

42. American Thoracic Society Board of Directors. Standards for the diagnosis and care of patients with chronic obstructive pulmonary disease (COPD). Am Rev Respir Dis 1987; 136:225–244.

43. Kraft M, Cassell GH, Henson JE, Watson H, Williamson J, Marmion BP, Gaydos CA, Martin RJ. Detection of Mycoplasma pneumoniae in the airways of adults with chronic asthma. Am J Respir Crit Care Med 1998; 158:998–1001.

44. Williamson J, Marmion BP, Worswick DA, Kok TW, Tannock G, Herd G, Harris RJ. Laboratory diagnosis of Mycoplasma pneumoniae infection. 4. Comparison of

antigen detection of M. pneumoniae in respiratory isolates. Epidemiol Infect 1992; 109:519–537.

45. Williamson J, Marmion BP, Kok TW, Antic R, Harris RJ. Confirmation of fatal Mycoplasma pneumoniae infection by polymerase chain reaction detection of adhesin gene in fixed lung tissue (letter). J Infect Dis 1994; 170:1052–1053.

46. Marmion BP, Williamson J, Worswick PA, Kok TW, Harris RJ. Experience with newer techniques for the laboratory detection of Mycoplasma pneumoniae infection: Adelaide, 1978–1997. Clin Infect Dis 199317:S90–S99.

47. Chirgwin K, Roblin PM, Gelling M, Hammerschlag MR, Schachter J. Infection with Chlamydia pneumoniae in Brooklyn. J Infect Dis 1991; 163:757–761.

48. Hammerschlag MR. Chlamydia pneumoniae infections. Pediatr Infect Dis J 1992; 12:260–261.

49. Karvonen M, Tuomilehto J, Pitkaniemi J, Naukkarinen A, Saikku P. Importance of smoking for Chlamydia pneumoniae seropositivity. Int J Epidemiol 1994; 23:1315–1321.

50. Verkooyen RP, Hazenberg MA, Van Haaren GH, Van Den Bosch JM, Snijder RJ, Van Helden HP, Verbrugh HA. Age-related interference with Chlamydia pneumoniae microimmunofluorescence serology due to circulating rheumatoid factor. J Clin Microbiol 1992; 30:1287–1290.

51. Routes JM, Nelson HS, Noda JA, Simon FT. Lack of correlation between Chlamydia pneumoniae antibody titers and adult-onset asthma. J Allergy Clin Immunol 2000; 105:391–392.

52. Gaydos CA, Quinn TC, Eiden JJ. Identification of Chlamydia pneumoniae by DNA amplification of the 16S r RNA Gene. J Clin Microbiol 1992; 30:796–800.

53. Yuan Y, Zhang YX, Watkins NG, Caldwell HD. Nucleotide and deduced amino acid sequence for the four variable domains of the major membrane proteins of the 15 Chlamydia trachomatis serovars. Infect Immun 1989; 57:1040–1049.

54. Gaydos CA, Roblin PM, Hammerschlag MR, Hyman C, Eiden JJ, Schachter J, Quinn TC. Diagnostic utility of PCR-enzyme immunoassay, culture, and serology for detection of Chlamydia pneumoniae in symptomatic and asymptomatic patients. J Clin Microbiol 1994; 32:903–905.

55. Hahn DL. Treatment of Chlamydia pneumoniae infection in adult asthma: a before-after trial. J Fam Pract 1995; 41:345–351.

56. Hahn DL, Bukstein D, Luskin A, Zeitz H. Evidence for Chlamydia pneumoniae infection in steroid-dependent asthma. Ann Allergy Asthma Immunol 1998; 80:45–49.

57. Kraft M, Cassell GH, Pak J, Martin RJ. Mycoplasma pneumoniae and Chlamydia pneumoniae in asthma: effect of clarithromycin. JAMA 2001; submitted.

58. Szefler SJ, Brenner M, Jusko WJ, Spector SL, Flesker KA, Ellis EF. Dose- and time related effect of troleandomycin on methylprednisolone elimination. Clin Pharmacol Ther 1982; 32:166–171.

59. Yanagihara K, Tomono K, Sawai T, Hirakata Y, Kadota J, Koga H, Tashiro T, Kohno S. Effect of clarithromycin on lymphocytes in chronic respiratory Pseudomonas aeruginosa infection. Am J Respir Crit Care Med 1997; 155:337–342.

60. Eryaud, A, Descotes J, Lombard JY, Laschi-Loquerie A, Tachon P, Veysseyre C, Evreux JC. Effects of erythromycin, josamycin and spiramycin on rat polymorphonuclear leukocyte chemotaxis. Chemotherapy 1986; 32:379–382.

61. Ianaro A, Ialenti A, Maffia P, Saute L, Rombola L, Carnuccio R, Iuvone T, D'Acquisto F, Di Rosa M. Anti-inflammatory activity of macrolide antibiotics. J Pharm Exp Therapeut 2000; 292:156–163.
62. Miyatake H, Taki F, Taniguchi H, Suzuki R, Takagi K, Sakate T. Erythromycin reduces the severity of bronchial hyperresponsiveness in asthma. Chest 1991; 99: 670–673.
63. Wildfeuer A, Laufen H, Zimmerman T. Distribution of orally administered azithromycin in various blood compartments. Int J Clin Pharm Therapeut 1994; 32:356–360.
64. Mufson MA. Mycoplasma pneumonia. In: Gorbach SL, Bartlett JG, Blacklow NR, eds. Infectious Diseases. 2nd ed. Philadelphia: W. B. Saunders, 1998:597–600.
65. Hammerschlag, MR. Chlamydia pneumonia. In: Gorbach SL, Bartlett JG, Blacklow NR, eds. Infectious Disease. 2nd ed. Philadelphia: W. B. Saunders, 1998:622–628.
66. Martin RJ, Chu HW, Honour JM, Harbeck RJ, Henson PM. M. pneumoniae infection in a murine model and bronchial hyperresponsiveness (BHR). Am J Resp Crit Care Med 2000; 161:A606.
67. Campbell LA, Melgosa MP, Hamilton DJ, Kuo CC. Detection of Chlamydia pneumoniae by polymerase chain reaction. J Clin Microbiol 1992; 30:434–439.

14

Sleep Disorders in Severe Asthma

ROBERT D. BALLARD

National Jewish Medical and Research Center
Denver, Colorado

I. Introduction

During the past 3 decades those interested in the interaction between sleep and breathing have focused their attention on obstructive sleep apnea (OSA). However, it is clear that sleep can alter breathing in a variety of ways that may occur independently of sleep apnea. Edward Smith reported in 1860 that ventilation is reduced during sleep in apparently healthy subjects (1). This has been confirmed multiple times in recent years, with the decrement in ventilation apparently resulting from a sleep-associated reduction in tidal volume (2,3).

Although such changes are usually of minimal importance in subjects with normal respiratory function during wakefulness, this is often not the case in patients with lung disease. Nocturnal bronchoconstriction has been well documented in the majority of patients with asthma (4,5), a pattern that appears to disrupt sleep in affected patients (6) and may explain previous reports of an excessive nocturnal death rate from asthma (7). Patients with chronic obstructive pulmonary disease (COPD) often demonstrate nocturnal worsening manifested by hypoxemia (8), disrupted sleep (9), and increasing airflow obstruction (10). Sleep-associated hypoxemia is also commonly observed in patients with cystic fibrosis (11).

323

It is now widely accepted that these nocturnal patterns of respiratory dysfunction are widespread and clinically important, but there continues to be no unifying hypothesis that explains these phenomena in a satisfactory fashion. One area of potential relevance is the role of sleep in modifying interactions between upper and lower airway function. Although data in this area remain incomplete, in this chapter we review current knowledge relating to the potential interaction between sleep-associated alterations in upper airway function and lower airway function.

II. Sleep and Upper Airway Function

Sleep onset leads to upper airway narrowing that occurs even in those without OSA (3,12,13). This narrowing apparently results from the combined effect of sleeping in the supine posture, a reduction in lung volume that occurs during sleep, and a sleep-associated reduction in pharyngeal dilator muscle activity (14,15). Such narrowing of the upper airway may actually constitute an intrinsic resistive load to breathing (16). As compensatory responses to resistive loading are decreased during sleep (17,18), upper airway narrowing may contribute to the sleep-associated reduction in ventilation. Previous work suggests this to be an important contributor to the reduced ventilation and associated hypoxemia previously demonstrated in patients with COPD (10) and cystic fibrosis (11).

Although sleep-associated upper airway narrowing appears to be of little importance in the majority of people, some have upper airways that are already significantly narrowed at one or more levels between the nasal choanae and epiglottis. A number of factors may contribute to this narrowing, including craniofacial characteristics (19), increased size and fat content of the soft palate and uvula (20,21), a large or posterior lying tongue (22), and vascular congestion plus edema of the pharyngeal mucosa (23). Affected persons apparently compensate for this anatomic narrowing during wakefulness by increasing upper airway dilator muscle activity (24). With sleep onset this ''compensatory'' response is reduced or lost, creating an imbalance between forces that promote collapse of the pharynx and those that support upper airway patency (25). This imbalance may lead to closure or critical narrowing of the airway, typically posterior to the palate, the tongue, or at both sites (26,27).

The subsequent reduction or absence of ventilation associated with airway narrowing or closure causes hypercapnia and hypoxia, leading to a progressive increase in inspiratory effort that eventually triggers arousal or awakening. The return to wakefulness restores the compensatory increase in upper airway dilator activity (14), subsequently deoccluding the airway and allowing resumption of normal ventilation until a return to sleep again allows airway narrowing or closure. This cycle can repeat itself hundreds of times during a single night, resulting in the syndrome of OSA.

III. Obstructive Sleep Apnea and Awake Airway Function in Patients Without Other Respiratory Disease

At least two reports have suggested that OSA may lead to altered lower airway function in otherwise healthy patients. Lin and Lin (28) observed that 4 of 16 patients with OSA had bronchial hyperreactivity demonstrated by an abnormal methacholine challenge, whereas none of 32 subjects with snoring alone had a positive methacholine challenge. Bronchial hyperreactivity was subsequently eliminated in the OSA patients after a 2- to 3-month trial with nasal continuous positive airway pressure (nCPAP). These investigators suggested several mechanisms by which OSA could induce reflex bronchoconstriction, including hypoxia-induced bronchoconstriction (29,30), the stimulation of glottic inlet and laryngeal mechanoreceptors by snoring (31), and vagal "hyperfunction" induced by repetitive Müller maneuvers during obstructive apneas (32). However, no mechanism whereby OSA could specifically increase bronchial reactivity was proposed.

Zerah-Lancner and colleagues (33) more recently evaluated pulmonary function abnormalities in 170 obese snorers with and without OSA. It was observed that forced expiratory flows (FEF_{50}, FEV_1, and FEV_1/FVC) decreased as OSA severity increased, findings that could not be explained by increasing levels of obesity. These findings suggested that OSA may be an independent risk factor for small airway disease. As $PaCO_2$ was observed to increase while PaO_2 and SaO_2 decreased with increasing severity of OSA, these researchers suggested that such small airway disease could play a role in the development of chronic hypoventilation in these patients. However, no potential explanation for the proposed effect of OSA on peripheral airway function was offered.

These two reports (28,33) therefore suggest that sleep apnea can promote heightened bronchial reactivity and increased airflow obstruction during wakefulness in nonasthmatic patients, although the mechanism(s) of this effect remain unclear. The implication for asthmatic patients could be substantial, as one would expect these effects to be much more pronounced in patients with preexisting bronchial hyperreactivity and airway obstruction.

IV. Obstructive Sleep Apnea and Asthma

Hudgel and Shucard (34) published the initial report of an asthmatic patient with coexisting OSA. This patient presented with nocturnal worsening of his dyspnea that evidently led to hourly awakenings, despite what was described as well-controlled asthma during the day. A sleep study confirmed severe OSA, with nocturnal oxygen desaturation to as low as 40%. Therapy with supplemental oxygen and medroxyprogesterone was ineffective, leading eventually to a tracheotomy. The tracheotomy resolved all symptoms of sleep apnea, although there was no mention of its effect upon asthma severity.

Chan and colleagues (35) subsequently suggested that OSA and snoring could be important triggers of nocturnal asthma attacks. They reported nine patients with asthma and concurrent OSA, noting that all patients had frequent nocturnal exacerbations of their asthma. When treated with nasal continuous positive airway pressure for OSA, these patients demonstrated marked improvement in their asthma, manifested by a decrease in symptoms, improved peak expiratory flow rate (PEFR), a reduced need for bronchodilator therapy, and resolution of the pattern of nocturnal worsening. Although no mechanism for this effect was clearly established, it was suggested that OSA may provoke asthma via apnea-associated hypoxemia, which could reflexly induce bronchoconstriction via the carotid bodies (29,30). However, review of their data reveals that nocturnal hypoxemia was actually quite mild in these patients, with only one of nine patients demonstrating transient desaturation to <85%. It was also previously noted by Hudgel and Shucard that supplemental oxygen was ineffective therapy for nocturnal dyspnea in their asthmatic patient with OSA (34).

Chan and co-investigators proposed that snoring and repetitive upper airway closures could stimulate neural receptors at the glottic inlet and in the laryngeal region, reflexly triggering bronchoconstriction. Nadel and Widdicombe (31) had previously demonstrated that mechanical stimulation of the larynx in anesthetized cats caused at least a twofold increase in total lung resistance. The afferent limb of this reflex appears to be the superior laryngeal nerve, while the efferent limb is apparently the vagus nerve. It was observed in the cat model that the triggered increase in total lung resistance occurred on the first subsequent breath, typically returning to baseline in less than a minute. This pattern appears to differ markedly from nocturnal exacerbations of asthma, which can sustain themselves and even progress after awakening (36,37) (Fig. 1).

Guilleminault and colleagues (38) subsequently reported findings from two separate populations of asthmatics: one group of middle-aged males with laboratory-confirmed moderate-to-severe OSA and another group of younger (age range 14–21 years) males with known nocturnal worsening of their asthma and a history of regular snoring. The middle-aged OSA patients were treated with nCPAP (range 10–15 cmH$_2$O) for 12–14 months, during which their previously frequent nocturnal asthma exacerbations were totally resolved. The younger males snored loudly, but did not have OSA of the severity demonstrated by the older patients. Lower levels of nCPAP (range 5–10 cmH$_2$O) resolved snoring and their intermittent OSA, while completely eliminating all nocturnal asthma attacks during a 6-month follow-up period.

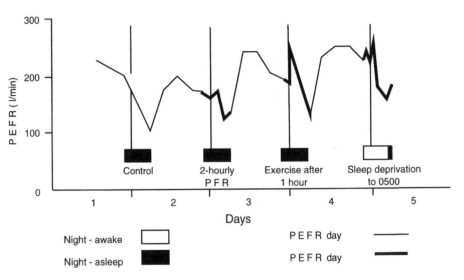

Figure 1 Overnight changes in PEFR (peak expiratory flow rate) in an asthmatic patient. On the third night he was awakened for a 1-h exercise period, which did not prevent the overnight fall in PEFR. On the fourth night he was maintained awake until 05:00, still demonstrating an overnight fall in PEFR. (From Ref. 36, with permission.)

These researchers also positioned esophageal balloons during sleep studies in four of the five younger male patients. They observed that at baseline, negative inspiratory esophageal pressures increased to a mean peak level of 47 ± 8 cmH$_2$O in association with snoring alone, an increase that was subsequently eliminated by the addition of nCPAP. This led to the proposal that complete or partial airway obstruction associated with snoring results in repetitive partial or complete Müller maneuvers. As already noted, this process may result in an increase in vagal tone, which could lead to subsequent increases in bronchomotor tone and airway narrowing (32,39). Therapy to prevent upper airway narrowing during sleep (nCPAP) would therefore eliminate this sleep-related pathological enhancement of vagal tone and the subsequent worsening of asthma. However, one would again expect this reflex-induced increase in bronchomotor tone to improve or resolve with arousal, whereas nocturnal exacerbations of asthma are often persistent or even progressive after awakening.

Martin and Pak (40) subsequently investigated the role of nCPAP in asthmatic patients with nocturnal worsening, but no snoring or known OSA. They reported that two of their seven patients demonstrated marked improvement in their nocturnal asthma when treated overnight with nCPAP at 10 cmH$_2$O. Although for the entire group there was no significant difference between overnight falls in FEV_1 on control and nCPAP nights (mean decrements of 29.3 ± 5.0% and 21.4 ± 5.1%, respectively, $P > 0.05$), it appears that, given the small sample size, a Type 2 error was possible. These investigators did note that the two patients who improved in response to nCPAP had more pronounced nocturnal oxygen desaturation than the other five patients, although their nocturnal asthma did not appear to be any more severe. These two patients could possibly have had an undetected upper airway resistance syndrome (41), which would have responded to nCPAP. Martin and Pak pointed out that the pattern of nocturnal asthma in these two patients also improved in response to nocturnal supplemental oxygen, suggesting that hypoxemia had induced bronchoconstriction via a carotid body-mediated reflex (29), augmented bronchial responsiveness (42), a direct action on bronchial smooth muscle (30), or the release of bronchoconstricting mediators (43). Whatever the potential mechanism(s) of this pattern of nocturnal worsening, these investigators observed that nCPAP was not well tolerated in their patients, who demonstrated reduced sleep efficiency and decreased REM sleep when treated in this fashion.

V. Sleep, Airflow Resistance, Lung Volume, and Intrapulmonary Blood Volume in Asthmatics with Nocturnal Worsening

To better assess the effect of sleep on airflow resistance in asthmatics with nocturnal worsening, we initially performed overnight studies on five patients while monitoring esophageal pressure and airflow via a face mask with an attached pneumotachygraph (44). Using these data to calculate pulmonary resistance (R_L) on a breath-by-breath basis, we observed that R_L increased during sleep in all five patients, leading to a 51.8 ± 10.7% increase ($P < 0.01$) from bedtime to morning awakening (Fig. 2).

In a subsequent study of six asthmatics selected for having nocturnal worsening but no snoring or known sleep apnea, we combined these methods with the addition of a supraglottic pressure catheter (37). This allowed us to also measure the contribution of the upper airway (supraglottic resistance, or Rsg) to sleep associated changes in R_L. Lower airway resistance (Rla = R_L − Rsg) increased overnight whether patients slept or remained awake throughout the night, although the rate of increase was twofold greater while both mean and peak Rla were higher when patients were allowed to sleep (Fig. 3).

These observations confirm that asthma can worsen during the night in the absence of sleep (possibly via a circadian process), but sleep itself also clearly contributes to nocturnal increases in Rla. Although we intentionally selected patients without known snoring or sleep apnea, Rsg was still significantly greater when the patients slept. Given the previous observations of an association be-

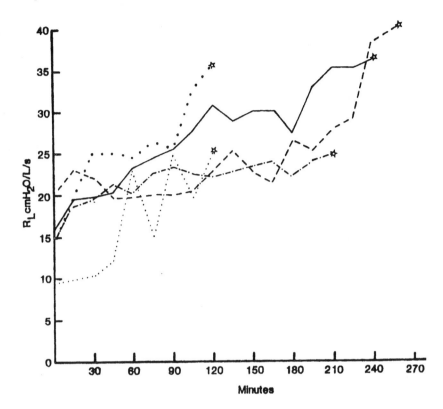

Figure 2   Changes in pulmonary resistance (R$_L$) measured at 15-min intervals in five asthmatic patients. Time 0 indicates time of sleep onset. Stars indicate final R$_L$ before awakening. (From Ref. 44, with permission.)

tween snoring and/or OSA and the nocturnal worsening of asthma, one can hypothesize that ''normal'' sleep-associated upper airway narrowing could also contribute to the nocturnal increases in Rla. However, these observations clearly do not yet confirm a causal relationship between sleep-associated changes in upper and lower airway resistance.

One sleep-related change that could possibly serve as an intermediary step between sleep associated changes in upper and lower airway resistance is the intrapulmonary pooling of blood. Using a horizontal body plethysmograph to study sleeping subjects, we previously demonstrated that sleep was associated with an impressive reduction in functional residual capacity (FRC) in asthmatics with nocturnal worsening (45). Although we found subsequent evidence that sleep-associated reductions in inspiratory muscle tonic activity could contribute

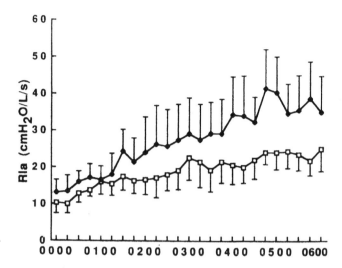

Figure 3 Nocturnal changes in lower airway resistance (Rla) during sleep (solid diamonds) and with prevention of sleep (open squares) in six asthmatic patients. (From Ref. 45, with permission.)

to these observed changes in lung volume (46), several observations led us to suspect that sleep promotes the intrapulmonary pooling of blood, which also contributes to a subsequent reduction in FRC. First, it has been previously documented that moving from the upright to the supine posture (the typical sleeping posture) increases venous return from peripheral vascular beds and augments pulmonary blood volume, an effect which likely contributes to the supine posture-dependent reduction in FRC (47). Additional findings from studies of the effects of general anesthesia (48) and submaximal paralysis (49) (two conditions that mimic many physiologic changes of sleep) also suggest that additional pulmonary blood pooling may occur during sleep.

The intrapulmonary pooling of blood could then worsen asthma by at least three mechanisms: (1) reflex bronchoconstriction triggered by the activation of intrapulmonary C-fiber nerve endings (50), (2) bronchial wall edema (51), and (3) an increase in bronchial responsiveness such as has been observed with the pulmonary vascular congestion associated with left ventricular dysfunction (52).

To qualitatively assess overnight changes in pulmonary blood volume, we subsequently employed a technique utilizing repetitive measures of diffusion capacity (DL CO) at differing alveolar PO_2s to estimate pulmonary capillary volume (Vc), as described by Roughton and Forster (53). We observed that asthmatic patients with nocturnal worsening demonstrated a significant overnight increase in Vc (54) (Fig. 4), suggesting that pulmonary blood volume could also be in-

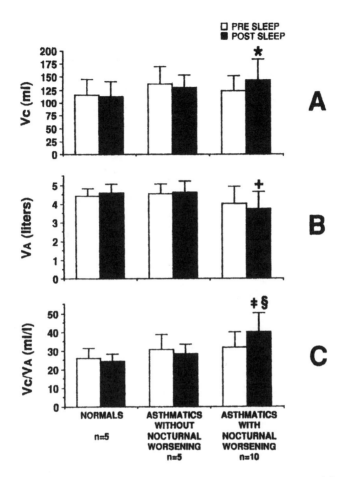

Figure 4 Changes in pulmonary capillary volume (Vc) and as corrected for alveolar volume (Vc /Va) in 5 normal controls and 15 asthmatic patients, 10 with and 5 without nocturnal worsening. Open bar, presleep measurements; solid bar, postsleep measurements. *$P = 0.02$ for presleep versus postsleep; $^+P = 0.0035$ for presleep versus postsleep; $^\pm P = 0.003$ for presleep versus postsleep; other, $P = 0.0095$ for postsleep subjects with asthma versus all other subjects. (From Ref. 54, with permission.)

creased in these patients. However, no such changes were observed in healthy controls or in asthmatic patients without nocturnal worsening.

Although there are many potential causes for increased Vc and pulmonary blood volume in the sleeping asthmatic, it was previously reported that the imposition of an inspiratory resistance in awake subjects can trigger similar changes

(55). In fact, this has been offered as an explanation for the observed increase in DLCO often measured in asthmatic patients (56). We, therefore, hypothesized that sleep-associated narrowing of the upper airway could augment intrapulmonary pooling of blood, even in the absence of snoring or frank OSA.

To explore this possibility, we evaluated the effect of applying progressive inspiratory resistance to healthy controls and asthmatic patients without snoring or OSA in the following sequence: hour 1, 9.0 cmH$_2$O/L/sec; hour 2, 17.0 cmH$_2$O/L/sec; and hours 3 and 4, 21.5 cmH$_2$O/L/sec. Ten of the asthmatic patients had been previously documented by PEFR and FEV$_1$ measurements to have a pattern of recurrent nocturnal worsening. Nine of these 10 patients demonstrated >20% reduction in FEV$_1$ (mean decrease in FEV$_1$ of 29.9 ± 5.7%, P = 0.0025) after the period of resistive loading, an overall decrement in FEV$_1$ that was similar to that previously observed overnight in these same patients (57). These nine patients also demonstrated a 16.0 ± 7.0% increase (P = 0.039) in Vc after the period of resistive loading. However, neither healthy controls nor asthmatic patients without nocturnal worsening demonstrated a significant change in either FEV$_1$ or Vc after the period of progressive inspiratory resistance. These observations suggest that sleep-associated upper airway narrowing (mimicked by our extrinsic resistive load) in the absence of snoring and OSA could play a role in the nocturnal worsening of asthma, and such an effect could be mediated by an associated increase in pulmonary blood volume. However, this link has yet to be firmly established.

These observations provide compelling evidence for a role of sleep-associated narrowing of the upper airway in both the nocturnal worsening and diurnal severity of asthma. This is of particular concern given the observation that asthmatics snore more frequently and find their sleep less refreshing than nonasthmatic controls (75,85). In the setting of severe asthma, and particularly in the presence of PEFR evidence of nocturnal worsening, one should question the patient carefully about signs and symptoms predictive of OSA: frequent, loud snoring; witnessed apneas; nonrestorative sleep and daytime somnolence; obesity and/or a neck circumference ≥17 in. in males or 16 in. in females; male gender; coexistent hypertension; and advancing age. If such predictors are present, one should proceed to nocturnal polysomnography to evaluate for OSA or upper airway resistance syndrome.

VI.   The Effect of Sleep and Circadian Rhythms on Rhinitis: Implications for Asthmatic Patients

As discussed elsewhere in this volume, there is strong evidence for a pathophysiologic link between rhinitis and asthma. Allergic rhinitis has been reported to occur in up to 57% of asthmatic adults (58), while up to 38% of patients with allergic rhinitis may have asthma (59). The onset of rhinitis and asthma symptoms is also often temporally linked (58,60). Finally, bronchial hyperreactivity to aerosolized methacholine and histamine can often be demonstrated in allergic rhinitis alone, with up to 32% of allergic rhinitis patients demonstrating bronchial responsiveness in the range of that observed in frankly asthmatic patients (61).

Other studies have assessed the effect of therapy with rhinitis-specific antiinflammatory medications upon asthma severity. Corren and colleagues (62) observed that the intranasal administration of beclomethasone to patients with seasonal rhinitis and asthma blocked their usual seasonal increase in methacholine responsiveness. In a similar study, Watson and associates (63) found that 4 weeks of intranasal therapy with beclomethasone significantly reduced bronchial responsiveness in patients with concurrent allergic rhinitis and asthma. Aubier and colleagues (64) demonstrated that intranasal administration of beclomethasone to asthmatic patients with rhinitis improved bronchial responsiveness, whereas intrabronchial administration of the same steroid had no effect on bronchial reactivity.

These studies suggest that the nasal inflammation associated with allergic rhinitis may play a significant role in modulating lower airway responsiveness in asthmatic patients. Several potential mechanisms have been offered to explain this relationship. The existence of a nasal-bronchial reflex has been suggested by the observation that application of silica particles to the nasal mucosa can trigger an immediate marked increase in lower airway resistance (65). This effect can be blocked by systemic atropine (65) or resection of the trigeminal nerve (66). Corren and associates (67) reported that nasal allergen challenge in patients with seasonal allergic rhinitis and asthma triggered an immediate increase in nonspecific bronchial responsiveness to methacholine. The rapidity of these changes clearly suggests the involvement of a neural reflex.

Another potential mechanism by which rhinitis could modulate bronchial responsiveness is that nasal obstruction resulting from mucosal swelling and secretions can promote a switch to oral breathing. Oral breathing has been demonstrated to aggravate exercise-induced bronchospasm (68). Finally, the postnasal drainage of cellular and biochemical inflammatory mediators with subsequent pulmonary aspiration has also been suggested to augment lower airway responsiveness (69).

Whichever mechanisms link nasal inflammation to lower airway function, there is substantial evidence that symptoms of allergic rhinitis increase at night and during the early morning. One study of "hay fever" sufferers suggested that in 75% of those sampled, symptoms (sneezing, nasal stuffiness, wheeze, and cough) were most severe while in bed at night or with morning awakening (70). Another study of nearly 1000 patients with perennial or seasonal rhinitis reported that 56% of those with seasonal rhinitis and 66% of those with perennial rhinitis had their most severe symptoms (sneezing, nasal stuffiness, and postnasal drainage) at the time of morning awakening (71). Reinberg and associates (72) also studied the day–night variation of allergic rhinitis symptoms in 765 patients. They observed that sneezing, nasal stuffiness, and rhinorrhea were all most severe in the early morning after awakening.

These studies all suggest that rhinitis increases in severity during the night and early morning hours. This may signify a nocturnal intranasal increase in inflammation, such as previously observed in the joints of patients with rheumatoid arthritis (73) and in the airways of asthmatic patients (74). As already discussed, evidence supports a link between nasal inflammation and lower airway function, and it is possible that a nocturnal or early morning increase in nasal inflammation could trigger subsequent worsening of asthma. One can therefore speculate that a sleep-induced or circadian rhythm-dependent early morning increase in nasal inflammation may contribute to the pattern of nocturnal worsening or "morning dipping" that is typical of asthma.

Another potential mechanism by which rhinitis could enhance asthma severity is by its effect upon nasal patency and the subsequent impact upon sleep and breathing. As already noted, nasal obstruction resulting from congestion and excessive secretions can promote a switch to oral breathing. Oral breathing has been widely observed to promote pharyngeal narrowing and even closure during sleep, presumably due to a drop of the mandible when the mouth opens. This allows for posterior movement of the tongue, which leads to hypoglossal narrowing of the airway and possibly even frank occlusion. Support for this sequence of events comes from reports that packing the nostrils of healthy subjects during the night triggers OSA (75,76,77).

In addition, the administration of topical anesthesia to the nasal mucosa has also been observed to provoke frank OSA in previously normal subjects (78). This latter observation suggests that receptors localized to the nasal airway play an important role in the maintenance of normal respiration during sleep. Whatever the mechanism, it is clear that inflammatory rhinitis can trigger snoring and OSA. This is perhaps best demonstrated by the observation of McNicholas and colleagues that allergic patients developed an increased frequency of obstructive apneas during allergy season (79). If such events occur in asthmatic patients, one would expect snoring and OSA to cause both nocturnal and diurnal worsening of asthma via the mechanisms already described. To interrupt this pathologic sequence of events, one should be prepared to utilize saline nasal washes, intranasal anti-inflammatory (steroid) agents, and antihistamines if indicated.

VII. Disturbed Sleep in Asthmatics

Although this chapter has focused primarily on the effects of sleep on asthma severity, it is also clear that asthma often disturbs sleep quality. Kales and co-investigators studied 12 young adult asthmatics in the sleep laboratory and observed them to have reduced sleep efficiency, more frequent awakenings, less stage 4 sleep, and earlier final awakenings than normal controls (80). Montplaisir and colleagues subsequently confirmed that nocturnal worsening of asthma is associated with a reduction in sleep efficiency (81). More recently, Fitzpatrick and co-investigators have reported not only a reduction in sleep efficiency in asthmatics with nocturnal worsening, but also impairment of daytime cognitive function (82).

Sleep disruption appears to be a common complaint in asthmatic patients. Turner-Warwick reported that 64% of 7729 asthmatic patients surveyed described awakening with worsening symptoms of asthma at least 3 nights weekly (4). Janson and colleagues surveyed 98 asthmatic patients, reporting that 51% complained of early morning awakening, 44% complained of difficulty maintaining sleep, while 44% also complained of daytime sleepiness (83). These complaints all increased with decreasing asthma control. In total, the prevalence rates of sleep complaints were approximately twofold greater in the asthmatic population than in healthy controls.

In a subsequent study of 1478 randomly selected adults, Fitzpatrick and co-investigators found that asthmatic patients of all ages found their sleep unrefreshing more often than controls (84). In logistic regression analysis, these investigators found asthma to be a positive independent predictor of unrefreshing nocturnal sleep, spending less time asleep at night, and having a perception of too little sleep at night. Janson and colleagues have recently reported from 2661 subjects (267 asthmatic patients) that asthmatic patients are about twice as likely to complain of difficulty initiating sleep and early morning awakenings than nonasthmatic subjects (85). Asthmatic patients were also about 50% more likely to complain of daytime sleepiness.

These studies all support the association between asthma and decreased objective and subjective quality of sleep. This has obvious implications for daytime cognitive function and quality of life in the asthmatic population. There may be even more serious consequences for the poorly controlled asthmatic patient with recurrent nocturnal exacerbations. We previously evaluated the effects of 36 h of sleep deprivation on ventilatory and arousal responses to induced bronchoconstriction during subsequent sleep in eight mild asthmatic patients (86). We found that ventilation was preserved in response to bronchoconstriction despite previous sleep deprivation. However, the "arousal threshold" to bronchoconstriction was markedly increased by prior sleep deprivation (mean maximal Rla of 8.3 ± 2.1 cmH$_2$O/L/sec tolerated during normal sleep vs. mean maximal Rla of 23.7 ± 2.1 cmH$_2$O/L/sec tolerated during sleep after sleep deprivation, $P < 0.01$ (Fig. 5). One could therefore theorize that an increased arousal threshold in asthmatics with chronically disrupted sleep might eventually prevent them from awakening and obtaining necessary treatment when severely bronchoconstricted.

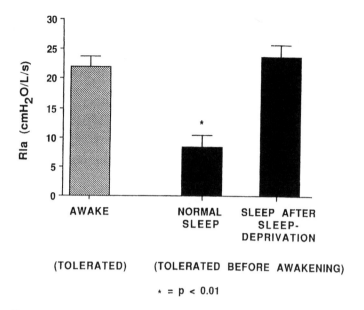

Figure 5 Mean maximum Rla attained by eight asthmatic patients before they asked the study to be terminated due to discomfort (awake) or were awakened spontaneously because of bronchoconstriction (normal sleep), awakened spontaneously because of bronchoconstriction (4), or awakened by researchers after exceeding Rla of 25 $cmH_2O/L/sec$ (4) (sleep after prior sleep deprivation). (From Ref. 86, with permission.)

VIII. Conclusion

Sleep alters respiratory function in a number of ways in those both with and without underlying respiratory disorders. One well-described effect leads to sleep-associated upper airway narrowing and even frank OSA. There is substantial evidence that upper airway narrowing and OSA can contribute to bronchial reactivity, airway obstruction, and increased severity of asthma via several potential mechanisms. The clinician must therefore be alert for the signs and symptoms of OSA in asthmatic patients, particularly in those with severe disease or recurrent nocturnal worsening.

Rhinitis is another inflammatory disorder that typically worsens during nocturnal sleep. This worsening of rhinitis appears to worsen coexisting asthma via several potential mechanisms. One must therefore be alert to rhinitis in the asthmatic patient and prepared to initiate appropriate anti-inflammatory therapy.

Finally, there is strong evidence that asthma itself can disrupt sleep in affected patients, leading to daytime fatigue and altered cognitive function. Such sleep disruption could place asthma patients at risk for not being able to respond appropriately to nocturnal bronchoconstriction. The clinician should therefore be guided to optimize asthma therapy to allow normal sleep.

References

1. Smith E. Recherches experimentales sur la respiration. J Physiol de l'Homme et des Animaux 1860; 3:506–521.
2. Douglas NJ, White DP, Pickett CK, Weil J, Zwillich C. Respiration during sleep in normal man. Thorax 1982; 37:840–844.
3. Hudgel DW, Martin RJ, Johnson B, Hill P. Mechanics of the respiratory system and breathing pattern during sleep in normal humans. J Appl Physiol 1984; 56:133–137.
4. Turner-Warwick M. Epidemiology of nocturnal asthma. Am J Med 1988; 85:6–8.
5. Connolly CK. Diurnal rhythms in airway obstruction. Br J Dis Chest 1979; 73:357–366.
6. Montplaisir J, Walsh J, Malo JL. Nocturnal asthma: Features of attacks, sleep, and breathing patterns. Am Rev Respir Dis 1982; 125:18–22.
7. Hetzel MR, Clark TJH, Branthwaite MA. Asthma: analysis of sudden deaths and ventilatory arrests in hospital. Br Med J 1977; 1:808–811.
8. Douglas NJ, Calverley PMA, Leggett RJE, Brash HM, Flenley DC, Brezinova V. Transient hypoxemia during sleep in chronic bronchitis and emphysema. Lancet 1979; 1:1–4.
9. Cormick W, Olsen LG, Hensley MJ, Saunders NA. Nocturnal hypoxemia and quality of sleep in patients with chronic obstructive lung disease. Thorax 1986; 41:846–854.
10. Ballard RD, Clover CW, Suh BY. Influence of sleep on respiratory function in emphysema. Am J Respir Crit Care Med 1995; 151:945–951.
11. Ballard RD, Sutarik JM, Clover CW, Suh BY. Effect of non-REM sleep on ventilation and respiratory mechanics in adults with cystic fibrosis. Am J Respir Crit Care Med 1996; 153:266–271.
12. Lopes JM, Tabachnik E, Muller NL, Levison H, Bryan AC. Total airway resistance and respiratory muscle activity during sleep. J Appl Physiol 1983; 54:773–777.
13. Hudgel DW, Hendricks C, Hamilton HB. Characteristics of the upper airway pressure-flow relationship during sleep. J Appl Physiol 1988; 64:1930–1935.
14. Remmers JE, de Groot WJ, Sauerland EK, Anch AM. Pathogenesis of upper airway occlusion during sleep. J Appl Physiol 1978; 44:931–938.
15. Tangel DJ, Mezzanotte WS, White DP. Influence of sleep on tensor palatini EMG and upper airway resistance in normal men. J Appl Physiol 1991; 70:2574–2581.
16. Skatrud JB, Jempsey JA. Airway resistance and respiratory muscle function in snorers during NREM sleep. J Appl Physiol 1985; 59:328–335.
17. Iber C, Berssenbrugge A, Skatrud JB, Dempsey JA. Ventilatory adaptations to resistive loading during wakefulness and non-REM sleep. J Appl Physiol 1982; 52:607–614.
18. Wiegand L, Zwillich CW, White DP. Sleep and the ventilatory response to resistive loading in normal men. J Appl Physiol 1988; 64:1186–1195.
19. Guilleminault C, Riley R, Powell N. Obstructive sleep apnea and abnormal cephalometric measurements: implications for treatment. Chest 1984; 86:793–794.

20. Horner RL, Mohiaddin RH, Lowell DG, Shea SA, Burman ED, Longmore DB, Guz A. Sites and sizes of fat deposits around the pharynx in patients with obstructive sleep apnea and weight matched controls. Eur Respir J 1989; 2:613–622.

21. Shelton KE, Woodson H, Gay S, Suratt PM. Pharyngeal fat in obstructive sleep apnea. Am Rev Respir Dis 1993; 148:462–466.

22. Ryan CF, Lowe AA, Li D, Fleetham JA. Three-dimensional upper airway computed tomography in obstructive sleep apnea. Am Rev Respir Dis 1991; 144:428–432.

23. Shepard JW, Pevernagie DA, Stanson AW, Daniels BK, Sheedy PF. Effects of changes in central venous pressure on upper airway size in patients with obstructive sleep apnea. Am J Respir Crit Care Med 1996; 153:250–254.

24. Suratt PM, McTier FR, Wilhoit SC. Upper airway muscle activation is augmented in patients with obstructive sleep apnea compared to with that in normal subjects. Am Rev Repir Dis 1988; 137:889–894.

25. Mezzanotte WS, Tangel DJ, White DP. Waking genioglossal electromyogram in sleep apnea patients: a neuromuscular compensatory mechanism. J Clin Invest 1992; 89:1571–1579.

26. Stein MG, Gamsu G, de Geer G, Golden JA, Crumley RL, Webb WR. Cine CT in obstructive sleep apnea. Am J Roentgenol 1987; 148:1069–1074.

27. Horner RL, Shea SA, McIvor J, Guz A. Pharyngeal size and shape during wakefulness and sleep in patients with obstructive sleep apnea. Q J Nucl Med 1989; 72: 719–735.

28. Lin CC, Lin CY. Obstructive sleep apnea syndrome and bronchial hyperreactivity. Lung 1995; 173:117–126.

29. Nadel JA, Widdicombe JG. Effect of changes in blood gas tensions and carotid sinus pressure on tracheal volume and total lung resistance to airflow. J Physiol 1962; 163:13–33.

30. Stephens NL, Kroger EA. Effects of hypoxia on airway smooth muscle mechanics and electrophysiology. J Appl Physiol 1970; 28:630–635.

31. Nadel JA, Widdicombe JG. Reflex effects of upper airway irritation on total lung resistance and blood pressure. J Appl Physiol 1962; 17:861–865.

32. Guilleminault C, Tilkian A, Lehrman K, Forno L, Dement WC. Sleep apnea syndrome: states of sleep and autonomic dysfunction. J Neurol Neurosurg Psych 1977; 40:718–725.

33. Zerah-Lancner F, Lofaso F, Coste A, Ricolfi F, Goldenberg F, Harf A. Pulmonary function in obese snorers with or without sleep apnea syndrome. Am J Respir Crit Care Med 1997; 156:522–527.

34. Hudgel DW, Shucard DW. Coexistence of sleep apnea and asthma resulting in severe sleep hypoxemia. J Am Med Assoc 1979; 242:2789–2790.

35. Chan CS, Woolcock AJ, Sullivan CE. Nocturnal asthma: role of snoring and obstructive sleep apnea. Am Rev Respir Dis 1988; 137:1502–1504.

36. Hetzel MR, Clark TJH. Does sleep cause nocturnal asthma? Thorax 1979; 34:749–754.

37. Ballard RD, Saathoff MC, Patel DK, Kelly PL, Martin RJ. Effect of sleep on nocturnal bronchoconstriction and ventilatory patterns in asthmatics. J Appl Physiol 1989; 67:243–249.

38. Guilleminault C, Quera-Salva MA, Powell N, Riley R, Romaker A, Partinen M,

Baldwin R, Nino-Murcia G. Nocturnal asthma: snoring, small pharynx and nasal CPAP. Eur Respir J 1988; 1:902–907.

39. Guilleminault C, Winkle R, Melvin K, Tilkian A. Cyclical variation of the heart rate in sleep apnea syndromes: mechanisms and usefulness of 24-hour electro-encephalography as a screening technique. Lancet 1984; 1:126–136.

40. Martin RJ, Pak J. Nasal CPAP in nonapneic nocturnal asthma. Chest 1991; 100: 1024–1027.

41. Guilleminault C, Stoohs R, Clerk A, Cetel M, Maistros P. A cause of excessive daytime sleepiness: the upper airway resistance syndrome. Chest 1993; 104:781–787.

42. Denjean A, Roux C, Herve P, Bonniot JP, Comoy E, Duroux P, Gaultier C. Mild isocapnic hypoxia enhances the bronchial response to methacholine in asthmatic subjects. Am Rev Respir Dis 1988; 138:789–793.

43. Peters SP, Lichtenstein LM, Adkinson NF. Mediator release from human lung under conditions of reduced oxygen tension. J Pharmacol Exp Ther 1986; 238:8–13.

44. Ballard RD, Kelly PL, Martin RJ. Estimates of ventilation from inductance plethys-mography in sleeping asthmatics. Chest 1988; 93:128–133.

45. Ballard RD, Irvin CG, Martin RJ, Pak J, Pandey R, White DP. Influence of sleep on lung volume in asthmatic patients and normal subjects. J Appl Physiol 1990; 68: 2034–2041.

46. Ballard RD, Clover CW, White DP. Influence of non-REM sleep on inspiratory muscle activity and lung volume in asthmatic patients. Am Rev Respir Dis 1993; 147:880–886.

47. Hamilton WF, Morgan AB. Mechanism of the postural reduction in vital capacity in relation to orthopnea and storage of blood in the lungs. Am J Physiol 1932; 99: 526–533.

48. Hedenstierna G, Lofstrom B, Lundh R. Thoracic gas volume and chest-abdomen dimensions during anesthesia and muscle paralysis. Anesthesiology 1981; 55:499–506.

49. Kimball WR, Loring SH, Basta SJ, DeTroyer A, Mead J. Effects of paralysis with pancuronium on chest wall statics in awake humans. J Appl Physiol 1985; 58:1638–1645.

50. Chung KF, Keyes SJ, Morgan BM, Jones PW, Snashall PD. Mechanisms of airway narrowing in acute pulmonary oedema in dogs: influence of vagus and lung volume. Clin Sci 1983; 65:289–296.

51. Regnard JP, Baudrillard P, Salah B, Dinh Xuan AT, Cabanes L, Lockhart A. Inflation of antishock trousers increases bronchial response to methacholine in healthy sub-jects. J Appl Physiol 1990; 68:1528–1533.

52. Cabanes LR, Weber S, Matran R, Regnard J, Richard MO, DeGeorges ME, Lockhart A. Bronchial hyperresponsiveness to methacholine in patients with impaired left ventricular function. N Engl J Med 1989; 320:1317–1322.

53. Roughton FJW, Forster RE. Relative importance of diffusion and chemical reaction rate in determining rate of exchange of gases in the human lung, with special refer-ence to true diffusing capacity of pulmonary membrane and volume of blood in the lung capillaries. J Appl Physiol 1957; 11:290–302.

54. Desjardin JA, Sutarik JM, Suh BY, Ballard RD. Influence of sleep on pulmonary

capillary volume in normal and asthmatic subjects. Am J Respir Crit Care Med 1995; 152:193–198.

55. Steiner SH, Frayser R, Ross JC. Alterations in pulmonary diffusing capacity and pulmonary capillary volume with negative pressure breathing. J Clin Invest 1965; 44:1623–1630.

56. Stewart RI. Carbon monoxide diffusing capacity in asthmatic patients with mild airflow limitation. Chest 1988; 94:332–336.

57. Sutarik JM, Suh BY, Ballard RD. Effect of flow-resistive load on airflow obstruction and capillary volume in asthmatics (abstr). Am J Respir Crit Care Med 1994; 149(suppl 4):A222.

58. Peckham C, Butler N. A national study of asthma in childhood. J Epidemiol Commun Health 1978; 32:79–85.

59. Blair H. Natural history of childhood asthma. Arch Dis Child 1977; 52:613–619.

60. Matternowski CJ, Mathews KP. The prevalence of ragweed pollinosis in foreign and native students at a midwestern university and its implications concerning methods for determining inheritance of atopy. J Allergy 1962; 33:130–140.

61. Ramsdale EH, Morris MM, Robers RS, Hargreave FE. Asymptomatic bronchial hyperresponsiveness in rhinitis. J Allergy Clin Immunol 1985; 75:573–577.

62. Corren J, Adinoff AD, Buchmeier AD, Irvin CG. Nasal beclomethasone prevents the seasonal increase in bronchial responsiveness in patients with allergic rhinitis and asthma. J Allergy Clin Immunol 1992; 90:250–256.

63. Watson WTA, Becker AB, Simons FER. Treatment of allergic rhinitis with intranasal corticosteroids in patients with mild asthma: effect on lower airway responsiveness. J Allergy Clin Immunol 1993; 91:97–101.

64. Aubier M, Clerici C, Neukirch F, Herman D. Different effects of nasal and bronchial glucocorticosteroid administration on bronchial hyperresponsiveness in patients with allergic rhinitis. Am Rev Respi Dis 1992; 146:122–126.

65. Kaufman J, Wright GW. The effect of nasal and oropharyngeal irritation on airway resistance in man. Am Rev Respir Dis 1969; 100:626–630.

66. Kaufman J, Chen JC, Wright GW. The effect of trigeminal resection on reflex bronchoconstriction after nasal and nasopharyngeal irritation in man. Am Rev Respir Dis 1970; 101:768–769.

67. Corren J, Adinoff AD, Irvin CG. Changes in bronchial responsiveness following nasal provocation with allergen. J Allergy Clin Immunol 1992; 89:611–618.

68. Shturman-Ellstein R, Zeballaos RJ, Buckley JM, Souhrada JF. The beneficial effect of nasal breathing on exercise-induced bronchoconstriction. Am Rev Respir Dis 1978; 118:65–73.

69. Irvin CG. Sinusitis and asthma: an animal model. J Allergy Clin Immunol 1992; 90:521–533.

70. Nicholson PA, Bogie W. Diurnal variation in the symptoms of hay fever: implications for pharmaceutical development. Curr Med Res Opin 1973; 1:395–401.

71. Binder E, Holopainen E, Malmberg H, Salo O. Anamnestic data in allergic rhinitis. Allergy 1982; 37:389–396.

72. Reinberg A, Gervais P, Levi F, Smolensky M, Del Carro L, Ugolini C. Circadian and circannual rhythms of allergic rhinitis: an epidemiologic study involving chronobiologic methods. J Allergy Clin Immunol 1988; 81:51–62.

73. Labrecque G. Inflammatory reaction and disease. In: Touitou Y, Haus E, eds. Biological rhythms in clinical and laboratory medicine. Berlin: Springer-Verlag, 1992:483–492.

74. Martin RJ, Cicutto LC, Smith HR, Ballard RD, Szefler SJ. Airways inflammation in nocturnal asthma. Am Rev Respir Dis 1991; 143:351–357.

75. Zwillich CW, Pickett C, Hanson FN, Weil JV. Disturbed sleep and prolonged apnea during nasal obstruction in normal men. Am Rev Respir Dis 1981; 124:158–160.

76. Olsen KD, Kern EB, Westbrook PR. Sleep and breathing disturbance secondary to nasal obstruction. Otolaryngol Head Neck Surg 1981; 89:804–810.

77. Millman RP, Acebo C, Rosenberg C, Carskadon MA. Sleep, breathing, and cephalometrics in older children and young adults. Part II—Response to nasal occlusion. Chest 1996; 109:673–679.

78. While DP, Cadieux RJ, Lombard RM. The effects of nasal anesthesia on breathing during sleep. Am Rev Respir Dis 1985; 132:972–975.

79. McNicholas WT, Tarlo S, Cole P, Zamel N, Rutherford R, Griffin D, Phillipson EA. Obstructive apneas during sleep in patients with seasonal allergic rhinitis. Am Rev Respir Dis 1982; 126:625–628.

80. Kales A, Beall GN, Bajor GF, Jacobson A, Kales JD. Sleep studies in asthmatic adults: relationship of attacks to sleep stage and time of night. J Allergy 1968; 41:164–173.

81. Montplaisir J, Walsh J, Malo JL. Nocturnal asthma: features of attacks, sleep and breathing patterns. Am Rev Respir Dis 1982; 125:18–22.

82. Fitzpatrick MF, Engleman H, Whyte KF, Deary IJ, Shapiro CM, Douglas NJ. Morbidity in nocturnal asthma: sleep quality and daytime cognitive performance. Thorax 1991; 46:569–573.

83. Janson C, Gislason T, Boman G, Hetta J, Roos BE. Sleep disturbances in patients with asthma. Respir Med 1990; 84:37–42.

84. Fitzpatrick MF, Martin K, Fossey E, Shapiro CM, Elton RA, Douglas NJ. Snoring, asthma and sleep disturbance in Britain: a community-based survey. Eur Respir J 1993; 6:531–535.

85. Janson C, De Backer W, Gislason T, Plaschke P, Bjornsson E, Hetta J, Kristbjarnarson H, Vermeire P, Boman G. Increased prevalence of sleep disturbances and daytime sleepiness in subjects with bronchial asthma: a population study of young adults in three European countries. Eur Respir J 1996; 9:2132–2138.

86. Ballard RD, Tan WC, Kelly PL, Pak J, Pandey R, Martin RJ. Effect of sleep and sleep deprivation on ventilatory response to bronchoconstriction. J Appl Physiol 1990; 69:490–497.

15

Allergen-Specific Therapy for Severe Asthma

TINA K. HATLEY, JUDITH A. WOODFOLK, GEORGE A. WARD, Jr. and THOMAS A. E. PLATTS-MILLS

University of Virginia Health Sciences System
Charlottesville, Virginia

I. Introduction

Asthma is an inflammatory disease of the lower airways in which common inhaled allergens, occupational agents, and viral and fungal elements, individually or in combination, play roles (1–6). The final common pathway is inflammation, bronchial hyperreactivity, and the well-known symptoms of airway obstruction (Fig. 1). The increase in mortality in some groups, and particularly among patients living in poverty in the United States, suggests that the severity of asthma and the prevalence have both increased. The persistent high prevalence and severity of asthma presents a challenge both to understanding the causes and to developing new modalities for treatment. Given the evidence for eosinophil-rich inflammation of the bronchi, it is logical to investigate patients to try to identify the antigens stimulating this immune response. However, it is clear that a large proportion of cases of severe asthma in adults do not have an obvious extrinsic (i.e., inhaled) cause for their disease. There are many other possible sources of foreign antigens, including colonizing organisms, viruses, and food, which have not been systematically investigated. The causes of extrinsic asthma have been more clearly defined, and it has become possible to focus on the patients among

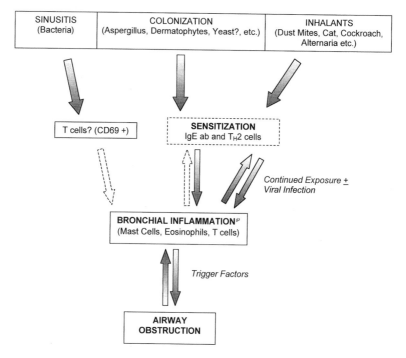

Figure 1   Etiology of bronchial reactivity in adults. Notes: $\wp$ = bronchial inflammation is related to bronchial hyperreactivity.

whom other causes of an inflammatory response of the bronchi should be investigated (7).

Severe asthma can present in several different forms (Table 1). Some patients suffer acute attacks that come on within minutes and require intubation. When these attacks are fatal postmortem examination of the lungs reveals open bronchi with inflammation but only minimal mucus or edema. These patients with sudden attacks are thought to contribute disproportionately to mortality. In the United States asthma mortality rates increased from 1.2/100,000 general population in 1979 to 2.1/100,000 in 1994 and 1995 (8,9,36). The reasons for this increase in mortality are not known. Possible causes include increased prevalence of asthma, increased indoor air pollution as a result of tighter construction of homes with an emphasis on energy conservation, and excessive exposure to allergen. Other patients have prolonged episodes of ''status asthmaticus'' (i.e., days of bronchospasm with mucus inspissation and extensive bronchial wall edema). A third type of severe asthma is chronically steroid-dependent, but not usually life-threatening in the short term. Severe steroid-dependent asthmatics have im-

Table 1 Different Forms of Asthma

Diagnosis	Evaluation	Sinus CT changes[a]	Eos	IgE	eNO	Specific treatment
Allergic asthma	Skin testing/RAST					
Perennial		0–++	>300	≥200	>10	Allergen avoidance
Seasonal		–	>300	≥100		Immunotherapy
Occupational	Specific challenge	–	100–300	>100		Prevent further exposure
Mycoses						
Aspergillus (ABPA)	IgE, skin testing, aspergillus precipitans, chest CT	0–++	>500	≥400	—	Itraconazole
Onychomycosis	Nail culture	++–+++	≥300	>200	—	Itraconazole
						Fluconazole
Aspirin-Sensitive asthma	History, IgE, sinus CT	+++	≥300	20–>300	>10 ppb	Aspirin desensitization
Eosinophilic asthma without allergy	Evaluation for collagen vascular disease	0–++	≥1000	<100	NK	Steroids plus immunosuppressants
Churg-Strauss						
Eosinophilic pneumonia						
Pseudoasthmas	Visualization of vocal cords, PFT's, exclude inflammation	0	<200	<100	<10	Behavior modification and speech therapy
Vocal cord dysfunction[b]						
Hyperventilation	PFT's					

[a] Sinusitis judged by mucosal thickening in each sinus. Scored on a scale from 0 to 35: ++, >12; +++, >20.

paired airflow despite maximal doses of conventional therapy with bronchodilators, cromolyns, ipratropium bromide, inhaled corticosteroids, and oral theophylline. They have generally progressed from multiple short courses of prednisone (or its equivalent) to daily oral steroids to maintain acceptable lung function. Oral steroids are effective at suppressing inflammation and maintaining airway patency, but the trade-off in toxicity is high; furthermore, steroids may have long-term deleterious effects on asthma. The sequelae of chronic steroid use have prompted trials of immunosuppressive agents such as methotrexate, Cyclosporin A, and gold, among others, in attempts to decrease steroid doses. These medicines may be helpful in some cases; however, they also have potentially severe side effects, and, like steroids, these "steroid sparing" agents do not address the specific cause. Understanding the triggers of the inflammatory response in severe asthmatics would allow for a more targeted approach to the treatment and decrease the need for broad spectrum anti-inflammatory agents with their multiplicity of systemic side effects. An obvious strategy is avoidance of agents that start the inflammatory cascade. In allergic asthma there is overwhelming evidence that prolonged exposure of sensitized individuals to aeroallergens is an important cause of bronchial hyperreactivity (10). In addition, patients with chronic severe asthma are tormented by exposure to multiple trigger factors, including passive smoke, and inadvertent inhalation of perfumes, soap odors, and so on; these reactions are presumed to reflect nonspecific bronchial hyperreactivity. This chapter (1) addresses the use of allergen avoidance as an arm of therapy for severe asthmatics, (2) reviews recent investigations on the role of sinusitis and fungal infections in severe asthma, and (3) discusses the limits of immunotherapy in severe asthma.

II. Inhalant Allergens

A. Indoor Allergens

Allergens are potent agents in initiating and prolonging pulmonary inflammation. It is thought that persistent allergen exposure through the interplay of allergen-specific IgE antibody, mast cells, T cells, and eosinophils results in symptomatic inflammation (10–13). Furthermore, it is generally accepted that this inflammatory response to common inhalants such as mite, cat, dog, and cockroach allergens is restricted to those individuals who have IgE antibodies and positive immediate hypersensitivity skin tests. Preventing the triggering protein from reaching the sensitized immune system in the lungs has been shown to decrease symptoms in patients with mild to moderate asthma. A thorough understanding of the sources of airborne particles that comprise allergen exposure is essential to develop a plan for reducing access of allergen to the lung. Changes in lifestyle over the past several decades have resulted in houses which are warmer, have lower ventilation rates, more furniture and carpets, and more pets indoors. These factors would all tend to increase indoor allergen levels. Accurate measurements of indoor allergen levels have become possible with the introduction of monoclonal antibody-based assays (14,15). Epidemiological studies have demonstrated that exposure to dust mite, cat, dog, and cockroach allergens are all relevant to asthma, the allergen of greatest importance depending on geographic location and socioeconomic level (16–19). Dust mite exposure and sensitization is common throughout the world and has been extensively studied, providing the best model for allergen avoidance in the treatment of asthma (20,21). Assessment of indoor allergen exposure has provided evidence for allergen levels associated with sensitization which may be used as goals for adequate allergen reduction as well as to provide the means to work out effective protocols for allergen reduction (22).

Allergen avoidance as a means of therapy for asthma was first proposed in 1929 by Storm van Leeuwen and more recently has been supported by studies on patients living in an allergen-free environment in England and the United States (23,24). These patients avoided allergen exposure by using a hospital room with filtered air as their bedroom and living room. The asthmatics in the allergen-free hospital environment showed reduced medication requirements, increased peak flow, and reduced bronchial reactivity as well as improvement in symptoms. This demonstrable improvement in well-being raised the awareness of allergen avoidance as a possible beneficial technique for the treatment of patients with moderately severe asthma. Subsequently, protocols for dust mite allergen reduction were devised that significantly lowered dust mite levels in homes (25,26,27). When these techniques were applied to the homes of dust mite allergic asthmatics, significant improvement in their symptoms ensued (28–31). In 1993, Ehnert et al. showed in a controlled trial that a dust mite avoidance protocol produced progressive decreases in allergen levels and bronchial hyperactivity which could be maintained for at least 1 year (29). The standard dust mite avoidance protocol concentrates on the patient's bedroom. Key elements in that protocol included covering the mattress, box spring, and pillows with impermeable encasings to seal in preexisting dust mite allergen or to prevent access of mites; washing the bed linens and blankets with hot water on a weekly and monthly basis, respectively, to kill dust mites in the bedding; and removing any other allergen-containing reservoirs from the patient's bedroom. Rugs and especially wall-to-wall carpets act as reservoirs which contain high levels of many allergens such as dust mite, cat, and cockroach per unit area, so the total allergen level in a home can be enormous (32,33). Removing a large source of allergen exposure like wall-to-wall carpet decreases the allergen load significantly yet is sometimes difficult for practical reasons. Removing other sources of dust mite allergen, such as upholstered furniture, stuffed animals, and down comforters, can also help to reduce the allergen levels (24,27,34,35).

None of the published studies on allergen avoidance have addressed the problem of severe asthma, and there is a general prejudice that allergen exposure is not directly relevant to the most severe cases. However, the highest incidence of fatal asthma occurs in areas and among age groups where many or most cases are extrinsic. Furthermore, in some fatal cases inhalant sensitization and exposure to relevant allergens had been demonstrated prior to death (36). In a recent study, steroid-dependent asthmatics were entered into a prospective study of an in-hospital allergen avoidance protocol for steroid dose tapering (36). The patients enrolled in the study were either on chronic steroid doses or on repeated tapering doses. Patients were admitted to an allergen-free research center and after several days steroid doses were tapered, without changes in other antiasthma medications. Peak flow responses and steroid doses were monitored. The results of the study showed that patients fell into two different categories in response to steroid dose tapering. Some of the patients with inhalant allergen sensitization were able to significantly reduce their steroid requirements, while maintaining or even improving their peak flow rates while in the unit. Another group of asthmatics was not able to tolerate steroid dose reductions without exacerbations of their asthma while in the allergen-free environment. The results suggested that even in severe steroid-dependent asthma, allergen avoidance could be beneficial in some cases, allowing reduced steroid requirement. Therefore, it is important to identify inhalant sensitization and to recommend specific avoidance protocols in severe as well as mild asthma.

B. Other Inhalant Allergens: Cat and Cockroach

Cat allergen is a potent stimulus for rapid reactions in the lungs, which may reflect its transport as small-sized particles, 2.0–5 μm, either because this allows deeper penetration into the lung or because it helps the allergen remain airborne for hours (37,38). Cat allergen avoidance is more difficult than mite avoidance due to the large quantities of allergen produced and to the aerodynamic nature of the allergen (35,37). Cat allergen has been found in houses without cats (15,16,39) and has been found in dust of schools in Sweden and in Atlanta, Georgia (40). Cat allergen is known to stick on the clothing of individuals handling cats and is thus transported to distant sites. Removal of cats from a patient's home without specific measures to remove residual allergen results in a slow reduction in allergen levels over a period of months (41). Washing cats on a weekly basis can decrease allergen levels; however, it appears that washing cats and removing the preexisting allergen are both necessary for there to be a clinically significant drop in allergen exposure (38). Furthermore, there is some debate as to the level of cat allergen reduction obtainable by washing the cat (42). Several recent studies have reported that children exposed to a cat at home have a decreased risk of asthma and sensitization to cat; suggesting that high exposure to cat allergen can induce a form of tolerance (22). However, in all these studies children who are sensitized to cat allergen are at increased risk of asthma. In addition some studies report sensitization to cat allergens is a risk factor for severe asthma (43).

There is evidence that sensitization to cockroach allergen is an important risk factor for asthma among children living in the large American cities (36,44). Further studies in Chicago and Baltimore have established that skin test reactivity to cockroach allergens is a risk factor for severity of asthma among African-American children (45,46).

Although controlled avoidance studies have not been performed with cat, dog, cockroach, or any indoor allergen other than dust mites, it seems reasonable to extend the principle of allergen avoidance in management of difficult cases. Certainly, some of the patients who responded to in-hospital care were cat- or cockroach-allergic.

C. Occupational Exposure

In most cases, occupational asthma does not reach the stage of steroid dependence and the primary treatment, i.e., avoidance of continued exposure in the work place, is generally successful. Clear examples of occupational asthma that are induced by inhaled antigen and are preventable by avoidance include the dust of red cedar in lumber mills, rat urinary allergen in animal houses, and "baker's asthma" from proteins in the flour or enzymes used in the baking process. The symptoms initially occur at work shortly after exposure and resolve when the person leaves the job site. With chronic exposure, however, symptoms begin to occur continuously and simply removing the exposure may produce only partial symptom remission. The implication is that continued exposure can lead to irreversible or partially irreversible changes, including bronchial hyperreactivity. The important point is that occupational asthma should be treated early with avoidance. By extension, it may be that similar "irreversible" elements develop in many cases of asthma which are induced by exposure to allergens in the indoor environment. It is also obvious that occupational exposure should be considered in all cases of allergic asthma that do not improve with conventional treatment.

Many patients with severe asthma report marked sensitivity to perfumes, chemicals, and passive smoke. While it seems unlikely that exposure to these irritants at work is actually a primary cause of the patient's asthma, they can become a dominant feature. Typical examples are passive smoke in a bowling alley, glutaraldehyde fumes in a dentist's office, and wood preservative in a furniture factory. The important principle is that many exposures which are relatively rare as a primary cause of occupational asthma can be extremely irritating to patients with severe asthma. Indeed, it is possible that irritants of this kind can increase the severity of symptoms sufficiently to push patients into steroid dependence. These problems can be very difficult to manage clinically. Ideally, sensitivity to chemicals would be established either by measuring serological responses or by provocation tests. In practice there are only a very few chemicals to which antibodies can be measured (e.g., TMA or isocyanates) and only a few centers have facilities suitable for carrying out provocation tests. Thus, in most cases the practitioner must rely on clinical history alone to make a recommendation about avoidance.

D. *Alternaria* and Other Outdoor Allergens

Although we now spend only 10% or less of our lives outside, inhaled allergens on pollen grains or fungal spores can still cause severe symptoms of hay fever and asthma (47,48). Seasonal asthma can be severe enough to require hospital admission, but in our experience it is unusual that chronic severe asthma can be attributed primarily to outdoor inhaled allergens. However, *Alternaria* appears to present an exception to the rule. Seasonal differences in asthma mortality and hospital admission rates, with high levels of asthma in autumn, have been described in several countries. A population-based study in Europe provides evidence that sensitization to *Alternaria alternata* is associated with severe asthma and life-threatening exacerbations (49). A major study from the upper Midwest reported that asthma patients with a positive skin test to *Alternaria* were at increased risk of severe and fatal attacks during the *Alternaria* "season" (50). We have identified severe asthmatics with sensitivity to *Alternaria* who appear to have perennial symptoms. At present, there is no evidence that these patients do better on immunotherapy; however, they should take all steps to decrease exposure to mold both growing within the house and coming in from outside.

III. Fungal Colonization and Sensitization as a Complication of (or Cause of) Severe Asthma

A. Dermatophytes of the Genus *Trichophyton*

Allergic and immunologic reactions to fungal proteins are well established and include immediate and delayed hypersensitivity responses (51,52); however, the protein constituents of fungi are poorly defined and are thought to vary depending on the conditions of growth and stage in the life cycle. Some proteins have been isolated from fungal extracts (Alt a 1) and these same proteins have been shown to elicit IgE antibodies and T-cell responses (51,53,54). It is known that foot infections with dermatophytes can cause acute urticaria and that in some cases eradication of the fungus will be followed by resolution of the urticaria (55). Subsequently, work by Ward et al. suggested that dermatophyte infection plays a role in a group of intrinsic, severe, steroid-dependent asthmatics (56). These predominantly male asthmatics had chronic fungal infection of their skin and nails and had unequivocal immediate skin test responses to proteins derived from *Trichophyton* (56,57,58). Some of these men, who would previously have been categorized as "intrinsic" (or idiopathic) asthmatics, had serum IgE antibodies to *Trichophyton*; they also responded to bronchial and nasal provocation with *Trichophyton*. In a controlled trial, long-term (≥ 1 year) oral antifungal therapy with fluconazole has been associated with improvement in breathing parameters (57). These studies are more interesting because the antifungal medications such as fluconazole and itraconazole have been used on a long-term basis without the severe side effects of ketoconazole or amphotericin B, which have previously prevented serious investigations of antifungal treatment. The safety profile of the new azoles is important, since dermatophyte colonization and asthma tend to reoccur after stopping treatment and may require prolonged therapy. The prevalence of dermatophyte-related asthma is not clear, but may represent as many as 20% of *intrinsic* male asthmatics in a tertiary referral clinic. This condition is also important because it strongly suggests that colonization with other organisms should be evaluated as possible treatable causes of severe asthma.

B. *Aspergillus fumigatus* as a Cause of Severe Asthma

A well-recognized form of severe asthma that is associated with fungal sensitization and colonization is allergic bronchopulmonary aspergillosis (ABPA). Fungal colonization of the airways leads to an immune response involving both IgG and IgE antibodies against proteins derived from *Aspergillus fumigatus*. Until recently, suppressing the inflammatory response with corticosteroids was the only well-recognized method of treatment and methods of titrating steroid dose against symptoms and total serum IgE are well established (6). Following case reports of treatment of ABPA with itraconazole, a recent controlled trial established that itraconazole can be helpful in the management of ABPA. (59). It has also been suggested that antifungals should be used in the treatment of *Aspergillus* colonization in patients with cystic fibrosis. Colonization is extremely common in CF, but only a minority of the patients are allergic to *A. fumigatus*. Thus, it has been suggested that specific antifungal therapy should be considered for both allergic and nonallergic CF patients who are colonized.

There are suggestions that immunological responses to other fungi could also contribute to disease. Allergic bronchopulmonary responses to several different fungi (e.g., *Curvularia* and *Candida*) have been reported in occasional cases. *Pitirosporium ovale* and *Candida albicans* are other colonizing fungi that have been shown to generate an IgE response (60). Asthma patients on chronic steroid therapy commonly have oropharyngeal, esophageal, and vaginal candidiasis; in some of these cases asthma has improved with prolonged antifungal treatment.

We need to ask whether, in addition to the well-recognized adverse consequences of steroid use, steroids might actually contribute to deterioration of asthma by inhibiting clearance of antigenic yeast and fungi.

IV. Sinusitis

In reported series of severe asthma, the prevalence of chronic sinusitis has been as high as 50% (61,62). This pairing of asthma and sinusitis could result if both conditions were different end-organ manifestations of one disease or if one condition led to the other. The improvement in asthma with the clearing of sinus disease by medical or surgical means suggests the latter possibility. There have been several, not necessarily exclusive, explanations of how sinusitis might exacerbate asthma. There is evidence for reflex bronchoconstriction after exposure of the nasopharynx to a variety of noxious stimuli. Studies using isotope tracers have cast doubt on the theory that infected or inflammatory secretions from the sinuses drain into the lung to cause worsening of asthma. A study by Newman et al. looked at patients with chronic sinusitis presenting for functional endoscopic sinus surgery (FESS) and found a strong relationship between the extent of the sinus disease on CT scan and wheezing and peripheral eosinophilia (63,64,65). The results suggested that the sinus inflammation was the source of the eosinophilia, and it is plausible to think that the activated eosinophils contribute to increasing the inflammatory process in the lung. However, the reasons for the eosinophilia remain unclear, and in this study it was not clearly related to atopy, as there was only a weak association with IgE antibodies and most patients had total IgE levels within the accepted normal range.

It has also been shown that nasal polyps and biopsies from sinus tissues have high levels of mediators and cellular infiltrate (66,67,68). This suggests that shared immune responses, which induce T cells and eosinophils, could represent the link between asthma and sinusitis. The specificity of the T-cell responses is unknown, but the colonizing bacteria are a possible source of antigen. Bacterial cultures taken from the sinuses at the time of surgery revealed over 90% prevalence of Gram-positive aerobes (63). No correlation between bacterial culture type and eosinophilia has been reported. At present it is not clear whether the aerobic bacteria cultured from the sinus tissue contribute to the inflammation. Certainly, it is not clear that attempts to eradicate these bacteria have long-term therapeutic effects. The question is important because optimal treatment of sinusitis has not been established. While studies have reported that improvement in sinus symptoms medically or surgically can result in improvement of asthma, the general experience is that in patients with severe asthma, relapse of sinusitis after treatment is common. Prolonged courses (i.e., 6 weeks to 3 months) of broad-spectrum antibiotics, decongestants, and steroids may lead to remission of sinus symptoms but not cure. Despite some good results, at present it is not clear what role FESS plays in the management of asthma.

V. Immunotherapy

Immunotherapy has been shown to be effective in the management of anaphylactic reactions to venom and in seasonal allergic rhinitis. Several controlled studies have also reported benefits in seasonal asthma. Immunotherapy for perennial asthma has resulted in symptomatic improvement in several studies; however, there are other investigators who have not found it to be useful (69,70). Immunotherapy for severe asthma is difficult for several reasons, but the main problem is that by definition the airways are very reactive. In order to derive the maximum benefit from immunotherapy, the highest tolerable dose should be used; however, in patients with asthma, the higher the dose, the more likely they are to have a severe reaction, including bronchoconstriction (71,72). A severe asthmatic may never be well enough to build up to an effective dose. In parallel, the risk of serious adverse reactions increases as FEV_1 decreases. Thus, Bousquet et al. concluded that immunotherapy should not be used for patients with FEV_1 <70% predicted (71). A review of deaths from immunotherapy strongly suggested that asthmatics with unstable asthma (e.g., requiring repeated courses of oral steroids or having made a recent emergency room visit) at the time of injection of allergen had the greatest risk (72). Oral immunotherapy in dust mite-sensitive asthmatics has been tried unsuccessfully in an attempt to reduce the reactions associated with conventional immunotherapy. Some investigators have successfully used rush immunotherapy protocols to build up the dose to a maintenance level while the patient is not wheezing, but this is primarily relevant to that minority of patients with seasonal asthma. Thus, although immunotherapy may be an option for a minority of cases of asthma; it is rarely useful in severe perennial asthma—it should be used with caution and only by experienced practitioners.

Assuming that the main risk of conventional immunotherapy is from interaction of allergen with IgE antibody on mast cells, it has been proposed that peptides that react with T cells might have a suppressive effect with less risk of severe reactions. Current studies are underway using T-cell reactive peptides derived from the cat allergen Fel d 1 and with peptides of mite allergen Der p 1 (73,74). However, no studies on severe asthmatics have been reported. Future therapies may also include recombinant humanized monoclonal anti-IgE antibody, which has potential as a treatment for subjects with moderate or severe allergic asthma (75). The interesting question is whether treatment with anti-IgE would make immunotherapy with conventional or modified antigens safer.

VI. Diet

There is considerable skepticism about the usefulness of allergy testing in the diagnosis of food sensitivity in patients with asthma. Certainly the positive predictive value of skin testing and RAST testing has not been convincingly demonstrated in relation to asthma. However, there are occasional cases of severe asthma where exclusion diets are helpful; a few cases have been demonstrated using double-blind placebo-controlled food challenges (76). One approach is to ask specific questions about food-related symptoms of all patients and to skin test a minority. If there is no evidence for other factors such as inhalants or fungal colonization, a 6-week trial of a modified exclusion diet is an option. The results are sufficiently gratifying in the few cases reported to make it worth a trial in severe cases who are not responding to other treatment.

VII. Conclusion

Asthma continues to be a major cause of mortality and morbidity throughout the world. Current treatment regimens, which include steroids and steroid sparing agents, contribute to the morbidity without always curing or controlling the disease process. Investigations of severe and fatal asthma have demonstrated that a proportion of these cases are sensitized and exposed to common inhalant allergens at home. This implies strongly that simple allergen avoidance measures should be considered for even the most severe cases. On the other hand, it is clear that many severe asthmatics are not allergic to common inhalant allergens and these cases generally do not improve in an allergen-free environment or with allergen avoidance at home. It is among these cases that colonization or infections with dermatophytes, yeasts, or *Aspergillus* have been demonstrated. Recent evidence suggests that some of these patients improve (with reduced steroid requirements) when treated with chronic antifungal therapy. In view of the low levels of toxicity of the newer antifungals relative to steroids this approach clearly needs to be considered. Allergen-specific therapy for asthma has increasingly focused on techniques for reducing exposure to foreign antigens, with allergen immunotherapy playing a smaller role. These methods are allergen-specific and thus are dependent on identifying the sensitivity (or sensitivities) of each patient. The overall conclusion is that the role of foreign antigens, either inhaled or "intrinsic," should be evaluated in all severe asthmatics.

Acknowledgments

The work presented in this chapter is supported by NIH Grants AI-20565 and AI-30840.

References

1. Hargreave FE, Ramsdale EH, Kirby JG, O'Byrne PM. Asthma and the role of inflammation. Eur J Respir Dis 1986; 147:16–21.
2. Liu MC, Hubbard WC, Proud D, Stealey BA, Galli SJ, Kagey-Sobotka A, Bleecker ER, Lichtenstein LM. Immediate and late inflammatory responses to ragweed antigen challenge of the peripheral airways in allergic asthmatics. Am Rev Resp Dis 1991; 144:51–58.
3. Glezen WP. Reactive airway disorders in children: role of respiratory virus infections. Clin Chest Med 1984; 5:635–643.
4. Frick WE, Busse WW. Respiratory infections: their role in airway responsiveness and pathogenesis of asthma. Clin Chest Med 1988; 9:539–549.
5. Selzer J, Bigby BG, Stulbarg M, et al. O_3-induced changes in bronchial reactivity to methacholine and airway inflammation in humans. J Appl Physiol 1986; 60:1321–1326.
6. Patterson R, Greenberger PA, Lee TM, Liotta JL, O'Neil EA, Roberts M, Sommers H. Prolonged evaluation of patients with corticosteroid-dependent asthma stage of allergic bronchopulmonary aspergillosis. J Allergy Clin Immunol 1987; 80:663–668.
7. Rakes GP, Arruda E, Ingram JM, Hoover GE, Zambrano JC, Hayden FG, Platts-Mills TA, Heymann PW. Rhinovirus and respiratory syncytial virus in wheezing children requiring emergency care: IgE and eosinophil analyses. Am J Res Crit Care Med 1999; 159:785–790.
8. Nelson Textbook of Pediatrics. 16th ed. Philadelphia: W. B. Saunders, 2000:679.
9. Lang, DM. Trends in US asthma mortality: good news and bad news. Ann Allergy Asthma Immunol 1997; 78:333–337.
10. Sporik RB, Chapman MD, Platts-Mills TAE. House dust mite exposure as a cause of asthma (editorial). Clin Exp Allergy 1992; 22:897–906.
11. Gleich GJ, Adolphson CR. The eosinophilic leucocyte structure and function. Adv Immunol 1986; 39:177–253.
12. Wegner CD, Torcellini CA, Clarke CC, Letts G, Gundel RH. Effects of single and multiple inhalations of antigen on airway responsiveness in monkeys. J Allergy Clin Immunol 1991; 87:835–841.
13. Tunnicliffe WS, Fletcher TJ, Hammond K, Roberts K, Custovic A, Simpson A, Woodcock A, Aytes JG. Sensitivity and exposure to indoor allergens in adults with differing asthma severity. Eur Res J 1999; 13(3):654–659.
14. Chapman MD, Heymann PW, Wilkins SR, Brown MJ, Platts-Mills TAE. Monoclonal immunoassays for the major dust mite (Dermatophagoides) allergens, Der p I and Der f I, and quantitative analysis of the allergen content of mite and house dust extracts. J Allergy Clin Immunol 1987; 80:184–194.
15. Pollart S, Smith TF, Morris EC, Gelber LE, Platts-Mills TAE, Chapman MD. Environmental exposure to cockroach allergens. Analysis with monoclonal antibody-based enzyme immunoassays. J Allergy Clin Immunol 1991; 87:505–510.
16. Call RS, Smith TF, Morris E, Chapman MD, Platts-Mills TAE. Risk factors for asthma in inner city children. J Pediatr 1992; 121:862–866.

17. Gelber LE, Seltzer LH, Bouzoukis JK, Pollart SM, Chapman MD, Platts-Mills TAE. Sensitization and exposure to indoor allergens as risk factors for asthma among patients presenting to hospital. Am Rev Resp Dis 1993; 147:573–578.

18. Custovic A, Simpson A, Woodcock A. Importance of indoor allergens in the induction of allergy and elicitation of allergic disease. Allergy 1998; 53(suppl 48):115–120.

19. Sporik R, Squillace SP, Ingram JM, Rakes GP, Honsinger RW, Platts-Mills TAE. Mite, cat, and cockroach exposure, allergen sensitization, and asthma in children: a case-control study of three schools. Thorax 1999; 54:675–680.

20. Shapiro GG, Wighton TG, Chinn T, Zuchrman J, Eliassen AH, Picciano JF, Platts-Mills TA. House dust mite avoidance for children with asthma in homes of low-income families. J Allergy Clin Immunol 1999; 103(6):1069–1074.

21. Carter M, Perzanowski M, Raymond A, Platts-Mills T. Allergen avoidance for asthmatic children in Atlanta (abstr). J Allergy Clin Immunol 1998; 101(1/2):S5.

22. Platts-Mills T, Vaughan J, Squillace S, Sporik R. Sensitisation, asthma, and modified Th2 response in children exposed to cat allergen: a population-based cross-sectional study. Lancet 2001; 357:752–756.

23. Platts-Mills TAE, Tovey ER, Mitchell EB, Moszoro H, Nock P, Wilkins SR. Reduction of bronchial hyperreactivity during prolonged allergen avoidance. Lancet 1982; 2:675–678.

24. Hayden ML, Perzanowki M, Matheson L, Scott P, Call RS, Platts-Mills TA. Dust mite allergen avoidance in the treatment of hospitalized children with asthma. Ann Allergy Asthma Immunol 1997; 79(5):437–442.

25. Luczynska CM, Arruda LK, Platts-Mills TAE, Miller JD, Lopez M, Chapman MD. A two-site monoclonal antibody ELISA for the quantification of the major dermatophagoides spp. allergens, Der p I and Der f I. J Immunol Methods 1989; 118:227–235.

26. Pauli G, Dietemann A, Ott M, Hoyet C, Bessot JC. Levels of mite allergens and guanine after use of an acaricidal preparation or cleaning solution in highly infested mattresses and dwellings (abstr). J Allergy Clin Immunol 1991; 887:321.

27. Platts-Mills TAE, Vervloet D, Thomas WR, Aalberse RC, Chapman MD. Indoor allergens and asthma: report of the Third International Workshop. J Allergy Clin Immunol 1997; 100(6/1):S2–24.

28. Dorward AJ, Colloff MJ, Mackay NS, McSharry C, Thomson NC. Effect of house dust mite avoidance measures on adult atopic asthma. Thorax 1988; 43:98–102.

29. Ehnert B, Lau S, Weber A, Buettner P, Schou C, Wahn U. Reducing domestic exposure to dust mite allergen reduces bronchial hyperactivity in sensitive children with asthma. J Allergy Clin Immunol 1992; 90:135–138.

30. Murray AB, Ferguson AC. Dust-free bedrooms in the treatment of asthmatic children with house dust or hose dust mite allergy: a controlled trial. Pediatrics 1983; 71:418–422.

31. Walshaw MJ, Evans CC. Allergen avoidance in house dust mite sensitive adult asthma. Q J Med 1986; 58:199–215.

32. Wood RA, Eggleston PA, Lind P, Ingemann L, Schwartz B, Graveson S, Terry D, Wheeler B, Adkinson NF, Jr. Antigenic analysis of household dust samples. Am Rev Resp Dis 1988; 137:358–363.

33. Platts-Mills TAE, Hayden ML, Chapman MD, Wilkins SR. Seasonal variation in dust mite and grass-pollen allergens in dust from the house of patients with asthma. J Allergy Clin Immunol 1987; 79:781–791.
34. Platts-Mills TAE, Chapman MD. Dust mites: immunology, allergic disease, and environmental control (rev). J Allergy Clin Immunol 1987; 80:755–775.
35. Wood RA, Mudd KE, Eggleston PA. The distribution of cat and dust mite allergens on wall surfaces. J Allergy Clin Immunol 1992; 89:126–130.
36. Call RS, Ward GW, Jackson S, Platts-Mills TAE. Investigating severe and fatal asthma. J Allergy Clin Immunol 1994; 94:1065–1072.
37. Luczynska CM, Li Y, Chapman MD, Platts-Mills TAE. Airborne concentrations and particle size distribution of allergen derived from domestic cats (Felis domesticus). Am Med Rev Respir Dis 1990; 141:361–367.
38. De Blay F, Chapman MD, Platts-Mills TAE. Airborne cat allergen (Fel d I). Am Rev Respir Dis 1991; 143:1334–1339.
39. Sporik R, Ingram JM, Price W, Sussman JH, Honsinger RW, Platts-Mills TAE. Association of asthma with serum IgE and skin-test reactivity to allergens among children living at high altitude. Tickling the dragon's breath. Am J Res Crit Care Med 1995; 151:1388–1392.
40. Munir AKM, Einarsson R, Schou C, Dreborg SKG. Allergens in school dust. J Allergy Clin Immunol 1993; 91:1067–1074.
41. Wood RA, Chapman MD, Adkinson NF, Jr., Eggleston PA. The effect of cat removal on allergen content in household-dust samples. J Allergy Clin Immunol 1989; 83:730–734.
42. Klucka CV, Ownby DR, Green J, Zoratti EM. Cat shedding of Fel d I is not reduced by washings, Allerpet-C spray, or acepromazine. J Allergy Clin Immunol 1995; 95(6):1164–1171.
43. Sarpong SB, Karrison T. Skin test reactivity to indoor allergens as a marker of asthma severity in children with asthma. Ann Allergy Asthma Immunol 1998; 80:303–308.
44. Rosenstreich DL, Eggleston P, Kattan M, Baker D, Slavin RG, Gergen P, Mitchell H, McNiff-Mortimer, K, Lynn H, Ownby D, Malveaux F. The role of cockroach allergy and exposure to cockroach allergen in causing morbidity among inner-city children with asthma. N Engl J Med 1997; 336:1356–1363.
45. Sarpong SB, Hamilton RG, Eggleston PA, Adkinson NF Jr. Socioeconomic status and race as risk factors for cockroach allergen exposure and sensitization in children with asthma. J Allergy Clin Immunol 1996; 97:1393–3401.
46. Togias A, Horowitz E, Joyner D, Guyson K, Malveaux F. Evaluating the factors that relate to asthma severity in adolescents. Int Arch Allergy Immunol 1997; 113:87–95.
47. Pollart SM, Chapman MD, Fiocco GP, Rose G, Platts-Mills TA. Epidemiology of acute asthma: IgE antibodies to common inhalant allergens as a risk factor for emergency room visits. J Allergy Clin Immunol 1989; 83:875–882.
48. Halonen M, Stern DA, Wright AL, Taussig LM, Martinez FD. Alternaria as a major allergen for asthma in children raised in a desert environment. Am J Res Crit Care Med 1997; 155:1356–1361.
49. Neurkirch C, Henry C, Leynaert B, Liard R, Bousquet J, Neukirch F. Is sensitization

to Alternaria alternata a risk factor for severe asthma? A population-based study. J Allergy Clin Immunol 1999; 103:709–711.

50. O'Hallaren MT, Yunginger J, Offord KP, Somers MJ, O'Connell EJ, Ballard DJ, Sachs MI. Exposure to an aeroallergen as a possible precipitating factor in respiratory arrest in young patients with asthma. N Engl J Med 1991; 324:359–363.

51. Deuell BL, Arruda LK, Hayden ML, Chapman MD, Platts-Mills TAE. Trichophyton tonsurans allergen I (Tri t I): characterization of a protein that causes immediate but not delayed hypersensitivity. J Immunol 1991; 147:96–101.

52. Lehrer SR, Lopez M, Butcher BT, Olson J, Reed M, Salvaggio JE. Basidiomycete mycelia and spore-allergen extracts: skin test reactivity in adults with symptoms of respiratory allergy. J Allergy Clin Immunol 1986; 78:478–485.

53. Slunt JB, Taketomi EA, Woodfolk JA, Hayden ML, Platts-Mills TAE. The immune response to Trichophyton tonsurans: distinct t-cell cytokine profiles to a single protein among subjects with immediate and delayed hypersensitivity. J Immunol 1996; 157:5192–5197.

54. Woodfolk JA, Sung SJ, Benjamin DC, Lee JK, Platts-Mills TAE. Distinct human T cell repertoires mediate immediate and delayed type hypersensitivity to Trichophyton antigen, Tri r 2. J Immunol 2000; 165:4379–4387.

55. Weary PE, Guerrant JL. Chronic urticaria in association with dermatophytosis: response to the administration of griseofulvin. Arch Derm 1967; 95:400–401.

56. Ward GW Jr., Karlsson G, Rose G, Platts-Mills TAE. Trichophyton asthma: sensitization of bronchi and upper airways to dermatophyte antigen. Lancet 1989; 1:859–862.

57. Ward GW Jr., Woodfolk JA, Hayden ML, Jackson S, Platts-Mills TA. Treatment of late-onset asthma with fluconazole. J Allergy Clin Immunol 1999; 104:541–546.

58. Platts-Mills TAE, Fiocco GP, Hayden ML, Guerrant JL, Pollart SM, Wilkins SR. Serum IgE antibodies to Trichophyton in patients with urticaria, angioedema, asthma, and rhinitis: development of a radioallergosorbent test. J Allergy Clin Immunol 1987; 79:40–45.

59. Denning DW, Van Wye JE, Lewiston NJ, Stevens DA. Adjunctive therapy of allergic bronchopulmonary Aspergillosis with Itraconazole. Chest 1991; 100:813–819.

60. Jensen-Jarolim E, Poulsen LK, With H, Kieffer M, Ottevanger V, Stahl Skov P. Atopic dermatitis of the face, scalp and neck: Type I reaction to the yeast P. ovale. J Allergy Clin Immunol 1992; 89:44–51.

61. Mings R, Friedman WH, Linford P, Slavin RG. Five year follow-up of the effects of bilateral intranasal sphenoethmoidectomy in patients with sinusitis and asthma. Am J Rhinol 1988; 71:123–132.

62. Rachelefsky GS, Katz RM, Siegel SC. Chronic sinus disease with associated reactive airway disease in children. Pediatrics 1984; 73:526–529.

63. Newman LJ, Platts-Mills TAE, Phillips CD, Hazen KC, Gross CW. Chronic sinusitis: relationship of computed tomographic findings to allergy, asthma and eosinophilia. J Am Med Assoc 1994; 271:363–367.

64. Crater SE, Peters EJ, Phillips CD, Platts-Mills TA. Prospective analysis of CT of the sinuses in acute asthma. Am J Roentgenol 1999; 173:127–131.

65. Hoover GE, Newman LJ, Platts-Mills TA, Phillips CD, Gross CW, Wheatley LM.

Chronic sinusitis: risk factors for extensive disease. J Allergy Clin Immunol 1997; 100:185–191.

66. Hamilios DL, Leung DYM, Wood R, Meyers A, Stephens JK, Barkans J, Meng Q, Cunningham L, Bean DK, Kay AB. Chronic hyperplastic sinusitis. J Allergy Clin Immunol 1993; 92:39–48.

67. Keith PK, Conway M, Evans S, Wong DA, Jordana G, Pengelly D, Dolovich J. Nasal polyps: effects of seasonal allergen exposure. J Allergy Clin Immunol 1994; 93:567–574.

68. Borish L, Arango P, Steinke JW, Baramki DF, Kountakis SE. Cytokine production in nasal polyposis tissue (abstr). J Allergy Clin Immunol 2001; 107:S168.

69. Bousquet J, Michel FB. Specific immunotherapy in asthma. J Allergy Clin Immunol 1994; 94:1–11.

70. Creticos PS. The consideration for immunotherapy in the treatment of allergic asthma. J Allergy Clin Immunol 2000; 105(2/2):S559–S574.

71. Bousquet J, Lockey R, Malling HJ, Alvarez-Cuestra E, Canonica GW, Chapman MD, Creticos PJ, Dayer JM, Durham SR, Semoly P, Goldstein RJ, Ishikawa T, Ito K, Kraft D, Lambert PH, Lowenstein H, Muller U, Norman PS, Reisman RE, Valenta R, Valovirta E, Yssel H. Allergen immunotherapy: therapeutic vaccines for allergic diseases. Ann Allergy Asthma Immunol 1998; 81(5/1):401–405.

72. Reid MJ, Lockey RF, Turkeltaub PC, Platts-Mills TAE. Surveys of fatalities from skin testing and immunotherapy 1985–90. J Allergy Clin Immunol 1993; 92:6–15.

73. Haselden BM, Kay AB, Larche M. Immunoglobulin E-independent major histocompatibility complex-restricted T cell peptide epitope-induced late asthmatic reactions. J Exp Med 1999; 189:1885–1894.

74. Norman PS. Immunotherapy: past and present. J Allergy Clin Immunol 1998; 102: 1–10.

75. Milgrom H, Fich RB Jr., Su JQ, Reimann JD, Bush RK, Watrous ML, Metzger WJ. Treatment of allergic asthma with monoclonal anti-IgE antibody. N Engl J Med 1999; 341:1966–1973.

76. James JM, Eigenmann PA, Eggleston PA, Sampson HA. Airway reactivity changes in asthmatic patients undergoing blinded food challenges. Am J Res Crit Care Med 1996; 153:597–603.

16

Aspirin, Nonsteroidal Anti-Inflammatory Drugs, and Preservatives as Causes for Severe Asthma

DONALD D. STEVENSON

Scripps Clinic
Scripps Research Institute
La Jolla, California

I. Introduction

A subset of asthmatic patients experience adverse respiratory reactions to aspirin (ASA) and nonsteroidal anti-inflammatory drugs (NSAIDs), including nasal and ocular mucosal swelling and bronchospasm. Such asthmatic patients have been classified as ASA sensitive (1), ASA intolerant (2), ASA idiosyncratic (3), or ASA-induced asthma (AIA) (4). All four descriptors refer to the same population of asthmatics. This chapter focuses on the clinical features of ASA respiratory disease; methods for diagnosis of ASA sensitivity; prevalence of ASA sensitive asthma; cross-reactions with NSAIDs; lack of cross-reactions with cyclooxygenase-2- (COX-2) inhibiting NSAIDs, as well as with other drugs and chemicals; the phenomenon of ASA desensitization; and treatment. Comments regarding the severity of asthma in ASA-sensitive asthmatics are focused in two areas: (1) respiratory reactions, which are sometimes life threatening and occur after ingesting ASA and NSAIDs; and (2) aspirin respiratory disease, particularly the relationship between active sinusitis and stimulation of asthma.

II. Concept and Clinical Features of Aspirin-Sensitive Respiratory Disease

Sensitivity to ASA and other NSAIDs occurs in patients with chronic rhinitis, sinusitis, nasal polyps, and asthma and continues in the absence of exposure to ASA/NSAIDs. Figure 1 outlines the usual clinical course of patients afflicted with this disorder. Onset is usually between 20 and 40 years of age. After having been in good health, undergoing uncomplicated upper respiratory tract infections (URIs) in the past, and having previously taken ASA without ill effects, the patient characteristically develops a respiratory virus infection. However, unlike past episodes of URIs, nasal and sinus symptoms persist and worsen and eventually the disease evolves into a chronic eosinophilic rhinosinusitis, usually with nasal polyps and secondary purulent pansinusitis (5). Either at the beginning of the inflammatory disease or later in the course, ingestion of ASA, or first-time exposure to any of the NSAIDs which inhibit cyclooxygenase-1 (COX-1), produces an episode of rapid-onset, intense rhinorrhea and asthma. Until an ASA-or NSAID-induced respiratory reactions occurs, one cannot establish this diagnosis, even though the clinical picture of the disease may appear to be identical to other ASA-sensitive asthmatic patients. Anosmia occurs with regularity in

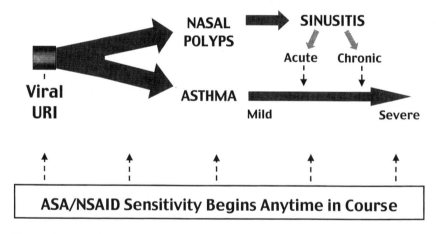

Figure 1   Natural history of aspirin respiratory disease. Patients acquire this disease in their adult life, frequently after a viral respiratory illness. Respiratory tract inflammation accelerates in severity over the years, with aggressive nasal polyp formation occluding sinus ostea and contributing to acute and then chronic sinusitis. Asthma exacerbations and then persistent severe asthma follow the course of sinusitis. Aspirin- or NSAID-induced respiratory reactions can begin at any time in the course of the illness and must occur before the diagnosis can be established.

patients afflicted with ASA respiratory disease (6), but bursts of systemic corticosteroids or sinus surgery will sometimes temporarily restore sense of smell. Ninety-six percent of ASA-sensitive patients have abnormal sinus X rays or CAT scans (7). The inflammatory disease may be limited to the upper airway (8), but more commonly lower respiratory tract inflammation with bronchospasm joins the upper airway disease. This "intrinsic" type of asthma progresses and usually becomes complicated by intractable pansinusitis, which frequently requires systemic corticosteroids to maintain bronchial or nasal function. Concomitant allergic respiratory disease can coexist.

Table 1 summarizes the clinical features of patients with ASA respiratory disease. Because of the frequent use of topical or systemic corticosteroids, nasal cytograms may be devoid of eosinophils. Peripheral blood eosinophilia is also significantly suppressed if systemic corticosteroids are required. The severity of respiratory disease can be mild, sometimes with rhino-sinusitis alone and without asthma (8), or the disease may be incapacitating, with severe systemic steroid-dependent asthma. Intermittent sinus infections almost always cause exacerbation of asthma activity and it is unusual to be able to clear such episodes without the addition of antibiotics and systemic corticosteroids. The evolution from acute to

Table 1 Clinical Features of Asthmatic Patients with Aspirin Respiratory Disease

Category	Feature
Age of onset	After age 10 to age 40
Rhinitis	Chronic vasomotor congestion (>90%)
	Associated IgE mediated (20%)
Nasal symptoms	Congestion, rhinorrhea, anosmia, paranasal headaches, sleep deprivation
Nasal examination	Pale, congested membranes polypoid tissue or frank polyps
Nasal smear	Eosinophils: variable[a]
	Mast cells: variable[a]
	PMNs: many
	Bacteria variable
Sinus radiographs (CT)	Abnormal with any pattern
	Pansinusitis most common
Sinusitis	Intermittent evolving to chronic
Prior sinus surgery	Very common; usually multiple operations (average: one sinus or polyp operation every 3 years)
Asthma	Intermittent and usually in remission if sinuses not infected
	Severe, persistent, particularly when associated with chronic sinusitis

[a] Topical and systemic corticosteroids substantially decrease numbers of eosinophils and mast cells. Bursts of systemic corticosteroids or sinus operations temporarily restore sense of smell.

chronic sinusitis is a poor prognostic event, with intractable steroid-dependent asthma following the evaluation into pansinusitis (see Fig. 1). Escalating use of systemic corticosteroids, with attendant side effects, then becomes necessary for the survival of the patient and much of the morbidity in these patients can then be ascribed to side effects of systemic corticosteroids.

III. Pathogenesis

Mechanisms which account for underlying ASA respiratory disease or respiratory reactions to ASA have been partly clarified (9–11). Immune recognition of ASA and the widely different NSAIDs seems unlikely and first exposure reactions to new NSAIDs occurs routinely, virtually eliminating the possibility of prior immune sensitization. Furthermore, IgE antibodies to ASA or NSAIDs have not been unequivocally identified in ASA-sensitive asthmatic patients.

Currently available data support the hypothesis that mast cells and eosinophils, infiltrating nasal and bronchial mucosa, significantly participate in the pathogenesis of ongoing inflammation in ASA respiratory disease. Both cells synthesize products of arachidonic acid. Eosinophils release major basic protein. Mast cells release preformed granule associated mediators (histamine and tryptase). Mast cells and eosinophils have been observed within the nasal cytograms, nasal tissue biopsies, bronchial biopsies, and bronchial alveolar lavage fluid from ASA-sensitive asthmatics (12–14). Sladik et al. (13) analyzed bronchial alveolar lavage fluid from ASA-sensitive asthmatics and found increased numbers of eosinophils and eosinophil cationic protein when compared to the bronchial alveolar lavage fluid from control asthmatics. PMNs, mast cells, and macrophages were found in the lavage fluid from both aspirin-sensitive and tolerant asthmatic patients. The fact that PMNs and macrophages are not preferentially increased in ASA-sensitive nasal and bronchial tissues does not exclude their potential participation in ASA disease, since both are capable of forming arachidonic acid products. Finally, bronchial lavage fluid contained increased leukotrienes (LTs) before introduction of ASA-lysine (15). Thus overproduction of these inflammatory mediators with their attendant biologic effects (eosinophil recruitment, vasodilation, bronchospasm, and mucus secretion) is characteristic of ASA respiratory disease and occurs in the absence of ASA or NSAIDs (see Fig. 2).

The above finding is further supported by urine sampling in ASA-sensitive asthmatics. When compared to that of control asthmatics and normals, urine from ASA-sensitive asthmatics contained higher levels of baseline leukotriene E_4 (LTE_4) and thromboxane B_2 (16–18). Thus, it appears that even before addition of aspirin, ASA-sensitive asthmatic patients synthesize substantially higher quantities of both cyclooxygenase and 5-lipoxygenase (5-LO) products. Indeed, the level of baseline urine LTE_4 roughly predicts the severity of subsequent ASA-

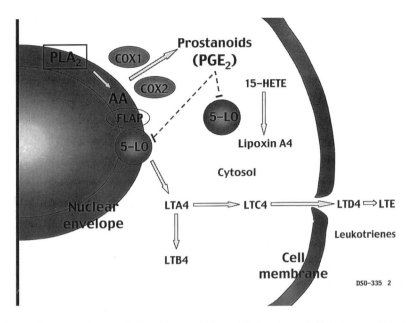

Figure 2 Excessive synthesis of prostanoids and leukotrienes (LTs) characterizes the metabolic activity of inflammatory cells, particularly mast cells and eosinophils. Prostaglandin E$_2$ (PGE$_2$) partially inhibits 5-lipoxygenase (5-LO) in the absence of exposure to ASA/NSAIDs. During ASA-induced respiratory reactions, inhibition of COX-1 reduces synthesis of PGE$_2$, which releases 5-LO, followed by rapid synthesis of LTs. Up-regulated cysLT$_1$ receptors augment the biologic effects of LTs. Simultaneously, histamine and tryptase are released from mast cells. During ASA desensitization, histamine release from mast cells stops and synthesis of phospholipase A$_2$ (PLA$_2$) declines, with subsequent reduction in LT synthesis. CysLT$_1$ receptors are down-regulated by ASA, thus diminishing the effect of LTs on target organs. High doses of ASA inhibit COX-2, the inflammatory COX enzyme, and one possible therapeutic effect of ASA may be regulation of the formation of COX-2 products. ASA distorts COX-2, altering its enzymatic activity to cease the formation of prostanoids and to generate 15-HETE instead. 5-LO converts 15-HETE to lipoxins, whose biologic activity is anti-inflammatory (inhibition of LT vasodilation and bronchoconstriction as well as inhibition of neutrophil chemotaxis, adhesion, and transmigration).

induced respiratory reactions, with the greatest bronchospastic responses occurring in those patients with the highest baseline LTE$_4$ levels (19).

Why such inflammation begins in the first place is an elusive question. Presumably there are several selective biochemical anomalies in cellular inflammatory enzymes which segregate in ASA-sensitive asthmatics. Professor Andrew Szczeklik (20) has suggested that ASA disease is a chronic or latent viral infection of the respiratory mucosa. The onset of ASA disease, following a viral URI, is compatible with this hypothesis. Professor Szczeklik has suggested that activated T lymphocytes or other cells, in the absence of negative feedback, secrete excessive quantities of cytokines and chemokines. These in turn up-regulate enzymes in the infiltrating inflammatory cells.

IV. Detection of Aspirin-Sensitive Respiratory Disease

Currently, an acceptable in vitro biochemical or immunological test for identification of ASA respiratory disease does not exist. Fortunately, reactions to the ingestion of ASA are dose dependent. Therefore, small doses of ASA (30 mg) rarely induce any respiratory symptoms, while 650 mg of ASA can cause such severe bronchospasm that hospitalization with intubation and ventilation are required to prevent death from asthma.

A. Oral ASA Challenges

The only definitive diagnostic test for identifying ASA sensitivity is ASA challenge. These challenges should be performed by trained personnel who are experienced in conducting oral ASA challenges and have rapid access to emergency resuscitative equipment in an intensive care unit. Several important observations regarding the safe and accurate performance of oral ASA challenges might be helpful. First, the more unstable or irritable the tracheobronchial tree at the time of challenge, the more likely that ASA will induce a severe bronchospastic response (21). At the start of the challenge, oral and inhaled corticosteroids, intranasal corticosteroids, theophylline, and long-acting oral bronchodilators should be continued, if they are already part of the patients ongoing treatment regimen. Following ASA ingestion, the onset of nasal and asthmatic reactions is usually between 15 min and 3 h. After a reaction is completed, there is a refractory period lasting 2–5 days, during which time the patient is tolerant to ASA or NSAIDs (22).

Table 2 summarizes our standard 3-day oral ASA challenge protocol and Table 3 summarizes the types of respiratory reactions which occur during these challenges. On the 1st day the patient ingests placebo capsules every 3 h. Spirometry, including expiratory and inspiratory flow/volume loops, are recorded every hour and forced expiratory volume in 1 sec (FEV_1) values should not change by more than 15% from baseline during the full day of placebo challenges. Some patients with laryngospasm, either before or during ASA challenges, can sometimes be identified by the flat, notched inspiratory loop seen in flow/volume curves.

Table 2 ASA Oral Challenge Protocol Used in the Scripps
Clinic General Clinical Research Center

Time	Day 1	Day 2	Day 3
7 A.M.	Placebo	30 mg	150 mg
10 A.M.	Placebo	45–60 mg	325 mg
1 P.M.	Placebo	60–100 mg	650 mg

Note. FEV_1 every hour for 3 h after each dose. Placebo day: FEV_1 baseline or first A.M. value >70% predicted; First A.M. FEV_1 value should be within 5% (up or down) from placebo; FEV_1 values should not change (i.e., <15%) during 9-h placebo challenges.

B. Inhalation Challenges with ASA-Lysine

In Europe and other parts of the world, inhalation challenges with ASA-lysine is routinely performed (23,24), but ASA-lysine has not been approved by the U.S. FDA for use in humans and, therefore, cannot be used in the United States. ASA-lysine inhalation challenges have the advantage of being performed with an increasing dose of ASA–lysine every 30 min. This allows the patient to complete the challenge within 4 h. Furthermore, the respiratory reactions are easier to control and the challenges can be performed as an outpatient.

In Europe, nasal challenges with ASA–lysine are also employed (25). Since upper airway reactions to ASA are present in over 95% of ASA-sensitive patients undergoing oral ASA challenges, the strategy of challenging nasal mucosa with ASA in solution makes good sense. The reactions are limited to the nasal passages, without obstructing essential airways, and the reaction can be observed

Table 3 Types of Respiratory Tract Signs and Symptoms Which Occur During Positive Oral ASA and NSAID Challenges

Reaction classification	Observed findings
No reaction	No symptoms and changes in FEV_1 <15%
Classic	Greater than 20% decrease in FEV_1 associated with naso-ocular reactions
Pure asthma	Greater than 20% decrease in FEV_1 values
Pure rhinitis	Naso-ocular reaction alone
Partial asthma	Decline of 15–20% in FEV_1 values combined with naso-ocular reaction
Laryngospasm	Crowing sounds in neck or upper chest; flow/volume curve: inspiratory loop flat and notched

and measured with relative ease. Specificity is 95.7% and sensitivity 86.7%, but a negative challenge result does not exclude ASA sensitivity (predictive value of a negative test result is 78.6%) (26). Unfortunately, about 20% of ASA-sensitive patients, with severe rhinosinusitis and nasal polyps, have such a profound degree of nasal obstruction that nasal inhalation of ASA-lysine is not possible and rhinometrict measurements of airflow cannot be recorded.

C. Comparing Inhalation Challenges with ASA-Lysine to Oral ASA Challenge

A study comparing the diagnostic accuracy and safety of bronchial inhalation and oral ASA challenges was conducted (27). In summary, both challenges accurately detected ASA-induced bronchospastic reactions and thus provided evidence that the patients had ASA respiratory disease. ASA inhalation challenge, because it is directed only at the bronchial tree, produced a limited and short bronchospastic reaction in almost all patients. By definition, bronchial challenge is not directed at the nasal or ocular mucosa and did not detect naso-ocular reactions. Therefore, to be confident that both upper and lower airway challenges were not reacting to ASA-lysine, ASA-lysine challenges would need to be performed twice, once by nasal inhalation and once by bronchial inhalation. Alternatively, oral challenge doses of 250 or 500 mg of ASA could be added if the highest inhaled ASA-lysine concentration of 25 mg/ml ×2, had failed to induce bronchospasm.

V. Prevalence of Aspirin-Sensitive Respiratory Disease

Prevalence of ASA-sensitive asthma varies, depending on the study population and the methods used to detect and thus report such individuals. Some reports present prevalence data based solely on the patients' history of reactions to ASA (28–30). Such studies underestimate ASA sensitivity, since many patients cannot correlate an asthma attack with ASA or NSAID ingestion or have avoided ASA/NSAIDs entirely, eliminating any chance of being able to report a reaction to one of these drugs. On the other hand, prospective oral ASA challenges in populations of asthmatics may overestimate the prevalence of the disease, since these studies were performed in medical centers that attract patients with severe asthma and were conducted by investigators who are known to be interested in this disorder.

Most ASA sensitivity begins after age 10 years and more commonly in young adults. In reviewing five studies of ASA sensitivity in children in which prospective single-blind oral-challenge studies were conducted to accurately identify ASA respiratory sensitivity (31–35), prevalence ranged from 0 to 28%. The study by Rachelefsky et al. (32), which reported a 28% prevalence of positive oral ASA challenges in their study population, included older children afflicted with more severe asthma and a high prevalence of chronic sinusitis.

Prevalence data for all asthmatics, without prescreening for specific clinical characteristics, range from 9 to 20% (3,36). Prevalence of ASA sensitivity in asthmatics with associated rhinosinusitis and/or nasal polyps, even without a history of ASA-induced respiratory reactions, increased significantly to 30–40% (37,38). Those studies of adult asthmatics who reported a prior ASA-induced respiratory reaction identified a prevalence of ASA sensitivity by oral ASA challenges ranging between 66 and 97% (3,37,39). Some patients who had an asthma attack in the past after ingesting aspirin or a NSAID would have had the asthma attack with drug exposure and incorrectly appropriated the attack to the drug.

VI. Reactions and Cross-Reactions Between ASA and Nsaids

A particularly dangerous event in the clinical course of these patients is the inadvertent ingestion of full doses of ASA or an NSAID that inhibits COX-1. Such a misfortunate ingestion can lead to life-threatening asthma attacks. If the patient survives long enough to reach an emergency medical facility, intubation and mechanical ventilation are needed to save the patient's life. These misadventures are not uncommon. Of 145 patients admitted to the hospital for severe asthma requiring mechanical ventilation, 25% were ASA-sensitive asthmatics (40). There are several problems in preventing such catastrophes. Reactions can occur upon first exposure to an NSAID or after ASA ingestion despite the fact that the patient's history indicates that prior exposure to ASA did not induce reaction. Since full therapeutic doses of the drugs are usually ingested, proximity to medical facilities and extent of reaction to ASA or on NSAID are important issues in the patient's survival. For example, if the event occurs too far from a medical facility or the patient hesitates to seek medical care, severe and untreated bronchospasm may claim the life of that individual. For those patients who survive the first exposure and reaction, several additional challenges are then in effect. First, some patients, and occasionally their physicians, fail to identify ASA or an NSAID as the cause of the first drug-induced reaction. Usually a series of reactions occurs before someone ascertains the association. Obviously, such individuals did not experience the most severe type of reaction because they survived. Second, ASA is frequently one of several drugs formulated in a single compound whose trade name does not contain the word "aspirin" (e.g., AlkaSeltzer). Third, some physicians and most patients are unfamiliar with the fact that, once sensitivity to ASA is established, cross-reactions will occur with any NSAID that inhibits cyclooxygenase-1.

VII. Pathogenesis of ASA- and NSAID-Induced Respiratory Reactions

Although the pathogenesis of ASA respiratory disease is not well defined, the biochemical events leading to ASA-induced respiratory reactions and cross-reactions are generally understood (11). Overproduction of all arachidonic acid products from mast cells, eosinophils, PMNs, and macrophages is associated with ASA disease (see Fig. 2). The 5-lipoxygenase enzymes are partly inhibited by a prostanoid from the cyclooxygenase pathway, namely, PGE_2. There are two COX isoenzymes, COX-1 (constitutive and involved in physiologic maintenance) and COX-2 (induced to participate in inflammatory responses to invading microorganisms and other noxious stimuli). COX-1 is found in most mammalian cells, including respiratory endothelial and epithelial cells. COX-2 is generally restricted to inflammatory cells. ASA and most NSAIDs preferentially inhibit or destroy COX-1, collapsing the enzyme channel and rendering it incapable of adding two oxygens, extracting a free radical from arachidonic acid, and forming a five-carbon ring, which is characteristic of prostaglandins (prostanoids). Thus synthesis of all COX-1 products ceases, including prostaglandin E_2 (PGE_2) (see Fig. 2). Inhibition of 5-LO and mast cell membranes is withdrawn, histamine is discharged from mast cells, and leukotrienes are rapidly formed via the 5-LO pathway. All NSAIDs, which cross-react with ASA and each other in respiratory reactions, also preferentially inhibit COX-1. By contrast, drugs that preferentially inhibit COX-2, leaving COX-1 undisturbed, or drugs that do not inhibit either isoenzyme do not cross-react with ASA.

VIII. Cross-Reactions with Aspirin

A. Strong Inhibitors of Cyclooxygenase-1

All NSAIDs, which inhibit COX-1 in vitro, cross-react with ASA on first exposure in the respiratory reactions described above (39,41,42). Furthermore, NSAIDs which inhibited COX-1 in vitro, with the least concentration of drug, required the smallest doses of NSAID to induce respiratory cross-reactions with ASA (41). All NSAIDs that cross-react with ASA also participate in cross-desensitization (22). Table 4 contains a list of NSAIDs which cross-react with ASA.

B. Weak Inhibitors of Cyclooxygenase

Cross-reactivity between ASA and compounds that are weak inhibitors of COX-1, such as acetaminophen and salsalate, are also of interest because they tend to induce weak reactions. Based upon Szczeklik's original in vitro studies with

Table 4 Nonsteroidal Anti-Inflammatory Drugs (NSAIDs) That Inhibit COX-1 and Cross-React with Aspirin (ASA) in Respiratory Reactions

Generic	Brand names
Piroxicam	Feldene
Indomethacin	Indocin
Sulindac	Clinoril
Tolmetin	Tolectin
Ibuprofen	Motrin, Rufen, Advil
Naproxen	Naprosyn
Naproxen sodium	Anaprox, Aleve
Fenoprofen	Nalfon
Meclofenamate	Meclomen
Mefenamic acid	Ponstel
Flurbiprofen	Ansaid
Diflunisal	Dolbid
Ketoprofen	Orudis, Oruval
Diclofenac	Voltaren, Cataflam
Ketoralac	Toradol
Etodolac	Lodine
Nabumetone	Relafen
Oxaprozin	Daypro

acetaminophen, he predicted that acetaminophen would cross-react poorly, if at all (41).

Acetaminophen

Initial studies reported a low to absent rate of cross-reactivity between acetaminophen and ASA (3,43–45). In these studies, however, oral challenges were performed with doses of acetaminophen equal to or less than 650 mg. Delaney (37) challenged ASA-sensitive asthmatics with 500 mg of acetaminophen and induced no reactions. He then doubled the dose of acetaminophen to 1000 mg and repeated the acetaminophen oral challenges. This time, 28% of known ASA-sensitive asthmatic patients experienced respiratory reactions to acetaminophen. Henochowicz also reported greater and greater positive respiratory reactions to acetaminophen as the challenge doses of acetaminophen were increased (44). In a study of 50 known ASA-sensitive asthmatics, using challenge doses of acetaminophen of 1000 and then 1500 mg, we reported (46) that respiratory reactions were induced during acetaminophen challenges in 34% of our ASA-sensitive study subjects. The observed respiratory reactions were generally mild, easily treated, and occurred only in a minority of ASA-sensitive asthmatics.

Salsalate

Salsalate is a partly effective anti-inflammatory agent that is used in the treatment of arthritis. Salsalate is also a weak inhibitor of COX-1. Stevenson et al. (47) studied 10 ASA-sensitive asthmatics to evaluate cross-sensitivity to salsalate. Two of the 10 experienced bronchospastic reactions to salsalate, but only when large doses (2 g) of the drug were ingested. Repeat challenges with 2 g of salsalate reproduced the same reactions. Both patients then underwent ASA challenge and desensitization. The same principle, as seen with acetaminophen, seems to apply. Salsalate, a weak inhibitor of COX-1, behaved like ASA and NSAIDs in producing respiratory reactions, but only after large doses of drug were ingested and only in a minority of ASA-sensitive asthmatics.

IX. Lack of Cross-Reactions with Aspirin

A. Selective Inhibitors of Cyclooxygenase-2

Two selective inhibitors of COX-2 were introduced into the U.S. market in the spring of 1999. In therapeutic doses, neither celecoxib or rofecoxib inhibit COX-1, the constitutive COX enzyme. Therefore, in the presence of these drugs, production of PGE_2 in epithelial and endothelial cells as well as inflammatory cells in the lungs continues (48). The protective effect of the available pool of PGE_2 is not substantially altered by COX-2 inhibitors and therefore there is no theoretical reason why cross-reactivity between pure COX-2 inhibitors and ASA should occur. Double-blind, placebo-controlled challenge studies with celecoxib and rofecoxib at our institution have yielded negative responses to both drugs in the first 92 known ASA-sensitive asthmatic patients (32 patients challenged with celecoxib 200 mg and 60 patients challenged with rofecoxib 25 mg). However, these ongoing studies have not been completed or published. Nimesulide and meloxicam are NSAIDs prescribed in other countries but are not available in the United States. They preferentially inhibit COX-2 but partially inhibit COX-1, particularly at high doses. Therefore, most ASA-sensitive asthmatics can take nimsulide or meloxicam without adverse effect, but there is a low percentage of cross-reactivity between these NSAIDs and ASA (49–52).

B. Drugs and Dyes That Do Not Inhibit Either COX-1 or COX-2

Other chemicals, dyes, and additives have been reported to cross-react with ASA, even though these compounds have not been shown to inhibit either COX enzyme

(2,3,53,54). Such reported chemicals include azo and non-azo dyes, sulfites, monosodium glutamate, benzoates, methylprednisolone, and hydrocortisone succinate. One author presented the theory that ingestion of tartrazine in the diet causes ASA-sensitive subjects to have ongoing asthma and rhinitis, even though patients are avoiding aspirin (2). Some have reported that oral challenge studies with these compounds lead to asthma attacks and changes in pulmonary function tests (3,53,55). However, others have expressed serious doubts that there is any cross-reactivity between ASA and non-COX-inhibiting chemicals or drugs (56). The following section summarizes the evidence against cross-reactivity.

Tartrazine

The best known azo dye is Yellow No. 5 (tartrazine) because it has been promoted by some authors as being responsible for cross-sensitivity reactions in ASA-sensitive asthmatic patients (2,3,54,57). When reviewing these publications, where an apparent cross-sensitivity was reported, one is struck by the fact that studies were conducted when study patients' airways were unstable and anti-asthmatic therapy had been simultaneously withdrawn. Therefore, spontaneous decreases in lung function measurements occurred, perhaps suggesting to the uninitiated that tartrazine was responsible for the changes (21,58). Weber et al. (38) identified 13 ASA-sensitive asthmatics, via oral ASA challenges, of a study population of 44 patients with rhinosinusitis and asthma. After withholding morning bronchodilators, they challenged all 44 patients with oral tartrazine, 2.5–25 mg. Seven patients (16%) experienced a decrease in FEV_1 values of at least 20%. The same 7 patients were then rechallenged with tartrazine 1 week later, but this time, bronchodilators were continued during the morning of tartrazine challenge. All 7 patients then ingested tartrazine and follow-up FEV_1 values did not decline, suggesting that they were never sensitive to tartrazine in the first place. As is true with many severe asthmatics, withholding essential antiasthmatic medications leads to uncontrolled asthma and a decline in lung function values (21). These same 7 patients were also challenged with six other azo and non-azo dyes without any measurable changes in their lung function values.

In the largest study of tartrazine and ASA sensitivity (59), we challenged 150 known ASA-sensitive asthmatics with tartrazine at doses of 25 and 50 mg. Six (4%) experienced a 20% or more decrease in FEV_1 values during open screening challenges after ingesting tartrazine. Five of 6 patients were available for follow-up and were rechallenged using a double-blind, placebo-controlled protocol. All repeat challenges with tartrazine, using the same dose associated with declining FEV_1 values in the screening challenges, were negative. A second study of an additional 44 known ASA-sensitive asthmatics with tartrazine challenges also did not reveal any instances of cross-sensitivity in known ASA-sensitive asthmatics to tartrazine (60). Tartrazine has not been shown to inhibit COX enzymes in vitro and therefore would not be expected to cross-react with ASA and NSAIDs (61).

Whether or not tartrazine has ever induced respiratory reactions in asthmatics, or if investigators have only reported spontaneous declines in pulmonary function studies, which were unrelated to the simultaneously ingested tartrazine, is still being debated. Furthermore, some of us are suspicious that rare IgE-mediated reactions to tartrazine occur in any asthmatic population, including those who are ASA-sensitive (11,62). Such a coincidental event, however, should not be confused with cross-sensitivity reactions. In view of the current literature, it is difficult to recommend that ASA-sensitive asthmatics should avoid any azo or non-azo dyes, unless a properly controlled oral challenge test documents a reaction in a patient to a specific dye.

Sulfites

In 1981, Stevenson and Simon (63) reported six patients who gave a history of severe, life-threatening asthma attacks after eating restaurant meals containing sulfites. Sulfite salts of potassium or sodium are added as antioxidants to foods to prevent browning and spoiling. Lettuce in salad bars, shrimp and other seafoods, cut potatoes, and wine and beer are the usual sources of foods and drinks containing sulfites. With single-blind oral challenges, we reproduced the patients asthmatic responses to sulfites in the laboratory, using capsules containing 5–50 mg of potassium metabisulfite. Since 1986, the Federal Government has banned the use of sulfiting agents as an additive to raw fruits, vegetables, and most recently on fresh, peeled potatoes. Packaged foods containing greater than 10 ppm of sulfur dioxide equivalents must carry sulfite-specific labeling. In the United States, because of these public health interventions, the risk of sulfite-induced asthmatic reactions in sulfite-sensitive asthmatics appears to have declined. Yet evidence that ASA-sensitive asthmatics are at risk for reactions to ingested sulfites does not exist. In fact, at Scripps Clinic, we have challenged 200 consecutive known ASA-sensitive asthmatics with gelatin capsules containing potassium metabisulfite, with ascending doses up to 200 mg, and have never identified sulfite sensitivity in any ASA-sensitive asthmatic patient. Even in the year 2000, sulfite ingestion in food and drink can still occur, particularly in sulfited dried fruits, seafood, and wine. Sulfite-induced asthma attacks can be very severe and death from such reactions has occurred.

Monosodium Glutamate

Allen et al. (53) reported that 13/32 (41%) asthmatic subjects experienced bronchospasm 2–12 h after ingesting capsules containing 2.5 g of monosodium glutamate (MSG). Furthermore, the authors stated that ASA sensitivity was a risk factor for MSG-induced reactions because of a high prevalence of ASA sensitivity in their 13 patients. Because the amino acid glutamate is present in certain foods (tomatoes, mushrooms, and parmesan cheese) and is added as a flavor enhancer in the form of the L-monosodium salt of glutamate, Allen's report initially generated considerable interest, since daily ingestion of glutamate might account for intrinsic or nonallergic asthma. However, the idea that ingestion of glutamate causes asthma attacks has not attracted support within the scientific community. First, glutamate is a nonessential amino acid, synthesized in a number of body compartments, including the brain and liver. Glutamate participates in a number of physiologic functions as a nutrient, energy-yielding substrate, structural determinant, enzyme regulator, and brain excitatory molecule (64). Glutamate is too small to be an antigen and its availability in normal physiology does not make it a good candidate to participate as an allergen in IGE-mediated reactions, such as bronchospasm. Second, the study by Allen et al. (53) and a follow-up study by Moneret-Vautrin (65) have been criticized because of uncontrolled challenge protocols and discontinuation of essential antiasthmatic medications (66). Third, other investigators have not been able to reproduce the Allen and Moneret-Vautrin results (67–70). At Scripps Clinic, confirmed asthmatic reactions to MSG did not occur during single-blind oral challenges with capsules containing 2.5 g of MSG in 70 known ASA-sensitive asthmatics and 30 asthmatics who gave a history of asthma attacks in Asian restaurants (70). It seems likely that the two studies reporting reactions to MSG (53,65) did not provide us with reliable challenge data and that MSG does not induce asthmatic attacks.

Hydrocortisone and Methylprednisolone Succinate

Despite prior reports of an association between aspirin sensitivity and allergic reactions to intravenous hydrocortisone (71,72), our current thinking is that COX-1 inhibition does not occur and that cross-reactivity is unlikely. Feigenbaum et al. (73) identified 1 of 45 known ASA-sensitive asthmatics who experienced angioedema and a respiratory reaction to IV hydrocortisone succinate. However, unlike cross-reactions between the NSAIDs, cross-desensitization could not be achieved between hydrocortisone succinate and ASA in this patient. Furthermore, the same reaction occurred after IV methylprednisolone, which also has a succinate base. A reasonable explanation is that succinate itself functions as a drug hapten in inducing occasional IgE-mediated reactions. The only association with ASA-sensitive asthmatics is their excessive exposure to IV hydrocortisone and methylprednisolone succinate during severe bouts of asthma, a logical opportunity for prior IgE sensitization.

Other Salicylates That Do Not Inhibit COX-1 or -2

Sodium and choline salicylates and a number of natural food-derived salicylates do not inhibit COX enzymes and do not cross-react in ASA-sensitive asthmatics

(74,75). Therefore, following a "salicylate-free" diet in order to control ASA respiratory disease is not an effective avoidance therapy.

X. Aspirin Desensitization

As allergists we think of desensitization as an alteration in immune responses, engineered by repeated exposure to injected antigens, thus reducing IgE-mediated reactions. Since IgE-mediated mechanisms have not been established for ASA respiratory sensitivity and are considered to be unlikely perpetrators of this reaction (9), desensitization is used here in its broadest sense (22). The first report of successful ASA desensitization was published in 1922 by Widal et al. (76). In 1976, Zeiss and Lockey (77) independently reported a 72-h refractory period to ASA after an indomethacin-induced reaction in one ASA-sensitive asthmatic. In 1980, Stevenson et al. (1) reported two ASA-sensitive asthmatics who became refractory to ASA after single-blind oral challenges with ASA. After first achieving ASA desensitization, both patients experienced improvement in respiratory disease activity when they were then treated with daily ASA. All ASA-sensitive asthmatics can be desensitized to ASA. Since 1980, in our General Clinical Research Center, we have successfully desensitized 596 consecutive ASA-sensitive patients. After ASA desensitization, in the absence of further exposure to ASA, the desensitized state persists for 2 to 5 days with full sensitivity returning after 7 days (22). Also, cross-desensitization, between ASA and any of the NSAIDs which inhibit COX-1, occurs routinely (22).

XI. Mechanisms of Aspirin Desensitization

During acute desensitization, defined as the patient exhibiting no reaction for 3 h after the first ingestion of 650 mg of ASA, histamine and LTC_4 disappeared in the nasal secretions (78). Serum histamine and tryptase levels disappeared (79) and a 20-fold decrease in bronchial airway responsiveness to inhaled LTE_4 immediately following ASA desensitization occurred (80). In aspirin desensitization studies with ingestion of 650 mg of aspirin twice a day for at least 2 weeks, LTB_4 synthesis in monocytes declined substantially to the same levels found in normal control subjects (81). During chronic aspirin desensitization in ASA-sensitive asthmatic subjects, Naser et al. (82) reported that urine LTE_4 levels declined to lower values than baseline but not to values found in normals. Such experiments suggest that aspirin desensitization, particularly long-term treatment with higher doses of aspirin, continues to inhibit COX-1 and probably COX-2. Inhibition of COX-2 by ASA is complicated because ASA prevents COX-2 from generating prostaglandins but switches its function to synthesize 15-HETE and perhaps other mediators (83). ASA does not effect the function of 5-LO, which is available to convert 15-HETE to lipoxins (LXA$_4$ and LXB$_4$) in leukocytes (see Fig. 2). The bioactivity of lipoxins is anti-inflammatory, in that they counter the biologic effects of LTs (vasoconstriction and bronchodilation). ASA, in high doses, may directly or indirectly reduce synthesis of mRNA phospholipase A$_2$, potentially leading to diminished synthesis of both prostanoids and LTs. Mast cells are also inhibited by high doses of ASA, either directly or indirectly. Simultaneously, cysLT$_1$ bronchial receptors are down-regulated, further blunting the effects of any available LTs. The biochemical pattern after ASA desensitization is consistent with down-regulating inflammatory activities through a number of biochemical interventions. These appear to be interactive, complicated, and only partly understood.

XII. Treatment

Based on the information presented in this chapter and elsewhere, it should be apparent that some of the features of ASA sensitivity require special treatment strategies which are unique to the management of this subgroup of asthmatics. Therefore, this section is organized into prevention and treatment of ASA reactions and treatment of ASA respiratory disease. Table 5 outlines our current approach to the treatment of these patients.

A. Prevention of ASA/NSAID-Induced Respiratory Reactions

Avoidance of ASA and all cross-reacting NSAIDs is essential in preventing respiratory reactions to these medications in unprotected ASA-sensitive asthmatic patients. Such preventive measures can be life-saving. Patient education should include the following principles: a discussion of the adverse effects

Table 5   Treatment of Aspirin-Sensitive Rhinosinusitis and Asthma

Reactions to ASA and NSAIDs
  Prevention of reactions: avoidance of all ASA and NSAID products
  Treatment of ASA-induced respiratory reactions: inhaled β-agonists, antihistamines, decongestants, rarely intubation
Treatment of the underlying respiratory disease
  Corticosteroids: Topical and systemic
  Antihistamines
  Leukotriene modifying drugs
  Antibiotics and bursts of corticosteroids for sinusitis
  Functional endoscopic sinus/polyp surgery
  Aspirin desensitization, followed by daily treatment with ASA

which reexposure of ASA/NSAIDs might have upon the patient, emphasis on the complete cross-reactivity between ASA and all COX-1-inhibiting NSAIDs, and extensive investigation of over-the-counter and prescribed drugs for the hidden presence of ASA or a potential cross-reacting NSAID. Only with the continued vigilance of the patient, physician, nurse, and pharmacist can future disasters be avoided in this highly vulnerable subset of asthmatic patients.

Theoretically, drugs that either inhibit or antagonize LTs should be effective in protecting ASA-sensitive asthmatics from inadvertant exposure to ASA/NSAIDs and in treating ASA disease. With respect to protection, the current literature demonstrates that LT modifiers protect patients from bronchospasm during oral and inhalation ASA challenges when small provoking doses of ASA are used (usually 60–90 mg of ASA orally or 5 mg/ml of ASA–lysine by inhalation) (84–87). Unfortunately, protection is inconsistent in preventing respiratory reactions after exposure to larger (therapeutic) doses of ASA. In a study using pretreatment with zileuton, escalating doses of ASA eventually induced respiratory reactions in all six patients and urinary LTE_4 levels increased during their reactions, suggesting that zileuton was unable to effectively block enough LTs to prevent the reaction (88). Similarly, the $CysLT_1$ receptor antagonist, montelukast, was also inconsistent in blocking ASA-induced respiratory reactions (89). Therefore, even though patients are routinely taking LT modifiers as a part of their daily antiasthmatic regime, they may have a severe respiratory reaction after inadvertently ingesting ASA or NSAIDs that inhibit COX-1.

B. Treatment of ASA-/NSAID-Induced Respiratory Reactions

Treatment of ASA-induced reactions in the emergency room or physicians' offices should focus on the following protocols established from treatment of respiratory reactions provoked during controlled oral ASA challenges. For bronchospasm, inhaled β-agonists using a nebulizer, delivering no more than five inhalations every 10 min, is generally effective in providing bronchodilation while ASA-induced reactions gradually subside over a number of hours. For laryngospasm, epinephrine s.q. is effective as is inhaled racemic epinephrine. For nasal congestion with paranasal headache, topical nasal application of oxymetazoline is an effective rapidly acting decongestant and topical antihistamine/decongestant solutions can be instilled in the conjunctivae. For systemic reactions of flush, urticaria, and abdominal pain, intravenous diphenhydramine and ranitidine are very effective and have a rapid onset of action. If a patient fails to respond to maintenance of airway in the ER, transportation to an ICU should follow. Intubation with mechanical ventilation is sometimes required.

C. Medical and Surgical Treatment of Aspirin-Sensitive Respiratory Disease

ASA disease is the ongoing inflammation of both the upper and lower respiratory tract mucus membranes. There is, however, significant interdependence, since asthma activity clearly correlates with acute and chronic sinus infections (90). Therefore, a major goal in controlling ASA disease is to reduce mucosal inflammation, particularly in the upper airways. Only in this manner is it possible to prevent nasal polyp formation, secondary sinusitis, and worsening asthma. As we have already learned, there is considerable evidence that a major contributor to mucosal inflammation is overproduction of arachidonate products. It should not be surprising that corticosteroids, because they stimulate synthesis of PLA_2 inhibitor protein (lipocortin) (91,92) and perhaps through blocking effects on mRNA synthesis and posttranscriptional expression of PLA_2 inhibition (93), offer significant therapeutic effects to ASA-sensitive asthmatic patients. High-dose topical corticosteroids, by both nasal insufflation and oral inhalation, should be used to reduce inflammation and retard nasal polyp formation. In a well-controlled study, intranasal fluticasone treatment was shown to effectively decrease mucosal inflammation in ASA-sensitive asthmatics (94). Although fluticasone has been studied in a population of ASA-sensitive asthmatics, this should not be interpreted to mean that other topical corticosteroids are ineffective in this disease. Clinical experience would suggest that all the competing nasal corticosteroids are effective to some degree in this disease. Unfortunately, inflammation in some ASA-sensitive asthmatic patients is not controlled with topical corticosteroids alone and the sheer bulk of polypoid tissues can prevent intranasal penetration of insufflated corticosteroids. This is particularly the case when the patient experiences viral URIs, which invariably progress to secondary bacterial sinus infections. Because of the further degree of inflammatory obstruction in the nose and sinus ostia, topical corticosteroids rarely penetrate sufficiently into the areas of intranasal inflammation. Therefore, bursts of corticosteroids are usually required during such infectious episodes. Bursts of systemic corticosteroids are also helpful to shrink nasal polyps and the mucosa around the sinus ostea, which will reestablish temporary sinus drainage.

Antibiotic treatment is also important and long courses of broad-spectrum antibiotics are usually required to clear purulent nasal secretions (75). If medical treatment fails, patients should undergo sinus CAT scans and be referred to a competent ear, nose, and throat surgeon for consideration of operative intervention. The purpose of such surgery is to debulk sinuses and nasal passages of excessive and hypertrophic inflammatory mucosa, reestablish drainage for the sinus ostea, and remove as much infected mucosa as possible without injuring essential structures (95,96). Patients with ASA sensitivity have a poorer outcome with respect to long-term remissions after sinus surgery compared to ASA-insensitive patients (97). This may be due to the sheer mass of polypoid tissue at the time of surgery as well as the aggressive reformation of additional polypoid tissues after surgery (98). Nevertheless, the role of sinusitis in provoking asthma is generally accepted (90) and good surgical results in ASA-sensitive asthmatics after extensive sinus surgery have been reported (99,100). The fundamental issues surrounding the indications for sinus surgery in ASA-sensitive asthmatics are not related to the effectiveness of these procedures in removing masses of hypertrophic and infected nasal and sinus tissues. In fact, rapid improvement in both upper and lower airways is observed in the majority of patients shortly after surgery (99). Because of reformation of polypoid tissues, the indications for repeated surgical procedures become the main therapeutic consideration. In fact, it is difficult, if not impossible, to safely remove enough of the inflamed and infected mucosal tissues to prevent reoccurrence and with each subsequent operation surgical landmarks, scarring, and excessive bleeding become further obstacles to functional improvement. Furthermore, surgery does not influence the fundamental biochemical pathology of ASA disease: continued overproduction of arachidonate products, eosinophil proteins, preformed mast cell mediators, and COX-2 products.

Two leukotriene-modifying drugs have been studied in the ongoing treatment of ASA respiratory disease: zileuton and montelukast (101,102). Both drugs, using standard methods of assessment, in relatively short studies, significantly enhanced asthma control. After the short-term montelukast study, long-term open treatment for over 2 years with 10 mg hs of montelukast was conducted. At Scripps Clinic, 5/10 ASA-sensitive asthmatics who were in the short-term study and elected to be treated with daily montelukast in the open study appeared to gain significant benefit from long-term treatment with montelukast. However, the other 5 patients discontinued montelukast because of lack of efficacy. Since LT overproduction is characteristic of ASA disease, fine tuning of the proper therapeutic dosing with these products is likely to be more important than in other types of asthma. Since zileuton partially blocks 5-LO and montelukast is a competitive inhibitor of $cysLT_1$ receptor, it is theoretically useful to use both drugs in a recalcitant patient and clinical experience shows enhanced control of disease in some patients. However, combined therapy has not been studied to determine whether it is better than single-drug therapy. Furthermore, the tendency for some ASA-sensitive asthmatics to fail to respond to one or both of these drugs is readily apparent. Zafirlukast, which has not been formally studied for efficacy in ASA-sensitive asthmatics, nevertheless seems to be quite effective in the treatment of some ASA-sensitive patients.

D. ASA Desensitization Treatment

There are seven published studies that report efficacy of ASA desensitization followed by ASA treatment (6,8,103–107). In 1990 Sweet et al. (107) reported the clinical courses of 107 known ASA-sensitive rhinosinusitis asthmatic patients treated with ASA between 1975 and 1988. Forty-two patients avoided aspirin and served as the control group. Thirty-five patients were desensitized to ASA and treated continuously with ASA daily for as long as 8 years. Thirty patients were initially desensitized to ASA and treated with ASA but discontinued ASA after a mean of 2 years, usually because of gastric side effects. Retrospective analysis of the three groups showed that the patients treated with ASA enjoyed statistically significant reductions in hospitalizations, emergency room visits, outpatient visits, need for additional sinus surgery, need for additional nasal polypectomies, number of upper respiratory infections/sinusitis requiring antibiotics, and improved sense of smell. ASA-desensitized and treated patients were also able to significantly reduce systemic corticosteroid maintenance doses and corticosteroid bursts per year and the continuously treated group was able to reduce inhaled corticosteroids compared to the control group. In the patients who had to discontinue ASA treatment after several years, respiratory disease improved while being treated with daily ASA, but reverted back toward pretreatment status after discontinuing ASA treatment. This study, the largest and longest to date, showed that ASA desensitization followed by long-term ASA treatment improved ASA-sensitive asthma rhinosinusitis, prevented regrowth of polyps, and allowed a significant reduction in the use of systemic and inhaled corticosteroids.

In 1996, Stevenson et al. (6) analyzed the clinical courses of 65 ASA-sensitive asthmatics who underwent oral ASA challenges followed by ASA desensitization between 1988 and 1994. These patients, after ASA oral challenges and standard desensitization to ASA, were then treated with daily doses of ASA (650 mg b.i.d.) and followed for an average of 3.3 years (range 1–6 years). The following clinical parameters were significantly improved after long-term ASA desensitization treatment: number of sinus infections per year, number of hospitalizations for asthma per year, number of sinus operations per year, sense of smell, and in use of both nasal topical corticosteroids and systemic corticosteroids. After ASA desensitization treatment the number of emergency room visits for asthma per year and use of inhaled corticosteroids remained unchanged. This study showed that the main components of ASA disease, namely aggressive nasal polyp formation and sinusitis, were significantly reduced during long-term ASA desensitization treatment. Concomitantly, nasal and systemic corticosteroids were reduced or discontinued without the previously expected increase of the inflammatory respiratory disease.

Another potential treatment strategy is to combine ASA desensitization with 5-LO inhibitors or selective antagonists of cysLT$_1$. Thus several points in the arachidonate synthetic pathway may need to be interrupted in order to reduce inflammation. Cytokine inhibitors, particularly inhibitors of IL2–IL5, might also provide opportunities to interrupt cell signaling before synthesis of mediators is underway. Additional knowledge of the fundamental defects in ASA-sensitive asthmatics will be necessary to understand the disease, reactions, and how best to modify and control inflammation.

References

1. Stevenson DD, Simon RA, Mathison DA. Aspirin-sensitive asthma: tolerance to aspirin after positive oral aspirin challenges. J Allergy Clin Immunol 1980; 66:82–88.
2. Samter M, Beers R Jr. Intolerance to aspirin: clinical studies and consideration of its pathogenesis. Ann Intern Med 1968; 68:975–983.
3. Spector SL, Wangaard CH, Farr RS. Aspirin and concomitant idiosyncrasies in adult asthmatic patients. J Allergy Clin Immunol 1979; 64(6/1):500–506.
4. Szczeklik A. Mechanism of aspirin-induced asthma. Allergy 1997; 52:613–619.
5. Stevenson DD, Simon RA. Sensitivity to aspirin and nonsteroidal antiinflammatory drugs. In: Middleton EJ, Reed CE, Ellis EF, Adkinson NF Jr., Yunginger JW, Busse WW, eds. Allergy: Principles and Practice. Vol. 2. St. Louis: Mosby, 1993:1747–1765.
6. Stevenson DD, Hankammer MA, Mathison DA, Christensen SC, Simon RA. Long term ASA desensitization-treatment of aspirin sensitive asthmatic patients: clinical outcome studies. J Allergy Clin Immunol 1996; 98:751–758.
7. Stevenson D. Adverse reactions to nonsteroidal anti-inflammatory drugs. In: Tilles S, ed. Drug Hypersensitivity. Vol. 18. 4th ed. Philadelphia: W. B. Saunders, 1998: 773–798.
8. Lumry WR, Curd JG, Zieger RS, Pleskow WW, Stevenson DD. Aspirin-sensitive rhinosinusitis: the clinical syndrome and effects of aspirin administration. J Allergy Clin Immunol 1983; 71:580–587.
9. Stevenson DD, Lewis R. Proposed mechanisms of aspirin sensitivity reactions (editorial). J Allergy Clin Immunol 1987; 80:788–790.
10. Lee TH. Mechanism of bronchospasm in aspirin-sensitive asthma (editorial). Am Rev Resp Dis 1993; 148:1442–1443.
11. Szczeklik A, Stevenson, DD. Aspirin-induced asthma: advances in pathogenesis and management. J Allergy Clin Immunol 1999; 104:5–13.
12. Yamashita T, Tsuyi H, Maeda N, Tomoda K, Kumazawa T. Etiology of nasal polyps associated with aspirin-sensitive asthma. Rhinology 1989; 8:15–24.
13. Sladek K, Dworski R, Soja J, et al. Eicosanoids in bronchoalveolar lavage fluid of aspirin-intolerant patients with asthma after aspirin challenge. Am J Resp Crit Care Med 1994; 149:940–946.
14. Nasser SM, Pfister R, Christie PE, Sousa AR, Barker J, Schmitz-Schumann M, Lee TH. Inflammatory cell populations in bronchial biopsies from aspirin-sensitive asthmatic subjects. Am J Respir Crit Care Med 1996; 153:90–96.
15. Szczeklik A, Sladek K, Dworski R, Nizankowska E, Soja J, Oates J. Bronchial aspirin challenge causes specific eicosanoid response in aspirin-sensitive asthmatics. Am J Respir Crit Care Med 1996; 154:1608–1614.
16. Christie PE, Tagari P, Ford-Hutchinson AW, et al. Urinary leukotriene E4 concentrations increase after aspirin challenge in aspirin-sensitive asthmatic subjects. Am Rev Respir Dis 1991; 143:1025–1029.

17. Sladek K, Szczeklik A. Cysteinyl leukotrienes overproduction and mast cell activation in aspirin-provoked bronchospasm in asthma. Eur Respir J 1993; 6:391–399.

18. Smith CM, Hawksworth RJ, Thien FC, Christie PE, Lee TH. Urinary leukotriene E4 in bronchial asthma. Eur Respir J 1992; 5:693–699.

19. Daffern P, Muilenburg D, Hugli TE, Stevenson DD. Association of urinary leukotriene E4 excretion during aspirin challenges with severity of respiratory responses. J Allergy Clin Immunol 1999; 104:559–564.

20. Szczeklik A. The cyclooxygenase theory of aspirin-induced asthma (Review). Eur Resp J 1990; 3:588–593.

21. Stevenson DD. Oral challenges to detect aspirin and sulfite sensitivity in asthma. NE Region Allergy Proc 1988; 9:135–142.

22. Pleskow WW, Stevenson DD, Mathison DA, Simon RA, Schatz M, Zieger RS. Aspirin desensitization in aspirin sensitive asthmatic patients: clinical manifestations and characterization of the refractory period. J Allergy Clin Immunol 1982; 69:11–19.

23. Melillo G, Podovano A, Cocco G, Masi C. Dosimeter inhalation test with lysine acetylsalicylate for the detection of aspirin-induced asthma. Ann Allergy 1993; 71:61–65.

24. Phillips GD, Foord R, Holgate ST. Inhaled lysine-aspirin as a bronchoprovocation procedure with aspirin in aspirin-sensitive asthma. J Allergy Clin Immunol 1989; 84:232–241.

25. Pawlowicz A, Williams WR, Davies BH. Inhalation and nasal challenge in the diagnosis of aspirin induced asthma. Allergy 1991; 46:405–409.

26. Milewski M, Mastalerz L, Nizankowska E, Szczeklik A. Nasal provocation test with lysine-aspirin for diagnosis of aspirin-sensitive asthma. J Allergy Clin Immunol 1998; 101:581–586.

27. Dahlen B, Zetterstrom O. Comparison of bronchial and per oral provocation with aspirin in aspirin-sensitive asthmatics. Eur Respir J 1990; 3:527–534.

28. Chafee FH, Settipane GA. Aspirin intolerance I. Frequency in an allergic population. J Allergy Clin Immunol 1974; 53:193–199.

29. Falliers CJ. Aspirin and subtypes of asthma: risk factor analysis. J Allergy Clin Immunol 1973; 52:141–147.

30. Giraldo B, Blumenthal MN, Spink WW. Aspirin intolerance in asthma: a clinical and immunologic study. Ann Intern Med 1969; 71:313–316.

31. Fischer TJ, Guilfoile TD, Kesarwala HH. Adverse pulmonary responses to aspirin and acetaminophen in chronic childhood asthma. Pediatrics 1983; 71:313–321.

32. Rachelefsky GS, Coulson A, Siegel SC, Stiehm ER. Aspirin intolerance in chronic childhood asthma: detection by oral challenge. Pediatrics 1975; 56:443–448.

33. Schuhl JF, Pereyra JG. Oral acetysalicylic acid (aspirin) challenge in asthmatic children. Clin Allergy 1979; 9:83–88.

34. Towns SJ, Mellis CM. Role of acetyl salicylic acid and sodium metabisulfite in chronic childhood asthma. Pediatrics 1984; 73:631–637.

35. Vedanthan PK, Menon MM, Bell TD, Bergin D. Aspirin and tartrazine oral challenge: incidence of adverse response in chronic childhood asthma. J Allergy Clin Immunol 1977; 60:8–13.

36. McDonald J, Mathison DA, Stevenson DD. Aspirin tolerance in asthma—detection by challenge. J Allergy Clin Immunol 1972; 50:198–207.

37. Delaney JC. The diagnosis of aspirin idiosyncrasy by analgesic challenge. Clin Allergy 1976; 6:177–181.

38. Weber RW, Hoffman M, Raine DA, Nelson HS. Incidence of bronchoconstriction due to aspirin, azo dyes, non-azo dyes, and preservatives in a population of perennial asthmatics. J Allergy Clin Immunol 1979; 64:32–37.

39. Pleskow WW, Stevenson DD, Mathison DA, Simon RA, Schatz M, Zieger RS. Aspirin-sensitive rhinosinusitis/asthma: spectrum of adverse reactions to aspirin. J Allergy Clin Immunol 1983; 71:574–579.

40. Marquette C, Saulnier F, Leroy O, Wallaert B, Chopin C, Demarcq JM, et al. Long-term prognosis for near-fatal asthma: a 6-year follow up study of 145 asthmatic patients who underwent mechanical ventilation for near fatal asthma. Am Rev Resp Dis 1992; 146:76–81.

41. Szczeklik A, Gryglewski RJ, Czerniawska-Mysik G. Clinical patterns of hypersensitivity to nonsteroidal anti-inflammatory drugs and their pathogenesis. J Allergy Clin Immunol 1977; 60(5):276–284.

42. Mathison DA, Stevenson DD. Hypersensitivity to non-steroidal anti-inflammatory drugs: indications and methods for oral challenge. J Allergy Clin Immunol 1979; 64:669–674.

43. Falliers CJ. Acetaminophen and aspirin challenges in subgroups of asthmatics. J Asthma 1983; 20:39–49.

44. Henochowicz S. Acetaminophen-induced asthma in a patient with aspirin idiosyncrasy. Immunol Allergy Pract 1986; 60:43–47.

45. Szczeklik A, Gryglewski J. Asthma and anti-inflammatory drugs: mechanisms and clinical patterns. Drugs 1983; 25:533–543.

46. Settipane RA, Shrank PJ, Simon RA, Mathison DA, Christensen SC, Stevenson DD. Prevalence of cross-sensitivity with acetaminophen in aspirin-sensitive asthmatic subjects. J Allergy Clin Immunol 1995; 96:480–485.

47. Stevenson DD, Hougham A, Schrank P, Goldlust B, Wilson R. Disalcid cross-sensitivity in aspirin sensitive asthmatics. J Allergy Clin Immunol 1990; 86:749–758.

48. Hawley C. COX-2 inhibitors. Lancet 1999; 353:307–314.

49. Andri L, Senna G, Betteli C, Givanni S, Scaricabarozzi I, Mezzelani P, Andri G. Tolerability of nimesulide in aspirin-sensitive patients. Ann Allergy 1994; 72:29–31.

50. Asero R. Aspirin and parcetamol tolerance in patients with nimesulide-induced urticaria. Ann Allergy Asthma Immunol 1998; 81:237–238.

51. Bavbek S, Celik G, Ediger D, Mungan D, Demirel YS, Misirlig Z. The use of nimesulide in patients with acetylsalicylic acid and nonsteroidal anti-inflammatory drug intolerance. J Asthma 1999; 36:657–663.

52. DiFonso M, Romano A, Quaratino D, Papa G, Venuti A. Meloxicam as an alternative drug in patients reporting adverse reactions to non-steroidal antiinflammatory drugs (NSAIDs). J Allergy Clin Immunol 1999; 103:538.

53. Allen DH, Delohery J, Baker G. Monosodium L-glutamate-induced asthma. J Allergy Clin Immunol 1987; 80:530–537.

54. Freedman B. Asthma induced by sulfur dioxide, benzoate and tartrazine contained in orange drinks. Clin Allergy 1977; 7:407–411.

55. Samter M, Stevenson DD. Reactions to aspirin and aspirin-like drugs. In: Samter M, Talmage DW, Frank MM, Austen KF, Claman HN, eds. Boston: Little, Brown, 1988:1135–1147.

56. Simon RA. Adverse reactions to drug additives. J Allergy Clin Immunol 1984; 74: 623–630.

57. Juhlin L, Michaelsson G, Zetterstrom O. Urticaria and asthma induced by food and drug additives in patients with aspirin sensitivity. J Allergy Clin Immunol 1972; 50:92–102.

58. Stevenson DD. Oral challenge, aspirin, NSAID, tartrazine, and sulfites. N Engl Region Allergy Proc 1984; 5:111–110.

59. Stevenson DD, Simon RA, Lumry WR, Mathison DA. Adverse reactions to tartrazine. J Allergy Clin Immunol 1986; 78:182–191.

60. Stevenson DD, Simon RA, Lumry WR, Mathison DA. Pulmonary reactions to tartrazine. Pediatr Allergy Immunol 1992; 3:222–227.

61. Gerber JG, Payne NA, Oelz O, Nies S, Oates JA. Tartrazine and the prostaglandin system. J Allergy Clin Immunol 1979; 63:289–294.

62. Szczeklik A, Nizankowska E, Sanak M. New insights into the pathogenesis and management of aspirin-induced asthma. Clin Asthma Rev 1998; 2:79–86.

63. Stevenson DD, Simon RA. Sensitivity to ingested metabisulfite in asthmatic subjects. J Allergy Clin Immunol 1981; 68:26–20.

64. Young V, Ajami AM. Glutamate: an amino acid of particular distinction. J Nutr 2000; 130:892S–900S.

65. Moneret-Vautrin D. Monosodium glutamate induced asthma: a study of the potential risk in 30 asthmatics and a review of the literature. Alergie Immunol 1987; 19: 29–35.

66. Stevenson D. Monosodium glutamate and asthma. J Nutr 2000; 130(4):1067–1073.

67. Schwartzstein R, Kelleher M, Weingerger SE, Weiss JW, Drazen JM. Airway effects of monosodium glutamate in subjects with chronic stable asthma. J Asthma 1987; 24:167–172.

68. Germano P, Cohen SG, Hahn B, Metcalfe DD. An evaluation of clinical reactions to monosodium glutamate (MSG) in asthmatics, using a blinded placebo controlled challenge (abstr). J Allergy Clin Immunol 1991; 87:177.

69. Woods R, Weiner J, Thien F, Abramson M, Walters E. The effects of monosodium glutamate in adults with asthma who perceive themselves to be monosodium glutamate-intolerant. J Allergy Clin Immunol 1998; 101:762–771.

70. Woessner K, Simon RA, Stevenson DD. Monosodium glutamate sensitivity in asthma. J Allergy Clin Immunol 1999; 104:305–310.

71. Dajani BM, Sliman NA, Shubair KS. Bronchospasm caused by intravenous hydrocortisone sodium succinate (Solu-Cortef) in aspirin sensitive asthmatics. J Allergy Clin Immunol 1981; 68:201–204.

72. Szczeklik A, Nizankowska E, Czerniawska-Mysik G, Sek S. Hydrocortisone and airflow impairment in aspirin-induced asthma. J Allergy Clin Immunol 1985; 76: 530–536.

73. Feigenbaum BA, Stevenson DD, Simon RA. Lack of cross-sensitivity to IV hydrocortisone in aspirin-sensitive subjects with asthma. J Allergy Clin Immunol 1995; 96:545–548.

74. Szczeklik A, Nizankowska E, Dworski R. Choline magnesium trisalicylate in patients with aspirin-induced asthma. Eur Respir J 1990; 3:535–539.
75. Stevenson D, Simon RA. Sensitivity to aspirin and nonsteroidal antiinflammatory drugs. In: Middleton E Jr., Ellis EF, Yunginger JW, Reed CE, Adkinson NF Jr., Busse WW, ed. Allergy: Principles and Practice. Vol. 2. St. Louis: Mosby, 1998:1225–1234.
76. Widal MF, Abrami P, Lermeyez J. Anaphylaxie et idiosyncrasie. Presse Med 1922; 30:189–192.
77. Zeiss CR, Lockey RF. Refractory period to aspirin in a patient with aspirin-induced asthma. J Allergy Clin Immunol 1976; 57:440–448.
78. Ferreri NR, Howland WC, Stevenson DD, Spiegelberg HL. Release of leukotrienes, prostaglandins, and histamine into nasal secretions of aspirin-sensitive asthmatics during reaction to aspirin. Am Rev Resp Dis 1988; 137:847–854.
79. Bosso JV, Schwartz LB, Stevenson DD. Tryptase and histamine release during aspirin-induced respiratory reactions. J Allergy Clin Immunol 1991; 88:830–837.
80. Arm JP, O'Hickey SP, Hawksworth RJ, et al. Asthmatic airways have a disproportionate hyperresponsiveness to LTE4, as compared with normal airways, but not to LTC4, LTD4, methacholine, and histamine. Am Rev Respir Dis 1990; 142: 1112–1118.
81. Juergens UR, Christiansen SC, Stevenson DD, Zuraw BL. Inhibition of monocyte leukotriene B4 production following aspirin desensitization. J Allergy Clin Immunol 1995; 96:148–156.
82. Nasser SMS, Patel M, Bell GS, Lee TH. The effect of aspirin desensitization on urinary leukotriene E4 concentration in aspirin-sensitive asthma. Am J Respir Crit Care Med 1995; 115:1326–1330.
83. Claria J, Serhan CN. Aspirin triggers previously undescribed bioctive eicosanoids by human endothelial cell-leukocyte interactions. Proc Natl Acad Sci USA 1995; 92:9475–9479.
84. Christie PE, Smith CM, Lee TH. The potent and selective sulfidopeptide leukotriene antagonist, SK&F 104353, inhibits aspirin-induced asthma. Am Rev Respir Dis 1991; 144:957–958.
85. Dahlen BJ, Kumlin M, Margolskee D, et al. The leukotriene receptor antagonist MK-0679 blocks airway obstruction induced by bronchial provocation with lysine-aspirin in aspirin-sensitive asthmatics. Eur Resp J 1993; 6:1018–1026.
86. Israel E, Fischer AR, Rosenberg MA, et al. The pivotal role of 5-lipoxygenase products in the reaction of aspirin-sensitive asthmatics to aspirin. Am Rev Resp Dis 1993; 148:1447–1451.
87. Yamamoto H, Nagata M, Kuramitsu K, et al. Inhibition of analgesic-induced asthma by leukotriene receptor antagonist ONO-1078. Am J Respir Crit Care Med 1994; 150:254–257.
88. Pauls J, Simon RA, Daffern PJ, Stevenson DD. Lack of effect of the 5-lipoxygenase inhibitor zileuton in blocking oral aspirin challenges in aspirin sensitive asthmatics. Ann Allergy Asthma Immunol 2000; 85:40–45.
89. Stevenson D, Simon RA, Mathison DA, Christiansen SC. Montelukast is only partially effective in inhibiting aspirin responses in aspirin sensitive asthmatics. Ann Allergy Asthma Immunol 2000; 85:477–482.
90. Slavin RG. Asthma and sinusitis. J Allergy Clin Immunol 1992; 90:534–537.

91. Peers SH, Flower RJ. The role of lipocortin in corticosteroid actions. Am Rev Respir Dis 1990; 141:18–21.

92. Ambrose MP, Hunninghake GW. Corticosteroids increase lipocortin I in BAL fluid from normal individuals and patients with lung disease. J Appl Physiol 1990; 68: 1668–1671.

93. Nakano T, Ohara O, Teraoka H, Arita H. Glucocorticoids suppress group II phospholipase A2 production by blocking mRNA synthesis and post-transcriptional expression. J Biol Chem 1990; 265:12745–12748.

94. Mastalerz L, Milewski M, Duplaga M, Nizankowska E, Szczeklik A. Intranasal fluticasone propionate for chronic eosinophilic rhinitis in patients with aspirin-induced asthma. Allergy 1997; 52:895–900.

95. Lanza DC, Kennedy DW. Current concepts in the surgical management of chronic and recurrent acute sinusitis. J Allergy Clin Immunol 1992; 90:505–510.

96. Nishioka GJ, Cook PR, Davis WE, McKinsey JP. Functional endoscopic sinus surgery in patients with chronic sinusitis and asthma. Otolaryngol Head Neck Surg 1994; 110:494–500.

97. Schaitkin B, May M, Shapiro A, Fucci M, Mester SJ. Endoscopic sinus surgery: 4-year follow-up on the first 100 patients. Laryngoscope 1993; 103:1117–1120.

98. Kennedy DW. Prognostic factors, outcomes and staging in ethmoid sinus surgery. Laryngoscope 1992; 102:1–18.

99. Mings R, Friedman WH, Linford PA, Slavin RG. Five-year follow-up of the effects of bilateral intranasal sphenoidethmoidectomy in patients with sinusitis and asthma. Am J Rhinol 1988; 2:13–16.

100. McFadden EA, Kany RJ, Fink JN. Surgery for sinusitis and aspirin triad. Laryngoscope 1990; 100:1043–1050.

101. Dahlen BN, Nizankowska E, Szczeklik A, Zetterstrom O, Bochenek G, Kumlin M, et al. Benefits from adding the 5-lipoxygenase inhibitor zileuton to conventional therapy in aspirin-intolerant asthmatics. Am J Respir Crit Care Med 1998; 157: 1187–1194.

102. Dahlen S, Malstrom K, Nizankowska E, Dahlen B, Kuna P, Kowalski M, Lumry WR, Picado C, Stevenson DD, Bousquet J, Pauwels R, Holgate ST, Shahane A, Zhang J, Reiss TF, and Szczeklik A. Improvement of aspirin-intolerant asthma by montelukast, a leukotriene anatagonist: a randomised, double blind, placebo controlled trial. Lancet 2001; in press.

103. Chiu JT. Improvement in aspirin-sensitive asthmatic subjects after rapid aspirin desensitization and aspirin maintenance (ADAM) treatment. J Allergy Clin Immunol 1983; 71(6):560–567.

104. Lockey RF. Aspirin-improved ASA triad. Hosp Pract 1978; 13:129–133.

105. Lockey RF, Rucknagel DL, Vanselow NA. Familial occurrence of asthma, nasal polyps and aspirin intolerance. Ann Intern Med 1973; 78(1):57–63.

106. Nelson RP, Stablein JJ, Lockey RF. Asthma improved by acetylsalicylic acid and other non-steroidal anti-inflammatory agents. N Engl Reg Allergy Proc 1986; 7(2): 117–121.

107. Sweet JA, Stevenson DD, Simon RA, Mathison DA. Long term effects of aspirin desensitization treatment for aspirin sensitive rhinosinusitis asthma. J Allergy Clin Immunol 1990; 86:59–65.

17

Occupational Asthma
Spectrum of Severity
and Implications for Management

RON BALKISSOON

National Jewish Medical and Research Center
Denver, Colorado

I. Introduction

Occupational asthma is now the most common work-related respiratory disorder in the majority of industrialized countries, surpassing conditions such as silicosis, asbestosis, and occupational lung cancer (1–6). Estimates of the proportion of cases of adult-onset asthma due to occupational exposure range from 2 to 15% (7–10). More than 300 agents have been identified as potential causes of occupational asthma and the list continues to expand (11–14). There have been few case reports of actual fatalities related to occupational asthma (15–17); nonetheless, morbidity associated with occupational asthma can be quite substantial, with many affected individuals being required to change jobs and/or seek workers' compensation. Many workers with occupational asthma are unable to find employment with wages comparable to those of their previous job. Individuals with severe occupational asthma often do not return to gainful employment in any capacity and require long-term disability. Such outcomes point to the substantial socioeconomic consequences of occupational asthma.

II. Work-Related Asthma: Definitions and Classifications

Work-related asthma encompasses two categories of asthma related to the occupational setting: (1) work-aggravated asthma and (2) occupational asthma (11). Work-aggravated asthma is preexisting asthma that is aggravated by irritants or physical stimuli (e.g., temperature change, dust, and smoke) in the workplace. Occupational asthma is characterized by variable airflow limitation and/or airway hyperresponsiveness caused by exposures and conditions attributable to a particular occupational environment (12–14). Individuals with preexisting asthma may develop superimposed occupational asthma due to a specific workplace agent.

Occupational asthma has been further defined in terms of the presence or absence of a latency period between onset of exposure and the development of asthma (12–14). Occupational asthma with latency primarily refers to the "classic" immune response-induced form that usually occurs following a variable period of exposure to either a high- or low-molecular-weight antigen in the workplace. In addition, there are certain forms of occupational asthma with latency for which a precise immunological mechanism has not been identified (e.g., "meat wrapper's asthma" and "potroom asthma"). Occupational asthma without latency refers to irritant-induced asthma resulting from exposure to high concentrations of irritant gases, fumes, dust, or chemicals. Reactive Airways Dysfunction Syndrome (RADS), the prototype of irritant-induced asthma (18), was originally defined as asthma occurring after a single exposure to high levels of an irritant agent with consequent development of asthma symptoms, variable airflow limitation, and bronchial hyperresponsiveness within 24 to 72 h of initial exposure. It is now recognized that irritant-induced asthma can develop following irritant exposures on one or several occasions (19). Regardless of the mechanism or inciting agent, the final common pathway leads to a pattern of respiratory embarrassment that is clinically indistinguishable from nonoccupational asthma.

Finally, there are a group of "occupational asthmalike" disorders (12) which demonstrate variable airflow limitation with symptoms of chest tightness associated with cross-shift changes in forced expiratory volume in 1 sec (FEV_1) but without persistent bronchial hyperresponsiveness or eosinophilia. Byssinosis, an airway disease due to exposure to textile dusts from cotton, flax, hemp, jute, or sisal, is a classic example of this type of disorder (20). Such exposures can lead to chronic airflow limitation.

III. Reports of Severe and Fatal Asthma Attacks in the Work Environment

A number of workplace sensitizers have been noted to cause severe asthma and or anaphylactic episodes. Some of the more potent occupational sensitizers include isocyanates (17), latex (21,22), flour (16), and laboratory animals (23). More important than the antigenic properties of any specific agent, the duration and level of exposure, particularly after developing evidence of sensitization, likely play critical roles in determining the severity of occupational asthma.

There have been three published reports of occupational asthma-related deaths due to isocyanates. Fabbri et al. (17) reported a fatality due to toluene diisocyanate (TDI) in a 43-year-old car painter. He had worked as a car painter for over 26 years and was a lifelong nonsmoker. He had had work-related asthma symptoms for approximately 11 years and was diagnosed with isocyanate asthma 6 years prior to his death. Despite recommendations to change his job and/or avoid the use of polyurethane paints, he had continued to work in his garage as a car painter. He regularly used protective respiratory equipment and was able to start a regular exercise program. He was apparently reasonably well until the week before his death, when he used a paint product that he had never used before. Exposure to this paint led to severe prolonged bronchospasm despite treatment with his regular medications. Symptoms apparently subsided within 3 days, but repeated use of this paint product 7 days later led to a fatal asthma attack. Autopsy on gross inspection showed gray glistening mucous plugs in the airways. Microscopy revealed mucous plugging of small bronchi and bronchioles, sloughing and shedding of epithelium, and thickening of the basement membrane. Bronchial walls had mucosal edema with diffuse infiltration of mononuclear and polymorphonuclear leukocytes and prominent eosinophilic infiltration in the lamina propria. Bronchial smooth muscle was hypertrophic and disarrayed. These morphological abnormalities were noted at the bronchial and alveolar levels. The morphological features noted in this case are essentially pathognomonic for asthma-related deaths due to nonoccupational causes. An exceptional feature atypical for nonoccupational asthma deaths included the presence of alveolar wall destruction that appeared as fragments of septa floating in the alveolar spaces. Using an isocyanate monitor (MDA Model 7005; MDA Scientific Inc., Glenview, IL), the concentration level of isocyanate vapor on top of the can that caused the fatal attack was 4 ppb. In this report Fabbri et al. cite a personal communication regarding another fatality related to TDI exposure during specific inhalation challenge testing. A 1985 report (24) briefly documented another asthma fatality in a car painter.

Carino et al. (15) reported the death of a 39-year-old foundry worker due to exposure to resins containing diphenylmethane diisocyanate (MDI). The victim had been diagnosed with occupational asthma 5 years prior to his death. He apparently had worked in this area for 6 years and had symptoms for a few years prior to his diagnosis. Details of the exposures on the fatal day are not given other than to mention that he had a severe attack which was unresponsive to topical β-agonist and parenteral corticosteroids. Histological findings at time of autopsy were similar to those noted in the Fabbri case report, including the disarray of smooth muscle.

The only other published report of an occupational asthma fatality involved a 42-year-old bakery employee in South Africa (16). He had worked as an assistant baker for over 20 years and had a 6-year history of symptoms related to work exposures. He was diagnosed with flour-related asthma following positive skin prick testing to whole-grain wheat and whole-grain maize and a positive specific inhalation challenge with flour. Despite recommendations to change his job he continued to work there for 5 more years before his fatal asthma attack. The patient apparently developed a severe asthma attack after a work shift and spent the following day symptomatic at home. The next morning he was found dead outside his home with a bronchodilator inhaler in his hand. No autopsy was performed. In the absence of any other plausible explanation, asthma was deemed to be the cause of death.

These cases illustrate that indeed occupational asthma can be a severe and even fatal disease. It is quite likely that many more fatalities due to occupational asthma have gone unreported or unrecognized. Demers et al. (25) reviewed death certificates for those who died in Chicago between 1980 and 1988 with asthma cited as the cause of death or a contributing cause of death. Analysis by occupation indicated that bakers had 9 times the age- and race-adjusted rates for the city of Chicago and 41 times the national rate. Painters' and bus drivers' mortality rates were closer to the city rates, but these rates were still 14 and 11 times the national rate. Further, it is also likely that for individuals with poorly controlled nonoccupational asthma certain nonsensitizing irritant exposures can trigger severe attacks requiring increased treatment, medical attention, and/or work absenteeism. Hence, occupational asthma represents a potentially preventable form of severe and/or fatal asthma. Clinicians should be aware of the possibility of occupational asthma in any case of adult- (or working adolescent-) onset asthma. Early recognition and removal from exposure represents an opportunity to prevent asthma progression in the given subject and perhaps prevent asthma onset in others.

IV. Epidemiological Aspects of Occupational Asthma

A. Prevalence of Occupational Asthma

Population-Based Studies

There have been relatively few population-based studies to establish the prevalence of occupational asthma in the general population. Previous studies in the United States have suggested that the prevalence of asthma in the general population is between 3 and 10% (26) and that occupational exposures are the cause in 2 to 15% of adult asthmatics (27). Occupational asthma appears to be on the rise in many industrialized countries, including Japan (28), the United Kingdom (2,3), and Canada (29,30). The 1994 U.S. National Health Interview Survey (NHIS) (31,32) reported an estimated prevalence rate of asthma in 18- to 44-year-olds of 51.7 per 1000 (5.2%), totaling 5.6 million adults. This is higher than that reported in 45- to 64-year-olds (5.1%). Prevalence rates of asthma among the working-age population appear to be increasing, not unlike the increases seen in other sectors of the population. Between the years 1987 and 1994 there was a 42% increase in the U.S. prevalence rate in 18- to 44-year-olds from 36.5 to 51.7 per 1000 (32,33).

There are also data to support a gender difference in prevalence rates in the working population. NHIS data from 1990 to 1992 (34) showed a 40% difference in rates among 18- to 44-year-old females (48 per 1000) and males (34.2 per 1000). Between 1986/1988 and 1990/1992 there was a 20.6% increase among working-age females compared to a 3% increase in working-age males (31).

European data for working-age populations have presented prevalence rates similar to those estimates reported for the United States. The European Community Respiratory Health Survey of 22 countries (35) reported the median prevalence of asthma for those 20 to 44 years old from 1988 to 1994 to be 4.5%. Despite a slightly narrower age range and different criteria for the definition of asthma, this is similar to the NHIS U.S. estimate of 4.1% reported for the time period 1990–1992 for 18- to 44-year-olds.

V. Host Risk Factors

A. Atopy

The fact that not all exposed individuals develop occupational asthma suggests that there are host factors that render certain individuals more susceptible to workplace agents. Since specific IgE antibodies are considered to play a role in many cases of occupational asthma, investigators have studied the role of prior atopy as a risk factor. The data suggest that atopy is a risk factor only for those exposed to high-molecular-weight antigens. For example, there is a high prevalence of skin test-proven atopy among workers with laboratory animal allergy and health care workers who develop latex asthma (36–38). There is no increased prevalence of atopy among asthmatics who respond to the low-molecular-weight plicatic acid found in western red cedar (39) or isocyanates (40). In a study of nonsensitizing occupational asthma, irritant-induced asthma patients were less likely to be atopic (20%) than were asthma controls (58%) (19).

B. Tobacco Smoke

Tobacco smoke has been shown to increase the chance of developing specific IgE antibodies and asthma in the workplace. In a study of workers exposed to tetrachlorophthalic anhydride, a greater proportion of those with specific IgE antibodies to this compound were smokers compared to those who lacked the specific antibody (41). Similar results were observed in response to ispaghula, green coffee bean, and ammonium hexachloroplatinate (37,42). Conversely, a study of sawmill workers exposed to western red cedar indicated that smoking was not associated with increased asthma risk (39). Tobacco smoke may contribute to the risk of irritant-induced asthma, based on the finding of higher numbers of current smokers in this group compared to other asthmatics (19). A group reporting chemical intolerance did not show a higher proportion of smokers compared to asymptomatic normal controls (43).

C. Preexisting Asthma

While it may seem logical to expect patients who have preexisting airways hyperreactivity to be at higher risk of developing occupational asthma, two prospective studies suggest that this is not the case. In studies of TDI-manufacturing workers (44) and western red cedar workers (45), those both with and without prior nonspecific hyperresponsiveness were equally likely to develop occupational asthma.

VI. Socioeconomic Consequences of Occupational Asthma

Due to its effects on the working population, occupational asthma has major socioeconomic consequences. The 1992 NHIS study revealed that asthma was second only to specific musculoskeletal disorders (e.g., back pain) and mental retardation as a primary cause of work limitation (46). It was more likely than diabetes or hypertension to lead to work limitations (Table 1). Comparing NHIS data from 1983 to 1985 (270,000 cases) to those of 1992 (308,000 cases) revealed a 14% increase in the prevalence of asthma-related disability. Interestingly, there was a 24% increase in asthma-related disability the working female population, whereas the increase in the male population was only 6% (46,47). The reason for this gender difference remains unknown.

Table 1 Health Conditions as
Primary Cause of Work Limitation

Condition	Number affected
Back pain	1,051,000
Asthma	308,000
Hypertension	60,000
Diabetes mellitus	147,000

Source: From Ref. 34.

Sibbald and coauthors (48) found that young adults in the UK with current asthma ($n = 192$) or past history of asthma ($n = 1522$) were more likely to be unemployed, have more job changes, and have less full-time employment compared to nonasthmatics ($n = 2505$). In New Zealand, McClellan et al. (49) found that 46% of adult asthmatics felt their disease effected their work activities and that their condition had contributed to dismissal, decreased advancement, and/or poorer work standards. A Singapore study (50) found that 62% of 21- to 58-year-olds missed school or work more than 1 day per year and 21% missed more than 1 week per year.

It is extremely difficult to ascertain all costs, direct and indirect, related to occupational asthma. Based on data from 1985, Weiss et al. (51) estimated that the indirect cost of lost workdays was $684.7 million in 1990 dollars. Comparatively, inpatient care costs were estimated at $869.6 million (physician and hospital services) and total medication costs were $712.7 million. Smith and colleagues used the 1987 National Medical Expenditure Survey (52) to estimate the total indirect costs of asthma to lost labor productivity, including housework, at approximately $242.7 million in 1994 dollars. Barnes et al. (53) reviewed nine primary studies and in a metaanalysis ascertained that the UK and Sweden had high indirect costs, the United States and France had intermediate costs, and Canada and Australia had the lowest indirect costs related to lost work. Taitel et al. (54) estimated that the total lost income was equivalent to 50% of all indirect asthma costs, 17% of the direct medical costs, and 13% of the total costs.

VII. Etiological Agents of Occupational Asthma

There are a number of occupations that present considerable risks for occupational asthma. These include chemical workers, spray painters, plastic and rubber workers, farmers, laboratory workers, food processors, health care workers, textile workers, and leather and wood craftspersons (10). Knowledge of high-risk professions and exposures prepares the physician to ask more informed questions to ascertain a possible occupational cause. Common low-molecular-weight agents known to cause occupational asthma include diisocyanates, acid anhydrides, amine compounds, metals such as platinum and nickel, solder flux (colophony), and wood dust extracts (e.g., plicatic acid from western red cedar). The more common high-molecular-weight agents include various animal proteins from farm or laboratory animals and plant proteins from flour, natural rubber latex, enzymes, and drugs. Tables 2–4 summarize many of the commonly recognized agents and workplaces associated with occupational asthma. For a more complete listing of commonly recognized etiologic agents at present, readers are encouraged to consult one of several recent references (55–58).

Table 2 Selected Examples of High-Molecular-Weight Compounds Causing Occupational Asthma

Agent	Occupation
Animal antigens	
Laboratory animals	Laboratory workers
Chicken	Poultry workers
Pigeons	Bird breeders
Eggs	Bakery workers
Arthropods (arachnids and insects)	
Grain mites	Farmers, grain handlers
Northern fowl mite	Poultry workers
Grain weevil	Laboratory workers
Bean weevil	Seed house workers
Locusts	Laboratory workers
Carmine (*Coccus cactis*)	Cosmetic dye workers
Fruit fly	Laboratory workers
Honey bee	Honey processing plant workers
Daphnia	Fish-food-store workers
Mealworm	Grain, poultry workers
Shellfish and fish	
Crab	Crab processors
Hoya (sea-squirt)	Oyster farming
Prawn	Prawn processors
Trout	Trout processors
Wood dust, bark, plant and vegetable products	
Western red cedar	Woodworkers
	Millers, joiners, carpenters
Eastern white cedar	Woodworkers
Oak, mahogany	Sawmillers, patterns maker
Ash	Woodworkers
California redwood	Carpenters, woodworkers
Grain dust	Grain handlers
	Grain elevator workers
Flour (wheat, buckwheat, rye, and soya)	Bakery workers, millers
Gluten	Bakery workers
Green coffee bean	Food process workers
Tea	Tea processors
Tobacco leaf	Tobacco manufacture
Henna	Hairdressers
Vegetable gums	Printers, gum manufacture
	Carpet manufacturing
Enzymes	
α-Amylase	Bakery workers
Bacillus subtilis	Detergent industry workers
Pancreatic extract	Nurses, pharmaceutical workers
Papain	Pharmaceutical workers
Pepsin	Pharmaceutical workers
Trypsin	Plastics, pharmaceutical workers
Pharmaceuticals	
Ampicillin, penicillins	Pharmaceutical workers
Cephalosporins	Pharmaceutical workers
Isoniazid	Pharmacists
Penicillamine	Pharmaceutical workers
Tetracycline	Pharmaceutical workers
Psyllium	Laxative manufacture
Cimetidine	Pharmaceutical workers
Methyl dopa	Pharmaceutical workers
Hydralazine	Pharmaceutical workers

Table 3 Selected Examples of Low-Molecular-Weight Compounds Causing Occupational Asthma

Agent	Occupation
Amines (aliphatic, aromatic, heterocyclic)	
Ethyleneamines	Shellac, rubber, lacquer handling industries
	Photography
Ethanolamines	Solders
	Spray painters
Paraphenylene diamine	Fur dyers
Piperazine hydrochloride	Chemists, chemical manufacture
Anhydrides	
Phthalic anhydride	Paint, plastics manufacture
Tetrachlorophthalic anhydride	Epoxy resins, plastics manufacture, electronics factory workers
Trimellitic anhydride (TMA)	Paint, chemical workers
Diisocyanates	
Toluene diisocyanate (TDI)	Polyurethane manufacture; plastics, varnish; foam manufacture
Diphenylmethane diisocyanate (MDI)	Foam manufacture; foundry workers
Hexamethylene diisocyanate (HDI)	Spray painters
1,5-Naphthylene diisocyanate	Rubber manufacture
Fluxes	
Colophony	Electronics workers
Zinc chloride and ammonium chloride	Metal joiner
Metals and metal salts	
Aluminum pot room fumes	Pot room workers
Chromium	Electroplating, printers; tanners
Cobalt	Hard metal workers, diamond polishers
Nickel	Electroplating
Platinum	Platinum refiners
Tungsten carbide	Hard metal grinder
Zinc	Solderers, locksmiths
Other chemicals	
Chloramine T	Chemical manufacture
Polyvinyl chloride	Meatwrappers
Organophosphate insecticides	Chemical packaging plant,
Dyes	Textile industry workers, reactive dye manufacture
Persulfates	Hairdressers
Hexachlorophene	Health care workers
Formaldehyde	Health care workers
Urea formaldehyde	Resin manufacture, foam manufacture
Glutaraldehyde	Hospital endoscopy technician
Freon	Refrigeration workers
Styrene	Plastics manufacture
Acrylic	Plastics
Latex	Glove manufacturing, health care workers

Table 4 Selected Examples of Irritant Exposures
Causing Occupational Asthma

Agent	Occupation
Chlorine	Gas leak, pulp mill workers
Diesel exhaust	Railroad workers
Fire smoke	Accidental fire
Glacial acetic acid	Accidental spill
Hydrazine	Power plant worker
Hydrochloric acid	Pool cleaner
Hydrogen sulfide	Agricultural workers
Paints	Spray painters
Perchlorethylene	Dry cleaner
Sulfuric acid	House cleaning
Toluene diisocyanate	Painting
Uranium hexafluoride	Chemical plant worker
Welding fumes	Welders

The following list of the six major categories of agents allows the clinician to quickly screen any asthmatic patient for potential exposures in the workplace that may be causally related to the onset of asthma:

High-molecular-weight agents
    Animals, shellfish, fish, and arthropods
    Wood, vegetables, and plants (including natural rubber latex)
    Enzymes and pharmaceuticals
Low-molecular-weight agents
    Chemicals (including solder fluxes and dyes)
    Metals
Irritants
    Nonsensitizing dusts, fumes, and gases

VIII. Pathophysiology

An extensive review of the pathophysiology of occupational asthma is beyond the scope of this chapter; however, a brief summary of our current understanding will inform the discussion regarding current diagnostic methods and treatment strategies. Asthma is a clinical diagnosis likely having a variety of pathological mechanisms which lead to the final common pathway characterized by variable airflow obstruction and bronchial hyperresponsiveness. Airway inflammation is a critical feature in the pathogenesis of asthma. In occupational asthma substantial evidence indicates that there are both similarities and differences in the inflammatory response to high-molecular-weight and low-molecular-weight agents. High-molecular-weight agents operate, in part, through IgE-mediated mechanisms to produce an immediate, delayed, or dual response (11). Low-molecular-weight agents often act as haptens requiring conjugation to a host protein before initiating an immune response that can also lead to an early, dual, or late response (59). Low-molecular-weight agents likely work through a variety of mechanisms. For example, platinum salts and acid anhydrides commonly produce substantial IgE responses and positive skin prick tests in sensitized individuals, whereas the response in western red cedar- (plicatic acid) or diisocyanate-sensitized individuals is much less predictable (59).

In addition to classic immune response-mediated pathways, there are other mechanisms that are potentially operative in occupational asthma. Direct pharmacological effects on smooth muscle (60), airway microvascular leaks (61–64), or neurogenic inflammation (65–70) have all been suggested as alternative or concomitant pathological responses to workplace exposures. These may be the predominant pathways in irritant-induced asthma, but this remains unknown.

The histological features of occupational asthma with latency have been shown to be similar but not uniformly identical to those found in nonoccupational asthma. High- and low-molecular-weight agents can induce inflammatory cell infiltration with eosinophil, lymphocyte, and mast cell activation (71). Reticular basement membrane thickening has also been noted and this has been shown to be reversible following removal from exposure to occupational sensitizers (72). Epithelial disruption has also been well described in occupational asthma (73,74). The histopathological features of irritant-induced asthma or RADS remain poorly characterized; however, Brooks reported two cases with bronchial epithelial cell desquamation and bronchial wall inflammation including lymphocytes and plasma cells but not eosinophils. There was no mucous gland hyperplasia, basement membrane thickening, or smooth muscle hypertrophy (18). Bernstein et al. described more typical histopathological features of asthma, including denuded epithelium, submucosal chronic inflammation, and collagen proliferation below the basement membrane following anhydrous ammonia exposure (75).

In summary, although occupational asthma appears to share common pathophysiological mechanisms with nonoccupational asthma, there is evidence to suggest potentially unique features, particularly for nonlatent (irritant induced) occupational asthma.

IX. Clinical Assessment

A. History

There are four major goals in obtaining the occupational/environmental history: (1) to generate a list of past and present jobs, especially those jobs that coincide or precede with the onset of asthma symptoms; (2) to outline past and present work practices and exposures, including estimates of the extent of exposure; (3) to assess the likelihood that the asthma condition and the patient's work are linked; and (4) to rule out avocational activities and the home environment as causes or contributing factors for a patient's asthma. Several researchers have published occupational history questionnaire templates (76–83). Table 5 outlines useful aspects of the occupational history that help to identify patients with a high or low probability of having occupational asthma.

All asthmatic patients should be questioned regarding "work-related" patterns. Recognition that a patient is employed in a high-risk industry should lead to increased vigilance to rule out occupational exposures as a factor. Conventionally, we think of the patient with occupational asthma as having progressively worsening symptoms during the work week that improve during weekends and vacations. This pattern, however, is an "ideal" oversimplification and is infrequently practiced at present for several reasons: (1) The workplace sensitizer induces a late-phase reaction that produces the worst symptoms in the evening or at night. Patients with "nocturnal asthma" should be questioned carefully about daytime activities and exposures. (2) The asthmatic may react not only to the occupational antigen or irritant, but also to nonspecific irritants found outside the workplace, thus masking the work-related pattern. (3) If a patient has been symptomatic and remained in exposure for prolonged periods, he or she may lose off-work reversibility.

Significant improvement away from work is usually found during the early stages of occupational asthma but may be lost as the disease progresses with ongoing exposure. A common mistake made by clinicians is to assume that if the symptoms do not improve away from the workplace the asthma must not be

Table 5 Clues That May Improve the Predictive Value of the Occupational History in Asthmatics

1.	Recognition of high-risk jobs
2.	Asking the patient about symptomatic co-workers or co-workers who have left the job because of respiratory health
3.	Allergen effects on other organs, such as rhinitis, conjunctivitis, dermatitis, or urticaria in workers exposed to high-molecular-weight compounds
4.	Unusual events at the time of onset of symptoms, such as a new job assignment, use of a new chemical, or temporal association with accidental exposures to irritants
5.	Failure of the disease to respond to conventional asthma therapy, suggesting possible ongoing exposure to an environmental or occupational trigger
6.	Personal risk factors such as atopy and cigarette smoking

work-related. This error can have dire consequences for the continually exposed asthmatic worker.

B. Assessment of Pulmonary Physiology

The diagnosis of asthma should be confirmed prior to investigating occupational causes. Frequently patients who are referred for evaluation of possible occupational asthma in fact have other diseases that mimic asthma, including hypersensitivity pneumonitis, sarcoidosis, bronchiolitis, or congestive heart failure (84). Perkner et al. (84) have described a series of patients with the presumptive diagnosis of RADS refectory to steroid therapy and other pharmacological intervention, even following removal from ongoing exposure. These patients described subsequent symptoms following exposure to even low levels of nonspecific irritants. These patients demonstrated variable truncation of their flow–volume loops (Fig. 1) and laryngoscopic evidence of paradoxical vocal cord adduction consistent with vocal cord dysfunction (84–86). There are several measures of pulmonary physiology that the clinician has available to assess occupational asthma. The particular clinical scenario and availability of expertise will dictate the choice of appropriate tests.

C. Spirometry and Bronchodilator Response

One of the characteristic features of asthma is variable airflow obstruction. Hence an initial screening for airflow obstruction and bronchodilator response is standard; however, these features are not particularly specific for asthma and may not be present in all cases of occupational asthma. Individuals with early-stage occupational asthma may have normal-range spirometry and exhibit low bronchodilator response. In more severe chronic cases these parameters usually fall in the abnormal range. Additional testing, including nonspecific bronchial provocation testing and/or peak flow monitoring, during times at work and away from work should be conducted.

D. Nonspecific Bronchial Provocation Testing

If the patient with suspected occupational asthma is still working, nonspecific bronchial hyperresponsiveness (NSBH) to histamine or methacholine can be performed on a workday and then reassessed after at least 2 weeks away from work as another means of confirming the work relatedness of the asthma. A recent study by Lemiere et al. (87) suggests that many subjects may require 4 weeks or more away from work before there is a significant improvement in NSBH. If airway hyperresponsiveness improves while away from work, this suggests that something in the workplace is responsible for the hyperreactivity. A negative response to nonspecific bronchial provocation testing in an asthmatic who is still working reduces the likelihood of occupational asthma (88). It should be noted

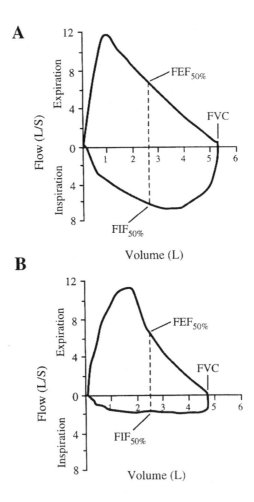

Figure 1 (A) A normal flow–volume loop. (B) Extrathoracic airflow obstruction with truncation of the inspiration loop. This is consistent with symptomatic VCD but may be seen in other laryngeal diseases. FVC, forced vital capacity; FIF_{50}, forced inspiratory flow at 50% forced vital capacity; FEF_{50}, forced expiratory flow at 50% forced vital capacity. (Reproduced with permission from Ref. 84; copyright American College of Occupational and Environmental Medicine.)

that some patients fail to respond to methacholine or histamine but will respond to specific antigen challenge (88).

E. Laryngoscopy

Consideration should be given to evaluating flow–volume loops while performing methacholine inhalation challenge tests to look for evidence of variable extrathoracic airway obstruction or vocal cord dysfunction. If there is any evidence of truncation or irregularity in the flow–volume loops one should perform laryngoscopy to look for evidence of paradoxical vocal cord adduction during the inspiratory and expiratory phases of the breathing cycle (Fig. 2) (84).

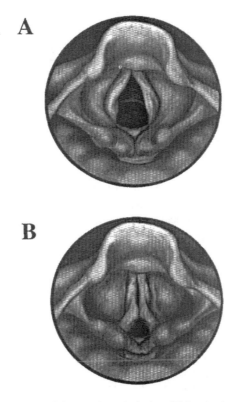

Figure 2 The appearance of the vocal cords during (A) inspiration in a healthy patient and (B) during inspiration in a patient with VCD, showing the adduction of the vocal cords with the characteristic posterior "chink" opening. Illustration by Leigh Landskroner. (Reproduced with permission from Ref. 84; copyright American College of Occupational and Environmental Medicine.)

F. Peak Expiratory Flow Monitoring

Since the late 1970s, peak expiratory flow (PEF) monitoring using portable peak flow meters has been utilized in the assessment of work-related patterns of airflow limitation (89,90). More recently, investigators have proposed the combined use of PEF monitoring plus measures of nonspecific bronchial hyperresponsiveness to assess asthma at work and away from work (91,92). Studies suggest that nonspecific bronchial reactivity does not add much to the sensitivity of PEF records in most circumstances (92,93). When measured under optimal conditions, PEF data can be instructive for the clinician in assessing the work-related patterns. Unfortunately, the quality of PEF varies greatly between individuals, and attention must be paid to the frequency and reproducibility of the measurements. PEF may either underestimate or overestimate the work-related pattern depending on a number of factors, including patient understanding and cooperation, effort, severity of asthma, and presence of nonspecific irritants in the work and nonwork environments (94). A recent study employing computerized peak flows demonstrated poor compliance and fabrication of results in over 40% of the subjects (95). When PEF records were compared with specific inhalation challenge tests (as the "gold standard"), they were 81 to 89% sensitive and 74 to 89% specific (92,93,96). Table 6 outlines general guidelines for optimal use of peak flow monitoring for occupational asthma.

PEF may be used as a screening tool for occupational asthma and in some cases to help confirm the diagnosis and to confirm the response to withdrawal from exposure. At best, PEF data help the physician and patient determine whether the problem is work-related. PEF cannot identify the specific agent or agents in the workplace that are causing the problem. Even if a causative agent is never identified, careful documentation of decreases in PEF related to place of employment is sufficient for recommending a change of the asthmatic's job duties, exposures, or place of employment.

Table 6 Recommendations for the Optimal Use of PEF in Assessing Occupational Asthma

1. Monitor for a minimum of 2 weeks both at work and away from work
2. Sample before, during, and after work on all days of the week, a minimum of four measurement points per day
3. Continue use of inhaled steroids and other medications in a stable fashion for the period of investigation
4. Keep an accompanying diary of information about work hours (especially important for shift workers) and unusual tasks or upset conditions at work or off work

Source: Ref. 91.

G. Temporary Work Restrictions

Temporary work restrictions may help confirm the relationship of the workplace to asthma if performed early in the illness and if adequate objective measures of disease severity are employed both prior to and after removal. Well-documented improvement following a trial removal or restriction may prove that the workplace caused or aggravated the disease. Failure to improve while off work should not be considered definitive evidence that the workplace is not the cause. Unless the patient has severe asthma, we generally advise them not to quit the job until the diagnosis is either excluded or confirmed by additional testing and investigation.

H. Specific Bronchoprovocation Testing

Specific challenge tests are considered the gold standard for diagnosis of occupational asthma (28,97,98). In the appropriate clinical setting, such as when the data gathered from the history of the present illness, the occupational history, pulmonary function tests, investigation of exposures, and PEF data are consistent, a confident diagnosis of occupational asthma can be made without specific challenge testing. In general, specific challenge testing should be reserved for (a) research investigations aimed at identifying possible new causes of asthma and (b) occasions when the patient may otherwise refuse to believe that the causative agent is causing his or her illness and refuses to leave exposure. Challenge testing for medical/legal purposes has been advocated; however, this is not, in and of itself, a sufficiently good reason to perform provocation testing. There is no benefit in using specific challenge testing when the asthma is due to a nonsensitizing exposure unless one is interested in using irritant challenges to elicit vocal cord dysfunction.

Testing should be performed only in specialized centers experienced in the administration of powders, aerosols, and gases; in the monitoring of dose; and in the monitoring and resuscitation of asthmatic patients. The method of administration depends on the suspected agent. One approach is to have the patient mimic his or her work exposure (e.g., pouring the powder) (99). This "Pepys challenge" is crude but often effective. Limitations of these type of challenges are that they are not quantitative and may lead to irritant reactions due to overexposure. More sophisticated testing can be performed using dust or aerosol generators that provide estimates of the dose delivered (100). Because of the possibility of selecting the wrong agent, a patient with true occupational asthma might not react to the specific challenge substance. A patient who is no longer in the workplace may lose antigen-specific reactivity over time (101). If the patient has asthma and the test substance is an irritant at the dose delivered, a false positive response may be observed that is not relevant to either the actual workplace exposure levels or to specific immunological reactivity.

Thus, both false negative and false positive responses can occur. In most centers a significant reaction is defined by a 20% decline in the FEV_1 from baseline/placebo.

When reactions occur, they usually fall into one of several patterns: (1) isolated immediate reactions (10 to 30 min after exposure), (2) isolated late reactions (onset of symptoms usually 1–2 or 4–8 h after exposure), and (3) dual reactions. The immediate and dual types are more commonly seen after exposure to high-molecular-weight agents, whereas isolated late reactions are more common in response to low-molecular-weight compounds, such as isocyanates (102). Some unusual reactions have also been described in response to low-molecular-weight agents, including a "progressive" reaction that starts within minutes and continues to crescendo for 8 h and an immediate reaction in which there is a prolonged recovery phase (102,103).

I. Assessment of Immune Response

The immunologic mechanisms and tests available for diagnosing occupational asthma have been reviewed elsewhere (104). Many workplace agents that cause occupational asthma have allergic properties, but there are multiple other pathogenic mechanisms operative in occupational asthma. In light of the apparent involvement not only of specific immunoglobulins, but also of cell-mediated immunity, chronic and acute inflammation, and other neurophysiological and pharmacological pathways (59), it is not surprising that immunological assessment has only a limited role in the diagnosis of occupational asthma.

High-molecular-weight compounds can induce allergic bronchoconstriction in part by producing specific IgE and in some circumstances specific IgG antibodies. Thus skin testing is often positive, as are some serologic tests, such as radioallergosorbent tests (RAST) and some precipitin tests. Serologic assays have been successfully employed to pinpoint the etiology of occupational asthma for cases involving *Bacillus subtilis* proteolytic enzyme (105), murine urine proteins (106), grain storage mites (107), and locusts (108). Low-molecular-weight compounds may act as haptens, combining with endogenous proteins as has been identified for anhydrides (109–111) and for reactive dyes (112). Establishing that a specific agent causes occupational asthma via an immunological mechanism requires integration with other clinical data. Serial immunological tests may be useful adjuncts for surveillance and possibly prevention of occupational asthma. While it has been shown that T-cell activation is evident in severe asthma (113), the utility of antigen-specific cell-mediated immune assays (CD25 for CD4+ lymphocytes, CD38 for CD8+ lymphocytes and CD69 after antigen stimulation) (114,115) has been studied to only a very limited extent and as yet has no clinical application.

X. Management

Accurate diagnosis has important medical, financial, and psychosocial consequences. Occupational asthma must be distinguished from aggravation of nonoccupational asthma. The latter may be worse at work because the inflammation in the bronchial airways renders them more sensitive to irritants such as smoke, dust, fumes, cold air, and exercise, leading to bronchoconstriction. The narrowing and resulting symptoms are a consequence of suboptimal or difficult-to-control asthma and not of exposure to irritants in the workplace, unless it is considered to be excessive.

It is important to differentiate latent (immune mediated) versus nonlatent (irritant induced) occupational asthma because the management of each is fundamentally different. The primary goal in management of occupational asthma with latency should be avoidance of further exposure to the offending agent. Avoidance can potentially cure this form of asthma. Respiratory protection, using masks, is inadequate protection and should not be considered an option. Low levels of ongoing exposure to antigen can perpetuate asthma in the sensitized individual. Pisati and colleagues (116) studied the medical outcomes for a group of 66 patients with TDI-induced asthma, some of whom remained in exposure. Despite use of respiratory protection, the 17 workers who remained assigned to jobs that had only an occasional risk of exposure to the chemical were compared to the 43 workers who were no longer exposed. The group with ongoing exposure were more symptomatic, required more medication, were considered clinically unstable, and demonstrated significant deterioration in FEV_1 and PC_{15} for methacholine. No worker who had been exposed to isocyanates for more than 10 years or who continued to work for more than 3 years after onset of asthma recovered. This study emphasizes the need to recognize occupational asthma early, the limitations of respiratory protection, and the central importance of eliminating further exposure.

Pharmacological treatment is the same as that for nonoccupational asthma, including the judicious use of systemic and inhaled steroids and bronchodilator medications (11). In rare circumstances, such as animal dander allergy, immunotherapy may be used as an adjunct in treatment (117); however, this should not be considered an option for chemical sensitizers, considering the unknown risks regarding toxicity and/or carcinogenicity. After a period of removal from the offending exposure, a minority of individuals will be able to discontinue all asthma medication, whereas the majority will need maintenance medication, perhaps at lower doses than initially prescribed.

In contrast, nonlatent (irritant induced) asthma or RADS patients may be able to remain in their job provided there have been changes that reduce the risk of further irritant exposure or industrial accident. Job process modifications may include substitution with safer substances, process isolation (i.e., enclosure), improved ventilation, and/or the use of personal protective equipment (respirators). Certain individuals will continue to report symptoms to even low-level exposures to the offending agent. In these circumstances attempts should be made to accommodate them in alternative locations or jobs. Respirators are uncomfortable and cumbersome to wear for a full work shift, making compliance a major problem. Pharmacological treatment is the same as that for latent (immune-mediated) occupational asthma. Some of these patients may have developed irritant-associated vocal cord dysfunction and may benefit from speech therapy instruction on throat relaxation, cough, and throat clearing suppression and breathing control techniques (84). Many of these individuals demonstrate evidence for gastroesophageal reflux disease and or rhinitis with postnasal drip. Treatment of these disorders will improve the vocal cord dysfunction.

Workplace aggravation of underlying asthma results usually from direct irritant effects by nonsensitizing stimuli such as smoke, dust, fumes, cold air, and exertion. Nonoccupational asthma aggravated by workplace exposure requires increased standard treatment with anti-inflammatory medication to better control the asthma and may or may not require a job change. Engineering controls to reduce exposure levels can benefit this group. These individuals may also develop irritant-associated vocal cord dysfunction and benefit from speech therapy.

Regardless of the type of asthma, one should always take the opportunity to discourage tobacco smoking, which is likely to exacerbate symptoms.

XI. Prognosis

The majority of patients with occupational asthma are left with some degree of permanent impairment. Several studies demonstrate that the majority of subjects fail to completely recover, even after leaving the site of exposure (116,118–120). Continued exposure after the onset of symptoms often leads to more severe asthma that persists even when exposure is eventually discontinued (11,55,116). These studies emphasize the need for early diagnosis, removal from the site of exposure, and appropriate treatment. To date, we do not know if there are significant differences in prognosis between latent and nonlatent occupational asthma. Brooks reported long-term persistent reactive airway disease in individuals who developed RADS (18).

XII. Prevention

When a case has been identified, employers should be informed that a worker has developed occupational asthma. Ideally, this should result in industrial hygiene efforts to prevent or minimize the risk for other workers becoming sensitized. Although it is recognized that sensitization can theoretically occur even at low-level exposures, there does seem to be an increased incidence of sensitization with higher level exposures (22,121). Threshold limit values (TLV) and peak exposure levels (PEL) are established to minimize toxic and irritant effects but are not a good standard to prevent sensitization. Employers need to know that if they use potential sensitizers in their workplace, no known level of exposure is absolutely protective against developing sensitization and that TLV and PEL values are irrelevant. The goal should be to reduce all exposures to the lowest possible levels for all workers. In cases where RADS develops as a result of an accidental spill, work procedures should be reviewed for any possible remedial strategies that might prevent a recurrence.

Even though prior atopy to common allergens appears to be a risk factor for high-molecular-weight antigen-induced asthma, it should not be used to exclude workers from employment. The positive predictive value of atopy for occupational asthma is insufficient to recommend its use in hiring and placement practices at work (36,122,123). Allergy skin tests should not be used to exclude workers from high-risk occupations. Knowledge of a person's atopic status can be used to help counsel employees that they are at a statistically higher risk of developing asthma on the job. This information can lead to appropriate precautions to minimize their exposure to high-molecular-weight antigens. It is prudent to closely monitor such workers for early signs of asthma.

In settings where medical surveillance for occupational sensitization and/or asthma is deemed appropriate, the physician can employ routine health surveys, serially monitor lung function, and consider the use of immunological markers of exposure. Although potentially helpful in identifying disease at early stages, these medical monitoring tools are less effective than those that reduce exposure (i.e., primary prevention).

XIII. Workers' Compensation

When a case of occupational asthma is confirmed, the physician should advise the patient that in the United States, as in many other industrialized countries, this is considered a work-related illness and that they are entitled to file for workers' compensation. Compensation will help cover medical expenses due to the illness and provide a reward commensurate with the degree of functional impairment and loss of past and future wage-earning potential due to the work-related illness.

XIV. Impairment and Disability Evaluations

Physicians may be called upon to assess whether the patient has reached "maximum medical improvement" before providing a permanent impairment rating.

This is defined as the point in time after which it is unlikely that the patient will improve further. At that juncture, the physician will be asked to assess the level of permanent impairment that has resulted from occupational asthma. Although most patients do not return to their premorbid status, progressive improvement may occur for up to 2 years after cessation of exposure (118). For this reason, it is advisable to wait 2 years before declaring the patient to be maximally medically improved (MMI) and assigning a permanent impairment rating (118). It remains somewhat debatable as to whether it is absolutely necessary to wait for 2 years to judge maximal medical improvement in every patient with occupational asthma. It may be practical and appropriate to declare the patient to be at MMI earlier than 2 years after ceasing exposure if the patient (1) has been removed from exposure for at least 6 months, (2) has relatively normal spirometry, (3) has minimal bronchodilator response or bronchial hyperresponsiveness, and (4) is clinically stable on minimum medication for at least 6 to 12 months. This decision ultimately rests on the clinical judgement of the attending physician.

Occupational asthma requires special evaluation when assessing impairment and disability. Strict adherence to the American Medical Association's *Guides to the Evaluation of Permanent Impairment* (124) is inadequate. The AMA guidelines place occupational asthma in a special category requiring special consideration based on the variable and somewhat unpredictable nature of the condition. The rating of impairment can range from 0%, if the patient has fully recovered and has no persistent airways hyperreactivity, to 100% impairment for the most severe, debilitating steroid-dependent asthma. Useful guidelines for assessing asthma impairment have been published by the American Thoracic Society (125). The important parameters to consider for assessment of impairment include (1) the postbronchodilator FEV_1, (2) the degree of bronchodilator response (%change in FEV_1) or nonspecific airway hyperresponsiveness (methacholine or histamine PC20), and (3) the minimum corticosteroid medication requirement to maintain clinical stability.

XV. Conclusions

Reversing the increasing prevalence of occupational asthma will require improved disease surveillance and improved physician recognition. This starts with the simple but often neglected question, "What type of work do you do?" The role of clinicians should be to work with industry, labor, government agencies, and specialists in the field of occupational health to prevent disease through early identification of old and new hazards. We should consider each patient with occupational asthma as a "sentinel health event" and seek consultation with those who can help initiate the investigative activities that will improve workplace conditions for all workers.

References

1. Lagier F, Cartier A, Malo JL. Statistiques medico-legales sur l'asthme professionel au Quebec de 1986 a 1988: medico-legal statistics on occupational asthma in Quebec between 1986 and 1988. Rev Mal Respir 1990; 7:337–341.
2. Meredith SK, Taylor VM, McDonald JC. Occupational respiratory disease in the United Kingdom 1989: a report to the British Thoracic Society and the Society and the Society of Occupational Medicine by the SWORD project group. Br J Ind Med 1991; 48:292–298.
3. Ross DJ, Keynes HL, McDonald JC. SWORD '96: Surveillance of work-related and occupational respiratory disease in the United Kingdom. Occup Med (Oxf) 1997; 47:377–381.
4. Reilly MJ, Rosenman KD, Watt FC, et al. Surveillance for occupational asthma: Michigan and New Jersey, 1988–1992. MMWR CDC Surveill Summ 1994; 43: 9–17.
5. Keskinen H, Alanko K, Saarinen L. Occupational asthma in Finland. Clin Allergy 1978; 8:569–579.
6. Contreras GR, Rousseau R, Chang-Yeung M. Occupational respiratory diseases in British Columbia, Canada in 1991. Occup Environ Med 1994; 51:710–712.
7. Brooks SM. Bronchial asthma of occupational origin: a review. Scand J Work Environ Health 1977; 3:53–72.
8. Kobayashi S. Different aspects of occupational asthma in Japan. In: Frazier CA, ed. Occupational Asthma. New York: Van Nostrand–Reinhold, 1980:229–244.
9. Syabbalo N. Occupational asthma in a developing country (Letter). Chest 1991; 99:528.
10. Fishwick D, Pearce N, D'Souza W, et al. Occupational asthma in New Zealanders: a population based study. Occup Environ Med 1997; 54:301–306.
11. Chan-Yeung M, Malo J-L. Current concepts: occupational asthma. N Engl J Med 1995; 333:107–112.
12. Bernstein DI, Korbee L, Stauder T, et al. The low prevalence of occupational asthma and antibody-dependent sensitization to diphenylmethane diisocyanate in a plant engineered for minimal exposure to diisocyanates. J Allergy Clin Immunol 1993; 92:387–396.
13. Bernstein IL, Bernstein DI, Chan-Yeung M, Malo J-L. Definition and classification of asthma. In: Bernstein IL, Chan-Yeung M, Malo J-L, Bernstein DI, eds. Asthma in the Workplace. New York: Marcel Dekker, 1993:1–4.
14. Bernstein IL, Chan-Yeung M, Malo J-L, Bernstein DI. Asthma in the Workplace. New York: Marcel Dekker, 1993:655.
15. Carino M, Aliani M, Licitra C, Sarno N, Ioli F. Death due to asthma at workplace in a diphenylmethane diisocyanate-sensitized subjects. Respiration 1997; 64:111–113.
16. Ehrlich RI. Fatal asthma in a baker: a case report. Am J Intern Med 1994; 26:799–802.
17. Fabbri LM, Danieli D, Crescioli S, et al. Fatal asthma in a subject sensitized to toluene diisocyanate. Am Rev Respir Dis 1988; 137:1494–1498.

18. Brooks SM, Weiss MA, Bernstein IL. Reactive airways dysfunction syndromes (RADS): persistent asthma syndrome after high level irritant exposures. Chest 1985; 88:376–384.
19. Tarlo SM, Broder I. Irritant-induced occupational asthma. Chest 1989; 96:297–300.
20. Merchant JA, Bernstein IL. Cotton and other textile dusts. In: Bernstein IL, Chan-Yeung M, Bernstein DI, eds. Asthma in the Workplace. New York: Marcel Dekker, 1993:551–576.
21. Palczynski C, Walusiak J, Ruta U, Gorski P. Occupational allergy to latex—life threatening reactions in health care workers. Report of three cases. Int J Occup Med Environ Health 1997; 10:297–301.
22. Baur X, Chen Z, Allmers H. Can a threshold limit value for natural rubber latex airborne allergens be defined? J Allergy Clin Immunol 1998; 101:24–27.
23. Watt AD, McSharry CP. Laboratory animal allergy: anaphylaxis from a needle injury. Occup Environ Med 1996; 53:573–574.
24. Anonymous. Terfenadine approved for allergic rhinitis. FDA Drug Bull 1985; 15:20.
25. DeMers MP, Orris P. Occupational exposure and asthma mortality. J Am Med Assoc 1994; 272:1575.
26. Becklake MR. Epidemiology: prevalence and determinants. In: Bernstein IL, Chan-Yeung M, Malo J-L, Bernstein DI, eds. Asthma in the Workplace. New York: Marcel Dekker, 1993:29–60.
27. Blanc P. Occupational asthma in a national disability survey. Chest 1987; 92:613–617.
28. Chan-Yeung M, Lam S. Occupational asthma: state of the art. Am Rev Respir Dis 1986; 133:686–703.
29. Malo J-L. Compensation for occupational asthma in Quebec. Chest 1990; 98:236S–239S.
30. Provencher S, Labreche FP, De Guire L. Physician-based surveillance system for occupational respiratory diseases: the experience of PROPULSE, Quebec, Canada. Occup Environ Med 1997; 54:272–276.
31. Blanc P. Characterizing the occupational impact of asthma. In: Weiss KB, Buist AS, Sullivan SD, eds. Asthma's Impact on Society. New York: Marcel Dekker, 2000:55–75.
32. Services USDoHaH. Vital and Health Statistics: Current Estimates from the National Health Interview Survey. Series 10, Data from the National Health Survey, No. 193. Hyattsville, MD: DHHS Publication No. PHS 96-1521, 1996.
33. Collins JG. Vital and Health Statistics: Prevalence of Selected Chronic Conditions: United States, 1986–1988. Series 10, Data from the National Health Survey, No. 182. Hyattsville, MD: DHHS, 1993.
34. Collins JG. Vital and Health Statistics: Prevalence of Selected Chronic Conditions: United States, 1990–1992. Series 10, Data from the National Health Survey, No. 194. Hyattsville, MD: DHHS, 1997.
35. Survey ECRH. Variations in the prevalence of respiratory symptoms, self-reported asthma attacks, and use of asthma medication in the European Community Respiratory Health Survey (ECRHS). Eur Respir J 1996; 9:687–695.

36. Slovak AJM, Hill RN. Does atopy have any predictive value for laboratory animal allergy? A comparison of different concepts of atopy. Br J Ind Med 1987; 44:129–132.

37. Venables KM, Dally MB, Nunn AJ, et al. Smoking and occupational allergy in workers in a platinum refinery. Br Med J 1989; 299:939–942.

38. Lagier F, Vervloet D, Lhermet I, Poyen D, Charpin D. Prevalence of latex allergy in operating room nurses. J Allergy Clin Immunol 1992; 90:319–322.

39. Chan-Yeung M, Lam S, Koener S. Clinical features and natural history of occupational asthma due to Western Red Cedar (Thuja plicata). Am J Med 1982; 72:411–415.

40. Grammer LC, Harris KE, Malo JL, Cartier A, Patterson R. The use of an immunoassay index for antibodies against isocyanate human protein conjugates and application to human isocyanate disease. J Allergy Clin Immunol 1990; 86:94–98.

41. Venables KM, Topping MD, Howe W, Luczynska CM, Hawkins R, Newman Taylor AJ. Interaction of smoking and atopy in producing specific IgE antibody against a hapten protein conjugate. Br Med J 1985; 290:201–204.

42. Zetterstrom O, Osterman K, McHardo L, Johansson SGO. Another smoking hazard: raised serum IgE concentration and increased risk of occupational allergy. Br Med J 1981; 283:1215–1217.

43. Baldwin CM, Bell IR, O'Rourke MK, Lebowitz MD. The association of respiratory problems in a community sample with self-reported chemical intolerance. Eur Epidemiol 1997; 13:547–552.

44. Butcher BT, Jones RN, O'Neill CE, et al. Longitudinal study of workers employed in the manufacture of toluene diisocyanate. Am Rev Respir Dis 1977; 116:411–421.

45. Chan-Yeung M, Desjardins A. Bronchial hyperresponsiveness and level of exposure in occupational asthma due to Western Red Cedar (Thuja plicata). Am Rev Respir Dis 1992; 146:1606–1609.

46. LaPlante MP, Carlson D. Disability in the United States: Prevalence and Causes, 1992. Washington, DC: National Institute on Disability and Rehabilitation Research, 1996.

47. LaPlante MP. Data on Disability from the National Health Interview Survey, 1983–1985: An InfoUse report. Washington, DC: U.S. National Insitute on Disability and Rehabilitation Research, 1988.

48. Sibbald R, Anderson HR, McGuigan S. Asthma and employment in young adults. Thorax 1992; 47:19–24.

49. McClellan VE, Garrett JE. Asthma and the employment experience. N Z Med J 1990; 103:399–401.

50. Goh L, Ng T, Hong C, Wong M, Koh K, Ling S. Outpatient adult bronchial asthma in Singapore. Singapore Med J 1994; 35:190–194.

51. Weiss KB, Gergen PJ, Hodgson TA. An economic evaluation of asthma in the United States. N Engl J Med 1992; 326:862–866.

52. Smith DH, Maline DC, Lawson KA, Okamoto LJ, Battista C, Saunders WB. A national estimate of the economic costs of asthma. Am J Respir Crit Care Med 1997; 156:787–793.

53. Barnes PJ, Jonsson B, Klim JB. The costs of asthma. Eur Respir J 1996; 9:636–642.

54. Taitel MS, Kotses H, Bernstein IL, Bernstein DI, Creer TL. A self-management program for adult asthma. Part II: cost–benefit analysis. J Allergy Clin Immunol 1995; 95:672–676.

55. Chan PC, Eustis SL, Huff JE, Haseman JK, Ragan H. Two-year inhalation carcinogenesis studies of methyl methacrylate in rats and mice: inflammation and degeneration of nasal epithelium. Toxicology 1988; 52:237–252.

56. Chan-Yeung M, Malo J-L. Aetiologic agents in occupational asthma. Eur Respir J 1994; 7:346–371.

57. Newman Taylor AJ, Pickering CAC. Occupational asthma and byssinosis. In: Parkes WR, ed. Occupational Lung Disorders. Oxford: Butterworth–Heinemann, 1994:710–754.

58. Chan-Yeung M, Malo J-L. Natural history of asthma. In: Bernstein IL, Chan-Yeung M, Malo J-L, Bernstein DI, eds. Asthma in the Workplace. New York: Marcel Dekker, 1993:299–322.

59. Fabbri LM, Ciaccia A, Maestrelli P, Saetta M, Mapp CE. Pathophysiology of occupational asthma. In: Bernstein IL, Chan-Yeung M, Malo J-L, Bernstein DI, eds. Asthma in the Workplace. New York: Marcel Dekker, 1993:61–92.

60. Kumar A, Busse WW. Eosinophils in asthma. In: Holgate ST, Busse WW, eds. Inflammatory Mechanisms in Asthma. New York: Marcel Dekker, 1998: Chapter 13.

61. Fabbri LM, Boschetto P, Zocca E, et al. Bronchoalveolar neutrophilia during late asthmatic reactions induced by toluene diisocyanate. Am Rev Respir Dis 1987; 136:36–42.

62. Lam S, LeRiche J, Phillips D, Chan-Yeung M. Cellular and protein changes in bronchial lavage fluid after late asthmatic reaction in patients with red cedar asthma. J Allergy Clin Immunol 1987; 80:44–50.

63. O'Byrne P. Mechanisms of Airway Hyperresponsiveness. In: Holgate ST, Busse WW, eds. Inflammatory Mechanisms in Asthma. New York: Marcel Dekker, 1998.

64. Persson C. Microvascular-epithelial exudation of bulk plasma on airway defense, disease and repair. In: Holgate ST, Busse WW, eds. Inflammatory Mechanisms in Asthma. New York: Marcel Dekker, 1998.

65. Barnes PJ, Baraniuk JN, Belvisi MG. Neuropeptides in the respiratory tract. Part II. Am Rev Respir Dis 1991; 144:1391–1399.

66. Barnes PJ, Baraniuk JN, Belvisi MG. Neuropeptides in the respiratory tract. Part I. Am Rev Respir Dis 1991; 144:1187–1198.

67. Nadel JA. Neutral endopeptidase modulates neurogenic inflammation. Eur Respir J 1991; 4:745–754.

68. Ollerenshaw SL, Jarvis D, Sullivan CE, Woolcock AJ. Substance P immunoreactive nerves from asthmatics and nonasthmatics. Eur Respir J 1991; 4:673–682.

69. Ollerenshaw LS, Jarvis D, Woolcock AJ, Sullivan CE, Scheibner T. Absence of immunoreactive vasoactive intestinal polypetide in tissue from the lungs of patients with asthma. N Engl J Med 1991; 320:1244–1248.

70. Mapp C, Boschetto P, Miotto D, De Rosa E, Fabbri LM. Mechanisms of occupational asthma. Ann Allergy Asthma Immunol 1999; 83:645–664.

71. Saetta M, DiStefano A, Maestrelli P, et al. Airway mucosal inflammation in occupational asthma induced by toluene diisocyanate. Am Rev Respir Dis 1992; 145:160–168.

72. Saetta M, Maestrelli P, Di Stefano A, et al. Effect of cessation of exposure to toluene diisocyanate (TDI) on bronchial mucosa of subjects with TDI-induced asthma. Am Rev Respir Dis 1992; 145:169–174.

73. Knobil K, Jacoby DB. Mediator functions and epithelial cells. In: Holgate ST, Busse WW, eds. Inflammatory Mechanisms in Asthma. New York: Marcel Dekker, 1998:Chapter 22.

74. White SR, Leff AR. Epithelium as a target. In: Holgate ST, Busse WW, eds. Inflammatory Mechanisms in Asthma. New York: Marcel Dekker, 1998.

75. Bernstein DI, Zeiss CR. Guidelines for preparation and characterization of characterization of chemical–protein conjugate antigens: report of the Subcommittee on Preparation and Characterization of Low Molecular Weight Antigens. J Allergy Clin Immunol 1989; 84:820–822.

76. Brooks SM. An approach to patients suspected of having an occupational pulmonary disease. Clin Chest Med 1981; 2:171–178.

77. Goldman RM, Peters JM. The occupational and environmental health history. J Am Med Assoc 1981; 246:2831–2836.

78. LaDou J. Approach to the diagnosis of occupational illness. In: LaDou J, ed. Occupational Medicine. Los Altos: Lange Medical Book, 1990:5–16.

79. Schwartz DA, Wakefield DS, Fieselmann JF, Berger-Wesley M, Zeitler R. The occupational history in the primary care setting. Am J Med 1991; 90:315–319.

80. Rosenstock L, Logerfo J, Heyer NJ, Carter WB. Development and validation of a self-administered occupational health questionnaire. J Occup Med 1984; 26:50–54.

81. Coye MJ, Rosenstock L. The occupational health history in a family practice setting. Am Fam Physician 1983; 28:229–234.

82. Frank AL, Balk SJ. Monograph 26: Case Studies in Environmental Medicine: Taking an Exposure History. Atlanta: U.S. Department of Health and Human Services, Public Health Service, Agency for Toxic Substances and Disease Registry and Centers for Disease Control and Prevention, National Institute for Occupational Safety and Health, 1992.

83. Levy BS, Wegman DH. The occupational history in medical practice: What questions to ask and when to ask them. Postgrad Med 1986; 79:301–311.

84. Perkner JJ, Fennelly KP, Balkissoon R, et al. Irritant-associated vocal cord dysfunction. J Occup Environ Med 1998; 40:136–143.

85. Hjörtsberg U, Orbaek P, Arborelius M Jr, Karlsson J-E. Upper airway irritation and small airways hyperreactivity due to exposure to potassium aluminum tetrafluoride flux: an extended case report. Occup Environ Med 1994; 51:706–709.

86. Sala E, Hytönen E, Tupasela O, Estlander T. Occupational laryngitis with immediate allergic or immediate type specific chemical hypersensitivity. Clin Otolaryngol 1996; 21:42–48.

87. Lemiere C, Pizzichinni M, Balkissoon R, et al. Diagnosing occupational asthma: use of induced sputum. Eur Respir J 1998.

88. Hargreave FE, Ramsdale EM, Pugsley SO. Occupational asthma without bronchial hyperresponsiveness. Am Rev Respir Dis 1984; 130:513–515.

89. Burge PS, O'Brien I, Harries M. Peak flow rate records in the diagnosis of occupational asthma due to colophony. Thorax 1979; 34:308–316.

90. Burge PS, O'Brien I, Harries M. Peak flow rate records in the diagnosis of occupational asthma due to isocyanates. Thorax 1979; 34:317–323.

91. Cartier A, Pineau L, Malo J-L. Monitoring of maximum peak expiratory flow rates and histamine inhalation tests in the investigation of occupational asthma. Clin Allergy 1984; 14:193–196.

92. Perrin B, Lagier F, L'Archeveque J, et al. Occupational asthma: validity of monitoring of peak expiratory flow rates and non-allergic bronchial responsiveness as compared to specific inhalation challenge. Eur Respir J 1992; 5:40–48.

93. Côte J, Kennedy S, Chan-Yeung M. Sensitivity and specificity of PC20 and peak expiratory flow rate in cedar asthma. J Allergy Clin Immunol 1991; 85:592–598.

94. Bérubé D, Cartier A, L'Archeveque J, Ghezzo H, Malo J-L. comparison of peak expiratory flow rate and FEV_1 in assessing bronchomotor tone after challenges with occupational sensitizers. Chest 1991; 99:831–836.

95. Quirce S, Contreras G, Moran O, et al. Laboratory and clinical evaluation of a portable computerized peak flow meter. J Asthma 1997; 34:305–315.

96. Coté J, Kennedy S, Chan-Yeung M. Sensitivity and specificity of PC_{20} and peak expiratory flow rate in cedar asthma. J Allergy Clin Immunol 1990; 85:592–598.

97. Cartier A, Malo J-L. Occupational challenge tests. In: Bernstein IL, Chan-Yeung M, Malo J-L, Bernstein DI, eds. Asthma in the Workplace. New York: Marcel Dekker, 1993:215–247.

98. Cartier A, Bernstein IL, Burge PS, et al. Guidelines for bronchoprovocation on the investigation of occupational asthma: report of the Subcommittee on Bronchoprovocation for Occupational Asthma. J Allergy Clin Immunol 1989; 84:823–829.

99. Pepys J, Hutchcroft BJ. Bronchial provocation tests in etiologic diagnosis and analysis of asthma. Am Rev Respir Dis 1975; 112:829–859.

100. Cloutier Y, Malo JL. Update on an exposure system for particles in the diagnosis of occupational asthma. Eur Respir J 1992; 5:887–890.

101. Cartier A, Malo J-L, Forest F, et al. Occupational asthma in snow crab-processing workers. J Allergy Clin Immunol 1984; 74:261–269.

102. Perrin B, Cartier A, Ghezzo H, et al. Reassessment of the temporal patterns of bronchial obstruction after exposure to occupational sensitizing agents. J Allergy Clin Immunol 1991; 87:630–639.

103. Zammit-Tabona M, Sherkin M, Kijek K, Chan H, Chan-Yeung M. Asthma caused by dimethyl methane diisocyanate in foundry workers: clinical, bronchial provocation, and immunologic studies. Am Rev Respir Dis 1983; 128:226–230.

104. Newman L, Storey E, Kreiss K. Immunologic evaluation of occupational lung disease. In: Rosenstock L, ed. Occupational Medicine: State of the Art Reviews. Philadelphia: Hanley and Belfus, 1987:345–372.

105. Pepys J, Wells ED, D'Souza M, Greenburg M. Clincial and immunological responses to enzymes of Bacillus subtilis in factor workers and consumers. Clin Allergy 1973; 3:143–160.

106. Newman Taylor AJ, Longbottom JL, Pepys J. Respiratory allergy to urine proteins of rats and mice. Lancet 1977; 2:847–849.
107. Ingram CG, Jeffrey IG, Symington IS, Cuthbert OD. Bronchial provocation studies in farmers allergic to storage mites. Lancet 1979; 2:1330–1332.
108. Tee RD, Gordon DJ, Hawkins ER, et al. Occupational allergy to locusts: an investigation of the sources of the allergen. J Allergy Clin Immunol 1988; 81:517–525.
109. Maccia CA, Bernstein IL, Emmett EA, Brookes SSM. In vitro demonstration of specific IgE in phthalic anhydride sensitivity. Am Rev Respir Dis 1976; 113:701–704.
110. Zeiss CR, Patterson R, Pruzansky JJ, Miller MM, Rosenberg M, Levitz D. Trimellitic anhydride-induced airway syndromes: clinical and immunologic studies. J Allergy Clin Immunol 1977; 60:96–103.
111. Howe W, Venables KM, Topping MD, et al. Tetrachlorophthalic anhydride asthma: evidence for specific IgE antibody. J Allergy Clin Immunol 1983; 71:5–11.
112. Luczynska CM, Topping MD. Specific IgE antibodies to reactive dye-albumin conjugates. J Immunol Methods 1986; 95:177–186.
113. Corrigan CJ, Kay AB. CD4 T lymphocyte activation in acute severe asthma: relationship to disease severity and atopic status. Am Rev Respir Dis 1990; 141:970–977.
114. Adelman DC, Functional assessment of mononuclear cells. Immunol Clin North Am 1994; 14:241–263.
115. Lopez-Cabrera M, Santis AG, Fernandez-Ruiz R, Esch F, Sanchez-Mateos P, Sanchez-Madrid F. Molecular cloning, expression, and chromosomal localization of the human earliest lymphocyte activation antigen AIM/CD69, a new member of the C-type animal lectin superfamily of signal transmitting receptors. J Exp Med 1993; 178:537–547.
116. Pisati G, Baruffini A, Zedda S. Toluene diisocyanate induced asthma: outcome according to persistence or cessation of exposure. Br J Ind Med 1993; 50:60–64.
117. Wahn Y, Siraganian RP. Efficacy and specificity of immunotherapy with laboratory animal allergen extracts. J Allergy Clin Immunol 1980; 65:413–421.
118. Malo JL, Cartier A, Ghezzo H, Lafrance M, McCants M, Lehrer SB. Patterns of improvement on spirometry, bronchial hyperresponsiveness and specific IgE antibody levels after cessation of exposure in occupational asthma caused by snow-crab processing. Am Rev Respir Dis 1988; 138:807–812.
119. Chan-Yeung M. State-of-the-art: Occupational asthma. Chest 1990; 98:148S–161S.
120. Lemiere C, Cartier A, Dolovich J, et al. Outcome of specific bronchial responsiveness to occupational agents after removal from exposure. Am J Respir Crit. Care Med 1996; 154:329–333.
121. Bernstein DI, Zeiss CR, Wolkonsky P, Levitz D, Roberts M, Patterson R. The relationship of total serum IgE and blocking antibody in trimellitic anhydride-induced occupational asthma. J Allergy Clin Immunol 1983; 72:714–719.
122. Venables KM. Prevention of occupational asthma. Eur Respir J 1994; 7:768–778.
123. Venables KM, Topping MD, Nunn AJ, Howe W, Newman Taylor AJ. Immunologic and functional consequences of chemical (tetrachlorophthalic anhydride) induced

asthma after 4 years of avoidance of exposure. J Allergy Clin Immunol 1987; 80: 212–218.

124. American Medical Association: Guides to the Evaluation of Permanent Impairment. Chicago: American Medical Association, 1993.

125. Chan-Yeung M, Malo J-L. Compendium I: Table of the major inducers of occupational asthma. In: Bernstein IL, Chan-Yeung M, Malo J-L, Bernstein DI, eds. Asthma in the Workplace. New York: Marcel Dekker, 1993:595–623.

18

Clinical Significance of Rhinosinusitis in Severe Asthma and Its Management

DANIEL L. HAMILOS

Washington University School of Medicine
St. Louis, Missouri

I. Introduction

Rhinosinusitis is common in patients with asthma, and there is a widely held view that it contributes to asthma severity. Many patients report that their asthma is primarily driven by their sinus symptoms. What actually accounts for these relationships? This controversial topic is the subject of this chapter.

II. Definition of Rhinosinusitis

Historically, inflammatory diseases of the upper airway, namely rhinitis and sinusitis, were regarded as distinct entities. In 1996, a Task Force was created by the American Association of Otorhinolaryngologists–Head and Neck Surgeons to develop a consensus definition of rhinosinusitis (1). One impetus for this effort was to focus greater attention on important interrelationships between nasal and sinus pathology. A second impetus was the general consensus that sinusitis is often preceded by rhinitis and rarely occurs without associated rhinitis. The Task Force recommended replacing the term "sinusitis" with "rhinosinusitis." Rhinosinusitis was defined as an inflammatory response involving the mucus membranes of the nasal cavity and paranasal sinuses and fluids within these cavities and/or underlying bone. As an extension of this definition, chronic rhinosinusitis was defined as rhinosinusitis lasting longer than 12 weeks.

Rhinosinusitis was defined as a clinical condition independent of physical examination or radiographic findings. Symptoms of rhinosinusitis most commonly include nasal obstruction, nasal congestion, nasal discharge, nasal purulence, postnasal drip, facial pressure and pain, alteration in the sense of smell, cough, fever, halitosis, fatigue, dental pain, pharyngitis, otologic symptoms (e.g., ear fullness and clicking), and headache (1).

There is little doubt that the future will see broader application of the term "rhinosinusitis" in clinical studies. However, prior to the year 2000 most studies relating upper airway disease to asthma classified patients as having either rhinitis or sinusitis. With this in mind, the studies of the potential relationships between rhinitis and sinusitis and asthma are reviewed.

III. Spectrum and Prevalence of Rhinosinusitis and Asthma

The clinical presentations of rhinosinusitis with or without asthma can be summarized as follows: allergic rhinitis (seasonal or perennial), allergic rhinitis (seasonal or perennial) with asthma, perennial nonallergic rhinitis [vasomotor or nonallergic rhinitis with eosinophilia (NARES)], perennial nonallergic rhinitis with nonallergic (intrinsic) asthma, chronic sinusitis, chronic sinusitis with asthma, and chronic sinusitis with nasal polyposis and asthma ("triad asthma" or Samter's syndrome).

While severe asthma may exist in association with any one of these conditions, certain generalities can be made (see Fig. 1). It is estimated that the prevalence of asthma in patients with allergic rhinitis is 17–38%, which exceeds that in the general population (approximately 5–8%) (2,3). Furthermore, nonspecific bronchial hyperresponsiveness has been reported with a prevalence of 20–30% in nonasthmatic patients with allergic rhinitis (3,4). Family studies in northern Sweden suggest a genetic linkage between allergic rhinitis and allergic asthma, which is consistent with current thinking about genetic factors in allergic disease (3). Perennial nonallergic rhinitis (PNAR) is diagnosed in approximately 20–30% of adult patients with rhinosinusitis (5). It is a poorly understood disease that may be broken down into "infectious rhinosinusitis," vasomotor rhinitis, and NARES. However, most epidemiologic studies have not broken down PNAR into subcategories. Asthma has been reported to be less prevalent in PNAR than in allergic rhinitis in one Swedish study (25% vs. 40%) (6) and one U.S. study (33%) (7). However, one recent study found that patients with PNAR had increased bronchial hyperresponsiveness to a degree similar to that of patients with allergic rhinitis (8). The NARES syndrome is rare and has been diagnosed in

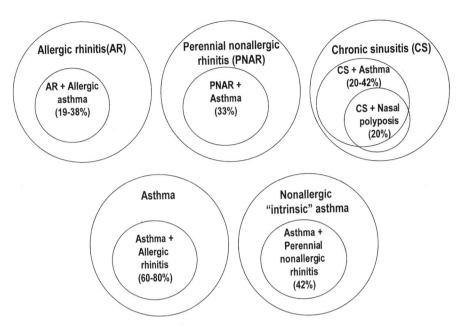

Figure 1 Venn diagrams illustrating important interrelationships between various subcategories of rhinosinusitis and asthma.

only 10–13.5% of cases in two series of patients with perennial nonallergic rhinitis (7,9). Moneret-Vautrin et al. (1990) found that 4 of 13 patients with NARES had the beginnings of nasal polyp formation and suggested that this syndrome may be a forerunner to the "aspirin triad." However, in their series of 13 patients, only 1 patient had nonspecific bronchial hyperresponsiveness and none of the patients had a history of asthma or aspirin sensitivity (9). Furthermore, in the original description of 52 patients with NARES reported by Jacobs, none of which had asthma (10), none of the patients demonstrated bronchial hyperresponsiveness to inhaled methacholine or ingested aspirin. Hence, NARES remains an enigma, and its relationship to asthma is equally obscure.

In patients with allergic asthma, the prevalence of rhinosinusitis has been estimated to be 60–80% (4,11). Nonallergic or "intrinsic" asthma accounts for approximately one-third of adult cases of asthma. There is still great speculation about the pathogenesis of intrinsic asthma, but recent studies have found significant similarities between allergic and intrinsic asthma in terms of increased numbers of IL-5 producing T lymphocytes in the lungs, overexpression of IL-5, and marked tissue eosinophilia (12,13). Furthermore, there is an increased prevalence of asthma in siblings of patients with intrinsic asthma, suggesting heritable factors in the disease (14). The prevalence of rhinosinusitis in patients with intrinsic asthma is lower than in those with allergic asthma and is reported to be approximately 40% (15).

The prevalence of asthma in patients with chronic sinusitis has been reported to be approximately 20% based on symptoms or medication use (16). These data were collected in an otolaryngologic clinic population. Based on this estimate, the prevalence of asthma was approximately fourfold higher than in the general population (17). However, the prevalence of asthma is even higher in the population of chronic rhinosinusitis patients who undergo endoscopic sinus surgery. Senior et al. reported that 42% of their patients undergoing FESS for chronic rhinosinusitis reported a history of asthma (18). Furthermore, in a series of 200 cases of sinusitis referred to an allergist's office, 57% of cases had asthma (19). In our own clinic, roughly 50% of the patients with severe chronic rhinosinusitis have a history of asthma.

Patients with chronic rhinosinusitis and nasal polyposis make up a distinct subgroup. This group of patients accounts for approximately 20% of all patients with chronic sinusitis (20). Asthma is present in approximately 50% of these patients, and approximately one-third of them have a history of bronchospastic-type sensitivity to aspirin. Furthermore, the subgroups of patients with chronic rhinosinusitis/asthma and chronic rhinosinusitis/nasal polyposis overlap highly, as shown in Fig. 1 (21).

IV. Inflammatory Mechanisms in Chronic Rhinosinusitis

Inflammation plays a key role in chronic sinusitis pathogenesis. One theory is that the immunopathology of chronic rhinosinusitis represents a spectrum of disease due to overlapping contributions from infectious and noninfectious processes (see Fig. 2). Patients have both infectious and noninfectious types of inflammation occurring at various times and to variable degrees depending on allergenic exposures, presence or absence of viral or bacterial infection, extent of sinus ostial obstruction, and extent of tissue eosinophilia.

Inflammation in rhinosinusitis may contribute to asthma as a result of inflammatory cells, cytokines, and mediators released into sinus secretions or systemically. Since the inflammation mechanisms involved in rhinosinusitis may impact on asthma, they are briefly reviewed. Mechanisms by which components of inflammation may impact asthma are covered in the following section.

A. Infectious Inflammation

The sinus mucosa is normally bathed by neutrophils even in the absence of infection. Hence, passage of neutrophils into sinus secretions is probably a part of the normal mucosal response mechanism to maintain sterility of the sinus cavity.

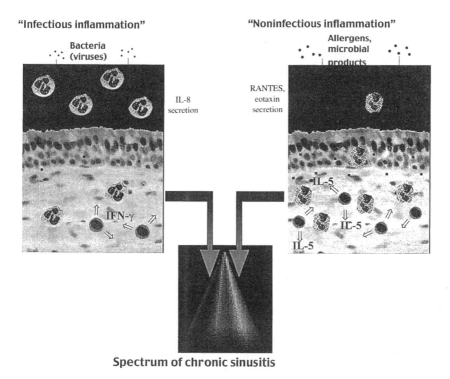

Figure 2 Two types of inflammation occur in sinusitis, contributing variably to the clinical expression of disease. Infectious inflammation is most clearly associated with acute sinusitis due to either bacterial or viral infection. Increased neutrophil influx into sinus secretions and IL-8 secretion has been implicated in this process. A ''Th1-type'' lymphocyte response is also likely to be involved. Noninfectious inflammation is so named due to the predominance of eosinophils and mixed mononuclear cells and the relative paucity of neutrophils commonly seen in chronic sinusitis. It is postulated that allergens and microbial products may drive this inflammatory response. It is associated with a ''Th2-type'' lymphocyte response, characterized by IL-5 producing T lymphocytes. RANTES and eotaxin secretion have also been implicated in this process. The clinical spectrum of chronic sinusitis is likely due to the variable overlap of ''infectious'' and ''noninfectious'' inflammatory components. (Reproduced with permission from Ref. 16.)

Lavage of the nasal cavity in normal, noninfected, and nonallergic subjects has the following distribution of cells: epithelial cells (50–60%); neutrophils (35–40%); and lymphocytes, macrophages, and eosinophils (<5%) (22). Similar studies using puncture of the maxillary antrum followed by lavage of the maxillary sinus in normal subjects have shown 63% epithelial cells, 28% neutrophils, 9% monocytes, and <1% eosinophils and mast cells (23). Data from nasal and sinus lavage are in contrast to results from nasal and sinus mucosal biopsies of normal subjects, since the latter show very few neutrophils (23,24). The cytokines or chemokines responsible for neutrophil passage into sinus secretions are unknown. However, there is evidence for a low level of IL-8 secretion (25) (see Fig. 2).

In patients with chronic sinusitis, maxillary sinus lavage fluid contains increased numbers of neutrophils and dramatically increased IL-8 levels (25). The highest levels of IL-8 and the highest percentages of lavage neutrophilia were seen in subjects classified as "nonallergic." In contrast, patients with chronic sinusitis and associated allergic rhinitis had a modest increased percentage of neutrophils and IL-8 in the lavage. In a related study, Rhyoo et al. found an increase in IL-8 in sinus tissue obtained at the time of sinus surgery (26). A correlation was also found between the amount of IL-8 detected in the sinus tissue and the radiographic extent of disease on preoperative sinus CT scans.

Studies in patients with acute sinus infection have detected IL-1β and IL-6 (and IL-8) in sinus tissues (27). Neutrophils were reported to be prominent in these tissues as well. Neutrophils are clearly the predominant inflammatory cell in nasal/sinus secretions (23). In contrast, GM-CSF and IL-5 were not elevated. An increase in the local elaboration of IL-8, IL-1β, and IL-6 as well as TNF-α would be expected in association with bacterial infection, owing to the capacity of airway epithelial cells to produce these cytokines in response to bacterial stimuli (28,29,30). These cells and inflammatory cytokines in postnasal drainage likely contribute to inflammation of the pharynx and pharyngobronchial reflexes (see below).

B. Noninfectious Inflammation

Chronic sinusitis inflammation can be associated with exuberant sinus mucosal thickening with little evidence for sinus pain or discomfort or other signs of infection. For this reason, this type of inflammation has been regarded as "noninfectious." The predominant sinus symptoms may be nasal congestion, facial pressure or fullness, postnasal drainage, and hyposmia or anosmia. At the extreme of "noninfectious" chronic sinusitis, patients have extensive bilateral mucosal thickening associated with nasal polyposis and are labeled "chronic hyperplastic sinusitis with nasal polyposis" (CHS/NP). At least 50% of the patients have associated asthma, and roughly 14–23% of cases have associated aspirin sensitivity (21,31). Nasal polyposis also occurs in >20% of patients with cystic fibrosis, but the pathogenesis of CF polyp formation is likely to be distinct from that of CHS/NP (32).

The cellular immunopathology of CHS/NP has been the focus of many studies. Since many of the features are relevant to the discussion of "shared pathogenesis" and "systemic amplification" in rhinosinusitis and asthma, they are briefly reviewed here. In comparison to normal control middle turbinate biopsies, NP contain a modestly increased number of inflammatory cells (CD45[+]), significantly increased numbers of eosinophils (MBP[+] or EG2[+]), and mildly increased numbers of tryptase[+] mast cells (24,33–35). The numbers of macrophages (CD68[+]), neutrophils (elastase[+]), and CD8[+] T lymphocytes are not increased above controls. The numbers of CD4[+] T lymphocytes are increased in CHS/NP subjects with positive allergy skin tests ("allergic CHS/NP") but not in subjects with negative skin tests ("nonallergic CHS/NP"). Altogether, between one-half and two-thirds of patients with CHS/NP are nonallergic based on the results of allergy skin tests (20,24,31). The levels of tissue eosinophilia are equal in allergic and nonallergic CHS/NP. The cellular features of NP are similar to those described in asthma with the exception that CD4[+] T lymphocytes have been found to be increased in both allergic and nonallergic asthma (13,36).

Our group found that cytokines promoting the activation and survival of eosinophils, namely GM-CSF, IL-3, and IL-5, were present in abundance in NP (24,33,35). The numbers of eosinophils in NP correlated with the density of GM-CSF and IL-3 mRNA[+] cells in both allergic and nonallergic CHS/NP (24). It is likely that much of the GM-CSF mRNA produced in NP represents autocrine production in eosinophils (37). On the other hand, most of the IL-5 produced in NP appears to come from T cells. We found that T cells accounted for roughly 68% of the IL-5-positive cells, and an increase in IL-5-producing T cells was a characteristic feature of both allergic and nonallergic CHS/NP (35). Furthermore, locally produced IL-5 has been shown to be the principal eosinophil survival-enhancing cytokine in NP (38). In our studies, the remainder of the IL-5 in NP was produced by eosinophils (18%) and mast cells (14%).

We also found that the C-C chemokines RANTES and eotaxin were strongly expressed in CHS/NP, particularly in epithelial cells and in some submucosal inflammatory cells (34,39). These chemokines facilitate the transendothelial migration of eosinophils and their movement into the epithelium. Increased mRNA expression of IL-8, a C-X-C chemokine, has also been reported in NP (40).

Other cytokines produced in abundance by inflammatory cells in NP include TNF-α, IL-1β, and IL-13 (34). In addition, IL-1, IL-6, and IL-8 are increased in nasal secretions in patients with allergic rhinitis (41).

With respect to the impact of rhinosinusitis on asthma pathogenesis or worsening, noninfectious inflammation is an important feature of "shared pathogenesis" and "systemic amplification." In addition, it could contribute to bronchospasm as a result of pulmonary aspiration of inflammatory mediators and may contribute to pharyngobronchial reflexes by virtue of the inflammatory cells and cytokines (particularly TNF-α and IL-1β) released into secretions that reach the posterior pharynx. Unfortunately, "noninfectious" and "infectious" inflammation have not been distinguished in terms of the cells and cytokines represented in postnasal drainage or nasal lavage.

V. Mechanisms of Association

There has been a long-held clinical view that disease in the upper airway indirectly exacerbates or amplifies disease in the lower airway, namely asthma. In this section, evidence in support of this theory is reviewed.

VI. Nasobronchial or Sinobronchial Reflexes in Bronchospasm

The nasobronchial or sinobronchial reflex theory asserts that stimulation of neural receptors in the nose and sinuses activates trigeminal afferent pathways and produces bronchoconstriction through a vagal efferent neural arc (42). This theory has been supported by a variety of studies showing that mechanical or chemical irritation of the nose could provoke bronchoconstriction (42–46) and that this response could be blocked by atropine (44). Furthermore, subjects with unilateral interruption of the second division of the trigeminal nerve develop irritant-induced bronchoconstriction only on the neurologically intact side of the face, suggesting that the afferent neuronal arc is carried in the maxillary division of the trigeminal nerve (45). Additional support for a nasobronchial reflex comes from studies of the effects of nasal exposure to bursts of cold, dry air which have found small but significant increases in lower airway resistance (47,48).

Despite this evidence, several studies in subjects with both nasal allergic disease and asthma have failed to demonstrate any bronchoconstrictive effect from nasal allergen challenges in subjects with seasonal nasal allergies (49–51). Using a similar model of nasal allergen challenge in allergic asthmatics, Corren and associates (52) also found no effect on pulmonary function. The nasal allergen challenge, however, did cause a mild increase in methacholine-induced bronchial hyperreactivity at 30 min and 4 h after the challenge. The significance of these findings appears to be borne out by a follow-up study that showed that use of intranasal beclomethasone caused a blunting of the seasonally induced increase in bronchial hyperresponsiveness in allergic asthmatics (53).

In contrast, a 10% reduction in lung function was found after nasal histamine challenge in patients with perennial allergic rhinitis and stable asthma (46). The results of this study suggest that nasobronchial or sinobronchial reflexes may be more significant in patients with more chronic inflammation (42). Hence, there is evidence for a role for rhinosinusitis inflammation in worsening of bronchial hyperresponsiveness but uncertainty about the role of sinobronchial reflexes in bronchospasm.

VII. Postnasal Drainage (Pulmonary Aspiration of Sinonasal Secretions)

Aspiration of sinonasal secretions into the tracheobronchial tree has long been postulated to contribute to lower airway disease in patients with rhinosinusitis and associated asthma. However, evidence for aspiration of sinus secretions is more compelling in animals than in humans.

Inflammatory mediators in sinonasal secretions have the potential to induce bronchoconstriction, cough, and possibly bronchial hyperresponsiveness. These include cysteinyl leukotrienes (LTC4) and platelet activating factor (PAF). The concentration of LTC4 in the sinus lavage of patients with chronic sinusitis (roughly 6 ng/ml) exceeded that found in nasal lavage of subjects with allergic rhinitis undergoing allergen challenge (54). Hence, if postnasal secretions were aspirated into the lungs during sleep, they might contribute to persistent bronchospasm, although this has not been demonstrated in clinical studies.

There are several other inflammatory substances in sinonasal secretions with the potential to induce bronchospasm or hyperresponsiveness if aspirated into the trachea. These include eosinophil basic proteins (such as MBP and ECP), IL-13, and possibly other cytokines. Elevated levels of eosinophil-derived ECP have been found in nasal secretions of patients with allergic rhinitis and nonallergic nasal polyposis (55). We found evidence for production of IL-13 in inflamed sinus tissues (34).

In a series of experiments performed in rabbits, Irvin and colleagues (56) found evidence for an effect of sinusitis on bronchial hyperresponsiveness. They first induced acute sinus inflammation by injecting the complement component C5a into the maxillary sinus. Rabbits so treated developed an increase in lower airway hyperresponsiveness (57). The hyperresponsiveness could be abrogated by strategies that prevented sinus exudate from draining below the level of the larynx, such as keeping the rabbits in an inverted position or preventing aspiration with an inflated endotracheal tube cuff. Hence, in the rabbit model direct passage of inflammatory mediators from the upper to the lower airways (i.e., aspiration of postnasal drainage) was found to best explain the effects on lower airway hyperresponsiveness. In contrast, a nasobronchial reflex could not be demonstrated (56).

Very few studies of this phenomenon have been conducted in humans. Huxley et al. (58) found that aspiration of pharyngeal secretions occurred in 45% of normal subjects during sleep and in 75% of subjects with a depressed sensorium. However, a study published by Bardin et al. (59) found no evidence for aspiration in normal subjects. In this study, aspiration of a radionuclide from the nasopharynx could be demonstrated in the bronchial tree in 2 of 4 patients with a depressed sensorium. However, when the isotope was injected into the maxillary sinus of 13 patients with sinusitis and tracked for 24 h, it could be demonstrated in the maxillary sinus, nasopharynx, esophagus, and lower gastrointestinal tract but not in the bronchial tree. This study has been taken as strong evidence against the ''postnasal drip'' theory to explain the relationship between sinusitis and asthma. However, certain questions could still be raised. First, is the volume of postnasal drainage a determinant in whether aspiration occurs? Second, are asthma patients with sinusitis at greater risk of aspiration than nonasthmatics? Until we have the answer to these questions, the postnasal drainage theory must be regarded as unsubstantiated in humans.

VIII. Pharyngobronchial Reflexes

Rhinosinusitis produces excessive mucus drainage down the posterior pharyngeal wall to the hypopharynx. Normal functioning of the hypopharynx prevents this drainage from entering the larynx or penetrating the vocal cords. However, the postnasal drainage may have significant irritational and inflammatory effects on the hypopharyngeal mucosa, rendering it erythematous and hypersensitive to constrictive stimuli.

Part of the difficulty in studying relationships between the upper (above the larynx) and lower airway physiology relates to the interpretation of physiologic measures of lower airway functioning. Typically, a histamine or methacholine bronchial challenge test is used to measure lower airways hyperresponsiveness (60). While these tests are considered ''gold standards'' of bronchial hyperresponsiveness, their results may be affected by lack of patient effort, variability in inspiratory effort and lung volume, or upper airway narrowing (61). An example of this is paradoxical inspiratory vocal cord closure (i.e., ''vocal cord dysfunction''), in which upper airway narrowing may confound the interpretation of lung function measurements, such as the FEV_1 or FVC.

The maximal midinspiratory flow rate is a simple measure that has been reported to be predictive of upper airway narrowing (62). In nonasthmatic patients with chronic sinusitis, sinusitis exacerbations were found to be associated with an exaggerated reduction in MIF_{50} in response to inhaled histamine, indicating a constrictive response at the level of the upper airway (61). A parallel increase in histamine-induced bronchial hyperresponsiveness was also observed in most patients. The drop in MIF_{50} was shown to occur earlier and to a greater extent than the reduction in FEV_1 in most patients, suggesting that the two responses were interrelated. Furthermore, treatment of the sinusitis exacerbation with antibiotics and inhaled corticosteroids was associated with a normalization of histamine-induced MIF_{50} and increase in methacholine PC_{20}, again in a closely related fashion. These studies have been interpreted as evidence that pharyngobronchial reflexes play a significant role in the exacerbations of asthma associated with episodes of sinusitis.

Postnasal drainage contains neutrophils and inflammatory mediators and proinflammatory cytokines, likely including TNF-α and IL-8. Biopsies of the pharynx in patients with chronic sinusitis have confirmed the presence of inflammatory changes, most prominent of which is thinning of the epithelial layer (63). These changes have been postulated to be associated with heightened stimulation of pharyngeal sensory neurons, leading to a pharyngobronchial reflex. However, to date no published studies have directly investigated this possibility.

IX. Shared Pathogenesis or "Common Mucosal Susceptibility"

Is it possible that rhinosinusitis and asthma symptoms are triggered concurrently rather than sequentially? This possibility would be most plausible if the upper and lower airway mucosae shared a common mucosal (genetic) susceptibility to exogenous stimuli. There is substantial evidence to support this concept, which also has been dubbed the concept of "one airway, one disease" (64,65). It is based on the premise that the upper and lower airways are affected by common inflammatory processes and that the diseases may also share underlying genetic susceptibility factors (4).

Supporting evidence for this concept includes (a) the finding that, if carefully questioned, approximately 90% of patients with asthma report symptoms of rhinosinusitis (66)*; (b) prospective studies that show that patients with allergic rhinitis have a higher risk of developing asthma over a 23-year period (67); and (c) the observation that patients with asthma and rhinitis have worse upper airway disease when compared to individuals with rhinitis alone (66). Other supportive evidence includes the very strong association between asthma and chronic hyperplastic sinusitis, the upper airway disease associated with the most intense eosinophil-predominant inflammation.

There are strong similarities between the respiratory mucosa and the inflammatory processes found in allergic asthma, allergic rhinitis, and chronic hyperplastic sinusitis. Even the nonasthmatic patients with allergic rhinitis demonstrate a low-level inflammatory process with similar features to those described above, suggesting a subclinical level of allergic inflammation and airway remodeling (68). Furthermore, approximately 20–30% of nonasthmatic patients with allergic rhinitis show evidence of mild bronchial hyperresponsiveness which exceeds the 5% level in normal controls (4). These similarities suggest that the immunologic response is being triggered by a common mechanism rather than a reflex mechanism. The key shared elements in the inflammatory processes are

---

* This percentage exceeds that in previous studies likely due to the more careful methods used to elicit patient's history (66).

illustrated in Fig. 3. The most important features are chronic mononuclear cell infiltration of the mucosa by eosinophils, increased CD4+ T cells of the Th2 phenotype (producing at a minimum IL-5 and possibly IL-4 and GM-CSF) (13,69), production of C-C chemokines RANTES and eotaxin by epithelial and inflammatory cells (39,70), increased endothelial expression of the vascular cell adhesion molecule-1 (VCAM-1) (71), and increased expression of proinflammatory cytokine mRNA. These findings suggest a common type of immunologic response in the mucosae.

Intense infiltration of the mucosa with eosinophils is the most characteristic feature of upper and lower airway inflammation in rhinosinusitis and asthma. Eosinophils are critical effector cells in both conditions, owing to their capacity to secrete toxic basic proteins which damage respiratory epithelium and their role in secretion of leukotrienes, PAF, and numerous proinflammatory cytokines (72).

Since the Th2-type immunologic response is similar in the upper and lower airways, it is important to question whether it is being stimulated by the same immunologic process. The possibility of a common allergenic stimulus is plausible for allergic rhinosinusitis and allergic asthma, but a similar mucosal response is seen in nonallergic patients with rhinosinusitis or asthma despite the lack of a complete "Th2 profile" (which would include production of IL-4) and the lack of clinically demonstrable allergy in these patients. Furthermore, epidemiologic studies suggest that in allergic subjects, the allergens having the greatest association with upper and lower airway disease are different. For instance, in the National Health Survey NHANES II, allergic rhinitis was most commonly associated with pollen allergy, whereas allergic asthma was most commonly asociated with sensitization to house dust mite and cat allergen (73). However, patients with both allergic rhinitis and asthma tended to have the greatest association with sensitization to the mold *Alternaria*. Hence certain allergens may be more likely to simultaneously trigger both upper and lower airway disease in the same patient, but their capacity to do so undoubtedly depends on whether both sites receive a sufficient exposure to the allergen. Patients living in areas with extremely high ambient mold spore counts may be particularly susceptible to combined upper and lower airway allergic stimulation, and the author has observed this pattern of response in many patients with rhinosinusitis and asthma during periods of high heat and humidity in the St. Louis area.

Elaboration of inflammatory mediators is another shared feature of rhinosinusitis and asthma. Overproduction of cysteinyl leukotrienes is a characteristic feature of chronic asthma, and this category of mediators is the single most important class of mediators responsible for increased resting bronchial smooth muscle tone in asthma (74). Increased concentrations of cysteinyl leukotrienes (LTC4, D4, and E4) are released during nasal ragweed allergen challenge in ragweed-sensitive patients (75). Cysteinyl leukotrienes have also been detected during both the early and late phases of nasal allergic responses to allergen challenge, and

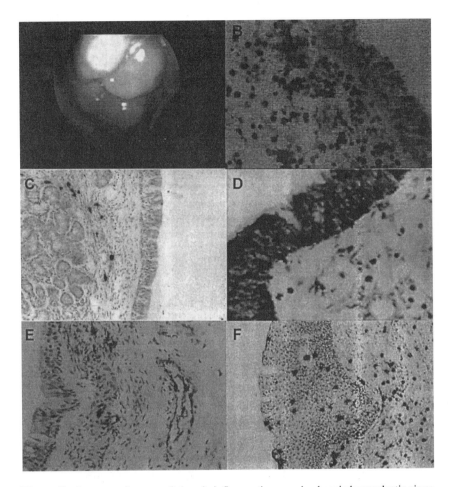

Figure 3 Important features of chronic inflammation seen in chronic hyperplastic sinusitis with nasal polyposis. (A) Extensive hyperplastic sinus mucosa ("polyposis") in the left anterior ethmoidal area. This area can be visualized due to previous surgery in this area. (B–F) The important inflammatory features in nasal polyps. (B) Extensive infiltration of the submucosa and epithelium with eosinophils immunostained for eosinophil cationic protein with EG2 antibody. (C) Double immunostain showing an increased number of IL-5-producing T lymphocytes. (D) Immunostain for eotaxin demonstrating intense staining of the epithelium and a few submucosal inflammatory cells. (E) Immunostain for VCAM-1 demonstrating staining of vascular endothelium. (F) In situ hybridization with an antisense probe for the proinflammatory cytokine TNF-α demonstrating numerous strongly positive cells. Similar features have been described in allergic asthma and allergic rhinitis. These findings suggest a common type of immunologic response in the mucosae. (Reproduced with permission from Refs. 34, 35, and 39.)

nasal provocation with LTD4 was found to cause an increase in nasal blood flow and increased nasal airway resistance but no increase in nasal secretions, sneezing, or pruritis (76). Furthermore, increased levels of cysteinyl LTs have been found in the sinus lavage of patients with chronic sinusitis (54). These mediators have some shared and some dissimilar effects on the upper and lower airways based on structural differences. For instance, edema formation may be induced in both the upper and lower airways, but only the lower airways contain smooth muscle and therefore respond with bronchospasm.

The shared pathogenesis hypothesis also offers a potential explanation for the increased prevalence and more intense representation of eosinophils in severe rhinosinusitis and nasal polyposis in patients with coexisting asthma. Many years ago, Harlin and Gleich observed that the number of eosinophils in inflamed maxillary and ethmoid sinus tissue were increased and that the most intense eosinophil infiltration was seen in patients with chronic sinusitis and asthma (77). We later studied eosinophils in chronic sinusitis patients with NP. Since all of our patients had NP, they may have had more chronic inflammation than those of Harlin and Gleich. We reported that eosinophils were increased in approximately 80% of NP and that this increase included patients without obvious asthma (78). However, in the author's clinic the highest levels of blood eosinophils are consistently seen in patients with coexisting asthma. Chronic rhinosinusitis patients with asthma had much higher levels of circulating eosinophils and a much higher prevalence of nasal polyposis and ASA sensitivity. Consistent with these observations, Newman et al. (79) found that the extent of sinus mucosal thickening on sinus CT scan correlated strongly with the presence of peripheral and tissue eosinophilia and was highly statistically associated with a history of wheezing. These data strengthen the link between eosinophils and the pathogenesis of rhinosinusitis associated with asthma. Eosinophils play the most prominent role when rhinosinusitis is associated with extensive sinus mucosal thickening and nasal polyp formation, a condition described as "chronic hyperplastic sinusitis."

A. The Special Case of Aspirin-Sensitive Asthma, Sinusitis, and Nasal Polyposis (Samter's Syndrome or "Triad Asthma")

This syndrome may represent the strongest case for a common pathogenesis of upper and lower airway disease. The common features include intense eosinophil infiltration of the respiratory mucosa and submucosa and increased production of cysteinyl leukotrienes (C4 and D4) in sinus and bronchial secretions. Furthermore, systemic administration of aspirin or topical exposure of either the nose or lungs to lysine-aspirin elicits an increase in LTC4 and an increase in eosinophils in nasal and bronchial secretions (80,81). In addition, such challenges result in an increase in tryptase in nasal secretions, suggesting concurrent mast cell activation (81). It is likely that eosinophils account for most of the cysteinyl leukotrienes produced in triad asthma, since eosinophils from asthmatic patients have been shown to produce greater than normal amounts of LTC4 (82). Furthermore, endobronchial biopsy studies have demonstrated a marked increase in the number of cells expressing the enzyme LTC4 synthase and much higher levels of airway eosinophils in aspirin-intolerant asthmatics than in aspirin-tolerant asthmatics (83).

Given the shared inflammatory features of these diseases and the paucity of evidence for (1) reflex neurally mediated bronchospasm in allergic rhinitis or chronic sinusitis/nasal polyposis or (2) direct postnasal drippage of mediators or cytokines into the lungs, the concept of common mucosal susceptibility emerges as a compelling argument to explain the link between rhinosinusitis and asthma. Furthermore, the fact that CHS/NP is the form of upper airway disease most strongly associated with asthma is entirely consistent with this concept, since the immunopathologic features discussed above are most intense in this form of upper airway disease.

X. Systemic Amplification

The prevalence of rhinosinusitis in asthmatics (60–80%) is much higher than the prevalence of asthma in patients with rhinosinusitis (13–38%) (3). Furthermore, as stated above, the severity of chronic rhinosinusitis is greater in the population of patients with asthma. These statistics suggest that, in addition to a ''shared pathogenesis,'' rhinosinusitis and asthma may affect each other by ''systemic amplification.'' Systemic amplification implies that the severity of rhinosinusitis and asthma may be influenced by bidirectional effects between the upper and lower airways, owing to systemically acting cytokines or chemokines.

Certain of the shared pathogenic features of rhinosinusitis and asthma are dependent on cells or cytokines that are mobilized systemically and which therefore may augment disease remote from the target organ. These include (1) cytokines promoting eosinophilopoiesis and mobilization of mature eosinophils and eosinophil progenitors cells from the bone marrow to the blood, (2) an increased level of circulating CD4+ T lymphocytes (in asthma) (84,85), and (3) chemokines or inflammatory mediators with potential for systemic actions.

Togias et al. have presented evidence that asthmatic patients with allergic rhinitis or chronic sinusitis have more severe upper airway disease than their nonasthmatic counterparts. Specifically, they found that subjects with allergic rhinitis and asthma demonstrate greater nasal responsiveness to cold, dry air in terms of symptomatology and biochemical markers of mast cell and glandular activation than subjects with allergic rhinitis alone (66). Similarly, as discussed previously, patients undergoing surgery for chronic sinusitis have a much higher prevalence of asthma than the group not undergoing surgery. Overall, the prevalence of asthma is approximately eightfold greater in patients undergoing surgery for chronic sinusitis than in the general population (17). These data are unlikely to represent reporter bias, since they represent a patient population seen by otolaryngologists rather than asthma specialists. Systemic amplification of upper airway eosinophilic inflammation is one way to explain these observations, namely, that asthmatic lower airway inflammation systemically amplifies the upper airway disease. Alternatively, asthma may be a phenotypic marker for a greater genetic risk for severe upper airway inflammatory disease.

The eosinophil represents an important common feature of asthma and chronic sinusitis, and elevated levels of blood eosinophils allow for a systemic mechanism for the sinusitis/asthma connection. Hence, inflammatory processes eliciting an eosinophilopoietic response in either the lungs or the sinuses may increase the eosinophil infiltration in the other organ. This is because local inflammatory factors in both the sinus and lung mucosa promote the selective local infiltration by eosinophils. Examples include the elaboration of C-C chemokines, such as RANTES and eotaxin, in the respiratory mucosa. RANTES and eotaxin are potent and selective eosinophil chemoattractants (86), but the extent to which they attract eosinophils into tissues is also dependent on the level of blood eosinophils. Hence, studies in the mouse showed that injection of eotaxin into the skin of mice induced only a very slight accumulation of eosinophils. In contrast, if the mice were first pretreated with IL-5, the eotaxin skin injection induced a strong eosinophil infiltration (87). The difference in tissue eosinophil infiltration is attributable to a 13-fold rise in blood eosinophils induced 1 h after intravenous IL-5. Furthermore, IL-5 elaboration in the lungs amplifies eotaxin-induced chemotaxis of eosinophils in the airways of mice (88). Similarly, in human subjects with mild asthma, IL-5 administration alone by inhalational challenge has been shown to increase eosinophils in bronchial mucosa and bronchoalveolar lavage (89).

Allergen inhalation challenge of the lungs in mild asthmatic patients induces an increase in bone marrow-derived CD34+ eosinophil progenitor cells within 24 h. These cells can be identified by their expression of the IL-5 receptor α-chain (90). The systemic stimulus for release of these cells is still debatable, but IL-5 is an obvious candidate. Increased circulating levels of IL-5 were shown to be required for systemic stimulation of bone marrow eosinophilopoiesis in a guinea pig model of antigen-induced airway eosinophilia (91). Recently, it was also discovered that eotaxin in guinea pigs promotes release of mature eosinophils and eosinophil progenitors from the bone marrow within 30 min (92). Hence, in addition to acting as a chemokine, eotaxin appears to function as a systemic cytokine.

Acute asthma is also associated with an increase in the number of CD4 T lymphocytes in bronchoalveolar lavage, bronchial mucosa, and blood expressing IL-5 mRNA (93). These "primed" lymphocytes have the potential to home to

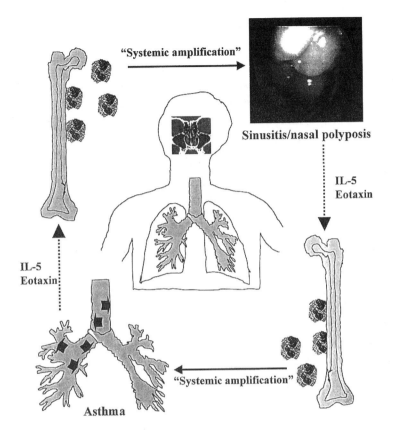

Figure 4 Interaction between rhinosinusitis and asthma through systemic amplification. The eosinophil is an important common feature of asthma and chronic sinusitis, and elevated levels of blood eosinophils allow for a systemic mechanism for the sinusitis/asthma connection. Inflammatory processes in either the lungs or the sinuses generate cytokines (e.g., IL-5) and chemokines (e.g., eotaxin) that stimulate eosinophilopoiesis and release of eosinophils and eosinophil progenitors from the bone marrow. The resulting increase in circulating eosinophils may allow for an increase in eosinophil infiltration in the other organ. This is because local inflammatory factors in the sinus and lung mucosa promote the selective local infiltration by eosinophils. Examples include the elaboration of C-C chemokines, such as RANTES and eotaxin. The extent to which RANTES and eotaxin attract eosinophils into tissues is dependent on the level of blood eosinophils.

areas of allergen exposure, as has been shown in the lungs after allergen challenge (94,95).

It is predicted that the intensity of the systemic stimulus from the upper and lower airways would be dependent on (1) the intensity of the mucosal inflammatory response and (2) the surface area affected in the target organ. Considering these factors, it seems unlikely that the "systemic interplay" between rhinosinusitis and asthma would be balanced. Rather, the effect should favor an effect of asthma on rhinosinusitis, since the mucosal surface area of the lungs greatly exceeds that of the upper airway (96). Several corollaries should obtain if this theory is true. First, there should be an imbalance in the reported associations. This appears to be true. The prevalence of rhinosinusitis with asthma is approximately 80%, whereas the prevalence of asthma with rhinosinusitis is no more than 50%. Second, there should be a difference in the degree of systemic eosinophilia in association with isolated rhinosinusitis as opposed to asthma. This also is true, as previously mentioned (see Fig. 4).

In contrast to cytokines and circulating blood cells, most inflammatory mediators released in rhinosinusitis and asthma, such as histamine, prostaglandins, leukotrienes, and platelet-activating factor, are either locally degraded in the tissues or rapidly inactivated in the bloodstream and therefore unlikely to exert systemic effects.

XI. Therapeutic Interventions in Rhinosinusitis and Their Impact on Severe Asthma

A. Effect of Allergic Rhinitis Treatment on Asthma

Studies demonstrating an impact of treatment of seasonal allergic rhinitis on seasonal changes in bronchial hyperresponsiveness were discussed under Nasal and Sinobronchial Reflexes. In general, these studies suggest that antiinflammatory therapy directed at the upper airway has a modest effect to reduce bronchial hyperresponsiveness. For instance, the study by Corren et al. (53) showed that treatment of allergic rhinitis with intranasal beclomethasone caused a blunting of the seasonally induced increase in bronchial hyperresponsiveness in allergic asthmatics.

Unlike results from studies of nasal allergen challenge, studies of asthma symptoms during ragweed season have shown worsening of asthma symptoms, although lung function was unaffected during the pollen season (53,97). Although it could be argued that the increased symptoms were due to allergen reaching the lower airways, the effect was shown to be attenuated by intranasal corticosteroids (53,97). It was also shown that the effects of the intranasal corticosteroid were not due to systemic absorption, since studies employing radiolabeled drug failed to show significant deposition in the lower airways (98).

Subjects with perennial allergic rhinitis and chronic inflammatory changes have been shown to have a marked increase in nasal airway resistance and a decrease in FEV_1 greater than 10% in response to intranasal inhalation of histamine (66). The effects could not be ascribed to systemic absorption of histamine (80). One study even found a greater effect of intranasal budesonide to reduce bronchial hyperresponsiveness to carbachol than the same dose of budesonide given by inhalation to patients with perennial rhinitis but no asthma (99). Similarly, Togias et al. found that some subjects with asthma demonstrate acute reductions in FEV_1 and FVC after nasal exposure to the neural stimulant capsaicin (66). Nasal airway hyperresponsiveness is a well-known feature of active allergic disease (100,101). These data have been interpreted to suggest that the chronic inflammation associated with perennial rhinitis might be sufficient to induce a sinobronchial reflex. However, it is unclear whether effects in the upper airway, i.e., pharyngobronchial reflexes, may have contributed to these ''lower airway'' effects of nasal histamine challenge. Similar to studies of seasonal allergic rhinitis, Watson et al. (98) showed that intranasal aqueous 200 μg of beclomethasone administered twice daily for 4 weeks significantly reduced lower airways bronchial hyperresponsiveness in subjects with perennial allergic rhinitis and asthma (although no significant improvement in asthma symptoms was seen). Again, the extent to which these effects were due to a reduction in pharyngobronchial reflex were not examined.

Hence, the results from several studies of seasonal or perennial allergic rhinitis have failed to show a significant effect of upper airway inflammation on bronchoconstriction but do suggest that upper airway inflammation may give rise to an increase in bronchial hyperresponsiveness. Unfortunately, the extent to which this apparent increase in bronchial hyperresponsiveness could be due to pharyngobronchial reflexes cannot be determined.

B. Effect of Sinusitis Treatment on Asthma

The best evidence for a causal or contributing role of sinusitis in asthma comes from studies in which treatment of sinusitis has been shown to reduce asthma severity and/or medication use. Rachelefsky and associated (102) assessed 48 children before and after medical therapy for sinusitis and reported a marked improvement in asthma symptoms, normalizations of pulmonary function tests (PFTs) in 67% of patients, and discontinuation of bronchodilator use in 79% of patients. In a similar study of 80 asthmatic children, Businco et al. (103) treated asthmatic children with baseline abnormal maxillary radiographs with ampicillin, phenylephrine, or triprolidine (if purulent postnasal drainage was present) or topical beclomethasone drops alone. Improvement in sinus radiographs and asthma were noted in both treatment groups. Cummings et al. (104) treated a group of children with asthma and sinusitis with either a program of topical corticosteroids, antibiotics, and oral decongestants or placebo. In this study, all children had marked thickening or opacification of the maxillary sinuses. Significant improvement in asthma symptoms and reduced need for inhaled bronchodilators or oral steroids were found in the active treatment group; however, no significant effects on pulmonary function or bronchial reactivity were seen. However, Friedman et al. (105) reported improvement in sinus radiographs, asthma, and pulmonary function tests in a group of 8 asthmatic children after medical therapy.

Comparable studies showing a benefit of medical treatment for adult asthmatic patients with sinusitis are notably lacking. However, the effects of surgical intervention have been reported in uncontrolled clinical trials.

C. Effect of Sinus Surgery on Asthma

Friedman and Slavin and colleagues (106–108) reported the use of aggressive surgical and medial management of sinusitis to treat an adult population with chronic sinusitis and severe asthma. Their population demographics were similar to those seen at our institution, namely two-thirds were nonallergic and approximately 50% had a clinical history of aspirin sensitivity. These patients had typically failed to respond to aggressive medical management and were corticosteroid-dependent. After bilateral intranasal sphenoethmoidectomy, 65% of the patients showed sustained improvement in asthma and nasal symptoms and reduction in medication usage (107). In most of these cases, the improvement was sustained even at 5 years (109). Since these results were reported, intranasal spenoethmoidectomy has been replaced in most surgeons' hands by functional endoscopic sinus surgery (FESS), as discussed below.

The effects of isolated nasal polypectomy on asthma have been reported in uncontrolled studies, the largest of which is the study of English (110). Subjective improvement and reduced use of asthma medications were reported in this study.

Functional endoscopic sinus surgery was developed in Germany by Messerklinger and Stammberger (111,112). Subsequently, it has been widely accepted as a major advance in sinus surgery. The main goal of FESS is to improve the function of the ostiomeatal complex, which includes the drainage pathways for the maxillary and anterior ethmoid sinuses. Since 1991, seven studies have commented on the effects of FESS on patients with coexisting asthma (Refs. 113–118; reviewed in Ref. 119). Most of the studies have used patient-based questionnaires to measure the impact of sinus surgery on asthma symptoms, hospitalizations, and medication use. None of the studies incorporated a nonsurgical control group or mechanisms to control for other potential changes in asthma management, such as introduction of new drugs (e.g., higher potency inhaled steroids, long-acting β-agonists, or leukotriene antagonists). All of the studies reported a beneficial effect of FESS on asthma. None of the studies found evidence for a worsening of asthma after sinus surgery.

Senior et al. (18) performed a prospective follow-up study on a group of

120 adult patients who had undergone FESS for chronic rhinosinusitis which was refractory to medical management. Patients were followed for a mean of 6.5 years. Of this group, 42% (30 patients) reported a history of asthma. Using a symptom scoring severity scale, 90% of patients reported a reduction in the severity of their asthma after FESS with the percentage of improvement ranging from 49% at 1.1 years to 65% at 6.5 years. Reductions in asthma attacks and asthma medication use were also observed, and 65% of patients reported less use of oral steroids. The extent to which modifications in asthma treatment may have affected their results was not examined. However, it should be noted that during the time frame of this study (1985–1990), the use of higher doses of inhaled steroids was becoming more common among asthma specialists in the United States.

In the study by Manning et al. (116), 14 pediatric patients with a history of ''sinusitis aggravating asthma'' underwent bilateral endoscopic sinus surgery and were examined for asthma symptom severity, impact on school performance, and medication use for the period of 12 months prior to surgery and 12 months postoperatively. All patients had computed tomographic evidence of chronic sinus disease. Eleven of the 14 patients experienced a significant reduction in asthma hospitalizations and school days missed. Decreased use of systemic steroids was noted in 12 of the 14 patients. Pulmonary function tests before and after surgery showed no significant changes.

In the surgical series reported by Dunlop et al. (118), 50 asthmatic patients with chronic rhinosinusitis refractory to medical management underwent FESS and were followed prospectively for 12 months. After FESS, improvement in asthma control was reported in terms of the percentage of patients improving as follows: overall asthma control (40%), use of less inhaled corticosteroids (20%), and use of less bronchodilatory inhaler (28%). In addition, use of oral steroids decreased from 20 patients during the year prior to surgery to 8 patients over the 12 months postoperatively. A 38% reduction in the number of hospitalizations for asthma was also observed.

Despite the limitations of these studies, there is a consensus of opinion that sinus surgery may be of significant benefit to patients with asthma. The author is in agreement with this, although it is not necessarily true that sinus surgery would be any better than aggressive medical therapy at accomplishing these results. A prospective study of the benefit of aggressive medical therapy for sinusitis in adult asthmatic patients has not been reported.

XII. Management of Rhinosinusitis in Severe Asthma

For many patients in our clinic, controlling chronic rhinosinusitis is a key factor in controlling asthma. In order to optimally treat rhinosinusitis in a patient with severe asthma, several issues must be addressed. These include identifying allergic triggers to both upper and lower airway disease, making appropriate environmental control recommendations, eradicating chronic sinus infection, and controlling rhinosinusitis inflammation. A key symptom to control is postnasal drainage because it contributes to chronic cough and sputum production and probably triggers asthma via pharyngobronchial reflexes.

A recommended approach to managing the patient with chronic sinusitis was recently published (16) and is outlined below. Evaluation of the patient begins with a complete medical history, physical examination, and review of old medical records, including previous X rays and operative reports. In the author's clinic, the baseline evaluation includes a "limited" sinus CT scan and rhinoscopy. Many clinicians reserve the sinus CT scan for treatment failures or for patients referred for sinus surgery. The limited sinus CT scan offers the advantage of reduced cost and radiation exposure for the patient and is an excellent imaging study for chronic sinusitis (120–122). Contributing factors to sinusitis should be sought and treated. These include an evaluation for perennial allergic sensitivities and indoor allergenic exposures and, in selected cases, evaluation for hypogammaglobulinemia.

Certain conditions should raise suspicion for the presence of Gram-negative sinus infection. These include a history of extensive antibiotic use or a prior history of Gram-negative sinus infection. In such patients, persistent severe symptoms and evidence of mucopurulent sinus secretions warrant obtaining a sinus culture. If the baseline limited sinus CT scan shows evidence of high attenuation signaling or expansion of the sinus cavity, allergic fungal sinusitis should be considered.

Sinus mucosal thickening in chronic sinusitis is the result of both infectious or noninfectious inflammation. However, the contribution of each to the radiographic or rhinoscopic appearance of chronic sinusitis is difficult to judge. Even patients with advanced nasal polyposis often have superimposed infection; conversely, patients with definite purulent infection may have prominent polypoid mucosal thickening. For these reasons, the author's initial approach to management of chronic sinusitis combines treatment with antibiotics and systemic steroids (prednisone). Adult patients receive antibiotics for 4 weeks and prednisone during the first 10 days of antibiotics (20 mg po b.i.d. for 5 days followed by 20 mg daily for 5 additional days). Patients are also treated with nasal saline irrigations, intranasal steroids, and possibly oral decongestants. The use of systemic and topical corticosteroids for treatment of chronic sinusitis was recently reviewed (123). The rationale for topical corticosteroids is to control eosinophilic inflammation (78). Use of topical corticosteroids has also been advocated for treatment of chronic sinusitis as part of a "comprehensive" medical treatment program (19), although there are no controlled studies specifically addressing their value in chronic sinusitis.

Patients should be reevaluated after 1 month of treatment. This may include rhinoscopy and possibly a follow-up limited sinus CT scan. The extent to which bacterial infection persists is judged on the basis of these examinations. If purulent secretions and/or sinus ostial obstruction persist, infection is presumed to still be present. If dramatic improvement has occurred, antibiotics may be stopped, and nasal saline irrigations and intranasal steroids are continued. For patients demonstrating minimal improvement or worsening, a retreatment regimen is usually given which includes a second antibiotic regimen and possibly another short course of prednisone. Again, the possibility of a Gram-negative or an antibiotic-resistant Gram-positive infection should be considered which may justify obtaining a bacterial culture. The further empiric use of antibiotics at this point is clearly of unproven benefit. This is especially true for patients with advanced "noninfectious" chronic hyperplastic sinusitis with nasal polyposis. Nonetheless, some patients improve during the second month of empiric antibiotic treatment and show regression of sinus mucosal thickening. Nasal saline irrigations, intranasal steroids, and oral decongestants are continued, and the patient is again reevaluated 1 month later. Patients who fail to improve after the second month of treatment are referred for consideration of sinus surgery. In the author's clinic, only about 10% of cases fail to improve after 1 or 2 months of intensive medical treatment, but an additional 10–15% of cases relapse within a few weeks thereafter. This latter group of patients is also referred for consideration of sinus surgery.

It is known that patients with extensive hyperplastic sinus mucosal thickening have a poorer outcome with sinus surgery (124), and they may respond poorly to the medical treatment outlined above. Sinus tissues from these patients usually show a large number of eosinophils, and increased levels of eosinophil-derived ECP in nasal mucosal brushings have been associated with poor outcomes after FESS (125). Patients may also have a persistently elevated absolute blood eosinophil count (AEC) of >500/µl. At least 50% of these patients have associated asthma. We have found that AECs of >500/µl are associated with frequent exacerbations of chronic sinusitis, leading to repeated use of antibiotics and progressive mucosal thickening. Patients in this category may require prednisone beyond the initial 10-day "burst," generally at a dose of 5–10 mg/day, in order to maintain the AEC at <500/µl. Hence, in these patients the AEC is used as an indicator of the need for continued prednisone therapy (cf. 126).

XIII. The Special Case of Allergic Fungal Sinusitis and Associated Asthma

A distinct entity of allergic fungal sinusitis (AFS) was first proposed by Katzenstein et al. in 1982 (127). It is caused by an intense allergic and eosinophilic inflammatory response to a fungal species and represents an upper airway equivalent to allergic bronchopulmonary aspergillosis (ABPA). The implicated fungi colonize stagnant mucus and are noninvasive. The disease has been described in association with various fungal species, including *Aspergillus, Bipolaris spicifera, Curvularia, Alternaria,* and *Fusarium.* Diagnostic criteria for AFS include the presence of chronic sinusitis usually with chronic mucosal thickening on sinus radiographs and the presence of "allergic mucin" and fungal hyphae within the allergic mucin (128–130). Nearly all patients with AFS have nasal polyps, and many have peripheral blood eosinophilia. Allergic mucin is defined as thick sinus secretions loaded with degranulating eosinophils. Sinus mucosal tissue characteristically shows intense chronic inflammation with large numbers of eosinophils. A positive fungal culture of the allergic mucin help to confirm the diagnosis but is not required. Most patients with AFS have evidence of fungal allergy based on prick or intradermal skin tests or fungal-specific IgE measurements (128,130). Fungal precipitins have been demonstrated in some but not all cases.

Certain radiographic features may alert the clinician to the possible presence of AFS. AFS may present as a persistently opacified sinus cavity despite prolonged antibiotic therapy. Most commonly, AFS causes unilateral sinus opacification, owing to obstruction of the sinus ostium by thick, inspissated mucus. Sinus CT images reveal the presence of a persistently opacified sinus cavity that may be expansile. Sinus CT images may also reveal high-intensity signaling within the opacified sinus. This signaling is felt to be caused by thick allergic mucin of high protein concentration (131). The corresponding lesions have a characteristic "hypodense" appearance on T1- and T2-weighted images on sinus MR imaging (131). Such lesions are nearly pathognomic for AFS, but they are not always present.

The diagnosis of AFS is usually confirmed based on the surgical findings and examination (and possibly culture) of the allergic mucin. In rare cases, the diagnosis may be made by performing GMS staining of pathologic specimens from a previous surgery.

Treatment of AFS requires surgical removal of the allergic mucin that obstructs sinus drainage (130). However, systemic corticosteroids are also essential (130). Guidelines for the use of prednisone for adults with AFS are patterned after treatment of ABPA. Treatment is initiated with 0.5 to 1.0 mg/kg of prednisone daily for 2 weeks and then the same dose is given q.o.d. for an additional 2 weeks before initiating a gradual tapering. In many cases, it is necessary to continue a low daily or every-other-day dose of prednisone to maintain control of the disease. High-potency intranasal corticosteroids should also be used in AFS, preferably with the patient using the "head-down-forward" technique to maximize penetration of the drug into the OMU and ethmoidal area (132,133). The role of fungal specific immunotherapy for AFS remains controversial, but a recent controlled study suggested that it may be an important adjunct to medical and surgical therapy of AFS (134).

In addition to the above, patients with AFS should receive treatment for their chronic sinusitis as outlined above. It is important to remember that patients with AFS also experience exacerbations of their chronic sinusitis due to bacterial infections.

XIV. The Special Case of Aspirin Sensitivity/Nasal Polyposis and Asthma

For patients with rhinosinusitis and a history of aspirin-induced asthma, the addition of a leukotriene antagonist should be strongly considered, although there are no controlled studies of their efficacy in treatment of rhinosinusitis or nasal polyp disease. Leukotriene antagonists may help to reduce eosinophilic inflammation in the sinus tissues. Aspirin desensitization has also been advocated as a treatment for severe chronic hyperplastic sinusitis with nasal polyposis. However, most published experience with aspirin desensitization is in the form of small uncontrolled case series (135–137).

XV. Summary and Conclusions

Patients with severe asthma frequently have associated rhinosinusitis, and exacerbations of their rhinosinusitis symptoms are commonly associated with exacerbations of asthma. In addition, postnasal drainage secondary to rhinosinusitis produces chronic cough and sputum production, symptoms that overlap with asthma and possibly contribute to it. Over the past several decades, a great deal of attention has been given to a possible causal relationship between rhinosinusitis and asthma. Most attention was focused on potential nasal or sinobronchial reflexes or pulmonary aspiration of postnasal drainage. Recently, abnormal pharyngobronchial reflexes were described in rhinosinusitis that affect the flow of air through the upper airway (hypopharynx) and thereby impact the results of lower airway functional measurements. These pharyngobronchial reflexes may be very important in explaining the relationship between flares of rhinosinusitis and asthma. Several studies have demonstrated improvement in asthma symptoms, reductions in medication use, and reductions in bronchial hyperresponsiveness after treatment of rhinosinusitis. Unfortunately, it is not possible to determine whether these improvements were due to effects on sinobronchial reflexes or pharyngobronchial reflexes, but the latter could potentially account for most if not all of the observed effects. Perhaps the most compelling reason for treating rhinosinusitis in patients with asthma is the fact that two of the most bothersome symptoms, namely chronic cough and sputum production, overlap the symptoms of asthma and result in a substantial reduction in quality of life.

Until recently, relatively little attention has been given to the possibility that rhinosinusitis and asthma represent a similar disease process occurring in the upper and lower airways. The concept of "common mucosal susceptibility" or "one airway, one disease" has now emerged with compelling data to support it. Technically speaking, this concept is less supportive of a causal role of rhinosinusitis in asthma and more supportive of a common underlying pathogenesis. Based on immunopathologic data, there would appear to be little doubt that the concept has merit. However, acceptance of this premise should not diminish interest in the role of rhinosinusitis as a trigger for asthma. A hopeful view is that its acceptance will stimulate more enthusiasm for developing strategies to control inflammation in the upper airway, as has been engendered for lower airway inflammation over the past decade.

References

1. Lanza DC, Kennedy DW. Adult rhinosinusitis defined. Otolaryngol Head Neck Surg 1997; 117(3/2):S1–S7.
2. Pedersen PA, Weeke ER. Asthma and allergic rhinitis in the same patients. Allergy 1983; 38(1):25–29.
3. Lundback B. Epidemiology of rhinitis and asthma. Clin Exp Allergy 1998; 28(suppl 2):3–10.
4. Vignola AM, Chanez P, Godard P, Bousquet J. Relationships between rhinitis and asthma. Allergy 1998; 53(9):833–839.
5. Annesi-Maesano I. Epidemiological evidence of the occurrence of rhinitis and sinusitis in asthmatics. Allergy 1999; 54(suppl 57):7–13.
6. Lindberg S, Malm L. Comparison of allergic rhinitis and vasomotor rhinitis patients on the basis of a computer questionnaire. Allergy 1993; 48(8):602–607.
7. Enberg RN. Perennial nonallergic rhinitis: a retrospective review. Ann Allergy 1989; 63(6/1):513–516.
8. Witteman AM, Sjamsoedin DH, Jansen HM, van der Zee JS. Differences in nonspecific bronchial responsiveness between patients with asthma and patients with rhinitis are not explained by type and degree of inhalant allergy. Int Arch Allergy Immunol 1997; 112(1):65–72.
9. Moneret-Vautrin DA, Hsieh V, Wayoff M, Guyot JL, Mouton C, Maria Y. Nonallergic rhinitis with eosinophilia syndrome a precursor of the triad: nasal polyposis, intrinsic asthma, and intolerance to aspirin. Ann Allergy 1990; 64(6):513–518.
10. Jacobs RL, Freedman PM, Boswell RN. Nonallergic rhinitis with eosinophilia (NARES syndrome): clinical and immunologic presentation. J Allergy Clin Immunol 1981; 67(4):253–262.
11. Corren J. Allergic rhinitis and asthma: how important is the link? J Allergy Clin Immunol 1997; 99(2):S781–S786.
12. Humbert M, Durham SR, Ying S, Kimmitt P, Barkans J, Assoufi B, et al. IL-4 and IL-5 mRNA and protein in bronchial biopsies from patients with atopic and nona-

topic asthma: evidence against asthma being a distinct immunopathologic entity. Am J Respir Crit Care Med 1996; 154(5):1497–1504.

13. Bentley AM, Meng Q, Robinson DS, Hamid Q, Kay AB, Durham SR. Increases in activated T lymphocytes, eosinophils, and cytokine mRNA expression for interleukin-5 and granulocyte/macrophage colony-stimulating factor in bronchial biopsies after allergen inhalation challenge in atopic asthmatics. Am J Respir Cell Mol Biol 1993; 8(1):35–42.

14. Pirson F, Charpin D, Sansonetti M, Lanteaume A, Kulling G, Charpin J, et al. Is intrinsic asthma a hereditary disease? Allergy 1991; 46(5):367–371.

15. Sibbald B. Epidemiology of allergic rhinitis. Monogr Allergy 1993; 31:61–79.

16. Hamilos DL. Chronic sinusitis. J Allergy Clin Immunol 2000; 106(2):213–227.

17. Adams PF, Marano MA. The National Health Interview Survey, 1994. Vital Health Statistics 10:83–84, 1995.

18. Senior BA, Kennedy DW, Tanabodee J, Kroger H, Hassab M, Lanza DC. Long-term impact of functional endoscopic sinus surgery on asthma. Otolaryngol Head Neck Surg 1999; 121(1):66–68.

19. McNally PA, White MV, Kaliner MA. Sinusitis in an allergist's office: analysis of 200 consecutive cases. Allergy Asthma Proc 1997; 18(3):169–175.

20. Settipane GA. Epidemiology of nasal polyps. Allergy Asthma Proc 1996; 17(5): 231–236.

21. Settipane GA. Aspirin sensitivity and allergy. Biomed Pharmacother 1988; 42(8): 493–498.

22. Tedeschi A, Palumbo G, Milazzo N, Miadonna A. Nasal neutrophilia and eosinophilia induced by challenge with platelet activating factor. J Allergy Clin Immunol 1994; 93(2):526–533.

23. Demoly P, Crampette L, Mondain M, Campbell AM, Lequeux N, Enander I, et al. Assessment of inflammation in noninfectious chronic maxillary sinusitis. J Allergy Clin Immunol 1994; 94(1):95–108.

24. Hamilos DL, Leung DY, Wood R, Meyers A, Stephens JK, Barkans J, et al. Chronic hyperplastic sinusitis: association of tissue eosinophilia with mRNA expression of granulocyte-macrophage colony-stimulating factor and interleukin-3. J Allergy Clin Immunol 1993; 92(1/1):39–48.

25. Demoly P, Crampette L, Mondain M, Enander I, Jones I, Bousquet J. Myeloperoxidase and interleukin-8 levels in chronic sinusitis. Clin Exp Allergy 1997; 27(6): 672–675.

26. Rhyoo C, Sanders SP, Leopold DA, Proud D. Sinus mucosal IL-8 gene expression in chronic rhinosinusitis. J Allergy Clin Immunol 1999; 103(3/1):395–400.

27. Bachert C, Wagenmann M, Rudack C, Hopken K, Hillebrandt M, Wang D, et al. The role of cytokines in infectious sinusitis and nasal polyposis. Allergy 1998; 53(1):2–13.

28. Bedard M, McClure CD, Schiller NL, Francoeur C, Cantin A, Denis M. Release of interleukin-8, interleukin-6, and colony-stimulating factors by upper airway epithelial cells: implications for cystic fibrosis. Am J Respir Cell Mol Biol 1993; 9(4): 455–462.

29. Inoue H, Massion PP, Ueki IF, Grattan KM, Hara M, Dohrman AF, et al. Pseudomonas stimulates interleukin-8 mRNA expression selectively in airway epithelium,

in gland ducts, and in recruited neutrophils. Am J Respir Cell Mol Biol 1994; 11(6): 651–663.

30. Khair OA, Davies RJ, Devalia JL. Bacterial-induced release of inflammatory mediators by bronchial epithelial cells. Eur Respir J 1996; 9(9):1913–1922.

31. Slavin RG. Sinusitis in adults and its relation to allergic rhinitis, asthma, and nasal polyps. J Allergy Clin Immunol 1988; 82(5/2):950–956.

32. Rowe-Jones JM, Shembekar M, Trendell-Smith N, Mackay IS. Polypoidal rhinosinusitis in cystic fibrosis: a clinical and histopathological study. Clin Otolaryngol 1997; 22(2):167–171.

33. Hamilos DL, Leung DY, Wood R, Cunningham L, Bean DK, Yasruel Z, et al. Evidence for distinct cytokine expression in allergic versus nonallergic chronic sinusitis. J Allergy Clin Immunol 1995; 96(4):537–544.

34. Hamilos DL, Leung DY, Wood R, Bean DK, Song YL, Schotman E, et al. Eosinophil infiltration in nonallergic chronic hyperplastic sinusitis with nasal polyposis (CHS/NP) is associated with endothelial VCAM-1 upregulation and expression of TNF-alpha. Am J Respir Cell Mol Biol 1996; 15(4):443–450.

35. Hamilos DL, Leung DY, Huston DP, Kamil A, Wood R, Hamid Q. GM-CSF, IL-5 and RANTES immunoreactivity and mRNA expression in chronic hyperplastic sinusitis with nasal polyposis (NP). Clin Exp Allergy 1998; 28(9):1145–1152.

36. Walker C, Bode E, Boer L, Hansel TT, Blaser K, Virchow JC Jr. Allergic and nonallergic asthmatics have distinct patterns of T-cell activation and cytokine production in peripheral blood and bronchoalveolar lavage. Am Rev Respir Dis 1992; 146(1):109–115.

37. Moqbel R, Hamid Q, Ying S, Barkans J, Hartnell A, Tsicopoulos A, et al. Expression of mRNA and immunoreactivity for the granulocyte/macrophage colony-stimulating factor in activated human eosinophils. J Exp Med 1991; 174(3):749–752.

38. Simon HU, Yousefi S, Schranz C, Schapowal A, Bachert C, Blaser K. Direct demonstration of delayed eosinophil apoptosis as a mechanism causing tissue eosinophilia. J Immunol 1997; 158(8):3902–3908.

39. Minshall EM, Cameron L, Lavigne F, Leung DY, Hamilos D, Garcia-Zepada EA, et al. Eotaxin mRNA and protein expression in chronic sinusitis and allergen-induced nasal responses in seasonal allergic rhinitis. Am J Respir Cell Mol Biol 1997; 17(6):683–690.

40. Takeuchi K, Yuta A, Sakakura Y. Interleukin-8 gene expression in chronic sinusitis. Am J Otolaryngol 1995; 16(2):98–102.

41. Bachert C, Ganzer U. [The role of pro-inflammatory cytokines in recruiting inflammatory cells in the nose]. Laryngorhinootologie 1993; 72(12):585–589.

42. McFadden ER Jr. Nasal-sinus-pulmonary reflexes and bronchial asthma. J Allergy Clin Immunol 1986; 78(1/1):1–3.

43. Drettner B. Pathophysiological relationship between the upper and lower airways. Ann Otol Rhinol Laryngol 1970; 79(3):499–505.

44. Kaufman J, Wright GW. The effect of nasal and nasopharyngeal irritation on airway resistance in man. Am Rev Respir Dis 1969; 100(5):626–630.

45. Kaufman J, Chen JC, Wright GW. The effect of trigeminal resection on reflex

bronchoconstriction after nasal and nasopharyngeal irritation in man. Am Rev Respir Dis 1970; 101(5):768–769.

46. Yan K, Salome C. The response of the airways to nasal stimulation in asthmatics with rhinitis. Eur J Respir Dis Suppl 1983; 128(1):105–109.

47. Fontanari P, Burnet H, Zattara-Hartmann MC, Jammes Y. Changes in airway resistance induced by nasal inhalation of cold dry, dry, or moist air in normal individuals. J Appl Physiol 1996; 81(4):1739–1743.

48. Fontanari P, Zattara-Hartmann MC, Burnet H, Jammes Y. Nasal eupnoeic inhalation of cold, dry air increases airway resistance in asthmatic patients. Eur Respir J 1997; 10(10):2250–2254.

49. Hoehne JH, Reed CE. Where is the allergic reaction in ragweed asthma? J Allergy Clin Immunol 1971; 48(1):36–39.

50. Rosenberg GL, Rosenthal RR, Norman PS. Inhalation challenge with ragweed pollen in ragweed-sensitive asthmatics. J Allergy Clin Immunol 1983; 71(3):302–310.

51. Schumacher MJ, Cota KA, Taussig LM. Pulmonary response to nasal-challenge testing of atopic subjects with stable asthma. J Allergy Clin Immunol 1986; 78 (1/1):30–35.

52. Corren J, Adinoff AD, Irvin CG. Changes in bronchial responsiveness following nasal provocation with allergen. J Allergy Clin Immunol 1992; 89(2):611–618.

53. Corren J, Adinoff AD, Buchmeier AD, Irvin CG. Nasal beclomethasone prevents the seasonal increase in bronchial responsiveness in patients with allergic rhinitis and asthma. J Allergy Clin Immunol 1992; 90(2):250–256.

54. Georgitis JW, Matthews BL, Stone B. Chronic sinusitis: characterization of cellular influx and inflammatory mediators in sinus lavage fluid. Int Arch Allergy Immunol 1995; 106(4):416–421.

55. Kramer MF, Ostertag P, Pfrogner E, Rasp G. Nasal interleukin-5, immunoglobulin E, eosinophilic cationic protein, and soluble intercellular adhesion molecule-1 in chronic sinusitis, allergic rhinitis, and nasal polyposis. Laryngoscope 2000; 110(6): 1056–1062.

56. Irvin CG. Sinusitis and asthma: an animal model. J Allergy Clin Immunol 1992; 90(3/1):521–533.

57. Brugman SM, Larsen GL, Henson PM, Honor J, Irvin CG. Increased lower airways responsiveness associated with sinusitis in a rabbit model. Am Rev Respir Dis 1993; 147(2):314–320.

58. Huxley EJ, Viroslav J, Gray WR, Pierce AK. Pharyngeal aspiration in normal adults and patients with depressed consciousness. Am J Med 1978; 64(4):564–568.

59. Bardin PG, Van Heerden BB, Joubert JR. Absence of pulmonary aspiration of sinus contents in patients with asthma and sinusitis. J Allergy Clin Immunol 1990; 86(1): 82–88.

60. Chai H, Farr RS, Froehlich LA, Mathison DA, McLean JA, Rosenthal RR, et al. Standardization of bronchial inhalation challenge procedures. J Allergy Clin Immunol 1975; 56(4):323–327.

61. Bucca C, Rolla G, Scappaticci E, Chiampo F, Bugiani M, Magnano M, et al. Extrathoracic and intrathoracic airway responsiveness in sinusitis. J Allergy Clin Immunol 1995; 95(1/1):52–59.

62. Bucca C, Rolla G, Scappaticci E, Baldi S, Caria E, Oliva A. Histamine hyperresponsiveness of the extrathoracic airway in patients with asthmatic symptoms. Allergy 1991; 46(2):147–153.

63. Rolla G, Colagrande P, Scappaticci E, Bottomicca F, Magnano M, Brussino L, et al. Damage of the pharyngeal mucosa and hyperresponsiveness of airway in sinusitis. J Allergy Clin Immunol 1997; 100(1):52–57.

64. Grossman J. One airway, one disease. Chest 1997; 111(suppl 2):11S–16S.

65. Durham SR. Effect of intranasal corticosteroid treatment on asthma in children and adults. Allergy 1999; 54(suppl 57):124–131.

66. Togias A. Mechanisms of nose-lung interaction. Allergy 1999; 54(suppl 57):94–105.

67. Settipane RJ, Hagy GW, Settipane GA. Long-term risk factors for developing asthma and allergic rhinitis: a 23-year follow-up study of college students. Allergy Proc 1994; 15(1):21–25.

68. Chakir J, Laviolette M, Boutet M, Laliberte R, Dube J, Boulet LP. Lower airways remodeling in nonasthmatic subjects with allergic rhinitis. Lab Invest 1996; 75(5): 735–744.

69. Durham SR, Ying S, Varney VA, Jacobson MR, Sudderick RM, Mackay IS, et al. Cytokine messenger RNA expression for IL-3, IL-4, IL-5, and granulocyte/macrophage-colony-stimulating factor in the nasal mucosa after local allergen provocation: relationship to tissue eosinophilia. J Immunol 1992; 148(8):2390–2394.

70. Rajakulasingam K, Hamid Q, O'Brien F, Shotman E, Jose PJ, Williams TJ, et al. RANTES in human allergen-induced rhinitis: cellular source and relation to tissue eosinophilia. Am J Respir Crit Care Med 1997; 155(2):696–703.

71. Iademarco MF, Barks JL, Dean DC. Regulation of vascular cell adhesion molecule-1 expression by IL-4 and TNF-alpha in cultured endothelial cells. J Clin Invest 1995; 95(1):264–271.

72. Weller PF. The immunobiology of eosinophils. N Engl J Med 1991; 324(16):1110–1118.

73. Turkeltaub PC, Gergen PJ. Epidemiology of allergic disease and allergen skin test reactivity in the US population: data from the second National Health and Nutrition Examination Survey (1976–1980)-NHANES II. Arb Paul Ehrlich Inst Bundesamt Sera Impfstoffe Frankf A M 1992; 85:59–80.

74. Spector SL. Leukotriene activity modulation in asthma. Drugs 1997; 54(3):369–384.

75. Creticos PS, Peters SP, Adkinson NF Jr, Naclerio RM, Hayes EC, Norman PS, et al. Peptide leukotriene release after antigen challenge in patients sensitive to ragweed. N Engl J Med 1984; 310(25):1626–1630.

76. Naclerio RM, Baroody FM, Togias AG. The role of leukotrienes in allergic rhinitis: a review. Am Rev Respir Dis 1991; 143(5/2):S91–S95.

77. Harlin SL, Ansel DG, Lane SR, Myers J, Kephart GM, Gleich GJ. A clinical and pathologic study of chronic sinusitis: the role of the eosinophil. J Allergy Clin Immunol 1988; 81(5/1):867–875.

78. Hamilos DL, Thawley SE, Kramper MA, Kamil A, Hamid QA. Effect of intranasal fluticasone on cellular infiltration, endothelial adhesion molecule expression, and proinflammatory cytokine mRNA in nasal polyp disease. J Allergy Clin Immunol 1999; 103(1/1):79–87.

79. Newman LJ, Platts-Mills TA, Phillips CD, Hazen KC, Gross CW. Chronic sinusitis. Relationship of computed tomographic findings to allergy, asthma, and eosinophilia [published erratum appears in J Am Med Assoc 1994 Sep 21; 272(11):852]. J Am Med Assoc 1994; 271(5):363–367.

80. Ferreri NR, Howland WC, Stevenson DD, Spiegelberg HL. Release of leukotrienes, prostaglandins, and histamine into nasal secretions of aspirin-sensitive asthmatics during reaction to aspirin. Am Rev Respir Dis 1988; 137(4):847–854.

81. Kowalski ML, Grzegorczyk J, Wojciechowska B, Poniatowska M. Intranasal challenge with aspirin induces cell influx and activation of eosinophils and mast cells in nasal secretions of ASA-sensitive patients. Clin Exp Allergy 1996; 26(7):807–814.

82. Kohi F, Miyagawa H, Agrawal DK, Bewtra AK, Townley RG. Generation of leukotriene B4 and C4 from granulocytes of normal controls, allergic rhinitis, and asthmatic subjects. Ann Allergy 1990; 65(3):228–232.

83. Cowburn AS, Sladek K, Soja J, Adamek L, Nizankowska E, Szczeklik A, et al. Overexpression of leukotriene C4 synthase in bronchial biopsies from patients with aspirin-intolerant asthma. J Clin Invest 1998; 101(4):834–846.

84. Wilson JW, Djukanovic R, Howarth PH, Holgate ST. Lymphocyte activation in bronchoalveolar lavage and peripheral blood in atopic asthma. Am Rev Respir Dis 1992; 145(4/1):958–960.

85. Corrigan CJ, Hartnell A, Kay AB. T lymphocyte activation in acute severe asthma. Lancet 1988; 1(8595):1129–1132.

86. Alam R. Chemokines in allergic inflammation. J Allergy Clin Immunol 1997; 99(3):273–277.

87. Collins PD, Marleau S, Griffiths-Johnson DA, Jose PJ, Williams TJ. Cooperation between interleukin-5 and the chemokine eotaxin to induce eosinophil accumulation in vivo. J Exp Med 1995; 182(4):1169–1174.

88. Mould AW, Ramsay AJ, Matthaei KI, Young IG, Rothenberg ME, Foster PS. The effect of IL-5 and eotaxin expression in the lung on eosinophil trafficking and degranulation and the induction of bronchial hyperactivity. J Immunol 2000; 164(4):2142–2150.

89. Shi H, Qin S, Huang G, Chen Y, Xiao C, Xu H, et al. Infiltration of eosinophils into the asthmatic airways caused by interleukin 5. Am J Respir Cell Mol Biol 1997; 16(3):220–224.

90. Sehmi R, Wood LJ, Watson R, Foley R, Hamid Q, O'Byrne PM, et al. Allergen-induced increases in IL-5 receptor alpha-subunit expression on bone marrow-derived CD34+ cells from asthmatic subjects: a novel marker of progenitor cell commitment towards eosinophilic differentiation. J Clin Invest 1997; 100(10):2466–2475.

91. Wang J, Palmer K, Lotvall J, Milan S, Lei XF, Matthaei KI, et al. Circulating, but not local lung, IL-5 is required for the development of antigen-induced airways eosinophilia. J Clin Invest 1998; 102(6):1132–1141.

92. Palframan RT, Collins PD, Williams TJ, Rankin SM. Eotaxin induces a rapid release of eosinophils and their progenitors from the bone marrow. Blood 1998; 91(7):2240–2248.

93. Lai CK, Ho AS, Chan CH, Tang J, Leung JC, Lai KN. Interleukin-5 messenger

RNA expression in peripheral blood CD4+ cells in asthma. J Allergy Clin Immunol 1996; 97(6):1320–1328.

94. Crimi E, Gaffi D, Frittoli E, Borgonovo B, Burastero SE. Depletion of circulating allergen-specific TH2 T lymphocytes after allergen exposure in asthma. J Allergy Clin Immunol 1997; 99(6/1):788–797.

95. Borgonovo B, Casorati G, Frittoli E, Gaffi D, Crimi E, Burastero SE. Recruitment of circulating allergen-specific T lymphocytes to the lung on allergen challenge in asthma. J Allergy Clin Immunol 1997; 100(5):669–678.

96. Mygind N, Dirksen A, Johnsen NJ, Weeke B. Perennial rhinitis: an analysis of skin testing, serum IgE, and blood and smear eosinophilia in 201 patients. Clin Otolaryngol 1978; 3(2):189–196.

97. Welsh PW, Stricker WE, Chu CP, Naessens JM, Reese ME, Reed CE, et al. Efficacy of beclomethasone nasal solution, flunisolide, and cromolyn in relieving symptoms of ragweed allergy. Mayo Clin Proc 1987; 62(2):125–134.

98. Watson WT, Becker AB, Simons FE. Treatment of allergic rhinitis with intranasal corticosteroids in patients with mild asthma: effect on lower airway responsiveness. J Allergy Clin Immunol 1993; 91(1/1):97–101.

99. Aubier M, Levy J, Clerici C, Neukirch F, Herman D. Different effects of nasal and bronchial glucocorticosteroid administration on bronchial hyperresponsiveness in patients with allergic rhinitis. Am Rev Respir Dis 1992; 146(1):122–126.

100. Sanico AM, Philip G, Proud D, Naclerio RM, Togias A. Comparison of nasal mucosal responsiveness to neuronal stimulation in non-allergic and allergic rhinitis: effects of capsaicin nasal challenge. Clin Exp Allergy 1998; 28(1):92–100.

101. Sanico AM, Philip G, Lai GK, Togias A. Hyperosmolar saline induces reflex nasal secretions, evincing neural hyperresponsiveness in allergic rhinitis. J Appl Physiol 1999; 86(4):1202–1210.

102. Rachelefsky GS, Katz RM, Siegel SC. Chronic sinus disease with associated reactive airway disease in children. Pediatrics 1984; 73(4):526–529.

103. Businco L, Fiore L, Frediani T, Artuso A, Difazio A, Bellioni P. Clinical and therapeutic aspects of sinusitis in children with bronchial asthma Int J Paediat Otorhinolaryngol 1981; 3:287–294.

104. Cummings NP, Wood R, Lere JL, Adinoff AD. Effects of treatment of rhinitis/sinusitis on asthma: results of a double-blind study. Paediat Res 1983; 17:373–378.

105. Friedman R, Ackerman M, Wald E, Casselbrant M, Friday G, Fireman P. Asthma and bacterial sinusitis in children. J Allergy Clin Immunol 1984; 74(2):185–189.

106. Friedman WH, Katsantonis GP, Slavin RG, Kannel P, Linford P. Sphenoethmoidectomy: its role in the asthmatic patient. Otolaryngol Head Neck Surg 1982; 90(2): 171–177.

107. Slavin RG. Relationship of nasal disease and sinusitis to bronchial asthma. Ann Allergy 1982; 49(2):76–79.

108. Lawson W. The intranasal ethmoidectomy: an experience with 1,077 procedures. Laryngoscope 1991; 101(4/1):367–371.

109. Mings R, Friedman WH, Linford P, et al. Five year follow-up of the effects of bilateral intranasal sphenoethmoidectomy in patients with sinusitis and asthma. Am J Rhinol 1998; 71:123–132.

110. English GM. Nasal polypectomy and sinus surgery in patients with asthma and aspirin idiosyncrasy. Laryngoscope 1986; 96(4):374–380.

111. Stammberger H. Endoscopic endonasal surgery—concepts in treatment of recurring rhinosinusitis. Part II: surgical technique. Otolaryngol Head Neck Surg 1986; 94(2):147–156.

112. Stammberger H. Endoscopic endonasal surgery—concepts in treatment of recurring rhinosinusitis. Part I: anatomic and pathophysiologic considerations. Otolaryngol Head Neck Surg 1986; 94(2):143–147.

113. Wigand ME, Hosemann WG. Results of endoscopic surgery of the paranasal sinuses and anterior skull base. J Otolaryngol 1991; 20(6):385–390.

114. Jankowski R, Moneret-Vautrin DA, Goetz R, Wayoff M. Incidence of medicosurgical treatment for nasal polyps on the development of associated asthma. Rhinology 1992; 30(4):249–258.

115. Nishioka GJ, Cook PR, Davis WE, McKinsey JP. Functional endoscopic sinus surgery in patients with chronic sinusitis and asthma. Otolaryngol Head Neck Surg 1994; 110(6):494–500.

116. Manning SC, Wasserman RL, Silver R, Phillips DL. Results of endoscopic sinus surgery in pediatric patients with chronic sinusitis and asthma. Arch Otolaryngol Head Neck Surg 1994; 120(10):1142–1145.

117. Senior BA, Kennedy DW. Management of sinusitis in the asthmatic patient. Ann Allergy Asthma Immunol 1996; 77(1):6–15.

118. Dunlop G, Scadding GK, Lund VJ. The effect of endoscopic sinus surgery on asthma: management of patients with chronic rhinosinusitis, nasal polyposis, and asthma. Am J Rhinol 1999; 13(4):261–265.

119. Lund VJ. The effect of sinonasal surgery on asthma. Allergy 1999; 54(suppl 57): 141–145.

120. White PS, Cowan IA, Robertson MS. Limited CT scanning techniques of the paranasal sinuses. J Laryngol Otol 1991; 105(1):20–23.

121. Mafee MF. Modern imaging of paranasal sinuses and the role of limited sinus computerized tomography: considerations of time, cost and radiation. Ear Nose Throat J 1994; 73(8):532–534,536–538,540–542.

122. Wippold FJ, 2nd, Levitt RG, Evens RG, Korenblat PE, Hodges FJ, 3rd, Jost RG. Limited coronal CT: an alternative screening examination for sinonasal inflammatory disease. Allergy Proc 1995; 16(4):165–169.

123. Hamilos DL. Noninfectious sinusitis. Allergy Clin Immunol Int 2001; 13(1):27–32.

124. Kennedy DW. Prognostic factors, outcomes and staging in ethmoid sinus surgery. Laryngoscope 1992; 102(12/2,suppl 57):1–18.

125. Haruna S, Yoshikawa M, Iida M, Ohtori N, Shimada C, Ozawa M, et al. [A study on the concentration of eosinophil cationic protein in chronic sinusitis]. Nippon Jibiinkoka Gakkai Kaiho 1999; 102(9):1015–1021.

126. Appenroth E, Gunkel AR, Muller H, Volklein C, Schrott-Fischer A. Activated and nonactivated eosinophils in patients with chronic rhinosinusitis. Acta Otolaryngol (Stockh) 1998; 118(2):240–242.

127. Katzenstein AL, Sale SR, Greenberger PA. Pathologic findings in allergic aspergillus sinusitis: a newly recognized form of sinusitis. Am J Surg Pathol 1983; 7(5): 439–443.

128. deShazo RD, Swain RE. Diagnostic criteria for allergic fungal sinusitis. J Allergy Clin Immunol 1995; 96(1):24–35.

129. Cody DT, 2nd, Neel HB, 3rd, Ferreiro JA, Roberts GD. Allergic fungal sinusitis: the Mayo Clinic experience. Laryngoscope 1994; 104(9):1074–1079.

130. Kuhn FA, Javer AR. Allergic fungal rhinosinusitis: our experience. Arch Otolaryngol Head Neck Surg 1998; 124(10):1179–1180.

131. Manning SC, Merkel M, Kriesel K, Vuitch F, Marple B. Computed tomography and magnetic resonance diagnosis of allergic fungal sinusitis. Laryngoscope 1997; 107(2):170–176.

132. Mott AE, Cain WS, Lafreniere D, Leonard G, Gent JF, Frank ME. Topical corticosteroid treatment of anosmia associated with nasal and sinus disease. Arch Otolaryngol Head Neck Surg 1997; 123(4):367–372.

133. Canciani M, Mastella G. Efficacy of beclomethasone nasal drops, administered in the Moffat's position for nasal polyposis. Acta Paediatr Scand 1988; 77(4):612–613.

134. Folker RJ, Marple BF, Mabry RL, Mabry CS. Treatment of allergic fungal sinusitis: a comparison trial of postoperative immunotherapy with specific fungal antigens. Laryngoscope 1998; 108(11/1):1623–1627.

135. Sweet JM, Stevenson DD, Simon RA, Mathison DA. Long-term effects of aspirin desensitization—treatment for aspirin-sensitive rhinosinusitis-asthma. J Allergy Clin Immunol 1990; 85(1/1):59–65.

136. Schapowal AG, Simon HU, Schmitz-Schumann M. Phenomenology, pathogenesis, diagnosis and treatment of aspirin-sensitive rhinosinusitis. Acta Otorhinolaryngol Belg 1995; 49(3):235–250.

137. Stevenson DD, Hankammer MA, Mathison DA, Christiansen SC, Simon RA. Aspirin desensitization treatment of aspirin-sensitive patients with rhinosinusitis-asthma: long-term outcomes. J Allergy Clin Immunol 1996; 98(4):751–758.

19

Monitoring Activity of Severe Asthma

RICHARD LEIGH, MARGARET M. KELLY, and FREDERICK E. HARGREAVE

St. Joseph's Healthcare
McMaster University
Hamilton, Ontario, Canada

I. Introduction

The severity of asthma has traditionally been defined according to clinical measurements that assess symptomatic interference of daily activities or sleep, the need for use of a short-acting β_2-agonist, frequency of exacerbations, and variable airflow limitation (1). However, with appropriate therapy, many of these defining features are minimal or absent. Their presence, therefore, indicates a lack of asthma control rather than of asthma severity (Table 1) (2,3). Asthma severity is more appropriately defined by the minimum dose of corticosteroid anti-inflammatory treatment required to maintain control when control is defined as no symptoms, no limitation of activities, no need for rescue bronchodilator, and normal spirometry or peak expiratory flow (PEF). The severity can be graded into very mild, mild, moderate, severe, and very severe (Table 2) (3). In this context, controlled asthma is not synonymous with mild asthma, since in many patients severe asthma can be controlled. Alternatively, mild asthma can become poorly controlled and associated with a severe exacerbation but, when appropriate treatment is given, it may eventually require treatment with only low-dose inhaled steroid to maintain control.

Table 1 Indications of Acceptable Asthma Control

Parameter	Frequency
Daytime symptoms	<4 days/week
Nighttime symptoms	<1 night/week
Physical activity	Normal
Exacerbations	Mild, infrequent
Absence from work or school	None
Need for short-acting β_2-agonist	<4 doses/week[a]
FEV$_1$ or PEF	>85% of personal best, ideally 90%
PEF diurnal variation[b]	<15% of diurnal variation

Note: FEV$_1$ = forced expiratory volume in 1 sec; PEF = peak expiratory flow obtained with a portable peak flow meter.
[a] May use one dose/day for prevention of exercise-induced symptoms.
[b] Diurnal variation is calculated by subtracting the lowest PEF from the highest and dividing by the highest PEF multiplied by 100.
From Ref. 3.

Table 2 Levels of Asthma Severity Based on Treatment Needed to Obtain Control

Asthma severity	Symptoms	Treatment requirements[a]
Very mild	Mild/infrequent (controlled)	None or rarely inhaled short-acting β_2-agonist
Mild	Controlled	Occasional short-acting β_2-agonist and low-dose inhaled corticosteroids
Moderate	Controlled	Short-acting β_2-agonist and low- to medium-dose inhaled corticosteroid ± additional therapy
Severe	Controlled	Short-acting β_2-agonist and high-dose inhaled corticosteroid ± additional therapy
Very severe	May be controlled or uncontrolled	Short-acting β_2-agonist and high-dose inhaled + ingested corticosteroid ± additional therapy

[a] Daily doses of inhaled corticosteroid (approximate equivalent doses) are as follows:
low: beclomethasone diproprionate ≤500 μg, fluticasone ≤250 μg, and budesonide ≤400 μg; medium: beclomethasone diproprionate >500–1000 μg, fluticasone >250–500 μg, and budesonide >400–800 μg; high: beclomethasone diproprionate >1000 μg, fluticasone >500 μg, and budesonide >800 μg.
From Ref. 3.

In this chapter, therefore, we limit our discussion to severe asthma, which requires a high dose of inhaled corticosteroid (beclomethasone diproprionate >1000 µg/day or equivalent) and sometimes additional therapy (e.g., long-acting β_2-agonists or leukotriene antagonists) to maintain control, and to very severe asthma, which requires additional treatment with prednisone (Table 2) (3). In these groups of patients, control will be achieved by some but in others it is more appropriate to aim for what is called "acceptable control" (Table 1); in a few patients, acceptable control cannot be achieved.

In asthma in general, objective measurements are needed to confirm the diagnosis and to monitor treatment. While this has been advised in all guidelines (1,3), it is frequently not applied. Objective measurements are essential in treating severe asthma, where recognition of airflow limitation can be poor and it can be difficult to optimize corticosteroid and additional treatments. The monitoring of severe and very severe asthma should therefore include assessment of symptoms, spirometry or PEF, and sometimes PEF monitoring at home and assessment of airway responsiveness. Induced sputum cell counts and exhaled nitric oxide (ENO) also need to be considered. Before reviewing these measurements, we discuss some principles of monitoring.

II. Principles in the Monitoring of Severe Asthma

Severe asthma is sometimes confused with other conditions such as laryngeal dysfunction, hyperventilation, chronic obstructive pulmonary disease, or heart failure. It is therefore important that the diagnosis of asthma is objectively confirmed and that these other conditions are either excluded or, if also present, included in the management. It is also important that an assessment is made of the compliance with corticosteroid treatment; poor compliance is a common cause of difficult-to-control severe asthma (4).

The cause of severe asthma is considered to be airway inflammation which results in airway hyperresponsiveness, airflow limitation, and variable airflow limitation, either directly or secondarily through remodeling. It is therefore important to carefully investigate causes of airway inflammation, like allergens and chemical sensitizers, to exclude the possibility that drugs are being used which cause bronchoconstriction (such as nonsteroidal anti-inflammatory drugs and β-blockers) and to determine whether aggravating conditions are present, such as gastroesophageal reflux or rhinosinusitis. Appropriate avoidance strategies or treatment of aggravating conditions can then be implemented. Once this has been done, the occurrence of severe and very severe asthma seems to indicate either that the patient is relatively corticosteroid resistant compared to those with milder asthma or that the inflammatory response is more severe, since larger doses of corticosteroid are necessary to maintain control. Careful monitoring of treatment is then required to identify the minimum dose of corticosteroid and short-acting β_2-agonist necessary to maintain control or acceptable control and, if required, to introduce additional treatment. The additional therapy can also help to minimize the corticosteroid dose required.

Managing severe and very severe asthma therefore is best handled by specialists who are familiar with the condition and have the resources to monitor the patients carefully. Determining the most effective treatment usually takes many months, even when patients are seen at intervals of 1 month. Specialized asthma clinics can also more easily investigate new methods of monitoring asthma, such as induced sputum cell counts (5) and ENO, and the effects of new treatments. Side effects of corticosteroid treatment are also appropriately investigated and treated in these settings.

III. Symptoms

Assessing the symptoms of asthma is clearly an essential part of obtaining and maintaining control of the disease. In addition to chest tightness, wheezing, and dyspnea, symptoms can also include cough and sputum. The symptoms are directly produced by airway inflammation and by episodic airflow limitation. The former is characteristically illustrated when symptoms, particularly cough and sputum, are present when variable airflow limitation and airway hyperresponsiveness are absent (6–8). This can occur in patients who require high-dose inhaled steroid or additional prednisone to control their symptoms.

The presence of symptoms, except those due to strenuous exercise if pretreatment with a β_2-agonist is not given, indicates that a patient's asthma is not controlled. As mentioned above, they do not necessarily reflect asthma severity. Symptoms present upon waking in the morning or which disturb sleep, limit activities, need treatment with an inhaled short-acting β_2-agonist several times a day or at night, and/or require a visit to the emergency department or hospital admission indicate a marked lack of asthma control.

The presence of symptoms is usually a good indicator of the level of control but, especially in cases of severe and very severe asthma, this is not always reliable (9,10). Some asthma patients, called poor perceivers, fail to recognize symptoms until airflow limitation is more severe. Some symptoms are the results of eosinophilic bronchitis, which characterizes uncontrolled asthma (11), or indicate variable airflow limitation (10,12) and are often misinterpreted by patients and physicians. For example, in patients with asthma, cough with or without sputum can be due to infective bronchitis, postnasal drip, or gastroesophageal reflux. Also, the other symptoms of asthma can be associated with an infective bronchitis or other complicating condition, such as chronic airflow limitation or heart failure. Chronic airflow limitation is common in patients with severe asthma. For these reasons, and because the definition of control also includes normal or best airway function, objective measurements of variable airflow limitation and airway inflammation are necessary.

IV. Spirometry

Spirometry, which is used to measure the forced expired volume in 1 sec (FEV_1) and the FEV_1/forced vital capacity (FVC) or slow VC, is the best way to monitor the presence, severity, and reversibility of any airflow limitation, when carried out according to recommended standards (13,14). It should be performed at each visit and, therefore, because this is impractical in the office or clinic of the family physician or internist, patients with severe asthma should be seen by a specialist (15). In this setting, measurements can be made on equipment that is calibrated and maintained and carried out by trained staff in accordance with published standards (16).

In severe asthma, as in milder asthma, the FEV_1, FVC, and slow VC are better indicators of airflow than PEF, which is measured with a peak flow meter (17). The latter does not record absolute lung volumes, can be less sensitive in detecting airflow limitation, and is more dependent on a maximal expiratory effort than the FEV_1. Spirometry may be required to confirm the presence of asthma such that improvement in FEV_1 of $\geq 12\%$ (preferably 15%) 15 min after inhaled β_2-agonist or $\geq 20\%$ after 10–14 days of corticosteroid treatment is demonstrated (3). It is also necessary to assess the level of control of asthma, which requires that the FEV_1 be within 10% of predicted or personal best value and that the patient is using a minimum of medication. Lower measurements reflect suboptimal control, and FEV_1 values <60% of predicted or personal best indicate markedly uncontrolled asthma. While the objective assessment of airflow is important, normal airflow measurements at one time point do not exclude suboptimal asthma control, since uncontrolled symptoms with airway inflammation can occur with a normal FEV_1 (7). Variability in FEV_1 of >20% (>250 ml) over a period of days or weeks in patients whose symptoms are apparently stable and who have no airflow limitation present at a given time point is also considered indicative of suboptimal asthma control (13).

V. Peak Expiratory Flow

While measurements of PEF are not as sensitive or reliable as FEV_1 measurements, they do provide a useful objective assessment of the presence, severity, reversibility, and variability of airflow limitation (18). They can be used to monitor severe asthma when spirometry is not readily available. They are commonly used by physicians who treat patients with asthma and, like the FEV_1, should be performed at each visit. However, the measurements are dependent on maximal expiratory effort and must be performed optimally to accurately interpret results.

The patient's best PEF rate needs to be identified so that it can be used to identify and maintain control of asthma. As for FEV_1, PEF measurements provide a marker of asthma control rather than of asthma severity. Well-controlled asthma is evidenced by PEF measurements >90% of predicted or personal best values, with lower measurements reflecting suboptimal control (3). PEF measurements <60% of predicted or personal best values indicate markedly uncontrolled asthma. PEF measurements are particularly useful in the emergency department, where they can be used to rapidly identify and monitor patients with exacerbations of asthma.

PEF measurements also have the advantage that they can be used by the patient to monitor asthma at home. In this setting they can be used to identify best results, to determine increased variability for the diagnosis of asthma, or to monitor the effects of treatment. While the latter has not been shown to be of benefit in mild to moderate asthma, it may be useful in severe asthma, especially in patients who are for some reason unable to self-monitor worsening airflow limitation (19). Measurements can be made in the morning and in the evening and, at times of increased symptoms, before and after β_2-agonist administration. Diurnal variation can be calculated over a number of days by dividing the difference between the highest PEF and the lowest PEF by the highest PEF during that period and then multiplying by 100 [(highest PEF − lowest PEF) ÷ highest PEF × 100]. In asthma that is adequately controlled, diurnal variation in PEF should be less than 15%, and patients should be alerted to the fact that an increase in diurnal variation in PEF >20% indicates a loss of asthma control (3). However, because of the cumbersome calculations involved in determining diurnal variation, Reddel and coworkers (20) have recently proposed the use of a simpler measure. This measurement, called the lowest percentage personal best, is obtained from the lowest PEF, usually upon waking, over 1 or 2 weeks as a percentage of the patient's personal best measurement recorded on the same peak flow meter. Values <80% correlate strongly with airway hyperresponsiveness and to a lesser extent with asthma symptoms and airflow limitation.

While peak flow meters are cost effective and easy to use in the home setting, PEF measurements do have limitations. The meters tend to underestimate the degree of airflow limitation and the correlation between PEF measured with a portable peak flow meter and that measured with spirometers is poor (21). The results recorded by peak flow meters of the same brand may vary, and readings may change with extended use; the meters should therefore be checked regularly for accuracy and reproducibility of results (22). Furthermore, because their performance in the home setting is unsupervised, the accuracy of the measurements cannot be confirmed, and compliance with performing regular PEF measurements has been shown to be problematic (23).

Until recently, symptoms, PEF measurements, and spirometry have been the only measurements on which to base treatment decisions regarding the appropriate doses of anti-inflammatory medication. However, measurement of airway responsiveness and of airway inflammation also need to be considered.

VI. Airway Hyperresponsiveness

Measurements of airway responsiveness are not usually required in patients with severe asthma but they may be needed to validate the diagnosis of asthma and they might be useful to monitor treatment. Most investigators have used methacholine to measure airway responsiveness but some prefer indirect stimuli, such as exercise (24) or hypertonic saline (25).

The methacholine inhalation test is the most sensitive method to measure airway responsiveness and to validate the diagnosis of asthma. Normal values have been published for different methods of aerosol generation and inhalation (26–29). The test is of most use when symptoms are consistent with asthma and the FEV_1 is normal, which is most often the case when asthma is not present or is of very mild to moderate severity. However, it can be useful in severe or very severe asthma when treatment has controlled the asthma (and may have returned the airway responsiveness to mild or normal) to a point where an additional bronchodilator may not be required. Alternatively it can be useful to investigate the cause of excessive symptoms when treatment has returned the FEV_1 to normal. In this situation, the presence of mild or normal responsiveness would suggest that the excessive symptoms have another cause, such as hyperventilation, laryngeal dysfunction, gastroesophageal reflux, or heart failure.

While methacholine causes airway constriction by a direct effect on smooth muscle, bronchoprovocation tests with hypertonic saline and exercise (or eucapnic hyperventilation of dry air, which demonstrates similar responsiveness) are considered to act indirectly through the release of bronchoconstrictive mediators (30). Like methacholine, their effect is enhanced in the presence of eosinophilic airway inflammation (31). The indirect tests are less sensitive than methacholine, but more specific for symptomatic asthma. When these tests are used for diagnosis, the milder forms of hyperresponsiveness are usually not detected (32).

The methacholine test has also been used to monitor the effects of treatment. In a prospective randomized controlled trial, Sont and coworkers (33) have shown that an anti-inflammatory treatment strategy aimed at reducing airway hyperresponsiveness, measured at 3-month intervals, reduced the number of mild exacerbations as well as the extent of chronic airway inflammation present in patients with mild to moderate asthma compared to anti-inflammatory treatment based solely on symptoms and lung function. Since only a small proportion of participants in this study had severe asthma, as indicated by their maintenance dose of inhaled corticosteroids, it might be implied that the results are not generalizable to patients with severe asthma. However, in a recent study from Australia (34), patients with poorly controlled asthma were treated with high doses of inhaled budesonide (>1600 µg/day) for 8 weeks, after which the dose was reduced in a carefully titrated fashion. By week 16, airway hyperresponsiveness had decreased approximately three doubling doses.

These studies confirm that appropriate corticosteroid treatment can reverse the airway hyperresponsiveness and raise the possibility that the tests might be useful to monitor corticosteroid treatment, even in patients with severe and very severe asthma. However, this requires further investigation. Similar studies of patients who require additional prednisone would be useful to investigate the value of measuring airway responsiveness with both methacholine and an indirect stimulus, such as hypertonic saline.

VII. Measurement of Airway Inflammation

Airway inflammation is considered to be a cause of asthma and of a number of other airway diseases, exacerbations, and remodeling (35). The latter, as suggested by the development of chronic airflow limitation, seems to be particularly prevalent in patients with very severe asthma. The treatment of the inflammation is therefore the primary objective. As the assessment of symptoms and airway function principally evaluate airway patency and responsiveness, and as these measurements do not necessarily correlate closely with airway inflammation (36), measurements of airway inflammation are important in research and are likely to be useful in clinical practice (37).

A. Induced Sputum Examination

Measurements of airway inflammation have become more common in clinical practice since modified methods of sputum induction have been applied in patients with asthma (38,39) and the methods of processing the sputum have been refined (39,40). The measurements of sputum inflammatory nonsquamous cell counts are easy, reliable (41,42), valid (41), and responsive (5,43,44), all qualities of good measurements. However, it has been shown that the expectorate needs to be processed within 2 h [although this has now been extended to 9 h if it is stored at 4°C (45)] and the processing and assessment together take about 2 h. Furthermore, it is necessary for technologists to be fully trained and that quality control measures are observed to ensure accurate results. These issues have therefore limited their use, although these measurements are commonly performed at a number of academic centers. Their main use at present is still for research and, in this setting, other examinations of the cells (44,46–48) and fluid-phase components (39,41,49) can also be performed.

Sputum induction, when performed by trained technologists, can be safe, even in patients with very severe or uncontrolled asthma or when there is moderate to severe airflow limitation (5,50–53). The procedure is performed by having the patient inhale an aerosol of hypertonic saline using an ultrasonic nebulizer with either a relatively low (0.9 ml/min) (38) or higher output (39). Methods of induction have been described (41,54,55) and their safety has been examined (50,52,56). In one clinical study of 329 patients, 40% had very severe asthma and only 8% showed a fall in FEV_1 of >20%, which was not predicted from the baseline postbronchodilator FEV_1; the procedure was successful in more than 90% (53). However, the possibility of inducing episodes of more severe airway constriction, albeit infrequent, highlights the importance of being cautious and having resuscitation equipment available in the laboratory and a responsible physician in the building when the inductions are performed.

The processing of sputum is performed on the whole expectorate (with measures to reduce the amount of saliva) (54,55) or of the sputum selected from the saliva (40,57). A specimen is processed with dithiothreitol (DTT) in order to break up the mucus and disperse the cells and is then filtered. From the resulting suspension, a total cell count is measured using a hemocytometer and cytospins are prepared and stained for differential cell counts on 400 nonsquamous cells. Additional measurements can be made on the cells for research purposes (44,46–48). The suspension can be centrifuged and the supernatant removed and stored at $-70°C$ for future measurements of soluble mediators (39,41,49).

A number of observations have been made which are relevant to the use of sputum cell counts in the monitoring of airway inflammation in severe asthma.

1. Normal values have been reported; of particular relevance are a total cell count of <9.7% and proportions of eosinophils and neutrophils of <2% and <64.5%, respectively (Tables 3 and 4) (58). The total cell count indicates the intensity of any inflammatory response and is particularly high in some cases of neutrophilia (37). Eosinophilia is usually not associated with an increase in the total cell count.

2. The accuracy with which physicians can predict the presence, type, and severity of airway inflammation from symptoms and FEV_1 is poor (11). The extent to which sputum cell counts will influence the outcomes of treatment needs investigation.

3. Eosinophilia classically characterizes uncontrolled asthma and predicts benefit from added corticosteroid treatment (51,59).

Table 3 Normal Values of Sputum Total and Absolute Differential Cell Counts
($\times 10^6$ cells/mL)[a]

	Mean (SD)	Normal range		Median (IQR)	Percentiles	
		Mean (−2 SD)	Mean (+2 SD)		10	90
Total cell count	4.13(4.81)	−4.6	13.76	2.4(3.19)	0.67	9.73
Eosinophils	0.01(0.04)	−0.06	0.09	0.00(0.01)	0	0.04
Neutrophils	1.96(3.03)	−4.09	8.02	0.87(1.96)	0.1	4.86
Macrophages	2.13(2.03)	−1.93	6.18	1.64(1.87)	0.3	4.86
Lymphocytes	0.04(0.07)	−0.1	0.18	0.02(0.05)	0.01	0.09
Bronchial epithelial cells	0.01(0.04)	−0.06	0.09	0.01(0.01)	0	0.03

[a] From Ref. 58.

4. Mild eosinophilia can occur in patients with clinically controlled asthma (11) and it precedes clinical exacerbation associated with a reduction in prednisone (5) or inhaled corticosteroid (60) dose. Hence, the significance of mild eosinophilia with controlled asthma needs further study and the occurrence of an eosinophilia during corticosteroid reduction should indicate caution if further reduction in dose is contemplated.

5. Eosinophilia in patients with uncontrolled severe or very severe asthma should raise the possibility of noncompliance (61).

6. Eosinophilia can be associated with cough and sputum without variable

Table 4 Normal Values for Sputum Differential Cell Counts (%)[a]

	Mean(SD)	Normal range		Median (IQR)	Percentiles	
		Mean (−2 SD)	Mean (+2 SD)		10	90
Eosinophils	0.4(0.9)	−1.4	2.2	0.0(0.3)	0	1.1
Neutrophils	37.5(20.1)	−2.7	77.7	36.7(29.5)	11	64.4
Macrophages	58.8(21.0)	16.8	100.8	60.8(28.9)	33	86.1
Lymphocytes	1.0(1.1)	−1.2	3.2	0.5(1.8)	0.01	2.6
Metachromatic cells	0.0(0.0)	−0.1	0.1	0.0(0.0)	0	0
Bronchial epithelial cells	1.6(3.9)	−6.2	9.4	0.3(1.3)	0	4.4

[a] From Ref. 58.

airflow limitation or airway hyperresponsiveness (i.e., without asthma) but still requires a medium to high dose of inhaled corticosteroid (6–8) or additional prednisone (6,62) to control the symptoms.

7. The absence of eosinophilia in uncontrolled asthma should suggest other causes for the lack of control, such as variable airflow limitation requiring, for example, long-acting β_2-agonist or antileukotriene treatment, or laryngeal dysfunction, hyperventilation, gastroesophageal reflux, or heart failure; or could be due to misinterpretation of the "symptoms" as abnormal. The absence of eosinophilia predicts that benefit will not occur with added corticosteroid treatment (51,59).

8. Intense neutrophilia with purulent sputum suggests bacterial infection. Milder neutrophilia has been observed in influenza exacerbations of asthma (63).

There is increasing evidence that sputum cell counts will be useful to monitor the activity of airway inflammation in severe asthma. However, the procedure is still time consuming and prospective evidence is still needed to determine the relevance of these measurements in the clinical outcomes of treatment.

B. Exhaled Gases

Several volatile mediators in exhaled breath have been evaluated as potential noninvasive markers of airway inflammation in asthma. Of these, only ENO can be considered for use in monitoring severe asthma (64–69). The measurement of ENO has considerable appeal because of the direct nature of the reading, the totally noninvasive procedure, and the immediate availability of the test results. However, its usefulness is limited by the fact that the equipment used to conduct these tests is expensive (resulting in tests being available in only a few specialist centers), that it is possibly overly sensitive to corticosteroid treatment, and that is role in monitoring airway inflammation in severe asthma is as yet undetermined.

Measurement of ENO are usually made using chemiluminescence analyzers and are based on the photochemical reaction between NO and ozone generated in the analyzer. The specificity of ENO measurements by chemiluminescence has been confirmed using gas chromatography–mass spectrometry (70) and methods for the standardization of techniques have been established and published (71,72).

Interest in the role of ENO in asthma has focused on its use as a marker to guide therapy and a number of observations have been made to suggest that ENO measurements may be useful for monitoring patients with asthma. Patients with untreated uncontrolled asthma have elevated levels of ENO (64,65,68), which can increase further following allergen challenge (73). Several studies have demonstrated that the level of ENO and the degree of airway inflammation correlate reasonably well, and ENO has been validated against invasive measurements of inflammation by bronchoscopy (74) and sputum eosinophilia in asthma (75). While there is no clear relationship between ENO, FEV_1, and symptoms in mild steroid-naive asthma (64,65), there is increasing evidence of a correlation between ENO, symptom frequency, and rescue β_2-agonist use, with exhaled NO levels being significantly higher in patients with severe persistent asthma who are not using corticosteroids (64,66). ENO levels have also been shown to be increased during deterioration in asthma control and during acute asthma exacerbations, suggesting that measurement of ENO is a reliable determinant of loss of asthma control and of inadequate treatment of airway inflammation (75).

However, additional observations indicate that ENO measurements are unlikely to be useful in monitoring severe asthma. High levels of ENO are also present in chronic airflow limitation due to smoking and respiratory tract infections and the recent ingestion of nitrite- and nitrate-containing foods (73) and are thus nonspecific to asthma symptoms. ENO measurements are also extremely responsive to corticosteroid treatment (64) and, while it has been suggested that ENO may be used to monitor corticosteroid treatment in asthma (76–78), this might also limit its application in monitoring patients with severe asthma. A recent study from our group (79) demonstrated that while ENO levels showed significant but weak correlations with sputum eosinophil counts in steroid-naive asthmatic subjects, ENO levels were significantly lower in asthmatic subjects who were using corticosteroids compared with those who were not, despite there being no difference in sputum eosinophil counts. These data suggest that ENO is likely to have limited utility as a surrogate clinical measurement for either the presence or severity of eosinophilic airway inflammation in asthma, except in steroid-naive subjects. Since most patients with severe asthma are treated with corticosteroids, it is unlikely this test will be used to monitor such patients. Prospective studies examining longitudinal changes in exhaled NO and their impact on clinical management (67) need to be conducted to determine the best times to administer ENO tests.

C. Bronchoalveolar Lavage and Biopsy

Flexible fiberoptic bronchoscopy with endobronchial biopsy followed by histological assessment is still considered the "gold standard" for evaluating airway inflammation. However, bronchoscopy performed for either bronchoalveolar lavage or endobronchial biopsy is too time consuming and invasive (with an associated risk of morbidity) to be commonly used to monitor severe asthma. These procedures may be suitable for monitoring asthma patients within well-designed, carefully supervised research studies (80), provided they are performed according to published guidelines (81).

VIII. Conclusions

Monitoring the activity of severe asthma must include objective measurements to identify the degree of clinical control and to establish the minimum medications required to maintain control. Of these measurements, spirometry is the best but PEF is more readily available. Measurements of airway responsiveness can be useful to confirm the diagnosis of asthma when spirometry is normal. While its use in monitoring the effects of treatment has been found to be beneficial, it is for the most part an impractical method. Monitoring airway inflammation is now possible by assessing induced sputum cell counts and exhaled nitric oxide levels. However, sputum examination is time consuming and the equipment used for measuring ENO is expensive; therefore their role in monitoring severe asthma requires further investigation.

References

1. National Heart, Lung and Blood Institute. Guidelines for the Diagnosis and Management of Asthma. Bethesda, MD: Department of Health and Human Services, NIH publication no. 97–405, 1997.
2. Cockcroft DW, Swystun VA. Asthma control versus asthma severity. J Allergy Clin Immunol 1996; 98:1016–1018.
3. Boulet LP, Becker A, Berube D, Beveridge R, Ernst P. Canadian Asthma Consensus Report, 1999. CMAJ 1999; 161:S1–S61.
4. Barnes PJ, Woolcock AJ. Difficult asthma. Eur Respir J 1998; 121:209–218.
5. Pizzichini MMM, Pizzichini E, Clelland L, Efthimiadis A, Pavord I, Dolovich J, Hargreave FE. Prednisone-dependent asthma: inflammatory indices in induced sputum. Eur Respir J 1999; 13:15–21.
6. Gibson PG, Dolovich J, Denburg JA, Ramsdale EH, Hargreave FE. Chronic cough: eosinophilic bronchitis without asthma. Lancet 1989; 1:1346–1348.
7. Gibson PG, Wong BJO, Hepperle MJE, Kline P, Girgis-Gabardo A, Guyatt G, Dolovich J, Denburg JA, Ramsdale EH, Hargreave FE. A research method to induce and examine a mild exacerbation of asthma by withdrawal of inhaled corticosteroid. Clin Exp Allergy 1992; 22:525–532.
8. Brightling CE, Ward R, Goh KL, Wardlaw AJ, Pavord ID. Eosinophilic bronchitis is an important cause of chronic cough. Am J Respir Crit Care Med 1999; 160(2): 406–410.
9. Kikuchi Y, Okabe S, Tamura G, Hida W, Homma M, Shirato K, Takishima T. Chemosensitivity and perception of dyspnea in patients with a history of near-fatal asthma N Engl J Med 1994; 330:1329–1334.
10. Kendrick AH, Higgs CM, Whitfield MJ, Laszlo G. Accuracy of perception of severity of asthma: patients treated in general practice. Br Med J 1993; 307:422–424.
11. Parameswaran K, Pizzichini E, Pizzichini MMM, Hussack P, Efthimiadis A, Hargreave FE. Clinical judgement of airway inflammation versus sputum cell counts in patients with asthma. Eur Respir J 2000; 15:486–490.

12. Adelroth E, Hargreave FE, Ramsdale EH. Do physicians need objective measurements to diagnose asthma? Am Rev Respir Dis 1986; 134:704–707.

13. American Thoracic Society. Lung function testing: selection of reference values and interpretative strategies. Am Rev Respir Dis 1991; 144:1202–1218.

14. Klein RB, Fritz GK, Yeung A, McQuaid EL, Mansell A. Spirometric patterns in childhood asthma: peak flow compared with other indices. Pediatr Pulmonol 1995; 20:372–379.

15. Shim CS, Williams MHJ. Relationship of wheezing to the severity of obstruction in asthma. Arch Intern Med 1983; 143:890–892.

16. American Thoracic Society. Standardization of spirometry, 1994 update. Am J Respir Crit Care Med 1995; 152:1107–1136.

17. Killian KJ. Pulmonary function tests In: O'Byrne PM, Thomson NC, eds. Manual of Asthma Management. 2nd ed. New York: W. B. Saunders, 2000; 81–89.

18. Beasley R, Cushley M, Holgate ST. A self management plan in the treatment of adult asthma. Thorax 1989; 44:200–204.

19. Grampian Asthma Study of Integrated Care (GRASSIC). Effectiveness of routine self-monitoring of peak flow in patients with asthma. Br Med J 1994; 308:564–567.

20. Reddel H, Jenkins C, Woolcock A. Diurnal variability—time to change asthma guidelines? Br Med J 1999; 319:45–47.

21. Sly PD, Cahill P, Willet K, Burton P. Accuracy of mini peak flow meters in indicating changes in lung function in children with asthma. Br Med J 1994; 308:572–574.

22. Miles JF, Bright P, Ayres JG, Cayton RM, Miller MR. The performance of Mini Wright peak flow meters after prolonged use. Respir Med 1995; 89:603–605.

23. Cote J, Cartier A, Malo JL, Rouleau M, Boulet LP. Compliance with peak expiratory flow monitoring in home management of asthma. Chest 1998; 113:968–972.

24. Crapo RO, Casaburi R, Coates AL, Enright PL, Hankinson JL, Irvin CG, MacIntyre NR, McKay RT, Wanger JS, Anderson SD, et al. Guidelines for methacholine and exercise challenge testing—1999 (This official statement of the American Thoracic-Society was adopted by the ATS Board of Directors, July 1999). Am J Respir Crit Care Med 2000; 161:309–329.

25. Smith CM, Anderson SD. Inhalational challenge using hypertonic saline in asthmatic subjects: a comparison with responses to hyperpnoea, methacholine and water. Eur Respir J 1990; 3:144–151.

26. Juniper EF, Cockcroft DW, Hargreave FE. Histamine and Methacholine Inhalation Tests: A Laboratory Tidal Breathing Protocol, 1994. 2nd ed. Lund, Sweden: Astra Draco AB.

27. Ryan G, Dolovich MB, Roberts RS, Frith PA, Juniper EF, Hargreave FE, Newhouse MT. Standardization of inhalation provocation tests: two techniques of aerosol generation and inhalation compared. Am Rev Respir Dis 1981; 123:195–199.

28. Yan K, Salome CM, Woolcock AJ. Rapid method for measurement of bronchial responsiveness. Thorax 1983; 38:760–765.

29. Woolcock AJ. Expression of results of airway hyperresponsiveness. In: Hargreave FE, Woolcock AJ, eds. Airway Responsiveness: Measurement and Interpretation. Mississauga: Astra Pharmaceuticals Canada Ltd, 1985; 80–85.

30. Pauwels RA, Joos G, Van Der Straeten M. Bronchial hyperresponsiveness is not bronchial hyperresponsiveness is not bronchial asthma. Clin Allergy 1988; 18:317–321.

31. O'Byrne PM, Dolovich J, Hargreave FE. Late asthmatic responses. Am Rev Respir Dis 1987; 136:740–751.

32. Hargreave FE, Pizzichini MMM, Pizzichini E. Airway hyperresponsiveness as a diagnostic feature of asthma. In: Johansson SGO, ed. Progress in Allergy and Clinical Immunology. Toronto, Ontario: Hogrefe & Huber, 1995; 63–67.

33. Sont JK, Willems LN, Bel EH, van Krieken JH, Vandenbroucke JP, Sterk PJ. Clinical control and histopathologic outcome of asthma when using airway hyperresponsiveness as an additional guide to long-term treatment. The AMPUL Study Group. Am J Respir Crit Care Med 1999; 159:1043–1051.

34. Reddel HK, Jenkins CR, Marks GB, Ware SI, Xuan W, Salome CM, Badcock C-A, Woolcock AJ. Optimal asthma control, starting with high doses of inhaled budesonide. Eur Respir J 2000; 16:226–235.

35. Homer RJ, Elias JA. Consequences of long-term inflammation: airway remodeling. Clin Chest Med 2000; 21:331–343.

36. Crimi E, Spanevello A, Neri M, Ind PW, Rossi GA, Brusasco V. Dissociation between airway inflammation and airway hyperresponsiveness in allergic asthma. Am J Respir Crit Care Med 1998; 157:4–9.

37. Jayaram L, Parameswaran K, Sears MR, Hargreave FE. Induced sputum cell counts: their usefulness in clinical practice. Eur Respir J 2000; 16:150–158.

38. Pin I, Gibson PG, Kolendowicz R, Girgis-Gabardo A, Denburg J, Hargreave FE, Dolovich J. Use of induced sputum cell counts to investigate airway inflammation in asthma. Thorax 1992; 47:25–29.

39. Fahy JV, Liu J, Wong H, Boushey HA. Cellular and biochemical analysis of induced sputum from asthmatic and from healthy subjects. Am Rev Respir Dis 1993; 147:1126–1131.

40. Pizzichini E, Pizzichini MMM, Efthimiadis A, Hargreave FE, Dolovich J. Measurement of inflammatory indices in induced sputum: effects of selection of sputum to minimize salivary contamination. Eur Respir J 1996; 9:1174–1180.

41. Pizzichini E, Pizzichini MMM, Efthimiadis A, Evans S, Morris MM, Squillace D, Gleich GJ, Dolovich J, Hargreave FE. Indices of airway inflammation in induced sputum: reproducibility and validity of cell and fluid-phase measurements. Am J Respir Crit Care Med 1996; 154:308–317.

42. Spanevello A, Migliori GB, Sharara A, Ballardini L, Bridge P, Pisati P, Neri M, Ind PW. Induced sputum to assess airway inflammation: a study of reproducibility. Clin Exp Allergy 1997; 27:1138–1144.

43. Claman DM, Boushey HA, Liu J, Wong H, Fahy JV. Analysis of induced sputum to examine the effects of prednisone on airway inflammation in asthmatic subjects. J Allergy Clin Immunol 1994; 94:861–869.

44. Gauvreau GM, Lee JM, Watson RM, Irani AA, Schwartz LB, O'Byrne PM. Increased numbers of both airway basophils and mast cells in sputum after allergen inhalation challenge of atopic asthmatics. Am J Respir Crit Care Med 2000; 161:473–478.

45. Efthimiadis A, Jayaram L, Weston S, Carruthers S, Hussack P, Hargreave FE. In-

duced sputum: time from expectoration to processing. Am J Respir Crit Care Med 2001. In press.

46. Hansel TT, Braunstein JB, Walker C, Blaser K, Bruijnzeel PLB, Virchow JCJ, Virchow C. Sputum eosinophils from asthmatics express ICAM-1 and HLA-DR. Clin Exp Immunol 1991; 86:271–277.

47. Kidney JC, Wong AG, Efthimiadis, A, Morris MM, Sears MR, Dolovich J, Hargreave FE. Elevated B cells in sputum of asthmatics: close correlation with eosinophils. Am J Respir Crit Care Med 1996; 153:540–544.

48. Olivenstein R, Taha R, Minshall EM, Hamid Q. IL-4 and IL-5 mRNA expression in induced sputum of asthmatic subjects: comparison with bronchial wash. J Allergy Clin Immunol 1999; 103:238–245.

49. Kelly MM, Leigh R, Evans S, Efthimiadis AE, Gleich GJ, Horsewood P, Hargreave FE. Induced sputum: validity of fluid-phase IL-5 measurement. J Allergy Clin Immunol 2000; 105:1162–1168.

50. de la Fuente PT, Romagnoli M, Godard P, Bousquet J, Chanez P. Safety of inducing sputum in patients with asthma of varying severity. Am J Respir Crit Care Med 1998; 157:1127–1130.

51. Pizzichini MMM, Pizzichini E, Clelland L, Efthimiadis A, Mahony J, Dolovich J, Hargreave FE. Sputum in severe exacerbations of asthma: kinetics of inflammatory indices after prednisone treatment. Am J Respir Crit Care Med 1997; 155:1501–1508.

52. Hunter CJ, Ward R, Woltmann G, Wardlaw AJ, Pavord ID. The safety and success rate of sputum induction using a low output ultrasonic nebuliser. Respir Med 1999; 93(5):345–348.

53. Vlachos-Mayer H, Leigh R, Sharon RF, Hussack P, Hargreave FE. Sputum induction for inflammatory indices: safety and success. Eur Respir J 2000; 16:997–1000.

54. Gershman NH, Wong HH, Liu MC, Mahlmeister MJ, Fahy JV. Comparison of two methods of collecting induced sputum in asthmatic subjects. Eur Respir J 1996; 9: 2448–2453.

55. Keatings VM, Nightingale JA. Induced sputum: whole sample In: Rogers DF Donnelly LE, eds. Methods in Molecular Medicine: Human Airway Inflammation: Sampling Techniques and Analytical Protocols. London: Humana Press, 2001:56.

56. Wong HH, Fahy JV. Safety of one method of sputum induction in asthmatic subjects. Am J Respir Crit Care Med 1997; 156:299–303.

57. Kelly MM, Efthimiadis A, Hargreave FE. Induced sputum: selection method. In: Rogers DF, Donnelly LE, eds. Methods in Molecular Medicine: Human Airway Inflammation: Sampling Techniques and Analytical Protocols. London: Humana Press, 2001:56.

58. Belda J, Leigh R, Parameswaran K, O'Byrne PM, Sears MR, Hargreave FE. Induced sputum cell counts in healthy adults. Am J Respir Crit Care Med 2000; 161:475–478.

59. Pavord ID, Brightling CE, Woltmann G, Wardlaw AJ. Non-eosinophilic corticosteroid unresponsive asthma. Lancet 1999; 353:2213–2214.

60. Jatakanon A, Lim S, Barnes PJ. Changes in sputum eosinophils predict loss of asthma control. Am J Respir Crit Care Med 2000; 16:64–72.

61. Parameswaran K, Leigh R, Hargreave FE. Sputum eosinophil count to assess compli-

ance with corticosteroid therapy in asthma. J Allergy Clin Immunol 1999; 104:502–503.

62. Hargreave FE, Leigh R. Induced sputum, eosinophilic bronchitis and COPD. Am J Respir Crit Care Med 1999; 160:S53–S57.
63. Pizzichini E, Pizzichini MMM, Johnston S, Hussack P, Efthimiadis A, Mahony J, Dolovich J, Hargreave FE. Asthma and natural colds: inflammatory indices in induced sputum: a feasibility study. Am J Respir Crit Care Med 1998; 158:1178–1184.
64. Kharitonov SA, Yates D, Robbins RA, Logan-Sinclair R, Shinebourne EA, Barnes PJ. Increased nitric oxide in exhaled air of asthmatic patients. Lancet 1994; 343:133–135.
65. Alving K, Weitzberg E, Lundberg JM. Increased amount of nitric oxide in exhaled air of asthmatics. Eur Respir J 1993; 6:1368–1370.
66. Stirling RG, Kharitonov SA, Campbell D, Robinson DS, Durham SR, Chung KF, Barnes PJ. Increase in exhaled nitric oxide levels in patients with difficult asthma and correlation with symptoms and disease severity despite treatment with oral and inhaled corticosteroids: Asthma and Allergy Group. Thorax 1998; 53:1030–1034.
67. Berlyne G, Barnes N. No role for NO in asthma? Lancet 2000; 355:1029–1030.
68. Paredi P, Leckie MJ, Horvath I, Allegra L, Kharitonov SA, Barnes PJ. Changes in exhaled carbon monoxide and nitric oxide levels following allergen challenge in patients with asthma. Eur Respir J 1999; 13:48–52.
69. Paredi P, Kharitonov SA, Barnes PJ. Elevation of exhaled ethane concentration in asthma. Am J Respir Crit Care Med 2000; 162:1450–1454.
70. Leone AM, Gustafsson LE, Francis PL, Persson MG, Wiklund NP, Moncada S. Nitric oxide is present in exhaled breath in humans: direct GC-MS confirmation. Biochem Biophys Res Common 1994; 201:883–887.
71. Kharitonov SA, Alving K, Barnes PJ. Exhaled and nasal nitric oxide measurements: recommendations. The European Respiratory Society Task Force. Eur Respir J 1997; 10:1683–1693.
72. Recommendations for standardized procedures for the on-line and off-line measurement of exhaled lower respiratory nitric oxide and nasal nitric oxide in adults and children. Am J Respir Crit Care Med 1999; 160:2104–2117.
73. Kharitonov SA, O'Connor BJ, Evans DJ, Barnes PJ. Allergen-induced late asthmatic reactions are associated with elevation of exhaled nitric oxide. Am J Respir Crit Care Med 1995; 151:1894–1899.
74. Massaro AF, Mehta S, Lilly CM, Kobzik L, Reilly JJ, Drazen JM. Elevated nitric oxide concentrations in isolated lower airway gas of asthmatic subjects. Am J Respir Crit Care Med 1996; 153:1510–1514.
75. Jatakanon A, Lim S, Kharitonov SA, Chung KF, Barnes PJ. Correlation between exhaled nitric oxide, sputum eosinophils and methacholine responsiveness in patients with mild asthma. Thorax 1998; 53:91–95.
76. Kharitonov SA, Yates DH, Chung KF, Barnes PJ. Changes in the dose of inhaled steroid affect exhaled nitric oxide levels in asthmatic patients. Eur Respir J 1996; 9:196–201.
77. Lim S, Jatakanon A, John M, Gilbey T, O'Connor BJ, Chung KF, Barnes PJ. Effect

of inhaled budesonide on lung function and airway inflammation: Assessment by various inflammatory markers in mild asthma. Am J Respir Crit Care Med 1999; 159:22–30.

78. van Rensen EL, Straathof KC, Veselic-Charvat MA, Zwinderman AH, Bel EH, Sterk PJ. Effect of inhaled steroids on airway hyperresponsiveness, sputum eosinophils, and exhaled nitric oxide levels in patients with asthma. Thorax 1999; 54:403–408.

79. Berlyne GS, Parameswaran K, Kamada D, Efthimiadis A, Hargreave FE. A comparison of exhaled nitric oxide and induced sputum as markers of airway inflammation. J Allergy Clin Immunol 2000; 106:638–644.

80. Wenzel SE, Schwartz LB, Langmack EL, Halliday JL, Trudeau JB, Gibbs RL, Chu HW. Evidence that severe asthma can be divided pathologically into two inflammatory subtypes with distinct physiologic and clinical characteristics. Am J Respir Crit Care Med 1999; 160:1001–1008.

81. Workshop summary and guidelines: Investigative use of bronchoscopy, lavage and bronchial biopsies in asthma and other airway diseases. J Allergy Clin Immunol 1991; 88:808–814.

20

Psychosocial Aspects of Severe Asthma in Children

MARIANNE Z. WAMBOLDT and FREDERICK S. WAMBOLDT

National Jewish Medical and Research Center
and University of Colorado Health Sciences Center
Denver, Colorado

I. Introduction

Not only is asthma the most common chronic illness of childhood, but despite considerable improvement in many aspects of asthma treatment, the prevalence, severity, and mortality related to this illness are on the rise. The prevalence of asthma in American children 18 years or younger increased from 3.2% in 1981 to 4.3% in 1988—an increase of nearly 40% (1,2), with current estimates suggesting that asthma afflicts approximately 4.8 million children in the United States (3). Furthermore, across this same period of time, asthma hospitalization rates have increased by 6%, while the asthma mortality rate has increased 31%, from 1.3 to 1.7 per hundred thousand population. The greatest increase (42%) occurred in children under age 20, with the highest increase in poor, urban, minority children (4–6).

   A number of case reports and studies have suggested that psychosocial and family factors are powerful predictors of asthma deaths (7–14). Consider the case-controlled study of Strunk and associates (13). They compared 21 children with severe asthma who were previously hospitalized on a tertiary asthma care pediatric inpatient unit and who subsequently died of asthma with 21 still-living control children matched for age at time of hospitalization, sex, and asthma severity. Of the 57 physiologic and psychosocial variables evaluated by review of hospital records, only those presented in Table 1 were found to be significantly different across the groups. As can be seen, psychosocial risk factors were prominent in severely ill asthmatic children who subsequently died.

There is, however, one important question that arises when one contemplates the above-cited data of Strunk and colleagues; specifically, what are the underlying mechanisms whereby psychosocial factors such as emotional disturbance, interpersonal conflict, and family dysfunction adversely affect asthma outcome? In this chapter, we examine research that helps us to understand how psychosocial factors may have such profound influence on asthma treatment and outcome. Additionally, we discuss how this research directly leads to assessment and management guidelines. Four relevant literatures are reviewed: (1) current knowledge concerning the role of genetic and environmental factors in asthma; (2) the role of individual psychological factors in asthma outcome; (3) the role

Table 1 Variables That Distinguished Asthma Death Group from Control Group

| | No. of patients | | |
Variables	Death group	Control group	Statistical comparison (P)
Physiological variables			
History of seizures during asthma attack	9	1	.01
Inhaled beclomethasone dipropionate	13	6	.05
Prednisone decreased ≥50% initial dose during hospitalization	13	5	.01
More asthma symptoms in week prior to discharge compared with 4 weeks prior to discharge	8	2	.05
Psychosocial variables			
Disregard of perceived asthma symptoms	7	2	.06
Self-care in hospital not appropriate for age	15	5	.01
Emotional disturbance	18	9	.01
Depressive symptoms	16	9	.05
History of emotional/behavioral reactions to separation or loss	15	6	.01
Patient–staff conflict	15	6	.01
Parent–staff conflict	15	6	.01
Patient–parent conflict	12	5	.05
Manipulative use of asthma	19	12	.01
Family dysfunction	17	11	.05

Note. Adapted from Ref. 13.

of family functioning in asthma treatment outcome; and (4) the relationships among psychosocial processes, adherence to treatment, and treatment outcome. Finally, we make recommendations regarding psychosocial evaluation and management of the patient with severe asthma that may alleviate morbidity and potentially reduce mortality.

II. Genetic and Environmental Interplay in the Onset and Course of Asthma

A. The Genetics of Asthma Highlight the Centrality of Environmental Factors

Current consensus views asthma as a multifactorial illness with both genetic and environmental (i.e., infectious, allergic, mechanical, and psychosocial) factors involved in its development and course. Three points are particularly informative. First, although asthma is fairly heritable (there is a two- to fourfold difference in the concordance rates for monozygotic and dizygotic twins), the concordance rates in monozygotic twins is fairly low, about 20–40% (15–17). Hence, phenotypic expression of the genetic component for asthma appears dependent on substantial environmental influence. This conclusion remains unchanged, even accepting the argument that some propensity toward atopy (e.g., as reflected by total serum IgE level) is the major genetic risk factor for asthma (18,19).

Second, asthma (and probably atopy as well) is unlikely to be a single-gene disorder. Indeed, Mrazek and Klinnert (20) have proposed an oligogenetic model which provides a good fit for our current knowledge. Their three-gene model includes (1) an immunologic regulator, (2) an airway sensitivity regulator, and (3) an autonomic nervous system regulator. To the degree to which this assumption is true, one can expect that there are differing types of asthma which may have qualitative and quantitative differences in the influence of psychosocial factors. For example, children who either do not report clear allergic triggers for their asthma or report emotional and family stress triggers appear to have higher rates of psychosocial problems than those who report only allergic triggers (21–24).

There have been few prospective studies of the role of environmental factors in the initial onset of childhood asthma. Most of these have not found global psychosocial factors to be important influences, although they have supported the role of early infections with parainfluenza or respiratory syncytial viruses, parental smoking habits, and specific antigen exposure leading to clinical atopy as major risk factors (25,26). Conversely, one study suggests that more specific psychosocial factors may be of importance. Klinnert and associates (27) have demonstrated an interactive effect of quality of parenting and family stress on asthma onset by 3 years of age in a group of infants at high genetic risk to develop asthma. Specifically, high family stress only increased asthma incidence by age 3 when the stress occurred in the context of worse parenting practices.

Future efforts at understanding the role of genetic and environmental factors in asthma onset are likely to benefit by using models that consider more complex effects, such as gene–environment interactions (28). For example, one recent hypothesis suggests that the reason prevalence rates of asthma are particularly rising in inner city, minority youth is that these youngsters are exposed to high levels of trauma and negative life events. The theory postulates that high levels of stress at a critical developmental phase, i.e., in utero and/or infancy, may lead to high cortisol secretion, which in turn may deviate the immune system from a primarily Th1 type to a Th2 type (i.e., increase rates of atopy). Since atopy is a primary risk factor for the development of asthma, children who have some of the other genes making them susceptible to asthma may be "triggered" by having high levels of stress in early childhood.

B. Comorbid Psychiatric Genetic Risk May Differentiate a Subset of Severe Asthmatics

Patients with asthma have higher rates of depression and anxiety than patients without asthma (29,30), although in a population sample, the effect size is small. It is possible that this effect is driven by a subset of patients with asthma who also have a different set of genetic risk factors than the majority of asthmatics. For example, approximately 15–20% of asthmatic children report emotional triggers for their asthma, and these may form a unique subset (22). Psychiatric symptoms, particularly depression and anxiety, in asthmatic children and their parents have been shown to be risk factors for increased asthma morbidity and mortality (13,31). Several studies have demonstrated a higher rate of depression or "nervousness" symptoms in mothers of asthmatic children than mothers of non-ill children (32–34). Since major depression and certain forms of anxiety disorders (panic disorder and separation anxiety) are known to have a genetic component (35,36), it is possible that those patients with asthma who also have a genetic risk for anxiety or depression may have an illness that is more difficult to control.

Wamboldt and colleagues (37) have looked at a sample of 62 severely asthmatic adolescents using a semistructured psychiatric interview with their first-degree relatives. These adolescents were hospitalized at a tertiary care center for asthma with symptoms of steroid dependence, history of intubations or seizures due to asthma, and/or numerous hospitalizations and emergency visits for asthma. In addition to establishing that first-degree biologic relatives of these adolescents had higher rates of depression, mania, substance abuse, and antisocial disorder than relatives of non-ill probands, they also found that there were high rates for anxiety disorders, including post traumatic stress disorder. Since anxiety disorders were not included in the interview of the non-ill proband's relatives, rates could not be compared to a population sample. The time of onset of the psychiatric disorder was compared to the time of onset of asthma in the proband. The majority of relatives suffering from anxiety disorders, substance abuse, and/or antisocial disorder had the onset of the disorder prior to the onset of the proband's asthma. This finding suggests that the psychological symptoms noted in relatives were not simply a stress response to having a severely ill child or sibling.

This linkage could be explained by both environmental and genetic pathways. Environmental hypotheses include the following: (1) Families with members suffering from antisocial disorder and/or substance abuse could have significant family chaos with ensuing stress for the child, as well as less adaptive parenting practices, at a critical developmental period. This could create a vulnerability to severe asthma in genetically at-risk children, as was seen in the Klinnert et al. studies (27). (2) Potentially, such family interactional factors lead to more respiratory infections in the child's early years, as family stress often precedes upper respiratory infections in young children (38,39). Repeated respiratory infections during infancy are a risk factor for the late onset of asthma in children (40). (3) It may also be that the repeated stress leads to an immune deviation toward atopy, as discussed above. (4) Finally, children from families with "chaotic disorders" may receive less than optimal medical care early in life and be more likely to be nonadherent to medications over time. Indeed, in this sample, higher numbers of psychiatric disorders in family members were associated with higher rates of nonadherence, as documented by blood levels upon admission (41). Likewise, families with numerous stressful family life events and/or posttraumatic anxiety symptoms may have higher rates of nonadherence due to the effects of familial anxiety on asthma management (42). It is possible that allowing the airways of a young child to be chronically inflamed and repeatedly assaulted by viral infections may "remodel" the airways, thereby worsening respiratory function (43).

A second group of children may have a genetic risk for anxiety and/or depressive disorders. In the sample studied by Wamboldt et al. (37), 40% of the adolescent probands met criteria for an anxiety disorder themselves. These adolescents had significantly higher rates of anxiety disorders in their first-degree relatives than those adolescents without anxiety disorders. It may be the comorbid anxiety disorder in the patient with asthma that results in more difficult to control asthma. In several twin studies, the covariation of asthma and anxiety and/or depression symptoms was found to be due to common genetic effects, not common environmental effects (44,45). The effect size is small, but it has been consistently found in several large samples. Thus, it may be that a subset of patients with asthma have comorbid genetic risk for anxiety or depressive disorders. Conversely, since these studies were done on self-report of asthma symptoms, not clinical confirmation of asthma, it may be that the common genetic trait is awareness of, and reporting of, numerous symptoms, including both psychological as well as physical. Future studies, including a laboratory assessment of asthma, would be able to distinguish these possibilities.

The studies of Klinnert et al. and Wamboldt et al. suggest that although psychological factors may not have large, direct effects on asthma onset, both the psychiatric genetics and psychosocial environment of a patient may still have important, albeit potentially complex, effects on asthma onset, as well as the more thoroughly documented and larger effects on the course and outcome of childhood asthma discussed below.

III. The Role of Individual Psychological Factors in Asthma Outcome

As noted above, psychosocial comorbidity is common in patients with asthma. Support for this association can be dated back at least as far as Maimonides' (1190) *Book on Asthma* (46): "When in mental anguish, fear, mourning, or distress . . . his agitation affects his respiratory organs and he cannot exercise them at will . . . The Cure of such conditions . . . lies not in food recipes, neither in drugs alone, nor in regular medical advice . . . psychological methods are a greater help."

Although Maimonides' rhetoric may have gone too far out on a limb for more modern ears, in chronic severe asthma psychosocial issues do become important determinants of the course and outcome of the asthmatic illness. This can be labeled the *comorbidity* of psychosocial problems in severe chronic illness. Whether or not the psychosocial problem caused the initial onset of the asthma, once psychosocial problems are present they do appear to worsen the course and outcome of the illness. Since Maimonides' time, the medical literature is replete with anecdotal reports as well as a growing scientific literature linking psychosocial factors to asthma outcome.

A. Psychosocial Problems Make Asthma More Difficult to Control

Patients with concurrent asthma and psychosocial problems have been shown to be more difficult to treat medically in a variety of ways. Children with more psychosocial problems have been shown (1) to require more concurrent anti-asthma medication, especially corticosteroids (31); (2) to require a greater number of hospitalizations in the prior year (47,48); (3) to exhibit poorer compliance with oral theophylline (49); (4) to have longer hospitalizations (50); (5) to require a greater number of hospitalizations, emergency room and urgent office visits, and longer hospitalizations in the year postdischarge from an asthma treatment center (51); and (6) to more frequently die of asthma (13,14,52,53).

It is difficult to assess whether psychosocial problems are associated more with physiologically severe asthma as opposed to mild or moderate asthma, in part because the ratings for severity often include a functional component. The NHLBI guidelines for asthma severity (54) include information as to frequency and severity of symptoms as well as medication requirements. In fact, the number of symptoms reported by the patients (or their parents), the number of days missed from school or work, and the amount of "as needed" medications utilized may all have psychological components to them. Patients with difficulty identifying respiratory sensations may confuse anxiety for bronchoconstriction and report more symptoms. Patients who are depressed or having interpersonal difficulties may be more likely to miss school or work and attribute this to increased asthma symptoms. Patients less compliant with anti-inflammatory medications may utilize more rescue medications. When the physician assesses the need for medications, she/he may take these functional symptoms into account and prescribe more medications, thus making it appear that the patient requires more medication, another component of rating asthma severity (55). Until there is a set laboratory or physiologic "gold standard" of asthma severity (56) it will be difficult to definitively establish whether increased psychopathology is only associated with physiologic severe asthma.

Nonetheless, there is some evidence that psychosocial problems are increased in children and adolescents with severe asthma relative to comparison groups with no medical illness or milder asthma (29,57–60). A word of caution is that much of the work documenting psychosocial problems in children with asthma has used either clinical impressions or questionnaire measures of child psychosocial adjustment, such as the Child Behavior Checklist (CBCL) (61), which is rated by the parents. Parental psychological states are well known to influence their ratings of their children's behavior (62), and in cases where the parent is depressed, may falsely elevate their rating of the child's psychopathology. For example, in a study of over 300 children recruited from asthma camps and hospitals, asthma severity was correlated with parental ratings of childhood anxiety and depressive symptoms on the CBCL, but was *not* related to the children's own ratings of anxiety (63). The authors concluded that severe illness in a child is a major stressor for parents, and the parents' personal distress may affect their reports of their child's symptoms.

In determining covariance of psychiatric disorders with asthma, a particularly obvious weakness is the paucity of studies that have collected research-based psychiatric diagnostic information from direct observations or interviews of the child. The studies that have reported such information support the idea that psychopathology is more prevalent in children with severe asthma than in normal controls. One large-scale epidemiologic study of an entire population, the classic Isle of Wight study (58), reported a higher prevalence of various psychiatric disorders in children with severe asthma than among those with mild asthma. Mrazek and associates (64) found higher rates of depression in children with severe asthma than in healthy controls using a semistructured interview with the mothers of the children. Kashani and associates (65) have reported increased psychiatric symptoms, especially anxiety-related, in mixed-severity asthmatic children versus controls on the Diagnostic Interview for Children and Adolescents—Parent Version (66). Using a semistructured psychiatric interview, the Child and Adolescent Psychiatric Assessment (CAPA), Wamboldt et al. (37) found anxiety disorders in 28% of moderate and severe asthmatic children. Since these diagnostic instruments yield information on disorders, not just symptom profiles, they are useful to be able to determine whether there are genetic linkages between certain psychiatric disorders, e.g., separation anxiety or major depression, and asthma. Having more precise diagnostic profiles for psychiatric disorders may suggest new avenues of research into both underlying mechanisms and potentially different pharmacologic treatments.

B. Specific Psychological Difficulties in Severe Asthmatics

Although early clinical reports in this area focused almost exclusively on the search for *the* asthmatic personality type (67), there is now solid evidence documenting the heterogeneity of personality styles and psychosocial difficulties found in patients with asthma (57,68). Nonetheless, even though patients with severe asthma are not all psychological clones, some meaningful stylistic differences among groups of asthmatic patients are worth mentioning.

1. Anxiety is a key construct. Kinsman and his associates (50,68,69) developed an assessment of anxiety levels from the MMPI that they labeled the panic–fear profile. They have shown that asthmatics who were either low or high on this dimension had more hospitalizations for asthma than those who scored in the moderate range (69,70). They hypothesized that too little anxiety was associated with denial of symptoms and delay in seeking treatment. High levels of anxiety were associated with poor discernment of respiratory versus anxiety symptoms, leading to overutilization of medical treatment. This work has been replicated in children (47).

2. A similar but distinct line of research examines the ability of asthmatics to detect changes in their respiratory functions. Approximately 15% of patients with asthma are unable to detect marked changes in airway obstruction (71). Additionally, lack of perception of dyspnea has been associated with near-fatal attacks of asthma (72–74). Fritz et al. (75) have shown that children have a marked variability in their ability to perceive respiratory changes. Poor perception was associated with more days missed from school due to asthma as well (76). Likewise, in a community sample of adolescents, there was also a wide range of ability to detect methacholine induced bronchoconstriction (77). Whether anxiety, depression, and personality traits are associated with this perceptual trait is still controversial (78–83).

3. A final subtype of asthma-related psychologic difficulties is illustrated

by the "vocal cord dysfunction" (VCD) syndrome (84,85). This syndrome, at times described as "factitious asthma" or a "masquerader of asthma," is characterized by a paradoxical adduction of the vocal cords during inspiration. Patients with VCD have often received extensive medication regimens and hospitalizations for their symptoms. Initial surveys of adults with this disorder found high percentages of women who had been sexually abused, which corroborated the psychogenic hypothesis (86); however, more recent reviews suggest that this case is greatly overstated with much more observed heterogeneity of psychological health (84). The pediatric population appears to be similarly heterogeneous. Brugman et al. (87) reviewed 37 pediatric patients diagnosed as having VCD. The majority of the group (78%) had documented concurrent asthma. Only 11% had a documented history of sexual abuse, although another 16% had suspected abuse. In comparison, the majority were characterized as high achievers (84% academic scholars and 61% successful athletes). The children with VCD also had a higher occurrence of depression, anxiety, and family dysfunction than a general pediatric population. This syndrome is worth diagnosing even if there is comorbid asthma, for often hospitalizations and medication requirements (and thus functional severity of asthma) can be markedly reduced with the ancillary treatments of speech therapy and/or psychosocial intervention (84).

More recent research indicates that VCD may overlap with other anxiety disorders, in particular, panic disorder and chronic hyperventilation syndrome (88). In a controlled retrospective study of adolescents admitted to a tertiary inpatient service for presumed severe, intractable asthma, anxiety symptoms were greater in the subjects subsequently diagnosed with VCD than in the subjects who retained a primary discharge diagnosis of asthma. Furthermore, in the patients diagnosed with VCD, the anxiety symptoms preceded the onset of the VCD (89). To the degree that there are physiological linkages between panic disorder and VCD, treatments efficacious for panic, e.g., cognitive behavioral therapy and antidepressants, may well be useful in treatment of some cases of VCD (88,90).

C. Possible Mechanisms of Linkage Between Psychosocial Comorbidity and Severe Asthma

The links between increased rates of psychosocial problems in patients with severe asthma could arise from multiple levels of biopsychosocial influence. Genetically, the data of Wamboldt and colleagues described above suggest the existence of a linkage between severe asthma and anxiety disorders, substance abuse, and antisocial disorders. Neurophysiologically, the increased incidence of panic disorder in asthmatic patients has been related to common projections from the respiratory centers to hypothesized panic centers in the brain (91,92). Hormonally, the medications used to treat severe asthma, particularly oral corticosteroids, can directly alter CNS functioning, causing a variety of potential psychiatric problems ranging from sleep disturbance to mild–moderate cognitive dysfunction to frank affective disorders. Psychologically, breathing is a profoundly central aspect of living. It is not surprising that a disorder that can cause sudden, unpredictable, and hard-to-control breathlessness might cause psychological distress in a patient. Similarly, a serious, chronic illness often causes multiple losses, such as a loss of a sense of personal power, security and independence, and activity and educational restrictions, and tension and increased distress with friends and family members. Such multiple losses are clear risk factors for psychosocial problems (93,94).

In addition to the above issues, children who develop asthma at a young age are also at special risk for psychological problems due to the impact of the illness upon specific developmental processes. Frequent hospitalizations for asthma, especially those resulting in separation from primary caretakers during the toddler years, have been demonstrated to increase the risk of developing psychologic sequelae (95). Medical events and interventions can precipitate symptoms of posttraumatic stress disorder (96,97), particularly in younger children without the cognitive-emotional skills required to make sense of what has happened to them during such an intervention. In children with severe asthma, events such as respiratory failure and intubation may lead to such anxiety symptoms (98). In terms of the child's psychological reaction, retention of consciousness during intubation can mean remembering a living nightmare. Restriction of activities is not only a current loss for children, but deprives them of developing skills, particularly in the athletic and social arenas, that would enhance their development (99). For children with asthma severe enough to require oral steroids, with the ensuing Cushingoid side effects, development of a healthy body image, with concomitant good self-esteem, can be difficult. Finally, severe illness can place a stress on the entire family, such as financial burden, loss of routines due to disruption of the illness, disagreements between parents regarding how to treat the sick child, and difficulty disciplining the child due to the mixed and confusing feelings that often arise in the parent with a chronically ill child (100–102). The ensuing family conflict and stress level can in turn lead to child emotional problems.

IV. The Success of Treatment in Severely Ill Asthmatic Children Is Related to Family Functioning

Current consensus is that many family processes can influence the course of childhood asthma, yet little is written about the number (many versus few) and the specific characteristics of these family influences. How might specific family processes influence asthma treatment outcome? Two strands of research evidence speak to this question. First, there are the reports of improved asthma management after family interventions. Second, several recent methodologically sound studies relate increased family dysfunction to worse asthma treatment management and/or outcome.

A. Family Treatments Improve Asthma Treatment Outcome

Family treatments have shown considerable promise as adjunctive therapy in the treatment of certain cases of childhood asthma. The ability of family interventions to improve medical management of asthma can be traced back to Peshkin's observations over 60 years ago that a subgroup of children with seemingly intractable asthma dramatically enter remission once separated from their families and placed in a hospital setting, the so-called "parentectomy" treatment (103,104). In one of the most provocative studies in this area, Purcell and associates (105), on the basis of family interviews, classified 25 children, ages 5 to 13 years, with frequent, clinically active asthma into family-reactive versus non-family-reactive groups. For 2 weeks all children were then cared for by a parent surrogate in their own homes (parents and siblings were moved into local hotels). For the group of 13 children predicted to improve with separation, all measures of asthma, including such objective indices as peak expiratory flow rate and amount of medication required, improved promptly after the separation. In contrast, only daily report of asthma symptoms improved for the 12 children predicted to be non-family-reactive. Data collected during the 4 weeks after families were reunited revealed the fatal flaw of "parentectomy" as a treatment for severe asthma—asthma symptomatology in the family-reactive group gradually returned to baseline levels, with a timing strongly suggesting that processes embedded in family interaction were involved in symptom exacerbation and/or maintenance for a potentially large subgroup of asthmatic children. However, the specific mechanism of this family effect remains unknown.

Three studies of *family therapy* with severely asthmatic children all found the treatment effective and speak to possible mechanisms. The first study reported improvement in seven families with a child suffering from severe, steroid-dependent, "psychosomatic" asthma (106). Therapy first taught and monitored the use of effective asthma management techniques and then worked to change dysfunctional family interactional patterns that promoted tension in the child. Ten to 22 months after 5 to 10 months of therapy, each child's asthma was in remission, with 6 children no longer requiring steroids or further hospitalization and having normal school attendance. Unfortunately, the lack of a control group in what should be seen as a series of case reports severely limits the confidence warranted by this report. Lask and Matthew (107) in a randomly assigned, controlled trial gave 6 h of family therapy over 4 months to the families of 18 moderately to severely ill asthmatic children, ages 4–14 years. The treatment focused on improving the family's coping with acute asthma attacks and discussing emotional issues related to the asthma. The control group of 16 families, matched on severity of child's asthma, age, social class, and psychological health, were followed in routine pediatric care. One year after the completion of therapy the experimental group was significantly better than the control group on two of five outcome parameters, daily wheeze score and thoracic gas volume, the latter being interpretable as a measure of air trapping related to chronic bronchospasm.

Gustafsson and associates (108) also reported a randomly assigned clinical trial using a family therapy drawing heavily on the techniques of Liebman et al. The 17 most severely ill asthmatic children, ages 6–15 years, from a clinical population of 600 cases were studied for an 8-month baseline and then randomly assigned to family therapy ($N = 9$) or routine clinical management ($N = 8$). Eight months after treatment the experimental group showed greater cumulative clinical improvement in blind pediatric assessments than the controls. At this point the control families were offered family therapy, and four accepted. After all cases had completed therapy, treatment cases showed significant improvement from baseline on overall pediatric assessment, functional assessment, peak expiratory flow rate, β_2-agonist use, and rate of emergency hospitalization. No index was significantly improved in the remaining control families. In their discussion the authors note the remarkable infrequency of open conflicts in these families, the inhibition of strong emotions seemingly due to family members' worry of provoking an asthma attack, and the degree to which family life had become organized around the disease. It is of note that although these family processes appear to complicate the course of asthma, the family processes are most likely the result of families trying to cope with asthma. Gustafsson has done a large prospective study of infants at genetic risk for atopic disorders. The families of those who did and did not develop asthma were similar at the beginning of the study. However, the families of those children who developed asthma became more chaotic and disruptive over time. Gustafsson interpreted this to be a reaction of the family to having a child with a chronic medical illness (109).

These studies suggest that selected families of asthmatics, perhaps as a reaction to the stress and burden of a child with a chronic medical illness, (1) have deficits in problem solving and conflict resolution skills, (2) have disordered (especially inhibited) emotional expression, and (3) can directly or indirectly impede treatment adherence and medical management. Yet, a clearer understanding of the specific family processes influencing the course and outcome of asthma is obscured by the broad goals of these therapies, the lack of clear operational definition of the family patterns targeted for change, and the fact that no valid measures of family functioning were collected during these studies.

B. Problematic Family Processes Are Found in Some Cases of Childhood Asthma

Four recent studies have found significant differences between families of asthmatic children and comparison families on directly *observed family processes.* Wikran et al. (110) compared the performance of 5 parents of children with severe asthma, ages 7–11, with 5 matched parents of children with congenital heart disease on a trick map reading task (unbeknown to the couple, one person's map had a crucial extra street). Whereas all of the parents in the heart disease group were able to discover the difference in their maps and successfully complete the task in the time allowed, 2 of the parents of asthmatics failed to complete the task. Given the small sample size, 12 additional parents of severely ill asthmatic children were recruited. Again, approximately one-third did not solve the problem. Qualitative examination of the taped discussions revealed that the reasons the couples could not solve the task were that they avoided statements that would indicate conflict or disagreement with what each other was saying and made very few attempts at understanding why the task could not be solved. This laboratory observation of "conflict avoidance" supported the theory stated by the family therapists that some asthmatic families have difficulty solving problems because they avoid all conflict.

Mrazek and colleagues (64) analyzed coded observations of a structured mother–child interaction paradigm, consisting of free play, play with a developmentally challenging toy, and a separation–reunion sequence, in mothers of 26 severely asthmatic, 36- to 72-month-old children and a comparison group of 22 healthy mother–child pairs. Active opposition was shown three times more often by the asthmatic children than by the controls, especially during the challenging task. Interestingly, persistent noncompliance with the mother's requests accounted for 57% of the oppositional interactions in the asthmatic group but only 34% of the interaction in the control group. Additionally, the asthmatic children were more frequently classified as insecurely attached to their mothers than the controls.

Third, Hermanns et al. (111) compared 25 mother–child pairs with moderately asthmatic 7- to 13-year-old children to 25 healthy, matched controls on three measures of maternal criticism and negative verbal exchange. They found that (1) on the Five Minute Speech Sample measure of expressed emotion [FMSS (112)] 10/25 mothers of asthmatics but only 2/25 control mothers made critical statements about their child; (2) during a mother–child discussion of a currently active family problem, mothers of asthmatics made more critical remarks to their child than the control mothers; (3) the asthma pairs showed longer negative verbal sequences (>5 lags) than the controls; and (4) those mothers showing more criticism had children with more severe asthma.

Fourth, Schöbinger, Florin et al. (113) repeated the overall design of Hermanns and colleagues (111) with the fathers of 27 asthmatic children (ages 6–
13) with 23 healthy controls. They similarly found that (1) significantly more
fathers of asthmatic children (9/27) than control fathers (2/23) made critical statements about their child on the FMSS; (2) fathers of asthmatics evidenced more
negative verbal behavior, including criticism of their child during a problem discussion with their child; and (3) the asthma pairs showed longer length sequences
of negative verbal behavior than the controls.

These studies provide an interesting comparison to the family therapy studies in three ways. First, although all four of these studies showed problem-solving
deficits in the family interaction of asthmatic children, three have revealed findings that appear diametrically opposed to the family therapy studies: The asthmatic groups showed increased opposition and criticism, not conflict avoidance.
Second, these studies suggest that three constructs proven to be very robust measures of family dysfunction—parental management problems, insecure attachment behavior, and high expressed emotion—are prevalent in certain asthmatic
families. Finally, these studies support the conception that asthma management
is more problematic if families are poorer at not only emotional regulation but
also behavioral and/or cognitive/conceptual regulation.

V. Treatment Adherence Is the Likely Mediator Between Psychosocial Factors and Asthma Treatment Outcome

Although a number of social scientists have rightly argued that nonadherence to
prescribed medication may be interpreted as an adaptive coping attempt on the
part of patients and their parents to take control of their illness and their lives
(114,115), the preponderance of research evidence clearly indicates the tremendous costs of nonadherence with prescribed asthma treatment due to compromised treatment effectiveness, including increased morbidity, mortality, health
care utilization costs, and sociovocational impairments (116).

A. Treatment Nonadherence Is Common in Childhood Asthma

Studies of medication adherence among asthmatic children suggest that medications are taken as prescribed less than 50% of the time (117,118). For example,
in the study of Eney and Goldstein (119), only 5 of 43 children presenting to the
Pediatric Allergy Clinic at Johns Hopkins Hospital had serum theophylline levels
in the therapeutic range (i.e., 10–20 mg/ml), despite all having been prescribed
reasonable daily dosages. Ten patients had no detectable level of theophylline at
all. Coutts and colleagues (120) found similar results for the case of inhaled
corticosteroids: In a group of asthmatic children, inhaled steroids were underused
in 55% of study days. Recent technological advances in the measurement of

patient adherence, such as microchip-equipped devices that record the date and time of each dose taken of an aerosolized antiasthma medication, have shown that old estimates of adherence like diary cards, canister weights, and pill counts consistently overestimate patient adherence by a large margin (119–127). Furthermore, such electronic monitoring devices allow the conceptualization of patient adherence to develop beyond simple dichotomies of compliant/noncompliant to patterns of adherence such as consistent underusage, consistent overusage, binge (presumably rescue-only) usage, and "dumping" (typically defined as canister activation ≥100 times in a day, usually occurring right before a scheduled return visit).

Nonadherence with medication used to control chronic illnesses increases when the benefits of the medication are not immediately apparent after dosing and when the patient does not believe that use of the medication affects the course of the illness (115). Asthma medications such as aerosolized corticosteroids, which play an important role in treating the underlying inflammatory basis of asthma but do not provide immediate symptom relief, appear to be greatly underutilized (126). Seeking immediate relief, some patients may use bronchodilators to the exclusion of anti-inflammatory medications with more long-term benefits. Prolonged, excessive use of inhaled bronchodilator drugs may result in deterioration of symptom control possibly due to inhibition of natural anti-inflammatory mechanisms and thereby contribute to asthma morbidity and mortality (128–130).

B. Nonadherence Is Associated with Poorer Asthma Outcome

For asthmatic children, nonadherence contributes to poorly controlled asthma and has been associated with increased morbidity and risk of death due to asthma. One study reported that a group of noncompliant asthmatic children experienced significantly more wheezing days, greater variability in peak flow rates, and lower asthma control scores than a group of compliant asthmatic children (131). Another group found that 49 of 50 children admitted to an emergency room with a chief complaint of acute wheezing/asthma had subtherapeutic theophylline levels (132). Furthermore, 37 of the 50 children had been prescribed theophylline at adequate dosage (5–6 mg/kg/6 h); hence, for these children inadequate adherence rather than improper dosing by the physician appears the likely cause of their low serum levels. This was further supported by their finding that 87% (32/37) of these "nonadherent" children had extremely low serum levels ("<5 µg/mL, with many having zero or trace levels").

Numerous reports evaluating the cause of childhood asthma deaths from around the world consistently list treatment nonadherence with medication and/ or patient or family delay in seeking emergency care as major "avoidable" factors linked to these deaths (7,9,12,14,133). The likely link between nonadherence and asthma death is most clearly documented in an investigation of a cluster of five deaths of asthmatic adolescents in St. Louis (134). This study found that despite having been prescribed appropriate amounts of theophylline, all four children who died in an emergency room, and hence had theophylline levels examined at the time of the fatal attack, had extremely low, subtherapeutic serum levels.

C. Nonadherence Is Associated with Family Dysfunction

On one hand, many clinicians have discussed the need for solid social support from family to ensure optimal treatment adherence and outcome in a complex, chronic illness like asthma, especially in the more severe cases. Hence, good family functioning likely promotes better treatment adherence (14,126,135). On the other hand, family dysfunction is related to both poorer treatment adherence and greater asthma morbidity. In a study of 38 chronically ill asthmatic children, the degree of family conflict and the psychological adjustment of the child were together the most predictive variables of nonadherence to oral theophylline (49). Furthermore, Strunk and colleagues (51) reported that greater evidence of family dysfunction prior to discharge from a tertiary care inpatient asthma specialty unit was correlated with a greater number of hospitalizations, emergency room and urgent office visits, and longer hospitalizations in the year subsequent to discharge.

Concerning family dysfunction and asthma mortality, all of the reports cited in the paragraph above that evaluated factors related to childhood asthma deaths also mention the role of psychosocial, especially family, problems in these deaths (7,8,10,12,53,134,136). For example, in her review of 15 childhood asthma deaths, Kravis (9) reported an association between psychosocial problems and noncompliance including that "all patients who had psychosocial problems requiring intensive treatment were non-compliant." Her definition of psychosocial problems included both individual as well as family problems and treatment. Sears and colleagues (11) quote comments from general practitioners citing a variety of family problems, including "poor family care of children," "mobile family," "alcoholic mother," "neglected child," "non-compliant family," and "fatalistic attitude" of the family concerning their child. Furthermore, they noted, as many others have continued to observe, the high percentage of parents who smoke despite having a seriously asthmatic child—75% of the child deaths which they reported occurred in families in which at least one parent smoked regularly. Similarly, Fritz and colleagues (8) note a range of family dysfunction in their cases of asthma death from "Paul's critical, demanding and unaccepting parents" to "Kathy's chaotic and overly abusive home situation." Finally, Sears (12) noted that "the majority of young people dying of asthma showed evidence of rejection of parental and medical supervision and a reluctance to seek attention or attend for regular follow-up.''

D. Parental Criticism May Be a Key Marker of Family Dysfunction Associated with Noncompliance

In an effort to more closely described which family dynamics were most crucial in predicting poorer medical outcome of adolescent asthmatics, our laboratory has been studying adolescent asthmatics and their families using a structured protocol that involves both self-report and coded observations of family and individual psychodynamics. We have previously reported (137) how one observational measure of family functioning [parental criticism on the Five Minute Speech Sample (138)] correlated with asthma treatment adherence and outcome in a sample of 19 hospitalized, inpatient adolescents with severe, chronic asthma. Although parental criticism of the adolescent during this task was not associated with asthma severity or dose of corticosteroids at admission, high parental criticism was associated with (1) worse adherence at admission with oral theophylline and steroids, (2) greater improvement in asthma severity at discharge, (3) less steroid medication at discharge, and (4) a shorter length of stay in the hospital. Hence, our data suggest that one dimension of family process, parental criticism, is related to poorer medication adherence as well as to a clinical presentation of ''severe'' asthma that met criteria for hospitalization to a major tertiary center, but responded promptly and quite well to treatment in the hospital.

We subsequently have replicated these results in a sample of 84 children meeting the same inclusion criteria as the pilot group. In this sample, we have again found parental criticism to be associated with poorer treatment adherence at admission. Once again, although oral steroid medication requirements were significantly reduced for both parental criticism groups across the hospitalization, the high-parental-criticism group required significantly lower doses of oral steroids at both admission and discharge. Furthermore, this study also used hierarchical multiple-regression techniques to show that the admission treatment adherence scores mediated the association between parental criticism and steroid medication requirements.

Why should parental criticism be a marker for family dysfunction that is associated with poorer adherence and increased morbidity and mortality? Our experience suggests that just as an elevated erythrocyte sedimentation rate is a nonspecific indicator of systemic inflammation, parental criticism on the FMSS is a nonspecific indicator of an ''inflamed'' parent–child relationship. Accordingly, the clinical challenge is to identify which of a variety of interpersonal problems exists. For example, parental criticism often occurs in the context of overt family conflict. In other samples these dynamics are related to conduct disorder and oppositional behaviors in adolescents and children (139,140). In families with an asthmatic child, these dynamics may be associated with the child rebelling by becoming noncompliant with their treatment regimen. If parents have not established an effective means of disciplining their child, they may blame and criticize the child for not following the rules, which further incites their child, continuing the cycle of noncompliance. Clinically we notice that often such parents have not developed an effective means of coping with their child's asthma and fostering good medical care. There may be a history of family chaos and/ or neglect of the ill child leading to poor medication monitoring by parents, inadequate regular medical follow-up, and delays in receiving urgent care during crises. Finally, some authors hypothesize potentially direct effects of increased conflict and stress mediated through the central and/or autonomic nervous systems (141,142). In any case the clinician should listen carefully for the parent whose reports of their child frame the asthmatic as a ''bad'' rather than an ''ill'' person, as this appears to be a reliable indicator of a breakdown in the parent–child partnership required for successful asthma (54). Further education about asthma management, as well as direct psychosocial intervention, may be particularly helpful in such cases.

VI.   Evaluation and Management Issues

A.   Education Is Necessary, but Not Sufficient, to Ensure Compliance

Given that psychological issues can cloud the ''true'' physiologic severity of asthma, the first task of the physician evaluating a person with difficult-to-control asthma is to ascertain how much of the apparent severity is due to noncompliance and/or poor self-care, including under- or overuse of medications, exposure to known triggers and allergens, and poor understanding of how to track and manage changing symptomatology. Although asthma education will not always alleviate noncompliance, it is a vital and necessary first step (54,143). Therefore, the physician must ensure that the patient and family have an adequate understanding about the pathophysiology of asthma, the mechanism of action of the various medications, the appropriate techniques for using inhalers and nebulizers, how to use a peak flow meter to monitor and record symptoms, an up-to-date asthma ''action plan,'' and so on. There are many educational programs available, and a number have established outcome criteria (144–147). Overall, these programs are primarily recommended for children with moderate to severe asthma and in these populations with much functional disability have shown to decrease school absenteeism, medical utilization, and family stress. For children with asthma, it is important to recommend a program that is developmentally appropriate for the youngster, but also to involve the parents. Programs that include some material on appropriate problem solving and communication among family members are particularly helpful.

Once education is completed, a structure for monitoring adherence provides useful feedback to the patient and/or parents as well as information for the physician. Although electronic monitoring devices for MDIs and peak flow meters are now research tools, they may become available for clinical use. Providing feedback about a person's actual decision making and use of MDIs based on readings from the computerized peak flow meters and MDIs can improve adherence (148,149). Scheduled return appointments and monitoring of drug levels if appropriate are also helpful to maintain adherence. For children, asthma camp experiences, such as those sponsored by the American Lung Association or other groups around the country, provide an excellent structure in which to reinforce good self-care habits in an accepting and supportive social structure.

B. Development of a Collaborative Physician/Patient Relationship Is Key to Adherence

The most critical factor in long-term adherence to a treatment plan is the development of a patient/physician relationship wherein patients feel encouraged to tell the physician of difficulties they are having with specific recommendations, e.g., side effects, too frequent dosing, and avoidance of specific triggers (122,150–152). With any chronic illness, adherence fluctuates over time and usually in response to specific portions of the treatment plan and changes in routines in the patients' lives. Having a trusting physician/patient relationship where these difficulties are accepted and treatment plans are mutually developed is the main factor in promoting overall compliance over time. The physician should not act as though any suggestion or complaint of the patient should take precedence over a rational treatment plan, which would undermine the patient's respect for the physician and decrease compliance. Rather, the physician should actively encourage questions and concerns and encourage the patient to take over more and more of the day-to-day decision making regarding their illness. The physician's role is still that of someone with wider knowledge and experience about the illness who can offer important information and advice. However, the responsibility for the patient's overall life is his or her own. The art of forging such a collaborative physician/patient/family relationship over time lies in large part to the use of a positive, friendly, warm, and supportive approach.

If patients still do not adhere, it is unlikely that more education is helpful. The issue of patient nonadherence is a very complex one, and numerous issues need to be taken into consideration (122,151). For example, the issue may be that they do not perceive themselves (or their child, in the parents' case) to be at risk for the issues the physician has stressed. Moving to a model of understanding their individual idiosyncratic beliefs about how *their/their child's asthma* actually reacts to smoking, theophylline, and so on may be helpful (153,154). Additionally, understanding the stress level, social support systems, structural needs, and interpersonal relationships of the family may be key (155,156). Understanding the etiology and recommending treatment for a specific patient's nonadherence may require a psychosocial evaluation.

C. When to Refer for Psychosocial Evaluation or Treatment

If adherence remains inadequate or if the primary physician suspects his/her patient of having other significant psychological symptoms, how does s/he decide when to refer the patient for psychosocial consultation? There are several areas of "red flags," or warning signs, that indicate a need for a more thorough psychosocial evaluation.

Self-Care Is a Useful Benchmark

Especially for children, judging how many self-management skills they have mastered is a good rule of thumb to judge overall coping of the child and family. Either too much or too little responsibility for their age can indicate problems. In Table 2, Klinnert and Tedesco have delineated appropriate asthma management expectations for children of varying ages based on their developmental levels. Roughly, adolescents over 16 years of age can be expected to manage all of their day-to-day tasks; however, if their illness exacerbates, parents should be involved in deciding which extra medications to take or when to call the physician, as per a set home care plan. Parents should be providing structure via checking on whether the child actually took the medication or recorded the peak flow. Children younger than this age should have some, but not all, of these responsibilities. If younger children are taking on too many responsibilities it may indicate inappropriate parental expectations or parental neglect; if adolescents are doing too little, it may indicate an overall parental overprotective attitude, depression and/ or cognitive problems in the child, or secondary gain issues.

Functional Status

A child who is missing more than 15 days of school a year should also be referred for further evaluation. His or her illness may indeed be incapacitating them, and the risk of secondary psychosocial problems is high. Likewise, it is possible that anxiety or depression are contributing to some of the dysfunction.

Over Focus on the Illness

Another reason to refer is when the illness becomes the center of the patient or family's life such that many other important family developmental needs are taking second place. Examples of this include parents focusing on the sick child

Table 2 Suggested Levels of Self-Care Responsibility for Pediatric Age Groups

Ages 0–3 years: Cooperate in taking respiratory treatments and medications: respond to adult guidance to slow down or sit down.

Ages 3–5 years: Learn body awareness with verbal labels for wheezing/tightness; learn to swallow pills.

Ages 6–7 years: Take medications and respiratory treatments correctly when adults remind; use peak flow meter correctly with adult reminders; listen to body so can report wheezing to adults and stop asthma attacks early.

Ages 7–8 years: Request medications from adults within 30 min of scheduled time; request and use peak flow meter at schedules time; notice, report, and record early warning signs and triggers; request pretreatment before exercise if scheduled; clean and put away nebulizer.

Ages 8–9 years: Recognize and report wheezing/tightness; obtain and sip water at the first sign of wheezing/tightness; record peak flow meter values at times schedules; learn to take pulse at times scheduled; demonstrate and use breathing exercises; begin learning about medications.

Ages 9–10 years: Know medications, including dose, times taken, action, indications, contraindications, and side effects; parents and adults provide emotional back-up.

Ages 11–12 years: Prepare respiratory treatments with supervision; assess condition before and after respiratory treatments; take and record pulse before and after respiratory treatments when scheduled.

Ages 13–14 years: Practice waking (with alarm clock) for nighttime medications and treatments; prepare each dose of medication, take medications with parents' knowledge.

Ages 14–15 years: Record medications, peak flows, pulse; pack medications for 24-h period with supervision; keep written records of medications, peak flow, and pulse with supervision; Awaken for nighttime medications and treatments.

Ages 16+: Prepare and take medications and respiratory treatments independently; arrange for refill of medications when low; assess condition before and after respiratory treatments; keep accurate records of medications, respiratory treatments, pulse, peak flows, and symptoms diary.

Note. It is assumed that the child will master all previous levels of self-care before progressing to the next stage. Adapted from Klinnert M, Tedesco, 1985. Developmentally based self-care for asthmatic children. Unpublished manuscript, National Jewish Medical and Research Center.

to the neglect of siblings, repeated cancellation of family vacations or social events due to the illness, employment or education decisions made solely on the basis of the asthma, and extreme financial duress due to the illness. When the illness runs a family's life, there is a good chance that family conflict is high, although it may not be overt. Such families often are dealing with numerous loss issues, and the patient may be shouldering a huge portion of guilt for this. Unless these issues are brought out in the open and the family given permission to voice their feelings about them, the patient may decline for reasons that are not often clear (157).

Apparent Depression or Anxiety or Manifest Denial of Serious Symptoms

These problems are known to interfere with the course of asthma and put the child with severe asthma at greater risk of asthma death. Moreover, they usually can be readily treated with medications and/or psychotherapy. A note regarding some old and damaging cultural myths that impair psychosocial treatment and/ or referral, especially for depression in the medically ill. Some people think that with all the burdens of a chronic illness, "I'd be depressed, too." Even if the depression is thought to be due to the "stress of asthma," it nonetheless should and *can* be treated. The old distinction between primary and secondary depression has no predictive value for outcome (158). Pharmacologic and psychotherapeutic treatments are equally effective for depression thought to be primary or secondary to aversive life events, e.g., asthma. Overall, the treatment response rate for major depression is over 80%, so it is likely that the depressed asthmatic patient will be able to recover from the depression (159).

Likewise, individual styles of coping typical of Kinsman et al.'s (69) low panic–fear (overly self-reliant) or high panic–fear (anxious-complaining) patients deserve an evaluation since these coping styles are associated with worse asthma outcome. High anxiety can often be treated pharmacologically as well as with cognitive and behavioral techniques. Low anxiety, or denial, is often best dealt with within the family or support system context. It may be very salient to the parents of a denying patient that their child ignores warning symptoms, even though it does not (by definition) bother the child. Using the parents' concern and the strength of their relationship to confront the child's denial can be very effective and helpful. Similarly, parental denial of illness severity may require broadening the social system involved in treatment. In extreme cases this may mean involving child protective services and in less extreme cases the child's grandparents or other members of the family's social support system.

Overt Conflict Between Patient and Family or Between Patient/Family and Health Care Providers

Family conflict has been associated with both increased asthma morbidity and mortality as well as greater asthma treatment noncompliance in children and adolescents. Research suggests that overt family conflict in the presence of relative strangers (as in a clinical or research setting) is an underestimate of the level that likely occurs at home (160). Hence, such behavior should alert the clinician that potentially significant family problems may exist. Brief family therapy can be exceedingly useful to get the family working together again.

D. Case Example

A case illustrating several of the above signs was Brian, a bright and likeable 14-year-old from a working-class family in Virginia. Brian had several respiratory arrests requiring intubation early in childhood, resulting in his mother being very protective and watchful over him. His asthma was well controlled from age 4 through 12 years, however, and he maintained high academic achievement and extracurricular activities. Mother attributed this to the fact that she personally ensured that he took his medications and recorded his peak flows. When Brian began having numerous exacerbations and symptoms at age 13, his mother decided the problem was "too much stress" and required him to quit his extracurricular activities. His symptoms continued to increase, requiring several hospitalizations. As his mother grew more anxious, Brian became overtly oppositional, demanding that he be allowed to take on a paper route and other part-time jobs. Mother refused to allow this. Brian's asthma continued to worsen and his grades began to drop. At the time he was referred for a psychiatric evaluation, he was overtly depressed. He disclosed in therapy that he felt guilty that his asthma "ran the family." He believed his mother refused to go to work because she was so worried about him. He believed that her refusal to work, as well as the cost of his prescriptions, necessitated his father taking on a second job. With his father gone most of the week, marital problems developed, for which Brian also felt responsible. His solution was to stop taking his most expensive medications (without telling anyone) to "make them last longer" and to get a job to "pay for his own meds." He felt he could not express these concerns to his family because "they already feel bad enough about it." His family, until they entered family therapy, never noticed his noncompliance nor the intensity of his personal distress and guilt about his illness, all of which were central factors in his deteriorating clinical course.

E. How to Refer and to Whom

One concern physicians often have when suggesting a psychiatric referral is that their patient will take offense or object. In fact, some patients may feel relief that their concerns are acknowledged and hopeful that they will receive help. Other patients, however, fear the physician may be telling them the problem is "all in their head" and that the physician does not want to continue as their doctor. One way to counteract this is to communicate an attitude from the initial visit onward that the physician is willing to take a comprehensive or integrative stance with the patient and consider all aspects of how the illness may be affecting them. Additionally, reassuring the patient that the physician will continue to provide for medical needs alleviates the fear of rejection. Citing the evidence that chronic, especially severe, asthma is often associated with concomitant psychological difficulties is helpful. Explaining that the best treatment for severe asthma combines a holistic approach, encompassing both medical and psychological attention, is also useful.

How does one pick a helpful consultant? Clearly the range and diversity of psychosocial clinicians is wide, and not all are well prepared to take on a patient with severe medical illness. Rather than their professional degree, per se, the major indicator of success is that you and your patient see the consultant as someone who understands the problem and can communicate a solution to the problem that seems straightforward and sensible. Sometimes several consultants need to be tried out until such a "good fit" can be achieved. Also it is sometimes useful to have a "team" of consultants that offer different strengths for differing types of psychosocial problems.

In general, the following are some more specific abilities that a "good" consultant should have. First, it is important that the consultant has the ability to confront the self-damaging or neglectful patient. Such patients need not only empathy and sympathy, but also someone able to structure the treatment so as to get "business" done. All too frequently, out of fear or lack of knowledge, psychosocial consultants may take a "you poor dear" approach that never gets the needed work done. Second, the consultant should have good knowledge of child development and the ability to deal psychotherapeutically with issues of loss, altered developmental course, and the burden of the illness on family. Third, the consultant requires knowledge about the effects of asthma medications on mood and behavior as well as of the diagnosis of depression and anxiety in the medically ill. If the consultant is not a psychiatrist, having access and willingness to use psychiatric referral is crucially important. For many major psychiatric illnesses, even in the context of severe asthma, medication *and* psychotherapeutic treatment in combination are the treatment of choice.

The availability of specific treatments useful for asthma are also helpful. These may include speech therapy (for VCD), biofeedback and/or relaxation therapy for anxiety, and psychoeducation groups for children and parents (161). An additional useful skill is the ability to work with a multidisciplinary team, especially if the patient has prominent somatizing concerns. A consultant who is willing to meet with the physician, the teachers, and the family to develop a treatment plan and keep all persons concerned in a communication loop can get the patient through many therapeutic impasses.

In these times of medical cost containment, it is important not to forget the important role of referral to a specialty asthma medical/psychiatric center. For certain patients with extremely hard-to-manage asthma, the "time out for asthma" (162,163) that such hospitals can provide for both inpatients and outpatients have proven ability to help refocus the patient and their family in a fashion that breaks the downward spiral of out-of-control illness (164–166).

VII. Conclusion

From the earliest times in medical history, the association of psychological factors and asthma has been observed. In this chapter, we reviewed the fact that although asthma has genetic underpinnings, it also requires a variety of environmental factors for the onset of the illness. There is some evidence that psychosocial variables, such as stressful parenting or trauma early in life, may be involved in the onset of asthma. There is more evidence that psychosocial factors have a profound influence on the course of asthma. With more severe asthma there is an increased risk of depression and anxiety in the patient and changes in family functioning to adapt to the illness such that the family tends to be less flexible and less expressive of emotions and thus has more difficulty with problem solving. Both the individual symptoms and the changes in family function are associated with poorer adherence, which in turn exacerbates the symptoms of asthma and may lead to more chronic and irreversible lung remodeling. Fortunately, most patients with severe asthma do not have extreme difficulties with the emotional factors involved in the illness. For those who are hampered by these difficulties, psychological and/or psychopharmacologic treatments are often very successful. The best approach to the patient with severe asthma is to treat them as a whole person and acknowledge that while emotional distress can exacerbate asthma, so can asthma lead to emotional distress.

Acknowledgments

The writing of this chapter was supported by NIH Grants R01-HL53391, R01-HL45157, K08-MH01486, and M01-RR0051.

References

1. Taylor WR, Newacheck PW. Impact of childhood asthma on health. Peds 1992; 90:657–662.
2. Weitzman M, et al. Recent trends in the prevalence and severity of childhood asthma. J Am Med Assoc 1992; 268:2673–2677.
3. Adams P, Marano M. Current Estimates from the National Health Interview Survey, 1994. Hyattsville, MD: National Center for Health Statistics. 1995.
4. Evans IR. Asthma among minority children: a growing problem. Chest 1992; 101: 368S–371S.
5. Weiss KB, Wagener DK. Changing pattern of asthma mortality: identifying target populations at risk. J Am Med Assoc 1990, 264(13):1683–1687.
6. Weiss KB, Gergen PJ, Crain EF. Inner-city asthma: the epidemiology of an emerging U.S. public health concern. Chest 1992; 101:362S–367S.

7. Carswell F. Thirty deaths from asthma. Arch Dis Child 1985; 60:25–28.
8. Fritz GK, Rubenstein S, Lewiston NJ. Psychological factors in fatal childhood asthma. Am J Orthopsychiat 1987; 57:253–257.
9. Kravis LP, An analysis of fifteen childhood asthma fatalities. J Allergy Clin Immunol 1987; 80:467–472.
10. Rubinstein S, et al. Sudden death in adolescent asthma. Ann Allergy 1984; 53: 311–318.
11. Sears MR, et al. Deaths from asthma in New Zealand. Arch Dis Child 1986; 61: 6–10.
12. Sears M. Fatal asthma: a perspective. Immunol Allergy Practice 1988; 9:259–267.
13. Strunk R, et al. Physiologic and psychological characteristics associated with deaths due to asthma in childhood. J Am Med Assoc 1985; 254(9):1193–1198.
14. Strunk RC. Asthma deaths in childhood: identification of patients at risk and intervention. J Allergy Clin Immunol 1987; 80(3):472–477.
15. Duffy DL, et al. Genetics of asthma and hayfever in Australian twins. Am Rev Resp Dis 1990; 142:1351–1358.
16. Ober C. Do genetics play a role in the pathogenesis of asthma? J Allergy Clin Immunol 1998; 101(22):S417–S420.
17. Sanford A, Weir T, Pare P. The genetics of asthma. Am J Resp Crit Care Med 1996; 153:1749–1765.
18. Hopp RJ, et al. Genetic analysis of allergic disease in twins. J Allergy Clin Immunol 1984; 73:265–270.
19. Hopkin JM. Genetics of asthma. Arch Dis Children 1993; 68(8):712–723.
20. Mrazek DA, Klinnert M. Asthma: psychoneuroimmunologic considerations. In: Ader R, Felten DL, Cohen N, eds. Psychoneuroimmunology. New York: Academic Press, 1991:1013–1035.
21. Block JH, Block J, Morrison A. Parental agreement—disagreement on child-rearing orientations and gender-related personality correlates in children. Child Dev 1981; 52:965–974.
22. Purcell K, Turnbull JW, Bernstein L. Distinctions between subgroups of asthmatic children: psychological test and behavior rating comparisons. J Psychosom Res 1962; 6:283–291.
23. Mrazek D, Strunk R. Psychological adjustment of severely asthmatic preschool children: allergic considerations. Psychosom Med 1984; 46:85.
24. Mrazek DA, Klinnert MD. Asthma and serum levels of IgE. N Engl J Med 1989; 320:1696.
25. Horwood L, et al. Social and familial factors in the development of early childhood asthma. Pediatrics 1985; 75(5):859–868.
26. Arshad SH, Hide DW. Effect of environmental factors on the development of allergic disorders in infancy. J Allergy Clin Immunol 1992; 90(2):235–241.
27. Klinnert MD, Mrazek PJ, Mrazek DA. Early asthma onset: the interaction between family stressors and adaptive parenting. Psychiatry 1994; 57:51–61.
28. Plomin R. Genetics, environmental risks, and protective factors. In Turner J, Cardon L, Hewitt J, eds. Behavior Genetic Approaches in Behavioral Medicine. New York: Plenum, 1995.

29. Vamos M, Kolbe J. Psychological factors in severe chronic asthma. Aust N Z J Psychiat 1999; 33(4):538–544.
30. Cuffel B, et al. Economic consequences of comorbid depression, anxiety, and allergic rhinitis. Psychosomatics 1999; 40(6):491–496.
31. Fritz GK, Overholser JC. Patterns of response to childhood asthma. Psychosom Med 1989; 51:347–355.
32. Meijer A. A controlled study on asthmatic children and their families: synopsis of findings. Isr J Psychiatry Relat Sci 1981; 18(3):197–208.
33. Jessop DJ, Riessman CK, Stein REK. Chronic childhood illness and maternal mental health. J Dev Beh Pediatr 1988; 9:147–156.
34. Davis JB. Neurotic illness in the families of children with asthma and wheezy bronchitis: a general population study. Psychol Med 1977; 7:305–310.
35. Battaglia M, et al. Age at onset of panic disorder: influence of familial liability to the disease and of childhood separation anxiety disorder. Am J Psychiatry 1995; 152(9):1362–1364.
36. Kendler KS, Prescott CA. A population-based twin study of lifetime major depression in men and women. Arch Gen Psychiat 1999; 56(1):39–44.
37. Wamboldt M, et al. Psychiatric family history in adolescents with severe asthma. J Am Acad Child Adol Psychiat 1996; 35(8):1042–1049.
38. Beautrais AL, Fergusson DM, Shannon FT. Life events and childhood morbidity: a prospective study. Pediatrics 1982; 70:935–940.
39. Boyce WT, Jemerin JM. Psychobiological differences in childhood stress response. I. Patterns of illness and susceptibility. Dev Behav Pediatr 1990; 11(2): 86–94.
40. Busse WW. Respiratory infections: their role in airway responsiveness and the pathogenesis of asthma. J Allergy Clin Immunol 1990; 85:671–683.
41. Wamboldt MZ, Hewitt J, Wamboldt FS. Individual and family factors associated with medical nonadherence. Behav Genet 1999; 29(5):374.
42. Wamboldt, MZ, et al. Links between past parental trauma and the medical and psychological outcome of asthmatic children: a theoretical model. Family Syst Med 1995; 13(2):129–149.
43. Laitinen L, et al. Damage of the airway epithelium and bronchial reactivity in patients with asthma. Am Rev Resp Dis 1985; 131(4):599–606.
44. Wamboldt MZ, Schmitz S, Mrazek D. Genetic association between atopy and behavioral symptoms in middle childhood. J Child Psychol Psychiat 1998; 39(7): 1007–1016.
45. Wamboldt MZ, et al. Familial association between atopy and depression in adult Finnish twins. Neuropsychiat Genet 2000; 96(2):146–153.
46. Maimonides MB. Treatise on Asthma. 1190. English translation in Muntner S. The Medical Writings of Moses Maimonides. Philadelphia: Lippincott, 1963.
47. Baron C, et al. Psychomaintenance of childhood asthma: a study of 34 children. J Asthma 1986; 23(2):68–79.
48. Baron C, Marcotte J. Experience and reason—briefly recorded: role of panic attacks in the intractability of asthma in children. Pediatrics 1994; 94(1):108–111.
49. Christiaanse ME, Lavigne JV, Lerner CV. Psychosocial aspects of compliance in children and adolescents with asthma. Dev Behav Pediatr 1989; 10(2):75–80.

50. Dirks JF, et al. Panic-fear: a personalilty dimension related to length of hospitalization in respiratory illness. J Asthma Res 1977; 14:61–71.

51. Strunk RC, et al. Outcome of long-term hospitalization for asthma in children. J Allergy Clin Immunol 1989; 83:17–25.

52. Kravis LP, Kolski GB. Unexpected death in childhood asthma: a review of 13 deaths in ambulatory patients. Am J Dis Child 1985; 139:558–563.

53. Sears MR, Rea HH. Patients at risk for dying of asthma: New Zealand experience. J Allergy Clin Immunol 1987; 80:477–481.

54. Institute, NHLaB. Expert Panel Report 2: Guidelines for the Diagnosis and Management of Asthma. Bethesda, MD: National Institutes of Health, NIH publication no. 97-4051, 1997, xi, 146.

55. Dirks JF, et al. Patient and physician characteristics influencing medical decisions in asthma. J Asthma Res 1976; 15(4):171–178.

56. Stein REK, et al. Severity of illness: concepts and measurements. Lancet 1987; December 26:1506–1509.

57. Mrazek D. Asthma: psychiatric considerations, evaluation, and management. In Middleton E, et al., eds. Allergy Principles and Practice. Washington, DC: Mosby, 1988:1176–1196.

58. Graham PJ, et al. Childhood asthma: a psychosomatic disorder: some epidemiological considerations. Br J Prev Soc Med 1967; 21:78–85.

59. Bussing R, Burket RC, Kelleher ET. Prevalence of anxiety disorders in a clinic-based sample of pediatric asthma patients. Psychosomatics 1996; 37(2):108–115.

60. Vila G, et al. Assessment of anxiety disorders in asthmatic children. Psychosomatics 1999; 40(5):404–413.

61. Achenbach, TM. Manual for the Child Behavior Checklist/4–18 and 1991 Profile. Burlington, VT: Univ. of Vermont Department of Psychiatry, 1991.

62. Brody GH, Forehead R. Maternal perceptions of child maladjustment as a function of the combined influences of child behavior and maternal depression. J Cons Clin Psychol 1986; 54:237–240.

63. Wamboldt MZ, et al. The relationship of asthma severity and psychological problems in children. J Am Acad Child Adol Psychiat 1998; 37(9):943–950.

64. Mrazek DA, Casey B, Anderson I. Insecure attachment in severely asthmatic preschool children: is it a risk factor? J Am Acad Child Adol Psychiat 1987; 26(4):516–520.

65. Kashani JH., et al. Psychopathology and self-concept in asthmatic children. J Ped Psychol 1988; 13(4):509–520.

66. Herjanic B, Reich W. Development of a structured psychiatric interview of children: agreement between child and parent on individual symptoms. J Abn Child Psychol 1982; 10:307–324.

67. Sperling M. Asthma in children: an evaluation of concepts and therapies. J Am Acad Child Psychiat 1968; 4:44–58.

68. Kinsman RA, Dirks JF, Jones NF. Psychomaintenance of chronic physical illness. In Millon T, Green CJ. Handbook of Clinical Health Psychology 1982. New York: Plenum, 1982:435–465.

69. Dirks JF, Kinsman RA. Clinical prediction of medical rehospitalization: psycholog-

ical assessment with the battery of asthma illness behavior. J Pers Assessment 1981; 45:608–613.

70. Dirks JF, et al. Psycho-maintenance in asthma: hospitalization rates and financial impact. Br J Med Psychol 1980; 53:349–354.

71. Rubinfeld A, Pain M. Perception of asthma. Lancet 1976; 1(7965):882–884.

72. Kikuchi Y, et al. Chemosensitivity and perception of dyspnea in patients with a history of near-fatal asthma. N Engl J Med 1994; 330(19):1329–1334.

73. Zach MS, Karner U. Sudden death in asthma. Arch Dis Child 1989; 64(10):1146–50; discussion 1450–1.

74. Banzett RB, et al. Symptom perception and respiratory sensation in asthma. Am J Resp Crit Care Med 2000; 162(3):1178–1182.

75. Fritz GK, Overholser JD. Accuracy of symptom perception in childhood asthma. 1990; 11(2):69–72.

76. Fritz GK, et al. Symptom perception in pediatric asthma: relationship to functional morbidity and psychological factors. J Am Acad Child Adolesc Psychiat 1996; 35(8):1033–41.

77. Bihun J, Wamboldt MZ, Szefler S. Perception of induced bronchoconstriction in a community sample of adolescents. Am J Resp Crit Care Med 2000; 161(3/2): A55.

78. Boner AL, et al. Perception of bronchoconstriction in chronic asthma. J Asthma 1992; 29(5):323–330.

79. Brand PL, et al. Perception of airway obstruction in a random population sample: relationship to airway hyperresponsiveness in the absence of respiratory symptoms. Am Rev Respir Dis 1992; 146(2):396–401.

80. Kendrick AH, et al. Accuracy of perception of severity of asthma: patients treated in general practice. Br Med J 1993; 307(6901):422–444.

81. Isenberg S, Lehrer P, Hochron S. Defensiveness and perception of external inspiratory resistive loads in asthma. J Behav Med 1997; 20(5):461–472.

82. Spinhoven P, et al. Association of anxiety with perception of histamine induced bronchoconstriction in patients with asthma. Thorax 1997; 52(2):149–152.

83. Rietveld S. Symptom perception in asthma: a multidisciplinary review. J Asthma 1998; 35(2):137–146.

84. Newman KB, Dubester SN. Vocal cord dysfunction: masquerader of asthma. Semin Respir Crit Care Med 1994; 15(2):161–167.

85. Newman KB, Mason UG, Schmaling KB. Clinical features of vocal cord dysfunction. Am J Respir Crit Care Med 1995; 152:1382–1386.

86. Freedman MR, Rosenberg SJ, Schmaling KB. Childhood sexual abuse in patients with paradoxical vocal cord dysfunction. J Nerv Ment Dis 1991; 179:295–298.

87. Brugman SM, et al. The spectrum of pediatric vocal cord dysfunction. Am Rev Resp Dis 1994; 149:A353.

88. Wamboldt F, et al. Diagnoses associated with persistent shortness of breath and upper airway dysfunction in patients with and without occupational or environmental irritant exposure. Am J Resp Crit Care Med 2000; 161(3/2):A55.

89. Gavin LA, et al. Psychological and family characteristics of adolescents with vocal cord dysfunction. J Asthma 1998; 35(5):409–417.

90. Park SJ, Sawyer SM, Glaun DE. Childhood asthma complicated by anxiety: an

application of cognitive behavioral therapy. J Paed Child Health 1996; 32(2):183–187.

91. Yellowlees PM, Kalucy RS. Psychobiological aspects of asthma and the consequent research implications. Chest 1990; 97:628–634.

92. Klein DF. False suffocation alarms, spontaneous panics, and related conditions:an integrative hypothesis. Arch Gen Psychiatry 1993; 50(4):306–317.

93. Alt HL. Psychiatric aspects of asthma. Chest 1992; 101(6):415S–417S.

94. Moran MG. Psychiatric aspects of asthma. Semin Resp Crit Care Med 1994; 15(2): 168–174.

95. Mrazek DA. Pediatric hospitalization: understanding the effects from a developmental perspective. In Christie M. ed. The Psychosomatic Approach. Chichester: Wiley, 1985.

96. Kazak AE. Posttraumatic distress in childhood cancer survivors and their parents. Med Pediatr Oncol 1998; Suppl(1):60–68.

97. Walker AM, et al. Post-traumatic stress responses following liver transplantation in older children. J Child Psychol Psychiat 1999; 40(3):363–374.

98. Gavin LA, Roesler TA. Posttraumatic distress in children and families after intubation. Ped Emergency Care 1997; 13(3):222–224.

99. Nocon A. Social and emotional impact of childhood asthma. Arch Dis Child 1991; 66:458–460.

100. Eiser C, et al. Discipline strategies and parental perceptions of preschool children with asthma. Br J Med Psychol 1991; 64(1):45–53.

101. Kazak AE. Families of chronically ill children: a systems and social-ecological model of adaptation and challenge. J Consult Clin Psychol 1989; 57(1):25–30.

102. Parker G, Lipscombe P. Parental overprotection and asthma. J Psychosom Res 1979; 23:295–299.

103. Peshkin MM. Asthma in children. IX: role of environment in the treatment of a selected group of cases: a plea for a ''home'' as a restorative measure. Am J Dis Child 1930; 39:774.

104. Robinson G. The story of parentectomy. J Asthma Res 1972; 9(4):199–205.

105. Purcell K, et al. The effect of asthma in children of experimental separation from the family. Psychosom Med 1969; 31(2):144–164.

106. Liebman R, Minuchin S, Baker L. The use of structural family therapy in the treatment of intractable asthma. Am J Psychiat 1974; 131:535–540.

107. Lask B, Matthew D. Childhood asthma: a controlled trial of family psychotherapy. Arch Dis Child 1979; 54:116–119.

108. Gustafsson PA, Kjellman N-IM, Cederbald M. Family therapy in the treatment of severe childhood asthma. J Psychosom Res 1986; 30(3):369–374.

109. Gustafsson PA, Bjorksten B, Kjellman NI. Family dysfunction in asthma: a prospective study of illness development. J Pediatr 1994; 125(3):493–498.

110. Wikran R, Faleide A, Blakar RM. Communication in the family of the asthmatic child. Acta Psychiat Scand 1978; 57:11–26.

111. Hermanns J, et al. Maternal criticism, mother–child interaction, and bronchial asthma. J Psychosom Res 1989; 33:469–476.

112. Magana AB, et al. A brief method for assessing expressed emotion in relatives of psychiatric patients. Psychiat Res 1985; 17:203–212.

113. Schobinger R, et al. Childhood asthma: paternal critical attitude and father–child interaction. J Psychosom Res 1992; 36(8):743–750.

114. Deaton AV. Adaptive noncompliance in pediatric asthma: the parent as expert. J Ped Psychol 1985; 10(1):1–14.

115. Conrad P. The meaning of medications: another look at compliance. Soc Sci Med 1985; 20:29–37.

116. Creer TL, Bender BG. Pediatric asthma. In Roberts M, ed. The Handbook of Pediatric Psychology. New York: Plenum, 1994.

117. Bender B, Milgrom H, Rand C. Nonadherence in asthmatic patients: is there a solution to the problem? Ann Allergy Asthma Immunol 1997; 79(3):177–185.

118. Jonasson G, et al. Patient compliance in a clinical trial with inhaled budesonide in children with mild asthma. Eur Respir J 1999; 14(1):150–154.

119. Eney RD, Goldstein EO. Compliance of chronic asthmatics with oral administration of theophylline as measured by serum and salivary levels. Pediatrics 1976; 57:513–517.

120. Coutts JAP, Gibson NA, Paton JY. Measuring compliance with inhaled medication in asthma. Arch Dis Child 1992; 67:332–333.

121. Creer TL. Medication compliance and childhood asthma. In Krasnegor NA, et al., eds. Developmental Aspects of Health Compliance and Behavior. Hillsdale, NJ.: Erlbaum, 1993:303–332.

122. Eraker S, Kirscht JP, Becker MH. Understanding and improving patient compliance. Ann Intern Med 1984; 100:258–268.

123. Mawhinney H, et al. Compliance in clinical trials of two nonbronchodilator, antiasthma medication. Ann Allergy 1991; 66:294–299.

124. Mawhinney H, et al. As-needed medication use in asthma: usage patterns and patient characteristics. J Asthma 1993; 30:61–71.

125. Rand CC, Wise RA. Measuring adherence to asthma medication regimens. Am J Resp Crit Care Med 1994; 149:S69–S76.

126. Spector SL, Mawhinney H. Aerosol inhaler monitoring of asthmatic medication. In Cramer JA, Spilker B, eds. Patient compliance in medical practice and clinical trials. New York: Raven Press, 1991.

127. Weinstein AG, Caskey W. Theophylline compliance in asthmatic children. Ann Allergy 1985; 54:19–21.

128. Burrows B, Lebowitz MD. The β-agonist dilemma. New Engl J Med 1992, 326:560–561.

129. Page CP. One explanation of the asthma paradox: inhibition of natural anti-inflammatory mechanism by β2-agonists. Lancet 1991; 337:717–720.

130. Sears MR, et al. Regular inhaled beta-agonist treatment in bronchial asthma. Lancet 1990; 336:1391–1396.

131. Cluss PA, et al. Effects of compliance for chronic asthmatic children. J Clin Cons Psychol 1984; 52:909–910.

132. Sublett JL, et al. Non-compliance in asthmatic children: a study of theophylline levels in a pediatric emergency room population. Ann Allergy 1979; 43:95–97.

133. Miller BD, Strunk RC. Circumstances surrounding the deaths of children due to asthma: a case-control study. Am J Dis Child 1989; 143(11):1294–1299.

134. Birkhead G, et al. Investigation of a cluster of deaths of adolescents with asthma: evidence implicating inadequate treatment and poor patient adherence with medications. J Allergy Clin Immunol 1989; 84:484–491.

135. Spector SL. Is your asthmatic patient really complying? Ann Allergy 1985; 55: 552–556.

136. Lanier B. Who is dying of asthma and why? J Pediatr 1989; 115:838–840.

137. Wamboldt FS, et al. Parental criticism and treatment outcome in adolescents hospitalized for severe, chronic asthma. J Psychosom Res 1995; 39:995–1005.

138. Magana AB. Manual for Coding Expressed Emotion from the Five Minute Speech Sample. Los Angeles: UCLA Family Project, 1993.

139. Patterson GR. Coercive Family Process. Eugene, OR: Castalia, 1982.

140. Patterson GR, Banks L. Bootstrapping your way in the nomological thicket. Behav Assess 1986; 8:49–73.

141. Miller BD, Wood BL. Psychophysiologic reactivity in asthmatic children: a cholinergically mediated confluence of pathways. J Am Acad Child Adolesc Psychiat 1994; 33(9):1236–1245.

142. Miller BD, Wood BL. Influence of specific emotional states on autonomic reactivity and pulmonary function in asthmatic children. J Am Acad Child Adolesc Psychiatry 1997; 36(5):669–677.

143. Tal D, et al. Teaching families to cope with childhood asthma. Fam Systems Med 1990; 8(2):135–144.

144. Creer TL, et al. A critique of 19 self-management programs for childhood asthma. part II: comments regarding the scientific merit of the programs. Ped Asthma Allergy Immunol 1990; 4(1):41–55.

145. Howland J, Bauchner H, Adair R. The impact of pediatric asthma education on morbidity. Chest 1988; 94:964–969.

146. Klingelhofer EL. Compliance with medical regimens, self-management programs, and self-care in childhood asthma. Clin Rev Allergy 1987; 5:231–247.

147. Wigal JK, et al. A critique of 19 self-management programs for childhood asthma. Part I: development and evaluation of the programs. Ped Asthma Allergy Immunol 1990; 4(1):17–39.

148. Nides MA, et al. Improving inhaler adherence in a clinical trial through the use of the nebulizer chronolog. Chest 1993; 104:501–507.

149. Rand CS, et al. Metered-dose inhaler adherence in a clinical trial. Am Rev Resp Dis 1992; 146:1559–1564.

150. Garrity TF. Medical compliance and the clinician–patient relationship: a review. Soc Sci Med 1981; 15E:215–222.

151. Gillum RF, Barsky AJ. Diagnosis and management of patient noncompliance. J Am Med Assoc 1974; 228(12):1563–1567.

152. Ley P. Satisfaction, compliance and communication. Br J Clin Psychol 1982; 21: 241–254.

153. Doherty WJ, et al. Effect of spouse support and health beliefs on medication adherence. J Fam Prac 1983; 17(5):837–841.

154. Janz NK, Becker MH. The health belief model: a decade later. Health Educ Q 1984; 11(1):1–47.

155. Cohen S, Wamboldt F. The parent–physician relationship in pediatric asthma care. J Pediatr Psychol 2000; 25(2):69–77.

156. Gavin LA, et al. Treatment alliance and its association with family functioning, adherence, and medical outcome in adolescents with severe, chronic asthma. J Pediatr Psychol 1999; 24(4):355–365.

157. Gonzales S, Steinglass P, Reiss D. Putting the illness in its place: discussion groups for families with chronic medical illnesses. Fam Proc 1989; 28(1):69–87.

158. Cohen-Cole, SA, Harpe C. Diagnostic assessment of depression in the medically ill. In: Stoudemire A, Fogel BS, eds. Principles of Medical Psychiatry. New York: Grune & Stratton, 1987:23–36.

159. Davis JM, Glassman AH. Antidepressant drugs. In Kaplan HI, Sadock, BJ, eds. Comprehensive Textbook of Psychiatry/V. Baltimore, MD: Williams & Wilkins, 1989:1627–1654.

160. Gottman JM. Marital interaction: experimental investigations. New York: Academic Press 1979.

161. Wamboldt MZ, Levin L. Utility of multi-family psycho-educational groups for medically ill children and adolescents. Fam Syst Med 1995; 13(2):151–161.

162. Mason RJ, Katz JL, Bethel RA. Time out for asthma: rationale for a comprehensive evaluation. Semin Resp Crit Care Med 1994; 15(2):97–105.

163. Wamboldt MZ. Current status of child and adolescent medical/psychiatric units. Psychosomatics 1994; 35:434–444.

164. Gavin LA, Roesler T, Brenner AM. Day treatment for pediatrics patients with medical and psychiatric needs. Continuum Dev Ambul Ment Health Care 1996; 3(2): 95–102.

165. Weinstein AG, et al. Outcome of short-term hospitalization for children with severe asthma. J Allergy Clin Immunol 1992; 90:66–75.

166. Weinstein AG, et al. An economic evaluation of short-term inpatient rehabilitation for children with severe asthma. J Allergy Clin Immunol 1996; 98(2):264–273.

21

Growth Impairment Related to Severe Asthma

DAVID B. ALLEN

University of Wisconsin Children's Hospital
Madison, Wisconsin

I. Introduction

Normal childhood growth is a sensitive indicator of health, and there are few chronic diseases of childhood that do not adversely affect growth. Several mechanisms of growth suppression appear to be commonly involved in various diseases, although a clear understanding of which mechanisms are most important is still lacking. To evaluate the effects of any chronic disease on growth, three important aspects of the condition need to be considered: (1) how the natural history of the disease itself affects growth; (2) how medications required to treat the disease affect growth; and (3) the clinical relevance of the growth effect, i.e., whether the growth impairment results in merely a delay in the normal tempo of growth with attainment of normal final height or whether ultimate height is adversely affected.

The most common chronic disease of childhood is asthma, and various effects of asthma on growth have been described. However, the relative contributions to growth impairment of the disease process itself versus the medications required to treat the disease remain uncertain. Recently, attention has focused on the role of corticosteroids as both the most effective treatment for persistent asthma as well as likely growth-suppressing agent. This chapter discusses normal

505

physiology of growth during childhood, pathophysiology of growth suppression by chronic disease, abnormalities in growth and development observed in children with asthma, effects of oral and inhaled corticosteroids on growth, and the clinical relevance of an effect of severe asthma and its treatment on final adult height.

II. Normal Growth

Although first examination of a childhood growth curve may suggest a simple and rather linear process, the regulation of normal growth is complex and the variations in normal growth are substantial. Understanding the various factors involved in the control of growth is aided by a conceptual model which identifies three major periods of growth: infancy, childhood, and puberty (Fig. 1) (1). The infancy period (first 2–3 years of life) is characterized by the distinctive combination of rapid yet rapidly decelerating growth rates. Control of growth during this period is primarily by nutrition-dependent factors (e.g., insulin and insulinlike growth factors), which are also critical for normal intrauterine growth. Consequently, caloric deprivation during infancy has a more significant growth-retarding effect than during later childhood. This slowing of the normal tempo of growth is reflected in delay in skeletal maturation. Conversely, overfeeding

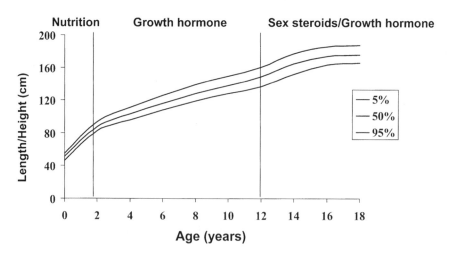

Figure 1   Phases of normal childhood growth (infancy–childhood–puberty) are depicted with the primary regulators of growth rate (nutrition–growth hormone–sex steroids plus growth hormone) during each phase. (Adapted with permission from Ref. 1.)

during this period can result in significant linear growth acceleration, which is accompanied by equal advancement in skeletal age.

During the early toddler years, a transition to dependency upon the endocrine system occurs, with the emergence of human growth hormone (GH) as the major growth-stimulating hormone. Accordingly, children who are severely GH deficient typically experience failure of growth toward the end of the first year of life. GH is secreted in pulsatile fashion from the anterior pituitary gland as a result of the interacting influences of hypothalamic growth hormone releasing hormone and somatostatin. Two important observations regarding the childhood GH-dependent phase of growth are relevant to a discussion of influences of asthma on growth. First, the efficiency of the transition from the nutrition-dependent to GH-dependent phase of growth appears to vary among children, with some demonstrating excessive slowing of growth and downward crossing of percentiles on the growth curve usually between 15 and 30 months of age. Normal growth along this lower part of the growth curve usually resumes by 3 years of age, but the delay in body maturation which accompanies the growth delay results in late pubertal development (i.e., ''late bloomers'') and prolonged growth, with attainment of normal adult height. As discussed below, this pattern of growth delay is commonly observed in children with moderate-to-severe asthma. Second, the phase of childhood GH-dependent growth is marked by a gradual but consistent decline in growth rate which reaches its nadir in the 2–3 years prior to puberty. Provocative testing of GH secretion often reveals an apparent GH deficiency at this time. This waning resiliency of a child's growth axis may make him/her unusually susceptible to growth-retarding effects of illness, medications, or psychological stress. Importantly, most studies of the effects of inhaled corticosteroids on growth in children with asthma have focused on children in the midst of this late-childhood phase.

Sex steroids, particularly low serum concentrations of estrogen, stimulate the production and secretion of GH. Combined with growth-promoting influences of rising levels of other hormones (insulin and androgens), these effects result in the growth rate acceleration associated with puberty (2). Since growth plate maturation proceeds in the presence of sex steroids (particularly estrogen), even when growth rates are reduced by disease or medications, significant reductions in final height can occur if growth failure is not corrected promptly during adolescence.

III. Chronic Disease and Growth: General Pathophysiology

Changes in endocrine function commonly occur during chronic illness. Although these changes represent an adaptation that benefits the individual in some way, the outcome in other systems (e.g., growth) is not always favorable. In general,

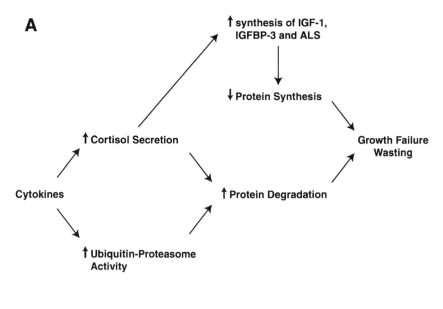

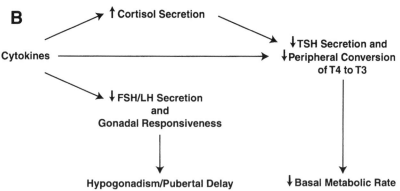

Figure 2 The effects of cytokines and glucocorticoids, both increased during chronic illness, on (A) protein degradation and synthesis and (B) thyroid and gonadal function. Abbreviations: IGF-1, insulinlike growth factor-1, IGFBP-3, IGF binding protein 3; ALS, acid-labile subunit. (Adapted with permission from Ref. 4.)

endocrine adaptations to chronic illness reflect a reduction in hypothalamic-pituitary output, peripheral conversion of hormones from inactive to more active forms, or development of some mechanism of peripheral hormone resistance that diminishes "nonessential" metabolic functions. As a result, growth, pubertal development, and peripheral thyroid hormone activity slow relatively early in the course of chronic illness, while adrenal function is maintained or even heightened (3).

Growth failure occurring during chronic illness can generally be attributed to factors related to both the primary illness and secondary disturbances in the endocrine growth axis (4). However, the mechanism through which asthma alone inhibits growth, and the relative importance of this effect, remains obscure. Physiologic stresses such as chronic hypoxia, infection, and poor nutritional status, thought to contribute to poor growth in children with cystic fibrosis, occur in only the most severe cases of intractable asthma. One attractive possibility is that a state of GH and insulinlike growth factor-1 (IGF-1) resistance develops during chronic illnesses such as severe asthma, which significantly reduces linear growth and other anabolic processes. Increased production of endogenous glucocorticoids observed during illness or stress has a direct inhibitory effect on protein synthesis in muscle and bone. In addition, protein degradation in chronic illnesses is enhanced by increased lysosomal activity and activity of the ubiquitin-proteasome pathway, mediated by the release of cytokines (5) and glucocorticoids (6), particularly in the midst of undernutrition (Fig. 2) (4).

Suppression of thyroid and gonadal function indirectly contributes to slowed growth during chronic illness by diminishing GH secretion and action. Illness-associated cytokines and glucocorticoids appear to exert suppressive effects on both central nervous system and peripheral control of these endocrine systems (Fig. 2). For instance, preferential conversion of thyroxine (T4) to relatively inactive reverse triiodothyronine (rT3) rather than to the most active thyroid hormone, triiodothyronine (T3), occurs early and to varying degrees during chronic illnesses (7). Disruptions in the hypothalamic-pituitary-gonadal axis are commonly observed during illness and manifest in delayed or arrested pubertal development or, in females, menstrual abnormalities. While these compromises initially represent beneficial adaptations to stress, allowing diversion of limited metabolic resources to vital functions, long-term disruption of thyroid and sex steroid activity has important adverse consequences for linear growth, bone mineralization, and body composition.

IV. Effects of Severe Asthma on Growth

When compared with the general population, children with asthma have been reported to have mean heights and height velocities during childhood and adolescence that are less than children without asthma (8). Although it is well recognized that daily and alternate-day administration of glucocorticoids can impair growth, shorter stature for age has been observed in children with asthma who have not been treated with glucocorticoids (9–12). Mechanisms other than the effect of glucocorticoid treatment proposed to explain the impaired growth of children with asthma include chronic hypoxia, diminished lung function, chronic infection, undernutrition, sleep disturbance, and long-term stress (13–15). An assessment of the degree to which these factors may affect growth in the absence of glucocorticoid treatment depends on early observations prior to the widespread use of glucocorticoid medications for asthma. One study revealed 77% of steroid-naïve children with severe asthma to be below the normal age-related mean for height, 30% >1 SD below the mean, and 8% >2 SD below the mean. By comparison, intermittent or continuous glucocorticoid treatment was associated with heights >2 SD below the mean in 15 and 30% of children, respectively (8). Others have reported 74% of asthmatic children below the 50th percentile for height, 37% below the 25th, 27% below the 10th, and 7% below the third percentile (16).

Severity of growth retardation has been associated with early onset of asthma symptoms (i.e., before 3 years of age), disease severity sufficient to cause chronic hypoxemia, and poor nutrition (17). As expected, in more severely asthmatic children, a higher incidence of growth retardation is observed (18,19). In fact, when children with asthma are separated according to disease severity, only the most severely affected group shows the development of a significant height deficit during adolescence (Fig. 3) (12). Several explanations for the association between asthma and growth delay have been proposed, but none have been verified consistently. Reduced GH secretion has not been documented in slow-growing children with asthma (also receiving inhaled corticosteroids) (20). Alterations in thyroid hormone metabolism have been observed by some investigators (21) but not by others (14). Deficient nutrient intake was suggested by earlier reports (14,17), but not confirmed by more recent studies (22). Energy expenditure in asthmatic children was reportedly increased by 14% compared to healthy matched controls, but concomitant eczema or use of β-agonist medications may have been confounding factors (22). The inability to identify mechanisms of asthma-related growth suppression most likely reflects failure to focus investigations on children with asthma of *sufficient severity to independently affect growth*. While such studies of severe asthma in the absence of glucocorticoid treatment are virtually impossible to ethically conduct today, information derived from children with cystic fibrosis are likely to be informative. That is, with disease of sufficient severity, cytokines and endogenous glucocorticoids released in response to chronic inflammation create an environment of GH resistance and reduced IGF-1 bioactivity, resulting in reduced protein synthesis and increased protein degradation (23).

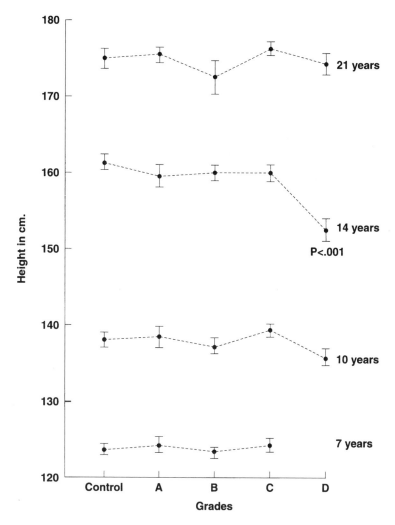

Figure 3 Growth of children with asthma (hatched bars) compared to controls (white bars), showing growth delay in peripubertal children with asthma. (Adapted with permission from Ref. 12.)

Invariably, significant declines in height-for-age are accompanied by delayed skeletal maturation, indicating a slowing of the normal *tempo* of growth, but not necessarily a reduced long-term height prognosis. Since the onset of puberty is more closely correlated with body maturation than with chronological age, delayed appearance of secondary sex characteristics is also observed more commonly in children with asthma (9). It is critical to account for this delayed growth pattern in assessing growth studies of children with asthma. As pointed out above, growth rates normally decline gradually throughout school-age years until pubertal growth acceleration occurs. Children experiencing a delayed growth pattern tend to show greater growth deceleration prior to puberty and exaggerated disparities in growth rates compared with pubertal peers. Consequently, this pattern of delayed growth is often misinterpreted as disease- or medication-induced growth failure. Because of the normal more prolonged prepubertal growth period in males compared to females, this period of growth slowing is often more pronounced in males and the susceptibility to further growth suppression by disease or medications enhanced. This difference between the sexes in the normal tempo of growth and development is a likely explanation for variations in male and female final height. One carefully designed study indicated that growth retardation observed in adolescent males with asthma was due to a delay in puberty but not to the prescription of 600 μg of inhaled BUD daily (24). In most cases, although transient reductions in growth rate can result in detectable height differences between children with asthma and peers, a more prolonged period of growth in the asthma group allows for "catch-up" and attainment of normal adult height appropriate for family (16,25).

Relatively few data are available regarding the final height of individuals with asthma who did not receive glucocorticoid treatment. One study reported that final measured heights of 95 patients with asthma not treated with glucocorticoids differed negatively from midparental height by 4.8 ± 5.8 cm for females (*P* = 0.18) and 3.6 ± 6.0 cm for males (p = 0.48). In the unmatched analysis of this data set, mean height of patients with asthma, after adjusting for sex and midparental height, was 0.15 cm taller than a nonasthmatic comparison group (*P* = *ns*), whereas the differences in measured height between asthmatic subjects and matched nonasthmatic subjects was 0.21 ± 9.42 cm (*P* = 0.95) (26). Reports of reduced final height of individuals with asthma tend to be confounded by prior long-term treatment with glucocorticoids (27). Consequently, while a delay in the growth process by severe asthma is well documented, it has not been shown that the disease of asthma itself, in the absence of glucocorticoid treatment, results in reduced final height (26).

V. Effects of Glucocorticoids on Growth

Growth retardation is commonly experienced by children who receive long-term treatment with glucocorticoids (GCs). While most disorders requiring such treatment are relatively rare, the expanding use of inhaled GC preparations for treatment of all degrees of persistent asthma has greatly increased the numbers of children chronically exposed to exogenous GCs. Consequently, physicians today are likely to care for children treated with GCs, and should be knowledgeable about potential growth effects of these medications.

The pathogenesis of growth suppression by GC is complex and multifactorial, involving several steps in the cascade of events leading to linear growth (Fig. 4) (28). During childhood, the primary known mediator of epiphyseal growth and maturation is GH. Pulsatile, primarily nocturnal release of pituitary GH (29) occurs under the influence of interwoven hypothalamic stimulation (via growth-hormone-releasing hormone, GHRH) and inhibition (via somatostatin). In late childhood and adolescence, GH secretion is augmented by sex steroids produced by the adrenal glands and gonads. Growth-promoting effects of GH in epiphyseal cartilage occur both directly and indirectly through insulin-like-growth-factor 1 (IGF-1). Linear growth also requires synthesis of new type 1 collagen, which can be assessed through determination of blood levels of its precursor, type 1 procollagen.

Multiple catabolic effects of GCs contribute to the profound impairment in linear growth associated with prolonged supraphysiologic GC therapy. Glucocorticoids interfere with nitrogen and mineral retention required for the growth process. Under the influence of GC excess, energy derived from protein catabo-

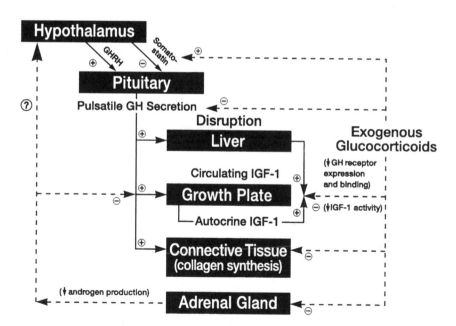

Figure 4 Mechanisms of growth suppression by glucocorticoids (derived from both in vivo and in vitro studies). (Adapted with permission from Ref. 28.)

lism is increased and the contribution from lipid oxidation is decreased (30). This effect leads to characteristic changes in body habitus that are frequently associated with GC excess. Glucocorticoids inhibit bone formation directly (31), through inhibition of osteoblast function, and indirectly, by decreasing sex steroid secretion (in older children and adolescents). They also decrease intestinal calcium absorption (partially reversible with vitamin D therapy), increase urinary calcium excretion, and promote bone resorption due to secondary hyperparathyroidism. Osteopenia is particularly prominent in trabecular bone, such as the vertebrae (32). Skeletal maturation is delayed by long-term GC therapy. Particularly in GC-treated boys, suppression of bone age advancement may exceed that of height age advancement (10).

Glucocorticoids are capable of both inhibiting and stimulating endogenous GH secretion, an effect which arises from dichotomous action at the level of the pituitary and/or hypothalamus. Cortisol facilitates pituitary GH synthesis by altering the affinity and density of pituitary GHRH receptors and interacting with a GC-responsive element on the GH gene (33). Thus, a minimum level of cortisol is essential for normal GH manufacture. Under conditions of eucortisolism, there is appropriate synthesis of GH as well as normal GHRH and somatostatin influence, resulting in the normal pulsatile release of GH. In the hypercortisolemic state, GH production is stimulated within the pituitary, but pulsatile release of GH is impaired, most likely through augmentation of hypothalamic somatostatin effect (34). Therefore, patterns of GH secretion in GC-treated children can resemble "neurosecretory GH deficiency," where stimulated GH levels are normal, but spontaneous secretion of GH is subnormal (35). In the clinical setting, this attenuation of GH secretion associated with exposure to exogenous GCs can be both rapid and profound (36).

In addition to altering GH output, GCs reduce GH receptor expression and uncouple the receptors from their signal transduction mechanisms (37). Hepatic GH receptor binding and plasma levels of GH binding protein (GHBP) are markedly reduced in dose-dependent fashion by GC treatment, an effect accompanied by growth failure in treated animals (37). GCs also exert a depressive effect on rat liver GH receptor mRNA levels; this suppression can be partially reversed by cotreatment with estrogen or continuous exposure to GH. However, it is not clear that these effects on GH receptor synthesis and expression occur in nonliver tissues such as chondrocytes or muscle. However, circulating levels of GH binding protein, which are derived from the extracellular domain of the GH receptor, are reduced in GC-treated children compared with age-matched controls (38).

Levels of IGF-1 can be decreased, normal, or increased in GC-treated patients. Although GCs do not consistently reduce circulating IGF-1 levels, they inhibit IGF bioactivity, possibly by increased production of IGF-1 inhibitors (39). IGF inhibitors, which have a molecular weight of 12 to 20 kDa and which clearly differ from IGF binding proteins, have been identified in in vitro investigations showing that cortisol increases IGF-I inhibitor release by liver explants (40). Precise characterization of these "somatomedin inhibitors," however, remains elusive. Alterations in IGF binding proteins may also play a role; IGFBP-3, an IGF-1 binding protein though to exert inhibitory effects on IGF-1 action, is increased in response to GCs (41). Glucocorticoids also antagonize GH effects at target tissues by inhibiting chondrocyte mitosis and collagen synthesis. GCs also interfere directly with posttranslational modifications of the precursor procollagen chains and increase collagen degradation (42).

Resumption of growth follows release of GC-induced growth inhibition. This "catch-up" growth has been hypothesized to result from a central nervous system mechanism which compares actual body size to an age-appropriated set point and adjusts growth rate accordingly (43). Recently, however, it was demonstrated that catch-up growth of a single growth plate exposed to locally administered GCs was restricted to the affected growth plate, suggesting a mechanism intrinsic to the growth plate (44). While anecdotal reports often suggest that catch-up growth is complete, resulting in normal adult height, controlled studies of animals and humans indicate that growth deficits are often not fully compensated (45).

VI. Growth of Asthmatic Children Treated with Oral Glucocorticoids

The adverse effects of systemically administered GCs on the growth of children with asthma has been well documented over the past 40 years (46). Dose, type of GC preparation, and timing of GC exposure each influence the degree of growth suppression observed. Large amounts of exogenous GC are not required for this adverse effect; relatively modest doses of prednisone (3–5 mg/m²/day) or hydrocortisone (12–15 mg/m²/day) can impair growth, particularly in prepubertal children (46,47). Alternate-day GC therapy reduces, but does not eliminate, the chances for growth failure. Children with asthma have reportedly received over 30 mg of prednisone (mean 41.8 ± 3.9 mg/day every other day for 6–50 months without experiencing growth suppression (48). However, in other more closely monitored studies, alternate-day doses of prednisone above 15 mg cause slowed growth velocity in many patients and resumption of normal growth was not observed when children with existing growth failure were switched from daily to alternate-day prednisone treatment (49). Growth-retarding effects of prednisone are greater than those of (equivalent doses of) hydrocortisone, most likely due to a comparatively longer half-life and sustained plasma concentration of prednisone.

The effects of oral GC therapy on final adult height have been variable, most likely reflecting variations in dose, compliance, length of continuous exposure, and other individual factors. Most children treated with oral GC have severe underlying illness, making it difficult to distinguish growth effects of GC from those of the illness itself. However, in one study examining asthmatic children already growth suppressed prior to GC therapy, more growth delay was observed with GC therapy, with the severity of increased retardation correlated to the dose and duration of GC exposure (50). Children exposed to GC excess just prior to puberty may be particularly susceptible to growth suppression; childhood growth velocity is at its slowest and endogenous GH secretion is often transiently reduced during this period. Suppression of adrenal sex steroid secretion (adrenarche) by exogenous GCs at this time may itself delay the activation of the hypothalamic-pituitary-gonadal axis and attenuate both the augmentation of GH release and direct growth stimulation by sex steroids normally observed in early puberty. Detrimental effects on final height, however, are more likely with GC treatment during puberty, since sex-hormone-mediated growth plate maturation can occur in the midst of suppressed linear growth (51). While some studies demonstrate that short-term (52) or intermittent (53) exposure to oral GC at supraphysiologic doses does not adversely affect final height, a meta-analysis of previous investigations found that long-term treatment of asthma with prednisone was significantly correlated with adult height reduction (54).

VII. Growth of Asthmatic Children Treated with Inhaled Corticosteroids

Inhaled corticosteroids (ICSs) offer several advantages over oral GCs in the treatment of asthma: delivery of high-potency GCs directly to the target site in high concentrations, reduced total dosage, and the opportunity for frequent dosing. Although physical properties shared by ICSs (e.g., rapid inactivation of absorbed drug) increase the ratio of topical anti-inflammatory to systemic activity, questions remain about the extent to which pulmonary effects of inhaled steroids may result from systemic actions.

Adverse effects from ICSs should be anticipated if daily systemic exposure exceeds normal endogenous cortisol production ($\sim$12 mg hydrocortisone equivalent/m^2/day) or if the pattern of drug bioavailability significantly disrupts normal diurnal hormonal rhythms. Systemic GC effect is determined not only by the amount of ICS delivered to the airway and absorbed into circulation, but also the binding affinity and plasma half-life of the corticosteroid, the drug's volume of distribution, the potency and half-lives of its metabolites, the patient's sensitivity to and metabolism of the medication, and newly described factors such as the duration of GC contact with the cell or the rate of rise in steroid concentration. Consequently, individual risk for adverse effects from ICSs varies widely and is difficult to predict.

Systemic bioavailability of ICSs results from a combination of oral (swallowed fraction) and lung components. Significant amounts of ICs are absorbed unaltered into the circulation following inhalation [e.g., ~70% for budesonide (BUD) (55) and ~30% for flunisolide (FLU) (56)], and the amount of drug available for absorption into the pulmonary vasculature is influenced by delivery vehicle (e.g., deposition following dry powder inhalation generally exceeds pressurized metered-dose inhalation) and technique. The bioavailability of swallowed drug varies significantly as follows: beclomethasone dipropionate (BDP), FLU, and triamcinolone acetonide (TA) 20–22%; BUD 10–15% (57); and fluticasone propionate (FP) 1% (58). These differences in inactivation of swallowed drug (which exerts little or no therapeutic effect) appear to be critical in determining a drug's therapeutic effect versus systemic effect profile. Plasma half-lives of most ICSs are brief (e.g., 1.5–2 h), due primarily to extensive first-pass hepatic metabolism. For some ICS (e.g., BUD), higher clearance rate and shorter plasma half-life have been shown in children when compared with adults, suggesting an increase in the ratio between local and systemic side effects (59). Intrapulmonary metabolism of ICS is also variable; BDP differs from other ICS because it is metabolized to potent active metabolites in the lung, which prolong the half-life of ''BDP-effect'' (~15 h) and account for most of the systemic GC effect of inhaled BDP (60).

Properties which make ICS extremely potent might increase risk for adverse effects as well. Two such factors are relative binding affinity for the glucocorticoid receptor compared with dexamethasone (e.g., 8:1 for racemic BUD and 20:1 for FP) and increased lipophilicity, which allows increased deposition in the lung lipid compartment, prolonged occupancy of the glucocorticoid receptor, and extended terminal elimination half-life with greater steady-state drug accumulation. The ranked order of lipophilicity among currently used ICSs is FP > BDP > BUD > TA > FLU, with FP being 3-fold and 300-fold more lipophilic than BDP and BUD, respectively (61). That receptor pharmacokinetics and lipophilicity are predictive of drug pharmacodynamics and potency is supported by the observed approximate 2–3:1 ratio in corticosteroid potency between FP and BDP when compared μg for μg. However, precise comparisons of different ICSs remain confounded by complexities of determining the *clinical therapeutic equivalence* of each compound and its delivery system. For instance, BUD delivered by metered-dose inhaler approximates BDP in potency, while delivery of BUD by dry powder inhaler may compare μg for μg in GC effect with FP, presumably due to greater lung deposition of the drug (62).

Consequently, well-designed studies are needed to more accurately assess the GC therapeutic equivalence of various ICS as well as dosing strategies designed to minimize adverse effects. Because the efficacy dose–response curve of ICSs flatten out at moderate-to-high doses after initial steepness at relatively low doses, comparisons of ICS-plus-delivery system therapeutic potency require determination of "minimal effective dosage" by step-down dosing within the steep part of the dose–response curve (62). While manipulations such as these may further reduce the relatively low risk of growth failure by ICS (compared to oral GC therapy), individual variations in absorption, responsiveness, and metabolism of ICSs will continue to place some patients at risk of toxicity, requiring ongoing vigilance by prescribing physicians.

Do inhaled corticosteroids impair growth? A critical analysis of this question is complicated by two central factors: first, children with chronic asthma frequently exhibit growth retardation, manifested primarily by delays in skeletal maturation and pubertal growth acceleration in proportion to either treatment with GCs or severity of pulmonary disease (19). Second, substantial pharmacodynamic differences exist between specific ICSs, and results obtained by studying one should not be extrapolated to another. In addition, nonsteroid asthma treatments (e.g., β2-receptor activation) may also inhibit the GH axis (63).

Although administering corticosteroids via inhalation is associated with fewer systemic effects compared to oral administration, the *potential* of ICSs to retard growth is clearly documented (64). This observation, however, is derived primarily from studies of BDP, whereas emerging data regarding BUD and FP suggest that ICS effects on growth might be reduced by the enhanced hepatic inactivation of swallowed drug exhibited by these preparations. Until recently, most studies of growth in asthmatic children treated with ICSs have suffered from flaws in study design. These include lack of evaluation of pubertal status, inappropriate stratification of pubertal status by age alone, lack of an adequate untreated control group, lack of baseline growth rate data, and baseline differences in age and height between treatment groups. However, during the past several years, prospective and, in some cases, well-controlled studies have overcome these confounding factors. In each case, growth inhibition by BDP was demonstrated.

Several recent studies have utilized knemometry, a sensitive technique of measuring growth of the lower leg, to assess short-term effects of higher dose ICSs therapy on growth. Studies using this technique have revealed dose-dependent inhibition of short-term lower leg growth (65) and reduced levels of type 1 procollagen (but not IGF-1, IGFBP-3, or osteocalcin) during ICS therapy >400 μg/day, suggesting a primary role for effects on collagen turnover in ICS-induced growth retardation (66). However, while accurate and reproducible, the predictive value of lower leg growth velocity determinations for either overall height velocity (67) or long-term future growth is poor (68). Consequently, proposed advantages of knemometry (e.g., shortened observation periods allowing for controlled and double-blinded studies) are essentially nullified by these constraints (69,70). Biochemical markers of growth also correlate poorly with total body linear growth over time. The predictive value of studies for assessing clinically relevant effects of ICSs on growth becomes more substantial with increasing duration of study (71) (Fig. 5). Consequently, prospective intermediate-to-long-term assessment of total body growth has yielded the most credible information regarding effects of ICSs on growth, and only these studies are discussed here.

Longer term prospective analysis of the effect of ICSs on growth is available predominantly for BDP, BUD, and, to a lesser extent, FP. A randomized clinical trial comparing BDP with oral theophylline in children, ages 6–17 years, with mild to moderately severe asthma demonstrated reduced growth in the BDP-treated children (72). A subsequent prospective parallel-group study compared growth effects of BDP (400 μg daily via dry powder device) to placebo in 94 prepubertal children (ages 7 to 9 years) with mild asthma. Over the 7-month study period, mean growth rate was significantly lower in the BDP group (0.79 mm/week, $P > 0.001$) and catch-up growth did not occur during the 4-month wash-out period (73). In another well-designed prospective and randomized study, growth was significantly slower in BDP-treated children compared to those treated with salmeterol, although asthma exacerbations were less frequent during ICS therapy (74) (Fig. 6). These findings were recently confirmed by a similar comparison of long-term controller medications in which mean linear growth was 3.96 cm/year in children receiving BDP compared with 5.40 cm/year in the salmeterol-treated group (75). Discontinuation of BDP in one trial restored a normal, but not accelerated, growth rate (73), highlighting the inconsistent occurrence of catch-up growth after cessation of GC therapy and a possible dampening of a supranormal growth recovery phase by persistent mild asthma. Taken together, these four prospective, controlled studies reveal a remarkably similar ef-

Sensitivity to detect systemic INS or ICS presence		
Short-term	Intermediate-term	Long-term
Knemometry Bone metabolism markers	Stadiometry (≥12 months)	Stadiometry (≥3 years)
Stadiometry (<6 months)		Final height analysis
Positive predictive value for important adverse effect		

Figure 5 Short-, intermediate-, and long-term tests of ICS on growth. Highly sensitive knemometry is a poor predictor of long-term growth, which is more accurately assessed by intermediate- or long-term stadiometry studies. (Adapted with permission from Ref. 71.)

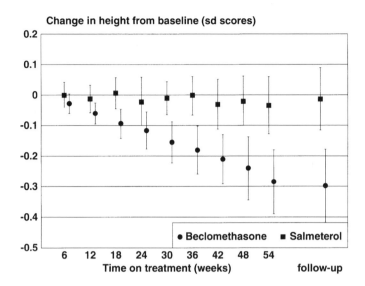

Figure 6 Decrease in rate of statural growth [shown as change in height SDS (standard deviation score), 95% confidence interval] observed in children with asthma treated for 1 year with inhaled BDP (400 μg/day). No significant change in rate occurred in children with asthma treated with inhaled salmeterol. (Adapted with permission from Ref. 74.)

fect of uninterrupted administration of 400 μg/day of BDP on growth: a reduction of ~1.5 cm gain in height per year. In other words, it has been clearly shown that conventional dose treatment with inhaled BDP, administered without interruption, is *capable* of suppressing linear growth.

Variations in the metabolism and pharmacokinetics of ICSs predict different degrees of pulmonary versus systemic effect; i.e., ICSs which have greater first-pass inactivation by the liver (e.g., BUD and FP) would theoretically be expected to have reduced effect on the growth axis for a given degree of airway anti-inflammatory effect. Several studies examining BUD in children with asthma have shown no adverse effects on growth. In a large controlled, prospective study, 216 children followed for 1 to 2 years while not receiving inhaled BUD and then for 3 to 6 years while receiving inhaled BUD (mean daily dosage decreased from 710 to 430 μg over the course of the study) showed no significant changes in growth velocity (76). While this and other studies (77) provide reassurance regarding the "real-world" experience with BUD, their conclusions are weakened by lack of control subjects, variations in dosage and delivery device, and poor documentation of consistency of drug administration.

One randomized, double-blind study examined 40 asthmatic adolescents (mean age 12.8 years) receiving salbutamol 600 μg daily and inhaled BUD 600 μg daily or placebo for a median period of 22 months. Growth rates were matched with those of 80 controls. Budesonide treatment was not associated with a significant effect on growth velocity compared to placebo. Interestingly, males treated with either BUD or placebo showed similar slowing of growth rates compared with controls, pointing again to a likely confounding effect of delayed puberty in the analysis of growth of children with asthma (24). With regard to FP, a recent double-blind, randomized, parallel-group multicenter study prospectively examined growth in 325 prepubescent children with persistent asthma treated with placebo or FP powder 50 or 100 μg administered twice daily. Over a period of 1 year, there was no significant difference in mean height increase (6.15 cm in the placebo group, 5.94 cm in the FP 50 μg BID group, and 5.73 cm in the FP 100-μg BID group) (Fig. 7). While the trend toward slower growth in the FP-treated children could have reflected drop-out of ill, poorly growing children from the placebo group, a small drug effect on growth could not be excluded. Compared with similarly designed studies administering clinically equivalent dosages of ICSs any potential growth effect of FP appeared to be 25–

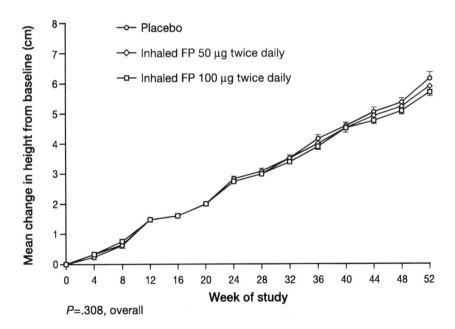

Figure 7 Mean (± SE) change in height in prepubescent patients after treatment with twice-daily doses of placebo, inhaled FP 50 μg or inhaled FP 100 μg for 1 year. For comparison between placebo-treated and FP 100-treated groups, $P = .313$, *ns*. (Adapted with permission from Ref. 78.)

30% that associated with BDP (78). It is important to point out that available information, regarding effects of ICSs on growth derives from studies using low-to-medium doses of ICSs. With the exception of anecdotal reports, there is a lack of information regarding the effect of high doses of ICSs, as recommended for the treatment of severe asthma, on growth rates and final stature.

In addition to drug properties that influence the degree of systemic effects observed at a given dosage, patient characteristics also affect susceptibility to growth suppression. These include age and growth pattern of the child, underlying disease severity, and timing of drug administration. In some children, susceptibility to growth suppression by a variety of influences is increased during transitions from one growth phase (i.e., infancy-to-childhood or childhood-to-adolescent growth) to another. This is particularly true in the 2 to 3 years prior to puberty, when growth rates are low and the resiliency of the growth hormone axis is transiently, physiologically low. Significantly, most studies of growth effects of ICSs have focused on children of this age, and results cannot confidently be extrapolated to infants or adolescents. As mentioned above, contributions of asthma itself can be over- and underestimated. Baseline characteristics of children with mild-to-moderate persistent asthma recruited into recent prospective trials shows them to have normal mean heights and skeletal ages for chronological age. Consequently, it appears that at least moderate-to-severe asthma is required to significantly slow the tempo of childhood growth and delay the onset of pubertal growth acceleration (12). With regard to dosing strategies, reducing the frequency of ICS administration to one inhalation per day might allow restoration of normal growth axis function between doses; although long-term growth studies have not examined this possibility, knemometry studies suggest that suppressed growth observed during b.i.d. intranasal steroid treatment was not observed when similar doses were administered once a day (79). Selectively eliminating night-time administration of ICSs might also avoid GC-mediated blunting of nocturnal pituitary GH secretion and/or ACTH-induced adrenal androgen production (80) (Fig. 8).

Little information is currently available regarding the influence of ICSs on growth during infancy and early childhood. Six-month treatment with BDP 200 μg daily, administered via a metered dose inhaler (MDI) and spacer plus mask (Aerochamber), had no effect on length/height in 12 very young children (mean age 1.22 years) (81). A subsequent study of children less than 3 years of age treated with nebulized BUD (1–4 mg/day) for 6–18 months showed no reduction in mean linear growth rates (82). Recently, a large study of children ages 6 months to 8 years treated with BUD inhalation suspension (0.5 mg once or twice daily) revealed a small, statistically significant decrease in growth velocity compared with children whose asthma was treated without the use of corticosteroids (83). Debate continues regarding the use of ICSs in children <3 years of age. Potential benefit of early intervention with ICSs is supported by one long-term study which

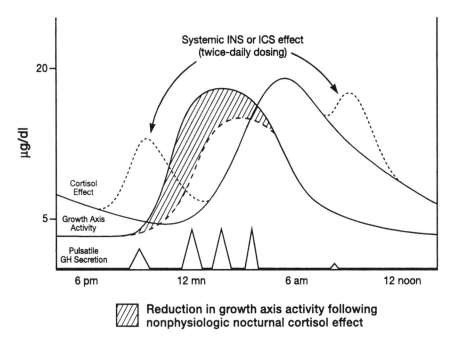

Reduction in growth axis activity following nonphysiologic nocturnal cortisol effect

Figure 8 Interaction of childhood growth axis and cortisol effect. Commencement of nocturnal growth hormone (GH) secretion normally coincides with the nadir in plasma cortisol concentrations. Consequently, administration and absorption of airway corticosteroids at bedtime may have a disproportionate suppressing influence on growth compared with early morning dosing. (Adapted with permission from Ref. 80.)

showed that improvement in lung function was significantly greater in children who started BUD treatment within 2 years of diagnosis of asthma compared with those who started later (84). Other studies have not shown evidence of deterioration in lung function in the absence of anti-inflammatory treatment.

Traditionally, the *clinical relevance* of growth suppression by ICS has been judged more on ultimate effect on final height than short-term reductions in growth rate. A 1986 study followed 66 asthmatic children (mean age 7.5 years at entry) for a mean of 13.1 years, 26 of whom were receiving inhaled BDP up to 600 μg/day. Eleven children whose dosage of BDP exceeded 400 μg/day showed decelerating growth velocity during a period of delayed onset of puberty, but later demonstrated catch-up growth and achieved their predicted adult height. There was no significant difference between the final heights of children receiving BDP and those not receiving inhaled corticosteroid (9). Similar results have been recently reported, although the number of patients followed to final height following ICS treatment *alone* was small (26) (Fig. 9). In two retrospective studies, final adult height was not significantly different in young adults treated with ICSs during childhood compared to those who were not treated with ICSs during childhood [actual mean numeric differences were 1.22 cm (26) and 1.4 cm (85), $P = ns$ for both]. However, there was also a small difference between the two groups for adult height minus target height (statistically significant in one study), suggesting mild permanent effects of growth retardation in ICS-treated patients. The authors could not exclude the possibility that differences in asthma severity accounted for this effect. A meta-analysis (of 21 studies in 810 asthma patients) of the effect of oral corticosteroid or inhaled BDP on growth showed a small but significant correlation between corticosteroid treatment in general and reduced final height. Growth impairment was linked to oral corticosteroid treatment, whereas inhaled BDP treatment was associated with reaching normal

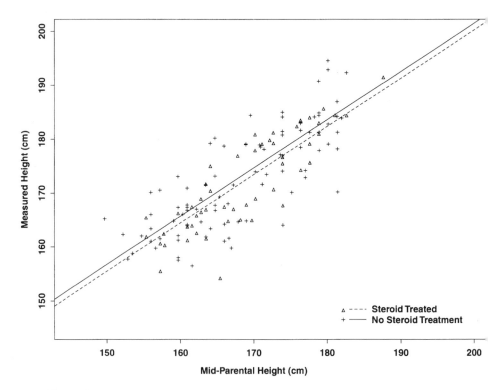

Figure 9   Adult height of patients with asthma who received oral or parenteral glucocorticoid therapy, *only* inhaled corticosteroids, or no corticosteroid therapy during childhood or adolescence. Individual data points and subgroup data regression lines are depicted. (Adapted with permission from Ref. 26.)

height. The statistical evidence did not suggest a link between growth impairment and BDP at higher doses, for more prolonged treatment durations, or among patients with more severe asthma (54).

Despite these encouraging long-term final-height data, these observations should be applied with caution to today's children receiving long-term treatment for asthma. ICS treatment is being prescribed earlier in life to children with milder asthma for longer duration and with greater consistency than in the past. Each of these factors could lead to a different growth outcome than that observed in the historical control population. It is likely that patients in the "real world," upon whom prior observational studies of final height were based, protected themselves from growth inhibition by ICSs by titrating dosage to symptoms, with resulting inconsistent ICS administration (86). The current trend toward placing greater emphasis on long-term treatment of inflammation, rather than symptom control, will increase the consistency of ICS administration to children with relatively healthy lungs, capable of efficient systemic absorption of ICSs (87). Finally, the criteria for "clinical relevance" of a growth-suppressing effect may require reevaluation as children with milder degrees of asthma are considered candidates for ICS treatment. Final-height prognosis notwithstanding, parents may express concern over a short-term decline in position on the growth curve when apparently mild but persistent asthma might be symptomatically alleviated by non-ICS medications.

How can recent prospective studies showing growth suppression by inhaled BDP be reconciled with retrospective studies showing minimal or no effect on growth rate or height? One likely explanation stresses the differences between therapeutic efforts to achieve constant *disease control* versus *symptom control* (87). Closely monitored clinical trials designed to achieve disease control with consistent dosing indicate that BDP inhaled at a dosage of 400 µg *every* day is capable of suppressing prepubertal growth. Most patients, on the other hand, reduce drug exposure by titrating medication to achieve symptom control rather than disease control (86), a fact which could account for the apparent absence of effect of "real-life" prescriptions of BDP 400 µg/day retrospective growth rates or final adult stature. It remains unknown whether long-term administration of ICSs at doses sufficient to maintain the clinician's definition of disease control could affect an asthmatic child's final height.

Studies cited above suggest the following conclusions regarding the effects of ICSs given in therapeutic doses on childhood growth: (1) detectable slowing of 1-year growth in prepubertal children can occur with continuous, twice-daily treatment with BDP (400 µg/day); (2) effects of ICSs on growth beyond 1-year of treatment or through adolescence remain unknown; (3) effects of ICS treatment during childhood on adult height appear minimal in retrospective analyses, but prospective study of growth effects of prolonged ICS use according to current asthma treatment guidelines is still needed; (4) in contrast, oral corticosteroid

treatment is associated with reduced adult stature; (5) administration of recommended doses of ICSs with more efficient first-pass hepatic inactivation of swallowed drug reduces risk of growth suppression; (6) because total systemic corticosteroid burden reflects absorption of exogenous corticosteroid administered by
any route, the risk for growth suppression is increased when ICS therapy is combined with intranasal or dermal steroid therapy; and (7) titration to the lowest
effective dose will minimize an already low risk of growth suppression by ICSs.

Important questions remain about the potential long-term effects of ICSs
on bone growth. It is possible, as suggested by one recent report, that growth
suppression is more prominent during early ICS treatment and that recovery of
normal growth occurs with longer term treatment (88). It is also possible that
ICS effects on growth observed during the prepubertal years will not persist into
puberty, during which the combined effects of sex steroids and increased growth
hormone secretion normally increase growth rate. Predictions that time of day
and/or frequency of dosing significantly affect risk of growth suppression by
ICSs require further confirmation. Finally, while studies examining bone metabolism in prepubertal children treated with moderate doses of ICSs have not found
a detrimental effect (89,90), treatment with higher dosages (mean 0.67 mg/m^2/
day) was associated with reduced acquisition of bone mineral (91). Long-term
study of pubertal (a critical period of bone mineral accretion and linear growth)
as well as prepubertal children treated consistently with ICSs is required to answer these questions.

VIII. Summary

Severe asthma, like all severe chronic diseases of childhood, can adversely affect
growth. Mechanisms underlying this effect remain obscure, but growth-suppressing influences of endogenous cytokines and glucocorticoids produced in response to illness and inflammation appear likely. Significant disease-related
growth suppression occurs only when asthma is persistent and of at least moderate
severity. Glucocorticoids are the most effective anti-inflammatory medications
for asthma, but also interfere with the normal process of linear growth at virtually
every site within the growth axis: secretion of GH, expression of GH receptors,
IGF-1 bioactivity, chondrocyte proliferation, collagen synthesis, accretion of
bone mineral, and maintenance of positive nitrogen balance. Long-term treatment
with oral glucocorticoids is associated with reduced growth rates and diminished
adult stature.

Inhaled corticosteroids have a high ratio of local to systemic activity, but *in
sufficient doses* are capable of suppressing growth, particularly during prepubertal
years. However, this effect on growth is markedly reduced when compared with
clinically equivalent doses of oral glucocorticoids, and available retrospective

final-height analysis of ICS-treated individuals suggests a negligible effect on ultimate height. Persistent addition of other topical steroid therapy (e.g., intranasal or dermal) could magnify growth suppression in individual cases. Finally, the possibility of *measurable* growth-suppressing effects of ICS must be weighed against the paramount objective of optimizing disease control and quality of life of the child with asthma. Only then can the clinical relevance of this potential systemic effect be placed in proper perspective.

References

1. Karlberg J, Engstrom I, Karlberg P, Fryer JG. Analysis of linear growth using a mathematical model. Acta Paediatr Scand 1987; 76:478–488.
2. Frank GR. Growth and estrogen. Growth Genet Horm 2000; 16(1):1–5.
3. VandenBerghe G, deZegher F, Bouillon R. Acute and prolonged critical illness as different neuroendocrine paradigms. J Clin Endocrinol Metab 1998; 83:1827–1834.
4. Zeitler PS, Travers S, Kappy MS. Endocrine complications of children with chronic illness. Adv Pediatr 1999; 46:101–149.
5. Vassilopoulou-Sellin R. Endocrine effects of cytokines. Oncology 1994; 8:43–49.
6. Umpleby AM, Russell-Jones DL. The hormonal control of protein metabolism. Baillieres Clin Endocrinol Metab 1996; 10:551–570.
7. Chopra IJ. Euthyroid sick syndrome: is it a misnomer? J Clin Endocrinol Metab 1997; 82:329–334.
8. Falliers CJ, Tan LS, Szentivanyi J, Jorgensen JR, Bukantz SC. Childhood asthma and steroid therapy as influences on growth. Am J Dis Child 1963; 105:127–137.
9. BalfourLynn L. Growth and childhood asthma. Arch Dis Child 1986; 61:1049–1055.
10. Morris HG. Growth and skeletal maturation in asthmatic children: effect of corticosteroid treatment. Pediatr Res 1975; 9:579–583.
11. Hauspie R, Susanne C, Alexander F. Maturational delay and temporal growth retardation in asthmatic boys. J Allergy Clin Immunol 1977; 59:200–206.
12. Martin AJ, Landau LI, Phelan PD. The effect on growth of childhood asthma. Acta Paediatr Scand 1981; 70:683–688.
13. Cogswell JJ, El-Bishti MM. Growth retardation in asthma: role of calorie deficiency. Arch Dis Child 1982; 57:473–475.
14. Sole D, Castro AM, Naspitz CK. Growth in allergic children. J Asthma 1989; 26:217–221.
15. Morris HG. Growth of asthmatic children. J Asthma 1989; 26:215–216.
16. Hauspie R, Susanne C, Alexander F. A mixed longitudinal study of the growth in height and weight in asthmatic children. Hum Biol 1976; 48:271–283.
17. Murray AB, Fraser BM, Hardwick DF, Pirie GE. Chronic asthma and growth failure in children. Lancet 1976; 24(2):197–198.
18. Chang KC, Miklich D, Barwise G, Chai H. Growth of chronic asthmatic children. J Allergy Clin Immunol 1978; 61:159.
19. Ninan T, Russell G. Asthma, inhaled corticosteroid treatment, and growth. Arch Dis Child 1992; 67:703–705.

20. Crowley S, Hindmarsh PC, Matthews DR, Brook CGD. Growth and the growth hormone axis in prepubertal children with asthma. J Pediatr 1995; 126:297–303.

21. Ferguson AC, Murray AB, Tze W-J. Short stature and delayed skeletal maturation in children with allergic disease. J Allergy Clin Immunol 1982; 69:217–221.

22. Zeitlen SR, Bond S, Wootton S, Gregson RK, Radford M. Increased resting energy expenditure in childhood asthma: does this contribute toward growth failure? Arch Dis Child 1992; 67:1366–1369.

23. Taylor AM, Bush A, Thomson A. Relation between insulin-like growth factor-1, body mass index, and clinical status in cystic fibrosis. Arch Dis Child 1997; 76: 304–309.

24. Merkus PJFM, VanEssenZandvliet EEM, Duiverman EJ, VanHouwelingen HC, Kerrebijn KF. Long term effect of inhaled corticosteroids on growth rate in adolescents with asthma. Pediatrics 1993; 91:1121–1126.

25. Sohat M, Sohat T, Kedem R, Mimouni M, Danon YL. Childhood asthma and growth outcome. Arch Dis Child 1987; 62:63–65.

26. Silverstein MD, Yunginger JW, Reed CE, Petterson T, Zimmerman D, Li JTC, et al. Attained adult height after childhood asthma: effect of glucocorticoid therapy. J Allergy Clin Immunol 1997; 99:466–474.

27. Oberger E, Engstrom I, Karlberg J. Long-term treatment with glucocorticoids/ ACTH in asthmatic children III. Effects on growth and adult height. Acta Paediatr Scand 1990; 79:77–83.

28. Allen DB, Julius JR, Breen TJ, Attie KM. Treatment of glucocorticoid-induced growth suppression with growth hormone. J Clin Endocrinol Metab 1998; 83:2824–2829.

29. Allen DB. Inhaled corticosteroids in children. In Middleton E, Reed CE, Ellis EF, Adkinson NF, Yunginger JW, Busse WW, eds. Allergy: Principles and Practice. St. Louis: Mosby Yearbook, 1993; 6–16.

30. Beaufrer B, Horber FF, Schwenk WF. Glucocorticoids increase leucine oxidation and impair leucine balance in humans. Am J Physiol 1995; 257:712–721.

31. Locascio V, Bonucci E, Imbimbo B. Bone loss in response to long term glucocorticoid therapy. Bone Miner 1990; 8:39–51.

32. Saville PD, Kharmosh O. Osteoporosis of rheumatoid arthritis: Influence of age, sex, and corticosteroids. Arthritis Rheum 1967; 10:423–430.

33. Moore DD, Marks AR, Buckley DI, Kapler G, Payvar F, Goodman HM. The first intron of the human growth hormone gene contains a binding site for glucocorticoid receptor. Proc Natl Acad Sci USA 1985; 82:699–702.

34. Guistina A, Wehrenberg WB. The role of glucocorticoids in the regulation of growth hormone secretion—mechanisms and clinical significance. Trends Endocrinol Metab 1992; 3:306–311.

35. Spiliotis BE, August GP, Hung W. Growth hormone neurosecretory dysfunction. J Am Med Assoc 1984; 257:2223–2226.

36. Kaufmann S, Jones KL, Wehrenberg WB, Culler FL. Inhibition by prednisone of growth hormone (GH) response to GH-releasing hormone in normal men. J Clin Endocrinol Metab 1988; 67:1258–1261.

37. Gabrielsson BG, Carmignac DF, Flavell DM, Robinson ICAF. Steroid regulation

of growth hormone (GH) receptor and GH-binding protein messenger ribonucleic acids in the rat. Endocrinology 1995; 136:209–217.

38. Tonshoff B, Mehls O. In: Tejani AH, Fine RN, eds. Pediatric Renal Transplantation. New York: Wiley, 1994:441–459.

39. Unterman TG, Phillips LS. Glucocorticoid effects on somatomedins and somatomedin inhibitors. J Clin Endocrinol Metab 1985; 61:618–626.

40. Binoux M, Lassarre C, Seurin D. Somatomedin production by rat liver in organ culture. II. Studies of cartilage sulphation inhibitors released by the liver and their separation from somatomedins. Acta Endocrinol 1980; 93:83–90.

41. Hokken-Koelega ACS, Stijnen T, deMuinckKeizer-Schrama SMPF, Blum WF, Drop SLS. Levels of growth hormone, insulin-like growth factor I (IGF-I) and -II, IGF binding protein-1 and -3, and cortisol in prednisone-treated children with growth retardation after renal transplantation. J Clin Endocrinol Metab 1993; 77:932–938.

42. Ristelli J. Effect of prednisolone on the activities of intracellular enzymes of collagen biosynthesis in rat liver and skin. Biochem Pharmacol 1977; 26:1295–1298.

43. Mosier HD. The determinants of catch-up growth. Acta Paediatr Scand 1990; 367: 126–129.

44. Baron J, Klein KO, Colli MJ, Yanovski JA, Novosad JA, Bacher JD, et al. Catch-up growth after glucocorticoid excess: a mechanism intrinsic to the growth plate. Endocrinology 1994; 135:1367–1371.

45. Tanner JM. Growth as a target-seeking function. In: Falkner F, Tanner JM, eds. Human Growth—A Comprehensive Treatise. Vol. 1. New York: Plenum, 1990: 167–179.

46. Van Metre TE, Pinkerton HL. Growth suppression in asthmatic children receiving prolonged therapy with prednisone and methylprednisolone. J Allergy 1959; 30: 103–113.

47. Kerribijn KF, DeKroon JPM. Effect on height of corticosteroid therapy in asthmatic children. Arch Dis Child 1968; 43:556–561.

48. Sadeghi-Nelad A, Semor B. Adrenal function, growth, and insulin in patients treated with corticoids on alternate days. Pediatrics 1969; 43:277–283.

49. Reimer LG, Morris HG, Ellis EE. Growth of asthmatic children during treatment with alternate-day steroids. J Allergy Clin Immunol 1975; 55:224–231.

50. Chang KC, Miklich D, Barwise G, Chal H, Miles EA, Lawrence R. Linear growth of chronic asthmatic children: the effects of disease and various forms of steroid therapy. Clin Allergy 1982; 12:369–378.

51. Allen DB. Growth suppression by glucocorticoid therapy. In: Rosenfield RL, ed. Growth and Growth Disorders. Philadelphia: Saunders, 1996; 699–718.

52. Lam CN, Arneil GC. Long-term dwarfing effects of corticosteroid treatment for childhood nephrosis. Arch Dis Child 1968; 43:589–594.

53. Foote KD, Brocklebank JT, Meadow SR. Height attainment in children with steroid responsive nephrotic syndrome. Lancet 1985; 2:917–976.

54. Allen DB, Mullen M, Mullen B. A meta-analysis of the effects of oral and inhaled glucocorticoids on growth. J Allergy Clin Immunol 1994; 93:967–976.

55. Ryrfelt A, Andersson P, Edsbacker S. Pharmacokinetics and metabolism of budesonide a selective glucocorticoid. Eur J Resp Dis 1982; 63(suppl 122):86.

56. Chaplin MD, Cooper WC, Segre EJ. Correllation of flunisolide plasma levels to eosinopenic response in humans. J Allergy Clin Immunol 1980; 65:445.

57. Ryrfeldt A, Edsbacker S, Pouwles R. Kinetics of epimeric glucocorticoid budesonide. Clin Pharmacol Therapeut 1984; 35:525–530.

58. Harding SM. The human pharmacology of fluticasone propionate. Respir Med 1990; 84(suppl A):25–29.

59. Pedersen S, Steffensen G, Ekman I, Tonnesson M, Borga O. Pharmacokinetics of budesonide in children with asthma. Eur J Clin Pharmacol 1987; 31:579–582.

60. Johansson SA, Andersson KE, Brattsand R. Topical and systemic glucocorticoid potencies of budesonide and beclomethasone dipropionate in man. Eur J Clin Pharmacol 1982; 22:523.

61. Johnson M. Pharmacokinetics and pharmacodynamics of inhaled glucocorticoids. J Clin Allergy Immunol 1996; 98:169–176.

62. Agertoft L, Pedersen S. A randomized, double-blind dose reduction study to compare the minimal effective dose of budesonide Turbuhaler and fluticasone propionate Diskhaler. J Allergy Clin Immunol 1997; 99(6):773–780.

63. Ghigo E, Valetto M, Gaggero L, Visca A, Valente F, Bellone J et al. Therapeutic doses of salbutamol inhibit the somatotropic responsiveness to growth hormone-releasing hormone in asthmatic children. J Endocrinol Invest 1993; 16:271–276.

64. Hollman GA, Allen DB. Overt glucocorticoid excess due to inhaled corticosteroid therapy. Pediatrics 1988; 81:452–455.

65. Wolthers OD, Pederson S. Controlled study of linear growth in asthmatic children during treatment with inhaled glucocorticoids. Pediatrics 1992; 89:839–842.

66. Wolthers OD, Hansen M, Juul A, Nielsen HK, Pederson S. Knemometry, urine cortisol excretion, and measures of insulin-like growth factor axis and collagen turnover in children treated with inhaled glucocorticoids. Pediatr Res 1997; 41(1):44–50.

67. Wales JKH, Milner RDG. Knemometry in assessment of linear growth. Arch Dis Child 1987; 62:166–171.

68. Agertoft L, Pedersen S. Relationship between short-term lower leg growth and long-term statural growth in asthmatic children treated with budesonide. Eur Respir J 1996; 9(suppl 23):294s–294s.

69. Hermanussen M, Burmeister J. Standards for the predictive accuracy of short-term body height and lower leg length measurements on half annual growth rates. Arch Dis Child 1989; 64:259–263.

70. Karlberg J, Gelander L, Albertsson-Wikland K. Distinctions between short- and long-term human growth studies. Acta Paediatr 1993; 82:631–634.

71. Allen DB. Limitations of short-term studies in predicting long-term effects of inhaled corticosteroids. Allergy 1999; 54(suppl 49):29–34.

72. Tinkelman DG, Reed CE, Nelson HS, Offord KP. Aerosol beclomethasone dipropionate compared with theophylline as primary treatment of chronic mild to moderately severe asthma in children. Pediatrics 1993; 92:64–77.

73. Doull IJM, Freezer NJ, Holgate ST. Growth of prepubertal children with mild asthma treated with inhaled beclomethasone dipropionate. Am J Resp Crit Care Med 1995; 151:1715–1719.

74. Verberne AAPH, Frost C, DipStat MA, Roorda RJ, van der Laag H, Kerribijn KF. One year treatment with salmeterol compared to beclomethasone in children with asthma. Am J Resp Crit Care Med 1997; 156:688–695.

75. Simons FER. A comparison of beclomethasone, salmeterol, and placebo in children with asthma. N Engl J Med 1997; 337:1659–1665.

76. Agertoft L, Pederson S. Effects of long-term treatment with an inhaled corticosteroid on growth and pulmonary function in asthmatic children. Resp Med 1994; 88:373–381.

77. Volovitz B, Amir J, Malik H, Kauschansky A, Varsano I. Growth and pituitary adrenal function in children with severe asthma treated with inhaled budesonide. N Engl J Med 1993; 329:1703–1708.

78. Allen DB, Bronsky EA, LaForce CF, Nathan RA, Tinkelman DG, Vandewalker ML, et al. Growth in asthmatic children treated with fluticasone propionate. J Pediatr 1998; 132:472–477.

79. Agertoft L, Pederson S. The importance of delivery system for the effect of Budesonide. Arch Dis Child 1993; 69:130–133.

80. Allen DB. Systemic effects of intranasal steroids: an endocrinologist's perspective. J Clin Allergy Immunol 2000; 106(October): in press.

81. Teper AM, Kofman CD, Maffey AF, Vidaurreta S, Bergadi I, Heinrich J. Effect of inhaled beclomethasone dipropionate on pulmonary function, bronchial reactivity and longitudinal growth in infants with bronchial asthma. Asthma 1995; 95:13–13.

82. Reid A, Murphy C, Steen HJ, McGovern V, Shields MD. Linear growth of very young asthmatic children treated with high-dose nebulized budesonide. Acta Paediatr 1996; 85:421–424.

83. Skoner DP, Szefler SJ, Welch M, Walton-Bowen K, Cruz-Rivera M, Smith JA. Longitudinal growth in infants and young children treated with budesonide inhalation suspension for persistent asthma. J Allergy Clin Immunol 2000; 105:259–268.

84. Pedersen S, Warner JO, Price JF. Early use of inhaled steroids in children with asthma. Clin Exp Allergy 1997; 27:995–1006.

85. Van Bever HP, Desager KN, Lijssens N, Weyler JJ, Du Caju MVL. Does treatment of asthmatic children with inhaled corticosteroids affect their adult height? Pediatr Pulmonol 1999; 27:369–375.

86. Milgrom H, Bender B, Ackerson L, Bowry P, Smith B, Rand C. Noncompliance and treatment failure in children with asthma. J Allergy Clin Immunol 1996; 98: 1051–1057.

87. Lemanske RF, Allen DB. Choosing a long-term controller medication in childhood asthma: the proverbial two-edged sword. Am J Respir Crit Care Med 1997; 156: 685–687.

88. Doull IJM, Campbell MJ, Holgate ST. Duration of growth suppressive effects of regular inhaled corticosteroids. Arch Dis Child 1998; 78:172–173.

89. Konig P, Hillman L, Cervantes C, Levine C, Maloney C, Douglas B et al. Bone metabolism in children with asthma treated with inhaled beclomethasone dipropionate. J Pediatr 1993; 122:219–226.

90. Agertoft L, Pedersen S. Bone mineral density in children with asthma receiving long-term treatment with inhaled corticosteroids. Am J Respir Crit Care Med 1998; 157:178–183.

91. Allen HDW, Thong IG, Clifton-Bligh P, Holmes S, Nery L, Wilson KB. Effects of high-dose inhaled corticosteroids on bone metabolism in prepubertal children with asthma. Pediatr Pulmonol 2000; 29:188–193.

22

Steroid-Induced Osteoporosis
Prevention and Management

DENNIS K. LEDFORD

Joy A. McCann Culverhouse Airway Disease Research Center
University of South Florida
and the James A. Haley VA Hospital
Tampa, Florida

I. Introduction

Corticosteroids (CSs) are the most effective anti-inflammatory medication for the treatment of asthma. Systemic CS therapy is associated with significant adverse effects, including the promotion of osteoporosis. In contrast to systemic CS therapy, inhaled corticosteroids (ICSs) provide effective therapy of asthma with few adverse effects (1). The effects of inhaled corticosteroid therapy on bone metabolism are not certain but are a concern with the increasing use of moderate and high doses for longer periods of time. The relative risk of osteoporosis for different inhaled corticosteroid preparations and dosages has not been defined. Research is delineating the best procedures for diagnosis, prevention, and treatment of osteoporosis (2,3). The goals of this chapter are to review what is known about osteoporosis risk factors and to recommend methods of prevention, diagnosis, and treatment of osteoporosis for the asthma specialist.

II. Definitions

Osteoporosis is a "disease characterized by low bone mass and microarchitectural deterioration of bone tissue, leading to enhanced bone fragility and a consequent increase in fracture risk'' (Fig. 1) (4,5). Similar to hypertension and athero-sclerosis, osteoporosis can be defined by an intermediate outcome decrease in bone mineral density (BMD) prior to fracture. Osteoporosis is a risk factor for fracture just as hypertension is for stroke. Osteoporosis is characterized by loss of both mineral and matrix from bone, with the ratio of the two remaining normal. This contrasts with osteomalacia, which is characterized by an increase in non-calcified osteoid in relation to normal bone.

Osteoporosis is the most common metabolic bone disease. The physiologic result of osteoporosis is decreased strength of bone and increased tendency to fracture from minimal trauma or stress. Skeletal bone with a greater proportion of trabecular bone, compared to cortical bone, is disproportionately affected. Osteoporotic fractures selectively occur in these trabecular-rich bone areas, which include vertebra, wrist, hip, proximal humerus, and pelvis. The clinical significance of osteoporosis is a product of the morbidity and mortality that accompanies these fractures.

Severe asthma and osteoporosis are potentially related by factors intrinsic to asthma and, more commonly, by factors related to its treatment, particularly CS therapy. Possible mechanisms by which severe asthma may increase osteoporosis

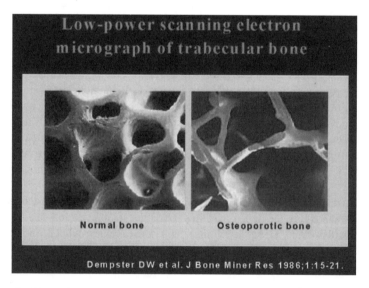

Figure 1 Photomicrograph of normal and osteoporotic trabecular bone. Normal bone is from a 75-year-old woman; osteoporotic bone is from a 47-year-old woman with multiple vertebral compression fractures. Note the increase in trabecular separation, decrease in trabecular width, and decrease in trabecular connectivity in osteoporotic bone. (From Ref. 5.)

include decreased physical activity and weight bearing, decreased outdoor activity and sun exposure, reduced calcium in diet related to avoidance of milk, reduced adrenal sex hormones, and systemic effects of chronic inflammation (6). None of these potential mechanisms definitely contribute to osteoporosis. In contrast, the effects of systemic CS therapy on bone metabolism are well documented. Effects of ICS therapy on development of osteoporosis are less clear.

III. Epidemiology

Osteoporosis is silent until fractures occur, but distinguishing osteoporotic fractures from other fractures may be difficult. Therefore, diagnostic testing of bone density is usually necessary to define the problem for epidemiologic studies. Unfortunately, there are no ideal diagnostic studies readily amenable to population surveys. The operational definition for postmenopausal women proposed by the World Health Organization is a bone density 2.5 s.d. below the young normal mean (Table 1) (7). The rationale for choosing a 2.5 s.d. decrease in bone density is the evidence that fracture rate doubles for each decrease in standard deviation of bone density. The relationship for fracture rate and bone density has only been investigated for postmenopausal osteoporosis, and it is unknown whether the same risk of fracture occurs with bone density decreases in other situations, including corticosteroid therapy.

Risk factors for osteoporosis are listed in Tables 2 and 3. Osteoporosis is three times more prevalent in women than in men because of lower peak bone mass and hormonal changes during menopause. Estrogens help preserve bone mass during adulthood, and sizable bone loss, as great as 3–10% or more per year, occurs during the perimenopausal decline in estrogen levels. In addition, women on average live longer than men and therefore are at greater risk of reduced skeletal mass and cumulative fracture risk (7). Women currently live on

Table 1 Definitions of Osteoporosis by Bone Mineral Density

The World Health Organization has established the following definitions based on bone mass measurement at any skeletal site in White women.

Normal: Bone mineral density is within 1 s.d. of a "young normal" adult (T score above -1).

Low bone mass (osteopenia): Bone mineral density between 1 and 2.5 s.d. below that of a "young normal" adult (T score between -1 and -2.5).

Osteoporosis. Bone mineral density is 2.5 s.d. or more below that of a "young normal" adult (T score at or below -2.5). Women in this group who have already experienced one or more fractures are deemed to have severe or "established" osteoporosis.

Table 2 Risk Factors for Osteoporotic Fracture

Nonmodifiable
  Personal history of fracture as an adult
  History of fracture in first-degree relative
  Advanced age
  Caucasian race
  Female gender
  Dementia
  Poor health/frailty
Potentially modifiable
  Current cigarette smoking
  Low body weight (<127 lbs)
  Estrogen deficiency
    Early menopause (age < 45 years) or bilateral ovariectomy
    Prolonged premenopausal amenorrhea (>1 year)
  Low calcium intake
  Alcoholism
  Diseases and drug therapy
  Impaired eyesight despite adequate correction
  Recurrent falls
  Inadequate physical activity
  Poor health/frailty

Note. The four items in boldface—personal history of fracture, family history of fracture, smoking, and low body weight—were demonstrated in a large, prospective U.S. study to be key factors in determining risk of hip fracture independent of bone density.

average a third of their lives after menopause and the number of postmenopausal women is increasing. Between the years of 1990 and 2025, the number of European women 50 years of age or greater will increase 30–40% (7). Life expectancy is increasing more rapidly for men than for women, so that in the same time frame the number of men over 50 years of age will increase by 50%. The increase in older adults is even larger in regions of the world other than Western Europe and North America. In 2025, the proportion of the population greater than 50 years of age will increase by 83% in Western Europe and North America and more than double in almost all other regions of the world. The greatest increases will occur in Africa, Asia, and Latin America.

These predictions concerning the aging of the general population are relatively secure since the people who will be older than 50 years in 2025 are already born. Thus, major catastrophes excluded, these forecasts are probably accurate in predicting future osteoporotic fracture risk. Estimates are that between 1.3 and 1.7 million hip fractures occurred worldwide in 1990 (8,9). The expected

Table 3 Diseases and Drug Therapies Associated with an Increased Risk of Generalized Osteoporosis in Adults

Diseases	
Acromegaly	Insulin-dependent diabetes
Adrenal atrophy/Addison's disease	Lymphoma/leukemia
Amyloidosis	Malabsorption syndromes
Ankylosing spondylitis	Mastocytosis
Chronic obstructive pulmonary disease	Multiple myeloma
Congenital porphyria	Multiple sclerosis
Cushing's syndrome	Nutritional disorders
Endometriosis	Osteogenesis imperfecta
Epidermolysis bullosa	Parenteral nutrition
Gastrectomy	Pernicious anemia
Gonadal insufficiency	Rheumatoid arthritis
Hemochromatosis	Severe liver disease
Hemophilia	Thalassemia
Hyperparathyroidism	Thyrotoxicosis
Hypophosphatasia	Tumor secretion of parathyroid hormone
Idiopathic scoliosis	
Drugs	
Aluminum	Corticosteroids and adrenocorticotropin
Anticonvulsants	Gonadotropin-releasing hormone agonists
Cigarette smoking	Heparin
Cytotoxic drugs	Lithium
Excessive alcohol	Tamoxifen (premenopausal use)
Excessive thyroxine	

population changes suggest that this number will conservatively increase to approximately 2 million by the year 2025. Hip fracture rates are increasing in some areas of the world faster than would be predicted by aging (9). The reasons for these changes are unknown with hypotheses including a decrease in regular physical activity or increase in physical stature. The number of hip fractures may be as great as 4 million by 2025, if these unknown factors as well as age continue to influence the fracture rate.

A large sample of U.S. residents demonstrated that 17% of postmenopausal White women had osteoporosis of the hip (8). Twelve percent of Latino women and 8% of African-American women were affected. The prevalence of osteoporosis increased as additional sites, such as the wrist or spine, were surveyed. Approximately a third of postmenopausal White women have osteoporosis of one of these sites. Less information is available about the prevalence of osteoporosis in men. Seven percent of White men, compared to 3% Latino men and 5%

African-American men, had a hip bone density 2.5 s.d. below the mean for young, normal men (8).

The social burden of osteoporosis is related to the frequency of fractures and their associated complications, pain, disability, hospitalization, surgery, dependence, and medical complications. Lifetime risk of fracture depends on both fracture incidence and life expectancy. The lifetime risk of hip fracture among 50-year-old British women is 14% compared to 3% for British men (10). The lifetime risk of hip, spine, or forearm fracture in the United States is estimated to be 40% in White women greater than 50 years of age and 13% in White men of the same age (10). These estimates are conservative, as no change in life expectancy is assumed. If life expectancy increases are factored in, the risk of hip fracture in Swedish men and women increases from 8.1 and 19.5% to 11.1 and 22.7% respectively (11).

Fractures have a significant negative effect on functional capacity and independence. Estimates are that 10% of women with a hip fracture become dependent in the activities of daily living. Four percent of women with vertebral fracture and 2% with distal forearm fractures suffer similar losses (12). Twenty percent of subjects with hip fractures die in the year following the fracture and only approximately one-third regain their prefracture level of function (12,13). Hip fracture rates are higher in White than in Black or Asian populations, although urbanization has resulted in increased fracture rates in these latter populations. The female preponderance in White populations is not detected in Blacks or Asians, in which males and females suffer equal number of hip fractures. The incidence of vertebral fracture is three times greater than hip fracture in postmenopausal, White women. However, the clinical diagnosis of fracture is only made in approximately 30% of these occurrences. Thus, the incidence of clinically diagnosed vertebral and hip fracture do not differ greatly. Radiographic surveys find 19–26% of postmenopausal White women to have vertebral deformity, primarily in the midthoracic or thoracolumbar region (14,15). In contrast to the prevalence of hip fractures, vertebral deformities are as common in Asian and White women but are less common in African-American and Latino populations (16–18). Vertebral fractures rarely result in hospitalization (e.g., 2% or less in the United Kingdom), but there is a significant negative effect on activities of daily living and quality of life (19). Early mortality does not increase following vertebral fracture as occurs with hip fracture. Survival worsens with the passage of time, probably secondary to decrease in activity and underlying diseases associated with osteoporosis (20). The direct medical expenditures for osteoporotic fractures in the United States were estimated to be $13.8 billion in 1995 (21).

There is limited data concerning the prevalence of osteoporosis in subjects with asthma, and these data are confounded by the treatments of the asthma, particularly the intermittent or chronic use of oral and inhaled CS therapy. A cross-sectional study of perimenopausal women in Finland shows that the lumbar and femoral bone density of asthmatic women, without treatment with inhaled or oral CSs, is statistically lower than that of a control group (22). This difference is eliminated by estrogen replacement therapy (Fig. 2). A study in Hong Kong demonstrates that asthmatic men and women have a lower BMD than controls, and the difference occurs in subjects not receiving inhaled or oral CS therapy (23). These differences are small and matching for all variables is difficult. Thus, asthma may result in a small decrement in BMD regardless of therapy.

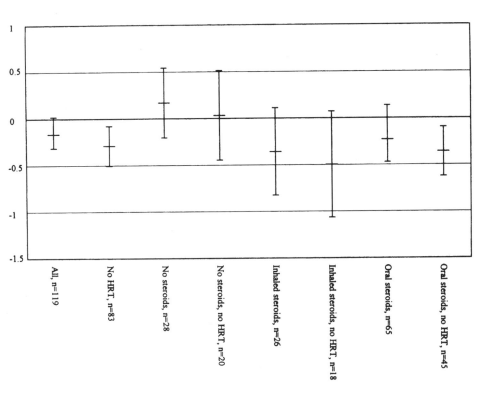

Figure 2 The Z score values with 95% confidence intervals are shown for spinal bone mineral density of asthmatics and different subgroups in a population study of perimenopausal Finnish women (age 47 to 56 years). The Z score is the standard deviation from the mean of the nonasthmatic, age-matched population. Asthmatic women had a slightly decreased bone mineral density with the difference statistically significant in women not receiving hormone replacement therapy (spinal bone mineral density 1.083 ± 0.150 (s.d.) vs. 1.128 ± 0.160 g/cm^2, $P < 0.05$). Although bone mineral density was not significantly decreased in the asthmatics who had used inhaled corticosteroid, the duration of inhaled corticosteroid use correlated negatively with spinal bone mineral density. (From Ref. 22.)

IV. Pathophysiology of Corticosteroid-Related Osteoporosis

Corticosteroid-induced osteoporosis has been recognized since 1932, when Cushing described bone loss and skeletal fracture in hypercortisolism. Corticosteroid-induced osteoporosis is primarily due to a decrease in bone formation with controversial effects on bone resorption. The various mechanisms by which corticosteroid therapy potentially affects bone and leads to osteoporosis are listed in Table 4. Bone is constantly being remodeled and 20% of trabecular bone is replaced each year. If formation and resorption change equivalently, the effects on bone density are probably minimal. Whenever the changes in bone formation or resorption are discordant, then there is a risk for bone loss. A number of serum biochemical markers have been described that may reflect bone formation or resorption (Table 5) (24–26). The clinical significance of changes in these markers is not known.

Bone remodeling occurs at a greater rate in children than in adults. The increase in bone mass during childhood is not at a constant rate but varies with age, season, and growth. Skeletal mass peaks in late adolescence or early adult life. The dynamic nature and variability of bone metabolism and bone density complicate the interpretation of studies of ICSs and osteoporosis.

Corticosteroids directly inhibit osteoblasts and reduce bone formation. The mechanisms of action include reduced protein synthesis resulting in a decrease in osteoid formation (27), inhibition of synthesis of bone collagen, and reduction of the conversion of precursor cells into functioning osteoblasts. In addition, CSs may modulate the response of osteoblasts to parathyroid hormone, prostaglandins, cytokines, growth factors, and 1,25-dihydroxyvitamin D.

The effects of CSs on bone resorption are less clear. Increase in parathyroid hormone levels, suspected to result from a decrease in calcium intestinal absorption and increased renal losses, are described in some studies. However, this apparent parathyroid hormone increase has been challenged as reflecting hormone fragments, and no change is detected when assaying the intact or midregion hormone molecule (28,29). The effects of corticosteroids on net intestinal calcium

Table 4 Mechanisms by Which Corticosteroids Potentially Affect Bone

Inhibition of osteoblast proliferation and function
Increase in urinary calcium excretion
Secondary hyperparathyroidism
Reduction of circulating estrogen and testosterone
Decrease in intestinal absorption of both calcium and phosphate

Note. Adapted from Ref. 23a.

Table 5 Selected Biochemical Markers of Bone Turnover

Markers of bone resorption	Markers of bone formation
Serum	
C-telopeptide of type I procollagen	Total and bone-specific alkaline phos-
Cross-linked N-telopeptide of type I	phatase
collagen	Carboxy terminal propeptide of type I
Deoxypyridinoline crosslinks	collagen
	Osteocalcin
Urine	
Deoxypyridinoline crosslinks	
Hydroxyproline	
Hydroxylysine glycosides	
Pyridinoline crosslinks	
Cross-linked N-telopeptide of type I	
collagen	
C-telopeptide of type I collagen	

Note. Adapted from Refs. 24–26.

absorption are also inconclusive, with studies showing increased, decreased, or unchanged calcium absorption (30–32). These contradictory effects may be the result of dose effects or variable effects on differing intestinal segments. Corticosteroids increase urinary calcium losses independent of any effects on gastrointestinal calcium absorption or parathyroid hormone levels. Variable effects of CSs on vitamin D metabolism have been reported. These include normal 1,25-dihydroxyvitamin D metabolism, reduction of vitamin D receptors, and reduced 1,25-dihydroxyvitamin D concentration (33–35). Corticosteroids reduce androgenic hormones by inhibiting pituitary gonadotrophin secretion, directly suppress the ovaries or testes, and reduce secretion of androstenedione and estrone from the adrenal gland. The net result of these hormonal changes might be to decrease bone resorption (36,37). In summary, the effects of corticosteroid therapy on bone resorption are unknown.

V. Diagnosis and Assessment

Osteoporosis is diagnosed by histology or bone density assessment, which requires techniques generally not acceptable for routine use. The end result of osteoporosis is a fracture occurring without significant trauma, generally affecting bone with a large content of trabecular bone. Depletion of bone mass is the physiologic process in osteoporosis which decreases fracture threshold. Ideally the diagnosis of osteoporosis should be made prior to fracture, since treatment is more effective if initiated prior to fracture. Bone mineral density measurements (BMD) correlate with bone mass. The most straightforward approach to the diagnosis of osteoporosis by BMDs is to define a fracture threshold, a cutoff for BMD that captures most subjects with osteoporosis fractures.

Conventional radiographs are insensitive to BMD changes, with 30% loss required before the process is recognized. The lateral chest radiograph provides an index of bone changes, particularly by the loss of trabecular striations and increased prominence of the vertebral endplates (Fig. 3). Change may be more apparent when comparative chest radiographs are available (Figs. 3A and 3B). The midthoracic to upper lumbar spine are the vertebral areas which first demonstrate discernable changes. Typically, perimenopausal osteoporosis is characterized by a greater loss of transverse vertebral trabeculae, resulting in apparently enhanced vertical striations. In reality the trabeculae are diminished both vertically and horizontally, with the apparent enhanced vertical striations appearing due to the selective decrease in the horizontal trabeculae. In contrast, the vertebral body in corticosteroid-induced bone loss demonstrates a ground-glass appearance without striations. This appearance is the result of generalized, progressive trabecular loss (Fig. 3). Vertebral height decrease is another clue to advanced bone loss, and this collapse may be subtle, evident only on comparative films (Fig. 3). The decrease in vertebral height and associated kyphosis are the major contributors to height loss associated with osteoporosis.

BMD testing techniques are listed in Table 6. Dual-energy X-ray absorptiometry (DEXA) and quantitative computed tomography (QCT) are the most widely utilized. Ultrasound techniques are improving. At present the DEXA is preferred over QCT because DEXA is less expensive, is more accurate, and requires less radiation exposure (2,38,39). The utility of a test to monitor a condition

---

Figure 3   Lateral chest radiograph in 1993 (A) and 1999 (B) of female with chronic asthma requiring high-dose inhaled corticosteroid therapy and intermittent systemic corticosteroid therapy. The patient did not complain of back pain. Anterior vertebral height of the 12th vertebral body has decreased in 1999, with a generalized decrease in density of vertebral bodies (arrows point to superior and inferior vertebral endplates of 12th vertebral body). Vertebral height in 1993 was 12 mm and in 1999 9 mm. The superior and inferior end plates of the vertebral bodies appear more distinct with the decline in bone density, and the vertebral bodies characteristically develop a ''haziness'' in osteoporosis (magnified inset). This ground glass appearance contrasts to the normal variegated appearance or vertical striations that are typical of postmenopausal osteoporosis. The reason for the latter is that the horizontal trabeculae are reduced preferentially in postmenopausal osteoporosis, leaving the vertical striations of the vertical trabeculae. In corticosteroid induced osteoporosis, the horizontal and vertical trabeculae are both reduced, resulting in a hazy appearance as the vertebral body becomes osteopenic.

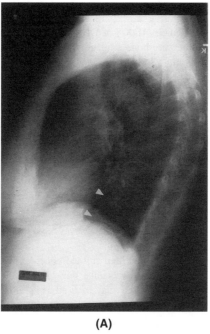

(A)

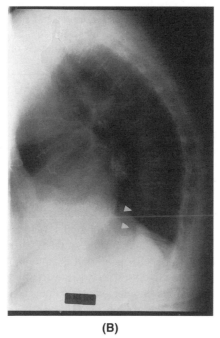

(B)

Table 6 Bone Marrow Density Testing Techniques

Dual-energy X-ray absorptiometry (DXA or DEXA)
    DEXA can be used to measure bone mineral density in the spine, hip or wrist.
    DEXA scans require only a few minutes and expose the tested subject to less radiation than one-tenth that of a standard X-ray.

Single-energy X-ray absorptiometry (SXA) and peripheral dual-energy X-ray absorptiometry (pDXA or pDEXA)
    These techniques measure bone density in the forearm, finger and sometimes heel. This method is affected by soft tissue density, limiting its application to the axial skeleton or proximal joints.

Radiographic absorptiometry (RA)
    RA is a technique based on a standard X-ray or computer-generated X-ray of the hand with a metal wedge in the same field. RA and SXA have similar accuracy and precision.

Quantitative computed tomography (QCT)
    QCT measures the sum of trabecular and cortical bone density at several sites but is most commonly used to measure trabecular bone density of the spine. QCT provides volumetric density data. QCT may be used as an alternative to DEXA for vertebral measurements.

Ultrasound densitometry
    Ultrasound assesses bone in the heel, tibia, patella or other peripheral sites where the bone is relatively superficial. Ultrasound measurements are not as precise as DEXA or SXA but predict fracture rates relatively well. Ultrasound may assess structural characteristics that provide additional estimates of fracture risk compared to radiographic density measurements.

is limited by the precision of the test. The magnitude of change in a monitored value must be 2.8 times the precision of the test before the change can be identified with a 95% confidence level. The precision of DEXA is 1 to 3%. Thus, if the rate of bone loss is 1–2% per year, repeat bone density assessments would not be of value any more often than 2–3 years. However, if the rate of loss is 5–10% per year, as sometimes occurs with low-dose systemic corticosteroid therapy, then repeat testing as often as every 6 months could be useful (40,41). Factors which may affect precision and accuracy of DEXA include bone marrow fat (resulting in falsely low bone density) and anatomical changes of the axial skeleton, such as compression fractures, scoliosis, osteophytes, intervertebral disk space narrowing, and previous laminectomy (resulting in falsely elevated bone density).

DEXA values are interpreted by comparing the number of standard deviations above or below the mean density to that of a young-adult, gender-matched population (*T* score) (Fig. 4). The *Z* score is the number of standard deviations above or below a population matched for age and gender. The *Z* score compares an individual to his or her peers; the *T* score compares an individual to his or her ideal. Osteoporosis is defined as a *T* score more than 2.5 standard deviations below the mean (38). Osteopenia is defined as a *T* score between −2.5 and −1.0. The relative risk for a fracture doubles in postmenopausal women for every decrease of 1 s.d. in bone mass of the hip or spine. Fracture thresholds currently apply to bone density measurements in postmenopausal women, as similar data have not been developed in other risk populations (42). It cannot be assumed that the risks of fracture are identical in different populations with the same bone density measurements. Some evidence suggests that the fracture threshold differs for GC-related osteoporosis and involutional osteoporosis (43).

Fracture rates or bone strength depend on factors other than mineral density. This is demonstrated by intervention studies that show a decrease in fracture rate prior to significant changes in BMD. These other factors are not well understood but probably include structural features of bone, noncalcified osteoid, and colla-

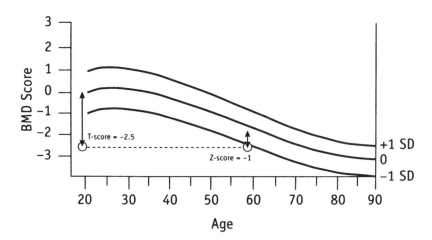

Figure 4 An example of bone mineral density (BMD) compared to age with the value of 59-year-old woman displayed. Compared to her age-matched average BMD (*Z* score) she is 1 standard deviation below the mean (*Z* score −1). Compared to a young normal population average (*T* score) she is 2.5 standard deviations below the mean (*T* score −2.5). Fracture rate approximately doubles for every standard deviation decrease in the *T* score. This comparison can be applied to any site but is generally used for the hip or spine.

gen. Ultrasound may assess these ultrastructural features of bone, such as bone stiffness and microarchitectural characteristics, more reliably than absorptiometry techniques.

There are a number of problems and limitations in the practical application of BMD measurements (44). BMD is only an index of bone density when bone is fully mineralized. The presence of osteomalacia, a complication of poor nutrition in the elderly, will lead to underestimation of bone mass. Osteoarthrosis and spondylosis of the hip or spine, common in the elderly, increase BMD measurement but not skeletal strength. Heterogeneity of BMD due to osteoarthrosis, previous fracture, or scoliosis can often be detected by the scan and in some cases excluded from the analysis. Adequately trained staff and quality control are essential in obtaining reliable BMD data.

The reference range used to determine normal or comparative BMD data should be obtained from appropriate populations. Recommendations made by the International Osteoporosis Foundation include a reference database for women ages 20 to 29 years (45). Suitable diagnostic cutoff values for men are less secure. Population studies and a prospective study suggest that BMD in women can be similarly applied to men (46–48). Thus, a BMD 2.5 s.d. below the average for women is applied to men, since the risk of hip and vertebral fractures are similar for men and women for any given BMD. These threshold values may not be suitable for all populations (48).

T scores for diagnostic criteria are most valid with DEXA at the hip and at the spine in younger individuals compared to results from test subjects. The use of *T* score cutoff at other sites and with other BMD techniques is less secure (45). For example, a *T* score of -1.0 at the heel with one ultrasound device is equivalent to a *T* score of -2.5 with DEXA at the hip. This difference is in part related to different rates of loss with age, different units of measurement, and differences in population variance (49). Errors of accuracy of different techniques also confound the ability to use *T* scores interchangeably between sites, even with the same technique (50). For these reasons, *T* score is best utilized for DEXA at the hip. In the case of other sites or techniques, it is preferable that deviations of measurement from normal values be expressed in units of measurement or units of risk (51).

Estimating fracture risk by BMD is comparable to the assessment of the risk of stroke by blood pressure readings. Blood pressure values are continuously distributed in the population, as is BMD. In the same way that a patient above a cutoff level for blood pressure is diagnosed as hypertensive, the diagnosis of osteoporosis is based on a value of BMD below a cutoff threshold. As with blood pressure, there is no absolute threshold of BMD that discriminates between those who will or will not fracture. The value of BMD in predicting fracture is, however, at least as good as that of blood pressure in predicting stroke and considerably better than the value of cholesterol in predicting coronary disease (38,52).

Normal BMD is no guarantee, however, that a fracture will not occur, only that the risk is decreased. If bone density is in the osteoporotic range, the risk of fracture is likely. Thus, the prediction of fracture with BMD has high specificity but low sensitivity.

Biochemical indices of bone turnover are divided into two groups: markers of resorption and markers of formation (Table 5) (24–26). Since BMD changes slowly, there has been interest in exploiting more rapid changes in markers as a means of diagnosing disease and monitoring treatment. Their utility is limited by precision errors. Several studies using these markers show a sustained increase in bone turnover in late postmenopausal and elderly women and in subjects treated with oral or inhaled CS. These changes are insufficiently discriminatory to provide a diagnostic test for osteoporosis. The greatest promise in the use of biochemical indices of skeletal metabolism has been in assessing fracture risk or in monitoring treatment response following intervention. In general, bone resorption markers change within 1 or 2 months of starting a bone treatment; formation markers require several more months before significant change is measurable. Prospective studies show an association of osteoporotic fractures with indices of bone turnover, independent of BMD (53–55). Hip fracture risk doubles in elderly women with values for resorption markers exceeding the reference range for premenopausal women. These studies suggest a combination approach, using BMD and biochemical markers of bone turnover to improve fracture prediction. Bone is continually being remodeled and changes in bone formation that are matched by appropriate, compensatory changes in bone resorption may not affect bone density. Thus, ideally measurements, particularly in clinical trials, should incorporate both types of markers. There is evidence, however, that bone tissue undergoing more active remodeling, even with formation and resorption in balance, may be more susceptible to fracture. The goal of a useful screening or monitoring blood test for osteoporosis remains elusive.

VI. Epidemiology of Systemic Corticosteroid Therapy and Osteoporosis

Approximately 30–50% of subjects chronically treated with systemic GCs develop osteoporosis (56). Prednisone dosages of less than 10 mg of prednisone per day result in a 10–12% annual reduction in the bone mineral content of the lumbar spine (40,41,57). Six milligrams of prednisone administered for 6 months results in significant osteopenia (58). The most rapid bone loss occurs during the first 6 to 12 months of GC therapy (59), but bone loss continues at a lower rate with more prolonged therapy (60). A retrospective, 15-year study examined bone loss in male asthmatic subjects treated with cumulative doses of systemic CS equivalent to 4 to 41 g of prednisone (61). Osteopenia occurred in 50% of subjects, 38% in the spine and 19% in the femoral neck. Regression analysis suggested that the largest cumulative GC dose without measurable bone loss was 5.6 g of prednisone. The National Osteoporosis Foundation recommends screening for osteoporosis if 7.5 mg prednisone or greater is administered for more than 1 month (62).

VII. Epidemiology of Inhaled Corticosteroid Therapy and Osteoporosis

Most of the literature concerning IGC and osteoporosis is with beclomethasone dipropionate (BDP), budsonide (BUD), and fluticasone (FLU). Conclusions concerning clinically significant effects are limited. There is convincing, consistent data showing that oral corticosteroid therapy has a greater effect on bone metabolism than therapeutically equivalent doses of IGC for asthma (63,64).

Data of IGC effects on biochemical markers of bone metabolism are inconclusive. Tartrate-resistant acid phosphatase (Table 5) levels are reduced in children receiving 300–800 μg/day of BDP (65). Doses of 800 μg/day of BUD in children were associated with reduced serum levels of procollagen type I carboxyterminal propeptide and cross-linked carboxyterminal telopeptide of type I collagen, suggesting a reduction in both formation and degradation of bone (Table 5) (66,67,68). Adult studies demonstrate a dose-dependent reduction in serum osteocalcin in subjects treated with 400–2000 μg/day of BDP (69,70). Serum osteocalcin was not suppressed by 1600 μg/day of BUD powered metered dose inhaler (pMDI) (71). BDP and BUD at doses of <800 μg/day had no effect on collagen propeptides (72). An increase in urinary hydroxyproline and a decrease in serum alkaline phosphatase occurs with 4 weeks of 2000 μg/day of BDP pMDI with a spacer but does not occur with 1800 μg/day of BUD (73). A comparison of 1-week therapy in healthy volunteers shows a decrease in collagen propeptide with both BUD and FLU at doses of 800–1600 and 750–1500 μg/day (74). In contrast, other reports show no effect in subjects with severe asthma treated with 1000 or 2000 μg/day of FLU or 1600 μg/day of BUD pMDI (75). A 3-year study of 51 subjects with asthma treated with high-dose ICS, mean 983 μg of BDP or BUD, shows no correlation with changes of bone density and a variety of bone metabolism markers (76). There is evidence that the relative potency of various CSs may vary for bone marker effects compared to adrenal suppression (64). Currently, serum bone turnover markers are not useful for making a diagnosis of osteoporosis or for selecting or screening high-risk, corticosteroid-treated subjects for BMD determination (77).

Interpretation of adult bone-density studies in subjects receiving ICS is complicated by intermittent systemic CS therapy before or during the study. Also, many of the comparisons are with normal, nonasthmatic adults, and this ignores any effect of asthma on bone density. The major studies in the medical literature addressing the issue of inhaled corticosteroid therapy and osteoporosis are summarized in Table 5 (78–92).

Published studies with ICSs are confusing, some showing reduced bone density (22,65,75,79,83,84,90) and others not (80,87,88). One report shows an effect only in women (86). A large cross-sectional study shows a decline in the bone density Z score of 0.5 standard deviations for each 1000 µg of ICS, BDP, or BUD via pMDI using a spacer (89). All postmenopausal women in the study received estrogen replacement therapy. Paradoxically, an increasing lifetime cumulative dose correlated with an increase in bone density and reduced fracture rate (Fig. 5). The suggested explanation was recovery of bone density because of reduced systemic GC therapy due to improved asthma control with IGCs. Two studies indicate that estrogen replacement therapy has a protective effect against ICS-induced bone loss (22,85). A cross-sectional study of asthmatic men and women, aged 20 to 40 years, demonstrates a reduction of T scores with increase

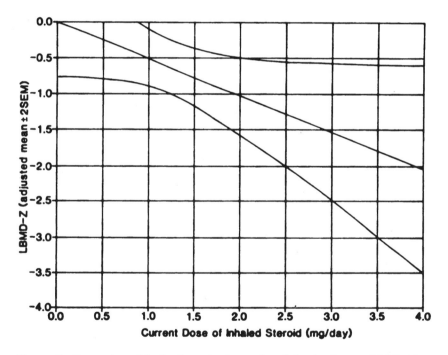

Figure 5 Regression of the lumbar spine bone mineral density Z score (LBMD-Z) (y axis) on the daily dose of inhaled corticosteroid (x axis). The values are adjusted to control for the effects of age, sex, years of estrogen use, physical activity, current daily dosage of prednisone, years of prednisone use, and cumulative lifetime dose of inhaled corticosteroid. The LBMD-Z declined significantly on the daily dosage of inhaled corticosteroid [$N = 0.013$, analysis of covariance (ANCOVA)]. (From Ref. 89.)

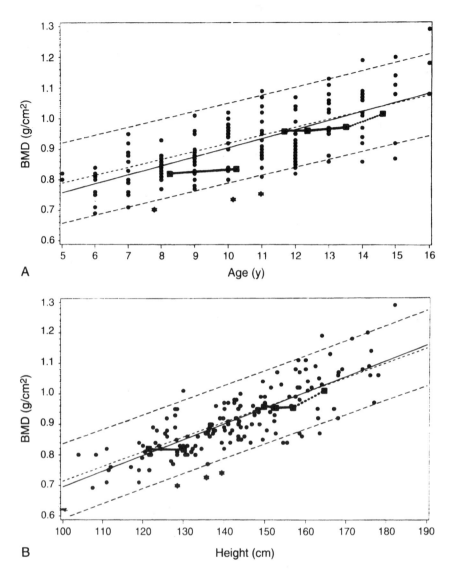

Figure 6 Individual bone mineral density (BMD) as a function of age (A) and height (B) in 157 children with asthma treated continuously for 3–6 years with inhaled budesonide (mean dosage 504 µg/day). The 95% prediction interval and mean regression lines from measurement in 111 children with asthma not treated with inhaled corticosteroids. Solid lines and squares represent measurements in two children receiving oral corticosteroid therapy. The dashed lines and squares indicate subsequent measurements in one child after discontinuation of oral prednisolone. Longitudinal measurement is depicted after systemic corticosteroid therapy was discontinued in one child (dashed line). (From Ref. 80.)

in ICS cumulative dosage (89a). A doubling of ICS cumulative dose reduces BMD by 0.16 SD at the lumbar spine, 8.14 SD at the femoral neck, 0.18 SD at Ward's triangle, and 0.13 SD at the trochanter. According to these results, a subject using 2000 μg ICS per day for 7 years would experience a decrease of 1 SD, probably doubling fracture risk (89a).

Data regarding osteoporosis secondary to IGCs in children are more limited compared to those of adults. Four cross-sectional studies (Fig. 6) (65,83,93,94) and two longitudinal investigations demonstrated no IGC effect on bone density (80,91). These six reports describe the changes in bone densitometry associated with 200–800 μg/day of BDP or BUD administered for 6 months to 4.5 years.

No increased occurrence of fractures has been detected in IGC-treated subjects without the presence of other osteoporosis risk factors. Two case reports describe fractures in two males treated 2 or more years with BDP at doses of 1500 μg to 3700 μg/day (95,96). Both of these individuals had other risk factors for osteoporosis. A radiographic, cross-sectional study of asthmatics shows a 56% occurrence of vertebral fractures in subjects receiving oral prednisone. There were significantly fewer fractures in a matched group treated with 600 μg/day of BDP (71).

These data are inconclusive concerning a causal relationship between IGC therapy and osteoporosis. It is likewise difficult to compare the various IGCs, although the majority of studies suggest that BDP has a greater effect, at equivalent efficacy doses, than BUD or FLU. Despite the lack of a consistent decrease in bone density with published studies of IGC, variable sensitivity among individuals limits the confidence that a given subject will not be affected by moderate-to high-dose IGC. This note of caution is supported by IGC effects on biochemical markers of bone metabolism.

VIII. Treatment of Osteoporosis

Effective pharmaceutical therapies for osteoporosis are available although optimal duration of treatment is not clear. Approved pharmacologic agents affect bone resorption without available agents specific for bone formation. Once osteoporosis develops it is unlikely normal BMD can be achieved, but fracture threshold may be improved even without significant improvement or normalization of BMD. Monitoring therapy to determine efficacy is another area of disagreement. Utilizing available data from treatment protocols for osteoporosis, subjects who do not improve in the 1st year of therapy improve during the 2nd year of treatment (97). Subjects who improve during the 1st year do not sustain the rate of increase in BMD during the 2nd year. The explanation for this phenomenon was a regression toward the mean for BMD testing. Thus, the utility of monitoring treatment with repeat BMD is open to question and to date no biochemical marker has been found to be useful for monitoring. Once pharmacologic therapy for osteopo-

Table 7 Summary Table of the Medical Literature Relating Inhaled Corticosteroid and Osteoporosis

Reference	Design	Treatment (dose and delivery device)	End points/outcomes
Wong et al. (2000)	Cross-sectional; 196 subjects, 119 women, age range 20–40 years; general practice recruitment; exclusion if systemic corticosteroid therapy in last 6 months or more than twice in lifetime	76% pMDI, 11% spacers; variable doses of beclamethasone (80%), budesonide (14%), fluticasone (6%); mean duration 6 years and median cumulative dose 876 mg	Negative correlation of cumulative inhaled corticosteroid and bone density—doubling dose decreased bone density 0.13–0.18 SD
Medici et al. (2000)	Double-blind, parallel group, multicenter; mild-to-moderate asthma; mean age 39 years; 67% men	Budesonide 800 or 1500 µg/day or Fluticasone 400–750 µg/day	Peripheral quantitative CT at baseline and q 6 months for 1 year; No effects on bone density
Laatikainen et al. (1999)	Cross-sectional; 3103 Finnish women 47–56 years of age compared to 119 women with asthma (28 without any corticosteroid therapy; 26 used inhaled only)	Belomethasone average dose 1100 µg/day (55 subjects); budesonide 800 µg/day (17 subjects); 8 used dry powder inhaler, 57 spacers	Subjects with asthma had lower DEXA BMD in spine and femoral head; inhaled corticosteroid duration of use correlated negatively with BMD; estrogen replacement was protective
Ebeling et al. (1998)	Cross-sectional; 53 subjects (34 female)	Oral corticosteroid >1 month during pass year and/or inhaled beclomethasone or budesonide ≥1500 µg/day	DEXA BMD decreased 1 s.d. with lumbar spine and femur; women affected more in spine with history of oral glucocorticoid, men affected more with hip; bone formation marker decreased, resorption normal

Lau (1998)	Cross-sectional; 146 subjects with asthma or COPD compared to 212 age-matched controls; 106/146 used inhaled glucocorticoid	Inhaled corticosteroid, current dose range 1400–4000 µg/day, mean dose 390–560 µg/day, cumulative dose 390–560 mg	DEXA BMD decreased in total body and spine in postmenopausal women with asthma DW not related to inhaled glucocorticoid; inhaled glucocorticoid negatively associated with BMD of femur in men; cigarette smoking associated with decreased BMD of femur, low calcium intake CT with spine
Agertoft and Pedersen (1998)	Cross-sectional; asthmatic children receiving inhaled steroid for 3–6 years (57); age-matched asthmatic steroid-naive controls (11)	Budesonide (0.2–1.3 mean, 0.5/spacer, DPI) for 4.5 years	DXA: lumbar/no difference in BMD between steroid and nonsteroid groups; bone density not related to treatment duration, accumulated or current dose of budesonide
Wisniewski et al. (1997)	Cross-sectional; receiving inhaled steroid (47); mean age, 32 years (28 women); unmatched asthmatic controls receiving no steroid (34); mean age, 28 years (15 women)	Beclomethasone dipropionate (n 41); budesonide (0.1–3.0); mean, 0.62/pMDI or DPI) for 7.8 years	DXA: lumbar, femur, radius/no difference in BMD between steroid vs. nonsteroid groups; cumulative inhaled dose associated with reduced lumbar BMD in women: no association with vertebral fracture

Table 7 Continued

Reference	Design	Treatment (dose and delivery device)	End points/outcomes
Luengo et al. (1997)	Longitudinal; receiving inhaled steroid (48); mean age 56 years (33 women); nonasthmatic controls (48)	Budesonide and/or beclomethasone (0.3–1.0, mean 0.66/device not specified) for 2 years	DXA: lumbar/no difference in BMD between asthmatics and nonasthmatics; no correlation with dose or duration of inhaled steroid; no difference between patients with or without course of oral steroid
Martinati et al. (1996)	Cross-sectional; receiving inhaled beclomethasone dipropionate (44); mean age, 6.7 years (prepubertal); matched asthmatic controls receiving cromolyn sodium (20)	Beclomethasone dipropionate (0.15–0.6); mean (0.32/device not specified) for 6.7 months	DXA: lumbar; DPA: radius/no effect of beclomethasone on BMD
Hanania et al. (1995)	Cross-sectional; receiving inhaled steroid (18); mean age, 37 years (12 women); matched asthmatic patients receiving no steroid (18)	Beclomethasone dipropionate and/or budesonide (0.8–2.0; mean 1.32/pMDI, spacer and DPI) for 30 months	DXA: lumbar, femur/inhaled dose and duration associated with reduced BMD in femoral neck; no reduction in BMD in lumbar spine or Wards triangle
Toogood et al. (1995)	Cross-sectional (69); mean age, 60 years (43 women, 41 postmenopausal) Taking inhaled steroid (69) Taking oral steroid (52)	Beclomethasone dipropionate and/or budesonide; mean, 1.3/spacer for 10.1 years Prednisone (mean, 3.0) for 10.7 years	DXA/DPA: lumbar/decreased BMD associated with daily dose of inhaled steroids and with years of prednisone therapy; increased BMD associated with years of supplemental estrogen therapy

Ip et al. (1994)	Cross-sectional; receiving inhaled steroid (30); mean age, 33 years (18 women); matched nonasthmatic controls (30)	Beclomethasone dipropionate and/ or budesonide (0.2–2.4, mean 1.1/device not specified) for 40 months	DXA: lumbar, femur/decreased BMD in asthmatic vs. nonasthmatic subjects, mainly women; association of daily inhaled dose and reduced lumbar BMD in women
Baraldi et al. (1994)	Longitudinal; receiving inhaled steroid (14); mean age, 9.1 years; matched asthmatic patients receiving no steroids (16)	Beclomethasone dipropionate (0.3–0.4/spacer) for 6 months	DXA: lumbar/no effects of beclomethasone on BMD
Herrala et al. (1994)	Longitudinal; women receiving inhaled steroids (19); mean age, 53 years (13 postmenopausal); matched nonasthmatic women (19; 13 postmenopausal)	Beclomethasone dipropionate (1.0/spacer) for 12 months	DXA: lumbar, femur/no effects of beclomethasone on BMD
Packe et al. (1992)	Cross-sectional receiving inhaled and intermittent systemic steroids (20); mean age, 38 years	Beclomethasone dipropionate (1.1–2.0/device not specified) for 3 years	CT: lumbar/reduced BMD in both beclomethasone and prednisolone groups vs. bronchodilator group
	Receiving inhaled and continuous systemic steroid (20); mean age, 39 years	Prednisolone (7 mg) for 8 years	
	Receiving no steroid (17); mean age, 36 years	Bronchodilators only	

Table 8 Recommended Daily
Calcium Intake

---

800 mg/day for 1–10 years of age
1200 mg/day for 11–12 years of age
1200 mg/day for pregnancy and lactation
1000 mg/day for adults >24 years of age
1500 mg/day for postmenopausal women

---

rosis is initiated the treatment may need to be for life, particularly if corticosteroid therapy cannot be discontinued.

Risk factors for osteoporosis have been identified, but many of these cannot be modified (Table 2). Furthermore, it is not consistently found that modification of risk factors always results in significant improvement. For example, lack of weight-bearing exercise is a known risk factor for osteoporosis, but it is not clear that starting a program of weight-bearing exercise significantly increases BMD. Thus, risk-factor reduction is based on good health practice and the hope that this will improve BMD.

A. Vitamin D and Calcium Supplements

Recommended daily intake of calcium is provided in Table 8. The National Osteoporosis Foundation recommends that all adults receive at least 1200 mg/day of elemental calcium; the average American diet provides less than 600 mg/day. Table 9 illustrates a simple method for estimating the calcium content of a diet. Increasing dietary calcium is the first-line approach, but calcium supplements should be used when an adequate dietary intake cannot be achieved. Vitamin D is required for absorption of oral calcium and physiologic supplementation (400

Table 9 Estimating Daily Dietary Calcium Intake

Product	No. of servings/day		Calcium content/ serving (mg)		Calcium (mg)
Step 1: Estimate calcium intake from dairy products[a]					
Milk (8 oz)	_____	×	300	=	_____
Yogurt (8 oz)	_____	×	400	=	_____
Cheese (1 oz)	_____	×	200	=	_____
Total					_____
Step 2: Dairy calcium + 250 mg for nondairy sources = Total dietary calcium					

[a] About 75 to 80% of the calcium consumed in American diets is from dairy products.

to 800 IU/day) is recommended. Vitamin D and oral calcium attenuate bone loss and reduce the general risk of fracture of the spine, hip, and other sites. However, these supplements do not increase bone mass in subjects with established osteoporosis. Optimizing daily calcium and vitamin D intake are recommended for all subjects with severe asthma.

A supraphysiologic dose of vitamin D, 50,000 units/week, was studied in the prevention of systemic CS-induced bone loss (98). Sixty-two subjects were included, a minority with asthma. High-dose vitamin D was of marginal benefit during the first 12 months but was of no value during the 2nd and 3rd years. High-dose vitamin D is associated with hypercalcemia and is not recommended for CS-induced bone loss.

B. Female Hormone Replacement

Oral estrogen hormone replacement (HRT) is proven effective for the prevention and treatment of postmenopausal osteoporosis (99–103). Transdermal estrogen is also effective (104). HRT is effective for CS-induced bone loss in one study of subjects with severe asthma treated with oral CS (103). Despite HRT's proven effectiveness, compliance with therapy is poor, with less than 20% taking HRT after 3 years (105). The rate of bone loss approximates that of menopause, 3–10% per year, if estrogen HRT is discontinued. Side effects of HRT include thromboembolic disease, increased risk of breast cancer, vaginal bleeding, and potential for uterine cancer if no previous hysterectomy. Reduction in cardiovascular disease risk with HRT has also been challenged.

C. Raloxifene

Selective estrogen receptor modulators are a new class of estrogen agonists and antagonists. Raloxifene, the only approved member of the class, increases BMD in postmenopausal osteoporosis without the associated treatment risk of increased uterine or breast cancer (106). However, raloxifene does not treat postmenopausal systemic symptoms and is associated with a two- to threefold increase in the risk of thromboembolism. Raloxifene has not been studied in CS-induced bone loss.

D. Bisphosphonates

Bisphosphonates inhibit bone resorption by suppressing osteoclast-mediated bone resorption. Etidronate, the first bisphosphonate to be approved in the United States for clinical use, should not be used continuously, as osteomalacia may occur. Therefore, etidronate is typically utilized cyclically, 2 weeks every 3 months. Etidronate is approved for Paget's disease but not osteoporosis. Alendronate and risedronate are the subsequently approved bisphosphonates with an indication for postmenopausal and CS-induced bone loss. All bisphosphonates tend to irritate the gastrointestinal tract, particularly the esophagus, and to be poorly absorbed with food.

Alendronate

Alendronate was studied in a double-blind, placebo-controlled prospective trial in CS-treated subjects with bone loss (107). The trial was of 1-year duration with 477 subjects; however, only 49 of these had airway obstruction with the majority having rheumatic conditions. The total group treated with both 5 and 10 mg/day of alendronate increased vertebral BMD by 2.1 and 2.9% respectively, $P <$ 0.0001, compared to placebo. The 49 subjects with airway disease increased vertebral BMD 1.9 and 3.7%, respectively. This study also demonstrated a reduction in vertebral fractures in postmenopausal women treated with alendronate, but there were insufficient numbers of postmenopausal women with airway disease to determine an effect in this subgroup. Another study showed alendronate added to HRT has a greater effect on vertebral BMD than estrogen alone, but this study did not include CS-treated subjects (108). Alendronate is approved for treatment of CS-induced bone loss.

Risedronate

Risedronate is approved in the United States for treatment and prevention of postmenopausal osteoporosis and CS-induced osteoporosis (oral prednisone or equivalent >7.5 mg/day). Risedronate has not been studied in asthma or COPD populations with CS-induced bone loss. Risedronate increased BMD in both axial and appendicular skeleton in CS-treated subjects. Vertebral fracture incidence after 1 year of CS-bone loss treatment decreased from 15% in the placebo group to 5% in the risedronate group, a relative risk reduction of 70% (109). Side effects are similar to placebo in the 5700 subjects treated up to 3 years in phase 3 trials. However, experience with risedronate is much less than with alendronate, and esophageal and gastrointestinal side effects have been reported after approval and widespread use.

Etidronate

Etidronate, administered in 2-week cycles every 3 months, has been extensively studied for treatment of CS-induced osteoporosis (110–116). Most of these studies are small, 39 to 68 subjects, and all but one include CS-treated subjects with rheumatic conditions. All of these studies show a beneficial effect in vertebral BMD compared to placebo but not necessarily increased from baseline. A prospective, 1.5-year study of asthmatic subjects treated with ICS (<1.5 g/day of BDP or BUD) demonstrated a 2.8% increase in spine BMD with etidronate plus calcium. However, the control group, treated with 1000 mg/day of calcium, also increased 2.2%, resulting in no statistical benefit of etidronate (116). This degree of improvement with calcium alone is atypical. The majority of studies demonstrate beneficial effects with etidronate therapy of CS-induced bone loss, including populations with airway disease. Etidronate is not approved for treatment of osteoporosis.

Clodronate

Clodronate is not approved for the treatment of osteoporosis in the United States. A 1-year, randomized, placebo-controlled trial showed increased BMD in 74 asthmatic subjects treated with oral corticosteroid (mean 8.3 mg/day prednisone or equivalent) and/or ICS (117). The control group had no change in BMD, whereas the clodronate treated group increased 3.0% at the lumbar spine and 4.3% at the femoral neck.

E. Calcitonin

Calcitonin is a polypeptide hormone which suppresses osteoclast activity and bone resorption. Intranasal (200 IU/day with one spray) and subcutaneous (100 IU) formulations of calcitonin are approved in the United States for prevention and treatment of postmenopausal osteoporosis. Calcitonin may be more effective for the axial than appendicular skeleton. One study is available investigating nasal calcitonin in CS-treated asthmatic subjects (118). A statistically significant 2.8% increase in spinal BMD was detected after 2 years of calcitonin therapy compared to 7.8% decrease in the placebo group. However, 35% of calcitonin-treated subjects withdrew due to side effects, primarily nausea and nasal irritation, or uncontrolled asthma. Other trials of CS-treated subjects without asthma have not detected such robust increases in spinal BMD. Vertebral fracture rate decreases with calcitonin therapy of postmenopausal osteoporosis, but no studies are available for fractures in CS-treated subjects.

F. Thiazide Diuretics

Thiazide diuretics and sodium restriction improve gastrointestinal absorption of calcium and reduce urinary excretion of calcium. Systemic CSs may reduce calcium absorption, which results in an increase in parathyroid hormone. The positive calcium balance effects of thiazide diuretics and sodium restriction would be predicted to ameliorate this possible secondary hyperparathyroidism resulting from CS therapy. Thiazide therapy has not been assessed in CS-treated individuals. However, thiazide diuretic therapy, 25 mg/day of hydrochlorothiazide, has been associated with higher bone density and a modest reduction in fracture risk in subjects not receiving corticosteroids (119). Thiazide diuretics, if indicated, should be used in combination with potassium-sparing diuretics, such as triamterene, to avoid hypokalemia.

G. Testosterone

Several studies demonstrate a decrease in serum testosterone in males treated with CS (120–122). A 1-year, unblinded study of monthly testosterone injections (250 mg/month) shows an increase in lumbar BMD and decrease in serum bone resorption markers in asthmatic males treated with CS (123). Assessment of serum testosterone levels is a consideration in males with osteoporosis or with an increased osteoporosis risk.

H. Fluoride

Fluoride salts are not approved in the United States for treatment of osteoporosis. Sodium fluoride stimulates bone formation, contrasting with the approved pharmacologic agents which interfere with absorption or bone loss. The long-term safety of oral fluoride is debated (124). BMD usually increases with therapy but this may not result in fracture reduction. The implication is that fluoride therapy leads to abnormally calcified bone. Fluoride compounds have been utilized in GC-induced bone loss. A group of 35 severe asthmatic subjects receiving chronic GC therapy were studied in a double-blind, placebo-controlled trial comparing fluoride plus calcium supplementation to calcium alone (125). After 2 years, the fluoride-treated group demonstrated a significant increase in lumbar spine BMD ($P = 0.05$). Fracture rates did not differ between the two groups. An 18-month study of CS-treated subjects, 44% with pulmonary diseases, showed an increase in lumbar spine BMD with fluoride therapy (7.8% increase) versus calcium supplementation alone (3.6% increase). The most common side effect reported with fluoride salt therapy is gastrointestinal discomfort. There remains a potential for fluoride therapy of osteoporosis, but a study showing fracture rate reduction is needed.

IX. Risk Stratification of Subjects with Asthma

The ideal strategy in asthma is to discontinue systemic GC, to use the lowest dose of IGC possible, and to utilize other measures to maximize bone density. These include sufficient calcium and vitamin D ingestion, regular weight-bearing exercise, avoidance of cigarette smoking, and minimizing ethanol ingestion and hormone supplementation in subjects deficient in sex hormones (126). Controlled treatment data with osteoporosis associated with ICS is generally lacking, with recommendations based on studies in systemically corticosteroid-treated subjects and perimenopausal osteoporosis. Consensus recommendations for physicians treating at-risk asthmatic populations have been published (126).

Physicians treating severe asthma may need to evaluate and treat patients of all ages. The prevalence of osteoporosis will increase with the aging of the population. Therefore, health providers should counsel all their patients concerning osteoporosis. The following are recommendations based on available medical literature review and consensus (see Table 10).

A. Low Risk

Subjects treated with inhaled corticosteroid dosages of no more than 800 μg/day of beclomethasone dipropionate or equivalent for adults and no more than 400 μg/day of BDP or equivalent for children have a risk of osteoporosis similar to the general population. Nasal corticosteroid doses should be added to the amount used to treat asthma for total corticosteroid load for both adults and children. No more than one other risk factor for osteoporosis should be present (Tables 1 and 2).

1. Maintain adequate calcium intake. Calcium intake is critical during the growing years, especially in adolescence, when bone growth is maximal (127). Calcium supplementation or increased dietary calcium is

Table 10 Summary of Risk Assessment and Treatment Recommendations

Risk	Recommendations
Low Adult ≤800 μg/day BDP Child ≤400 μg/day BDP	Adequate calcium, Vitamin D; weight-bearing exercise; no tobacco, limited alcohol; check TSH in patient with history of thyroid abnormality
Medium Adult >800 μg/day BDP Child >400 μg/day BDP	As above plus measure height annually; consider estrogen in postmenopausal women without contraindications; consider DEXA if inhaled corticosteroid dose >1200 μg/day for adults or >600 μg/day for children; alternative to DEXA in adults is alendronate or risedronate 5 mg/day if no contraindication
High Chronic systemic corticosteroid or systemic corticosteroid >4 Continuous weeks or more than 4–7 "bursts"/year	As above plus DEXA; consider 24-h urine for those receiving chronic systemic corticosteroid; measure free testosterone in men and consider replacement if low

Note. Adapted from Ref. 126.

important if milk and dairy products are to be avoided, such as with food allergy or intolerance. Detailed recommendations for patients can be found in *Boning Up on Osteoporosis. A Guide to Prevention and Treatment* (National Osteoporosis Foundation, 1997)

2. Encourage exercise, particularly weight-bearing exercise. Specific exercise recommendations are available in *Boning Up on Osteoporosis* (see Ref. 1).

3. Supplement diet with vitamin D, particularly if sunlight exposure is limited. Although vitamin D is found in egg yolks, salt-water fish, liver, and vitamin D fortified milk, milk is the only significant dietary source and not drinking milk is a risk factor for osteoporosis. Individuals who are ill with a chronic disease may have a greater need for vitamin D than normals.

4. Discourage cigarette smoking and excessive ethanol ingestion.

5. Ensure euthyroid status for patients on thyroid supplementation by measuring TSH at regular intervals.

6. Use the lowest effective corticosteroid dose and/or topical preparations whenever possible. As recommended by the 1997 NHLBI Guidelines (1), always try to lower the corticosteroid dosage when therapeutic goals have been met.

B. Moderate Risk

Adult subjects treated for more than 6 weeks with >800 μg/day or equivalent of inhaled beclomethasone dipropionate or children treated with >400 μg/day or equivalent of BDP have a potential risk of osteoporosis. Nasal corticosteroid dosages should be added to the amount used to treat asthma for total corticosteroid load for both adults and children. If two or more additional osteoporosis risk factors are present, consider evaluating as high risk (Table 1 and 2).

1. Follow low-risk recommendations. Review calcium and vitamin D intake and other risk factors (see Table 1).

2. Measure height annually. Asymptomatic vertebral compression fractures are common in subjects with osteoporosis. If an adult loses more than 1 in. of height, bone densitometry should be considered. Stadiometer is the preferred method of assessing height, since this technique will more likely be sensitive to early changes. A lateral thoracolumbar spine radiograph should be considered to evaluate compression fractures. If either height decreases or lateral spine radiograph is abnormal, evaluation as a high-risk subject is suggested. Children or adolescents

whose growth rate declines are a special concern. Evaluation for causes of growth delay and review of asthma therapy, particularly corticosteroid therapy, should occur. Bone densitometry may be indicated.

3. Consider estrogen replacement therapy for postmenopausal women who are without identified contraindications.
4. Consider bone densitometry.

C. High Risk

Subjects who are treated with chronic systemic corticosteroid therapy or systemic therapy for more than four contiguous weeks or who receive more than four 7-day bursts of systemic corticosteroids per year have an increased risk of osteoporosis. Some authorities would recommend the addition of low-dose alendronate (5 mg/day) or residronate (5 mg/day) in high-risk subjects pending bone densitometry studies or during intermittent systemic corticosteroid therapy. Bisphosphonate therapy is more strongly indicated if other osteoporosis risk factors are present (Tables 1 and 2).

1. Follow low-risk recommendations. Review calcium and vitamin D intake and other risk factors (see Table 1).
2. Assess bone density. If the T score is decreased more than 1 standard deviation below the mean, then initiate evaluation and treatment or refer to an authority in osteoporosis management.
3. Consider obtaining a 24-h urine collection for calcium and creatinine for individuals receiving chronic, systemic corticosteroid therapy (see below).

D. Evaluation

The following levels may need to be evaluated: serum calcium, creatinine, phosphorous, alkaline phosphatase, liver transaminases, TSH, estradiol in premenopausal women with change in their menstrual cycle, free testosterone in males, and 24-h urine for calcium and creatinine. Additional studies considered by osteoporosis specialists include determining the 25-OH vitamin D serum level in select cases (e.g., malabsorption, poor dietary intake, or chronic liver disease) and parathyroid hormone levels in cases of hypercalcemia.

E. Treatment

Estrogen replacement therapy for women who have no contraindications for such therapy and who are postmenopausal or with hypogonadal function. Evaluation for estrogen replacement therapy includes breast exam, pelvic exam, and mammography. Raloxifene (60 mg/day) is an alternative if breast or uterine cancer is a concern.

Testosterone therapy for men with low free testosterone levels should be considered. Pretreatment evaluation should include a digital examination of the prostate and a prostate-specific antigen (PSA) level.

An oral bisphosphonate or calcitonin is recommended for osteoporosis. The bisphosphonates available are cyclic etidronate (400 mg/day for 2 weeks every 3 months), oral alendronate (10 mg/day), or residronate (5 mg/day). Evaluation of suspected swallowing disorders may be necessary prior to alendronate or risedronate therapy. Alendronate or risedronate may be difficult to administer if there are any swallowing difficulties. Calcitonin at doses of 200 IU/day by nasal spray or 100 IU/day by subcutaneous injection is an alternative therapy. Nasal calcitonin may be mildly irritating to the nasal mucosa. Lower dose alendronate (5 mg/day) or risedronate (5 mg/day) is utilized by some authorities if BMD is decreased but not below -1.0 s.d. Dosage of alendronate would be increased to 10 mg/day if BMD is more severely decreased, but the dosage of risedronate is the same in both situations.

A thiazide combined with amiloride should be considered if the 24-h urine calcium level is more than 300 mg/24 h or if there is a history of ureterolithiasis. The serum potassium level should be monitored.

Additional assessments such as bone biopsy or additional treatment utilizing low-dose parathyroid hormone, growth hormone, fluoride therapy, high-dose vitamin D (greater than 800 U/day), or $1,25\text{-}(OH)_2\text{-}$vitamin D should be supervised by a bone disease specialist.

F. Special Consideration for Children and Adolescents

Long-term use of systemic corticosteroids is associated with osteoporosis in younger age groups (128,129). Furthermore, corticosteroid use in these age groups may result in failure to achieve peak bone mass, a risk for osteoporosis later in life (65,130–132). While alternate-day A.M. dosing of prednisone does not appear to protect against osteoporosis for any age group, such dosing in children is more likely to preserve normal linear growth (95). Whether or not the long-term use of inhaled steroids causes osteoporosis is an area for study (95,133,134).

X. Summary

Long-term use of ICS has a variably documented effect on BMD. Confounding interpretation of the studies are effects of previous or concurrent systemic CS therapy, variable study designs, limited population size, variable dosing and duration of multiple CSs, and differing severity of asthma among the published studies. The threshold for decrease in BMD may vary for the different ICSs. Suggested threshold doses for adverse effects on BMD based on available data are 800 to 1200 µg/day for BDP, 800–1000 µg/day for BUD, 750 µg/day for FLU, and >1000 µg/day for flunisolide. Data for triamcinolone are more limited but likely to be similar to those for flunisolide. Most of the data are derived from studies using metered dose inhaler delivery systems and the results may or may not apply to other systems, such as dry powder.

A small increase in the relative risk of osteoporosis would have important public health considerations. Inhaled CSs are widely prescribed [one of six subjects with asthma in the UK receive more than 800 µg/day (135)] and asthma is a common condition. Thus, any aggravating effect of CSs, either inhaled or systemic, upon osteoporosis could have significant repercussions. A cautious, cost-effective approach is a reasonable starting point, based on the information available. Risk stratification coupled with utilizing the lowest effective dose of CS may optimize the utilization of health care resources in containing this problem.

References

1. Expert Panel Report II. Guidelines for the Diagnosis and Management of Asthma. Bethesda, MD: Public Health Service, National Institutes of Health, 1997.
2. Raisz LG. The osteoporosis revolution. Ann Intern Med 1997; 126:458–462.
3. American College of Rheumatology Task Force on Osteoporosis Guidelines. Recommendation for the prevention and treatment of glucocorticoid-induced osteoporosis. Arth Rheum 1996; 39:1791–1801.
4. Consensus development conference: Diagnosis, prophylaxis and treatment of osteoporosis. Am J Med 1991; 91:1S–68S.
5. Dempster DW, Shone E, Horbert W, Lindsay R. A simple method for correlative light and scanning electron microscopy of human iliac crest bone biopsies: qualitative observations in normal and osteoporotic subjects. J Bone Miner Res 1986; 1: 15–21.
6. Weinstein RE, Lobocki CA, Gravett S, Hum H, Negrich R, Herbst J, Greenberg D, Peiper DR. Decreased adrenal sex steroid levels in the absence of glucocorticoid suppression in postmenopausal asthmatic women. J Allergy Clin Immunol 1996; 97:1–8.
7. Kanis JA and the WHO Study Group. Assessment of fracture risk and its application to screening for postmenopausal osteoporosis: synopsis of a WHO Report. Osteoporos Int 1994; 4:368–381.
8. Looker AC, Orwoll ES, Johnston CC Jr, Lindsay RL, Wahner HW, Dunn WL, Calvo MS, Harris TB, Heys SP. Prevalence of low femoral bone density in older U.S. adults from NHANES III. J Bone Miner Res 1997; 12:1761–1768.
9. Melton LJ, Atkinson EJ, O'Connor MK, O'Fallon WM, Riggs BL. Bone density and fracture risk in men. J Bone Miner Res 1998; 13:1915–1923.

10. Melton LJ III. Epidemiology of fractures. In Riggs BL, Melton LJ III, eds. Osteoporosis: Etiology, Diagnosis and Management. 2nd ed. Philadelphia: Lippincott–Raven, 1995:225–247.

11. Oden A, Dawson A, Dere W, Johnell O, Jonsson B, Kanis JA. Lifetime risk of hip fractures is underestimated. Osteoporosis Int 1998; 8:599–603.

12. Chrischilles EA, Butler CD, Davis CS, Wallace RB. A model of lifetime osteoporosis impact. Arch Intern Med 1991; 151:2026–2032.

13. Poor G, Jacobsen SJ, Melton LJ III. Mortality following hip fracture: Facts and research in gerontology. J Bone Miner Res 1994; 7:91–109.

14. Jones G, White C, Nguyen T, Sambrook PN, Kelly PJ, Eisman JA. Prevalent vertebral deformities: relationship to bone mineral density and spinal osteophytosis in elderly men and women. Osteoporos Int 1996; 6:233–239.

15. O'Neill TW, Felsenberg D, Varlow J, Cooper C, Kanis JA, Silman AJ and the European Vertebral Osteoporosis Study Group. The prevalence of vertebral deformity in European men and women: The European Vertebral Osteoporosis Study. J Bone Miner Res 1996; 11:1010–1018.

16. Lau EMC, Chan HHL, Woo J, Lin F, Black D, Nevitt M, Lenng PC. Normal ranges for vertebral height ratios and prevalence of vertebral fracture in Hong Kong Chinese: a comparison with American Caucasians. J Bone Miner Res 1996; 11:1364–1368.

17. Jacobsen SJ, Cooper C, Gottlieb MS, Goldberg J, Yahnke DP, Melton LJ III. Hospitalization with vertebral fracture among the aged: a national population-based study, 1986–1989. Epidemiology 1992; 3:515–518.

18. Bauer RL, Deyo RA. Low risk of vertebral fracture in Mexican American Women. Arch Intern Med 1987; 147:1437–1439.

19. Greendale GA, Barrett-Connor E, Ingles S, Haile R. Late physical and functional effects of osteoporotic fracture in women: The Rancho Bernardo Study. J Am Geriatr Soc 1995; 43:955–961.

20. Cooper C, Atkinson EJ, Jacobsen SJ, O'Fallon WM, Melton LJ III. Population-based study of survival after osteoporotic fractures. Am J Epidemiol 1993; 137:1001–1005.

21. Ray NF, Chan JK, Thamer M, Melton LJ III. Medical expenditures for the treatment of osteoporotic fractures in the United States in 1995: report from the National Osteoporosis Foundation. J Bone Miner Res 1997; 12:24–35.

22. Laatikainen AK, Kroger HPJ, Tukiainen HO, Honkanen RJ, Saarikoski SV. Bone mineral density in perimenopausal women with asthma: a population-based cross-sectional study. Am Respir Crit Care Med 1999; 159:1179–1185.

23. Lau EMC, Li M, Woo J, Lai C. Bone mineral density and body composition in patients with airflow obstruction—the role of inhaled steroid therapy, disease and lifestyle. Clin Exp Allergy 1998; 28:1066–1071.

23a. Lukert BP, Raisz LG. Glucocorticoid-induced osteoporosis. Rheum Dis Clin North Am 1994; 20:630–651.

24. Garnero P, Gineyts E, Riou JP, Delmas PD. Assessment of bone resorption with a new marker of collagen degradation in patients with metabolic bone disease. J Clin Endocrinol Metab 1994; 79:780–785.

25. Delmas PD. Clinical use of biochemical markers of bone remodeling in osteoporosis. Bone 1992; 13:517–521.

26. Hanson DA, Weis M-AE, Bollen A-M, Maslan SL, Singer FR, Eyre DR. A specific immunoassay for monitoring human bone resorption: quantitation of type I collagen crosslinked *N*-telopeptides in urine. J Bone Miner Res 1992; 7:1251–1258.

27. Peck WA, Brand J, Miller I. Hydrocortisone-induced inhibition of protein synthesis and uridine incorporation in isolated bone cells in vitro. Proc Natl Acad Sci USA 1967; 57:1599–1606.

28. Fucik RF, Kukreja SC, Hargis GK, Bowser EN, Henderson WJ, Williams GA. Effect of glucocorticoids on function of the parathyroid glands I man. J Clin Endocrin Metab 1975; 41:152.

29. Pearce G, Tabensky DA, Delmas PD, et al. Corticosteroid-induced bone loss in men. J Clin Endocrin Metabol 1998; 83:801–806.

30. Hahn TJ, Halstead LR, Strates B, Imbimbo B, Baran T. Comparison of subacute effects of oxazacort and prednisone on mineral metabolism in man. Calcif Tissue Int 1980; 31:109–115.

31. Lekkerkerker JF, Van Woudenberg F, Doorenbos HD. Influence of low dose of steroid therapy on calcium absorption. Acta Endocrinol (Copenh) 1972; 69:488–496.

32. Sjoberg HE. Retention of orally administered 47-calcium in man under normal diseased conditions: studies with a whole-body counter technique. Acta Med Scand 1970; 509:1–28.

33. Chesney RW, Mazess RB, Hamstra AJ, DeLuca HF, O'Reagan S. Reduction of serum 1,25-dihydroxyvitamin D in children receiving glucocorticoids. Lancet 1978; 2:1123–1125.

34. Godschalk M, Levy J, Downs RW. Glucocorticoids decrease vitamin D receptor numbers and gene expression in human osteosarcoma cells. J Bone Miner Res 1992; 7:21–27.

35. Kimberg DV, Baerg DV, Gershon E, Graudusius RT. Effects of cortisone administration on the metabolism and localization of 25-hydroxy-cholecalciferol in the rat. J Clin Invest 1971; 50:1309–1321.

36. Crilly RG, Cawood M, Marshall DH, Nordin BE. Hormonal status in normal, osteoporotic and corticosteroid-treated postmenopausal women. J R Soc Med 1978; 71:733.

37. Doerr P, Pirke KM. Cortisol-induced suppression of plasma testosterone in normal adult males. J Clin Endocrin Metabol 1976; 43:622–629.

38. World Health Organization. Assessment of fracture risk and its application to screening for post-menopausal osteoporosis. WHO Tech Rep Ser 1994; 843:5–6.

39. Johnston CC Jr, Slemenda CW, Melton LF III. Clinical use of bone densitometry. N Engl J Med 1991; 324:1105–1108.

40. Verstraeten A, Dequeker J. Vertebral and peripheral bone mineral content and fracture incidence in postmenopausal patients with rheumatoid arthritis: effect of low dose corticosteroids. Ann Rheum Dis 1986; 45:852–857.

41. Buckley LM, Leib ES, Cartularo KS, Vacek PM, Cooper SM. Effects of low dose corticosteroids on the bone mineral density of patients with rheumatoid arthritis. J Rheumatol 1995; 22:1055–1059.

42. Riggs BC, Wahner HW, Seeman E, Offord KP, Dunn WL, Mazess RB, et al. Changes in bone mineral density of the proximal femur and spine with aging. J Clin Invest 1982; 70:716–723.

43. Saito JK, Davis JW, Wasnich RD, Ross PD, Users of low dose glucocorticoids have increase bone loss rates, a longitudinal study. Calcif Tissue Int 1995; 57:115–119.

44. Kanis JA, Delmas P, Burckhardt P, Cooper C, Togerson D. Guidelines for diagnosis and management of osteoporosis. Osteoporosis Int 1997; 7:390–406.

45. Kanis JA, Gluer CC. An update on the diagnosis and assessment of osteoporosis with densitometry. Osteoporosis Int 2000; 11:192–202.

46. DeLaet CEDH, Van Hout BA, Burger H, Hofman A, Weel AEAM, Pols HAP. Hip fracture prediction in elderly men and women: validation in the Rotterdam Study. J Bone Miner Res 1998; 13:1587–1593.

47. DeLaet CEDH, Van Hout BA, Burger H, Hofman A, Pols HAP. Bone density and risk of hip fracture in men and women: cross sectional analysis. Br Med J 1997; 315:221–225.

48. Melton LJ, Atkinson EJ, O'Connor MK, O'Fallon WM, Riggs BL. Bone density and fracture risk in men. J Bone Miner Res 1999; 13:1915–1923.

49. Faulkner KH, von Stetten E, Steiger P, Miller P. Discrepancies in osteoporosis prevalence at different skeletal sites: impact on the WHO criteria. Bone 1998; 23: S194 [abstract].

50. Grampp S, Genant HK, Mathur A, Lang P, Jergas M, Takada M, Gluer CC, Lu Y, Chavez M. Comparisons of non-invasive bone mineral measurements in assessing age related loss, fracture discrimination and diagnostic classification. J Bone Miner Res 1997; 12:697–711.

51. Kanis JA. An update on the diagnosis of osteoporosis. Curr Rheumatol Rep 1999; 2:62–66.

52. Marshall D, Johnell O, Wedel H. Meta-analysis of how well measure of bone mineral density predict occurrence of osteoporosis fractures. Br Med J 1996; 312:124–159.

53. Riis BJ. The role of bone loss. Am J Med 1995; 98(suppl 2A):29–32.

54. Hansen M, Overgaard K, Riis B, Christiansen C. Role of peak bone mass and bone loss in postmenopausal osteoporosis: 12 year study. Br Med J 1991; 303:961–964.

55. Ganero P, Hause E, Chapuy MC, Marcelli C, Grandjean H, Muller C, Cormier C, Breard G, Meunier PJ, Delmas PD. Markers of bone turnover predict hip fractures in elderly women. The EPIDOS prospective study. J Bone Min Res 1996; 11:1531–1538.

56. Adinoff AD, Hollister JR. Steroid-induced fractures and bone loss in patients with asthma. N Engl J Med 1983; 309:265–268.

57. Ruegsegger P, Medici TC, Anliker M. Corticosteroid-induced bone loss: a longitudinal study of alternate-day therapy in patients with bronchial asthma using quantitative computed tomography. Eur J Clin Pharmacol 1994; 25:615–620.

58. Pearce G, Ryan PFJ, Delmas PD, et al. The deleterious effects of low-dose corticosteroids on bone density in patients with polymyalgia rheumatica. Br J Rheumatol 1998; 37:292–299.

59. Gennari C. Glucocorticoids and bone. In: Peck WA, ed. Bone and Mineral Research. Amsterdam: Elsevier; 1985:213–232.

60. LoCascio V, Bonucci E, Imbimbo B, Ballanti P, Adami S, Milani S, et al. Bone loss in response to long-term glucocorticoid therapy. J Bone Miner Res 1990; 8: 39–51.

61. Villareal MS, Kaustermeyer WB, Hahn TJ, et al. Osteoporosis in steroid-dependent asthma. Ann Allergy Asthma Immunol 1996; 76:369–372.

62. Johnston CC, Melton LJ, Lindsay R, et al. Clinical indications for bone mass measurements. J Bone Miner Res 1989; 4:1354–1350.

63. Hodsman AB, Toogood JH, Jennings B, et al. Differential effects of inhaled budesonide and oral prednisolone on serum osteocalcin. J Clin Endocrinol Metab 1991; 72:530–540.

64. Jennings BH, Andersen K-E, Johansson S-A. Assessment of systemic effects of inhaled glucocorticoids: Comparison of the effect of inhaled budesonide and oral prednisolone on adrenal function and markers of bone turnover. Eur J Pharmacol 1991; 40:77–82.

65. Konig P, Hillman L, Cervantes C, Levine C, Maloney C, Douglas R, et al. Bone metabolism in children with asthma treated with inhaled beclomethasone dipropionate. J Pediatr 1993; 122:219–226.

66. Sorva R, Turpeinen M, Juntunen Backmann K, et al. Effects of inhaled budesonide on serum markers of bone metabolism in children with asthma. J Allergy Clin Immunol 1992; 90:808–815.

67. Wolthers OD, Juul A, Hansen M, et al. Growth factors and collagen markers in asthmatic children treated with inhaled budesonide. Eur Respir J 1993; 6(suppl 17): 261S.

68. Wolthers OD, Juul A, Hansen M, et al. The insulin-like growth factor axis and collagen turnover in asthmatic children treated with inhaled budesonide. Acta Paediatr 1995; 84:393–397.

69. Pouw EM, Prummel MF, Oosing H, et al. Beclomethasone inhalation decreases serum osteocalcin concentrations. Br Med J 1991; 302:627–628.

70. Teelucksingh S, Padfield PL, Tibi L, et al. Inhaled corticosteroid, bone formation and osteocalcin. Lancet 1991; 338:60–61.

71. M, Del Rio L, Guanabens N, et al. Long-term effect of oral and inhaled glucocorticoids on bone mass in chronic asthma: a two year follow-up study. Eur Respir J 1991; 4:342s.

72. Kerstjen HA, Postma DS, van Doormaal JJ, et al. Effects of short-term and long-term treatment with inhaled corticosteroids on bone metabolism in patients with airways obstruction: Dutch CNSLD Study Group. Thorax 1994; 49: 652–656.

73. Ali NJ, Capewell S, Ward MJ. Bone turnover during high dose inhaled corticosteroid treatment. Thorax 1991; 46:160–164.

74. Grove A, Allam C, McFarlane LC, et al. A comparison of systemic bioactivity of inhaled budesonide and fluticasone priopionate in normal subjects. Br J Clin Pharmacol 1994; 8:527–532.

75. Ayres JG, Bateman ED, Lundback B, et al. High dose fluticasone propionate, 1 mg daily, versus fluticasone propionate, 2 mg daily, or budesonide, 1.6 mg daily, in patients with chronic severe asthma: International Study Group. Eur Respir J 1995; 8:579–586.

76. Boulet L-P, Milot J, Gagnon L, et al. Long-term influence of inhaled corticosteroids in bone metabolism and density: are biological markers predictors of bone loss: Am J Respir Crit Care Med 1999; 159:838–844.

77. Toogood JH, Hodsman AB, Fraher LJ, Markov AE, Baskerville JC. Serum osteo-calcin and procollagen as markers for the risks of osteoporotic fracture in cortico-steroid-treated asthmatic adults. J Allergy Clin Immunol 1999; 104:769–774.

78. Lipworth MJ. Systemic adverse effects of inhaled corticosteroid therapy: a system-atic review and meta-analysis. Arch Intern Med 1999; 179:941–955.

79. Ebeling PR, Erbas B, Hopper JL, Wark JD, Rubinfeld AR. Bone mineral density and bone turnover in asthmatic treated with long-term inhaled or oral glucocorti-coids. J Bone Miner Res 1998; 13:1283–1289.

80. Agertoft L, Pedersen S. Bone mineral density on children with asthma receiving long term treatment with inhaled budesonide. Am J Respir Crit Care Med 1998; 157:178–183.

81. Wisniewski AF, Lewis SA, Green DJ, Maslanka W, Burrel H, Tattersfield AE. Cross section investigation of the effects of inhaled corticosteroids on bone density and bone metabolism in patients with asthma. Thorax 1997; 52:853–860.

82. Luengo M, del Rio L, Pons F, Picado C. Bone mineral density in asthmatic patients treated with inhaled corticosteroids: a case-control study. Eur Respir J 1997; 10: 2110–2113.

83. Martinati B, Bertoldo F, Gasperi E, Micelli S, Boner AL. Effect on cortical and trabecular bone mass of different anti-inflammatory treatments in preadolescent children with chronic asthma. Am J Respir Crit Care Med 1996; 153:232–236.

84. Egan J, Kalra S, Adams J. A randomised double blind study comparing the ef-fects of beclomethasone dipropionate 2000 μg/day versus fluticasone propionate 1000μg/day on bone density over 2 years. Thorax 1995; 50(suppl 2):A78.

85. Hanania NA, Chapman KR, Sturtridge WC, et al. Dose-related decrease in bone density among asthmatic patients treated with inhaled corticosteroid. J Allergy Clin Immunol 1995; 96:571–579.

86. Marystone JF, Barrett Connor EL, Morton DJ. Inhaled and oral corticosteroids: their effects on bone mineral density in older adults. Am J Public Health 1995; 85: 1693–1695.

87. Herrala J, Puolifoki H, Impivaara O, et al. Bone mineral density in asthmatic women on high-dose inhaled beclomethasone dipropionate. Bone 1994; 15:621–623.

88. Medici TC, Grebski E, Hacki M, Ruegsegger P, Maden C, Efthimiou J. Effect of one year treatment with inhaled fluticasone propionate or beclomethasone dipropio-nate on bone density and bone metabolism: a randomised parallel group study in adult asthmatic subjects. Thorax 2000; 55:375–382.

89. Toogood JH, Baskerville J, Markov AE, et al. Bone mineral density and the risk of fracture in patients receiving long-term inhaled steroid therapy for asthma. J Allergy Clin Immunol 1995; 96:157–166.

89a. Wong CA, Walsh LJ, Smith CJ, et al. Inhaled corticosteroid use and bone mineral density in patients with asthma. Lancet 2000; 355:1399–1403.

90. Ip M, Lam K, Yam L, Kung A, Ng M. Decreased bone mineral density in premeno-pausal asthma patients receiving long-term inhaled steroids. Chest 1994; 105:1722–1727.

91. Baraldi E, Bolline MC, De Marchi A, Zacchello F. Effect of beclomethasone di-propionate on bone mineral content assessed by x-ray densitometry in asthmatic children: a longitudinal evaluation. Eur Respir J 1994; 7:710–714.

92. Packe GE, Douglas JG, McDonald AF, Robins SP, Reid DM. Bone density in asthmatic patients taking high dose inhaled beclomethasone and intermittent systemic corticosteroids. Thorax 1992; 47:414–417.

93. Agertoft L, Pedersen S. Bone densitometry in children treated for 3–6 years with high dose inhaled budesonide. Eur Respir J 1993; 6(suppl 17):261S.

94. Hopp RJ, Degan JA, Phelan J, et al. Cross-Sectional study of bone density in asthmatic children. Pediatr Pulmonol 1995; 20:189–192.

95. Chalkey SM, Chisholm DJ. Cushing's syndrome from an inhaled corticosteroid. Med J Aus 1994; 160:611–615.

96. Laroche M, Portea L, Caron P, et al. Osteoporotic vertebral fractures in a man under high-dose inhaled glucocorticoid therapy: a case-report with a review of the literature. Rev Rheum Engl Ed 1997; 64:267–270.

97. Cummings SR, Palermo L, Browner W, Marcus R, Wallace R, Pearson J, Blackwell T, Eckert S, Black D. Monitoring osteoporosis therapy with bone densitometry: misleading changes and regression to the mean: Fracture Intervention Trial Research Group. J Am Med Assoc 2000; 283:1318–1321.

98. Adachi JD, Bensen WG, Bianchi F, Cividino A, Pittersdorf S, Sebaldt RJ, Tugwell P, Gordon M, Steele M, Webber C, Goldsmith CH. Vitamin D and calcium in the prevention of corticosteroid induced osteoporosis: a 3 year follow up. J Rheumatol 1996; 23:95–100.

99. Ettinger B, Genant HK, Cann CE. Long-term estrogen replacement therapy prevents bone loss and fractures. Ann Intern Med 1985; 102:319–324.

100. Keil DP, Felson DT, Anderson JJ, et al. Hip fracture and the use of estrogens in postmenopausal women. N Engl J Med 1987; 817:1169–1174.

101. Weiss NS, Ure CL, Ballard JH, et al. Decreased risk of fractures of the hip and lower forearm with postmenopausal use of estrogen. N Engl J Med 1980; 303: 1195–1198.

102. The Writing Group for the PEPI. Effects of hormone therapy on bone mineral density: results from the postmenopausal estrogen/progestins interventions (PEPI) trial. J Am Med Assoc 1996; 276:1389–1396.

103. Lukert BP, Johnson BE, Robinson RG. Estrogen and progesterone replacement therapy reduces glucocorticoid-induced bone loss. J Bone Miner Res 1992; 7:1063–1069.

104. Lufkin EG, Wahner HW, O'Fallon WM, et al. Treatment of postmenopausal osteoporosis with transdermal estrogen. Ann Intern Med 1992; 112:1–9.

105. Ravnikar VA. Compliance with hormone therapy. Am J Obstet Gynecol 1987; 156: 1332–1334.

106. Delmas PD, Bjarnason NH, Mitlak BH, et al. Effects of raloxifene on bone mineral density, serum cholesterol concentrations and uterine endometrium in postmenopausal women. N Engl J Med 1997; 335:1641–1647.

107. Saag KG, Emkey R, Schnitzer TJ, et al. Alendronate for the prevention and treatment of glucocorticoid-induced osteoporosis. N Engl J Med 1998; 339:292–299.

108. Lindsey R, Cosman F, Cary DJ, et al. Effect of alendronate added to ongoing hormone replacement therapy in the treatment of postmenopausal osteoporosis. Osteoporos Int 1998; 8:12 [abstract].

109. Reid DM, Hughes RA, Laan RF, Sacco-Gibson NA, Wenderoth DH, Adami S, Eusebio RA, Devogelaer JP. Efficacy and safety of daily risedronate in the treatment of corticosteroid-induced osteoporosis in men and women: randomized trial. European Corticosteroid-Induced Osteoporosis Treatment Study. J Bone Miner Res 2000; 15:1006–1013.

110. Struys A, Snelder AA, Mulder H. Cyclical etidronate reverses bone loss of the spine and proximal femur in patients with established corticosteroid-induced osteoporosis. Am J Med 1995; 99:235–242.

111. Adachi JD, Granney A, Godsmith CH, et al. Intermittent cyclic therapy with etidronate in the prevention of corticosteroid-induced bone loss. J Rheumatol 1994; 21: 1922–1926.

112. Pitt P, Li F, Todd D, et al. A double-blind, placebo controlled trial to determine the effects of intermittent cyclic etidronate on bone mineral density in patients on long-term corticosteroid treatment. Thorax 1998; 53:351–356.

113. Skingle SJ, Moore DJ, Crisp AJ. Cyclical etidronate increases lumbar spine bone density in patients on long-term glucocorticosteroid therapy. Int J Clin Pret 1997; 51:364–367.

114. Adachi JD, Bensen WG, Brown J, et al. Intermittent etidronate therapy to prevent corticosteroid induced osteoporosis. N Engl J Med 1997; 337:382–387.

115. Roux C, Oriente P, Laan R, et al. Randomized trial of effect of cyclic etidronate in the prevention of corticosteroid-induced bone loss. J Clin Endocrinol Metab 1998; 83:1128–1133.

116. Wang WQ, Man MS, Tsang QWT, et al. Antiresorptive therapy in asthmatic patients receiving high-dose inhaled steroids: a prospective study for 18 months. J Allergy Clin Immunol 1998; 101:445–450.

117. Herrala J, Puolizjoki H, Liippo K, Raito M, Impivaairo O, Tala E, Nieminen MM. Clodronate is effective in preventing corticosteroid-induced bone loss among asthmatic patients. Bone 1998; 22:577–582.

118. Luengo M, Pons F, Martinez de Osaba MJ, et al. Prevention of further bone mass loss by nasal calcitonin in patients on long-term glucocorticoid therapy for asthma: a two year follow up study. Thorax 1994; 49:1099–1102.

119. Luengo M, Pons F, Martinez de Osaba MJ, et al. Prevention of further bone mass loss by nasal calcitonin in patients on long-term glucocorticoid therapy for asthma: a two year follow up study. Thorax 1994; 49:1099–1102.

120. Reid IR, Ibbertson HK, France JT, et al. Plasma testosterone concentrations in asthmatic men treated with glucocorticoids. Br Med J (Clin Res Ed) 1985; 291:574.

121. McAdams MR, White RH, Chipps BE. Reduction of serum testosterone levels during chronic glucocorticoid therapy. Ann Intern Med 1986; 104:648–651.

122. Pierce G, Tabensky A, Delmas PD, et al. Testosterone therapy induced bone loss in men. J Clin Endocrinol Metab 1998; 83:801–806.

123. Reid JF, Wattie DJ, Evans MC, et al. Testosterone therapy in glucocorticoid-treated men. Arch Intern Med 1996; 156:1173–1177.

124. Delmas PD, Dupuis J, Duboeuf F, et al. Treatment of vertebral osteoporosis with disodium monofluorophosphate: comparison with sodium fluoride. J Bone Miner Res 1990; 5:S143–S147.

125. Guaylelier-Souquieres G, Kotzki PO, Sabatier JP, et al. In corticosteroid-treated

respiratory disease, monfluorophosphate increases lumbar bone density: a double-masked randomized study. Osteopor Int 1996; 6:171–177.

126. Ledford DK, Apter A, Brenner AM, Rubin K, Prestwood K, Frieri M, Lukert B. Osteoporosis in the corticosteroid-treated patient with asthma. J Allergy Clin Immunol 1998; 102:353–362.

127. Norman ME. Juvenile osteoporosis. In: Favus MJ, ed. Primer on the Metabolic Bone Diseases and Disorders of Mineral Metabolism, 3rd ed. Philadelphia: Lippincott–Raven, 1996:75–82.

128. Warady BD, Linsley CB, Robinson RG, Lukert BP. Effects of nutritional supplementation on bone mineral status of children with rheumatic diseases receiving corticosteroid therapy. J Rheumatol 1994; 21:530–535.

129. Slemenda CS, Reister TK, Hui SL, Miller JZX, Christian JC, Johnston CC. Influences on skeletal maturation in children and adolescents: evidence for varying effects of sexual maturation and physical activity. J Pediatr 1994; 125:201–207.

130. Seeman E, Tsalamandris C, Formica C, Hopper JL, McKay J. Reduced femoral neck bone density in daughters of women with hip fractures: the role of low peak bone density in the pathogenesis of osteoporosis. J Bone Miner Res 1994; 9:739–743.

131. Ott SM. Bone density in adolescents. N Engl J Med 1991; 325:1647.

132. Reimer LG, Morris HG, Ellis EF. Growth of asthmatic children during treatment with alternate-day steroids. J Allergy Clin Immunol 1975; 55:224–231.

133. Kinberg KA, Hopp RJ, Biven RE, Gallagher JC. Bone mineral density in normal and asthmatic children. J Allergy Clin Immunol 1994; 94:490–497.

134. Martinelli LC, Bertoldo F, Gaspari E, et al. Effect on cortical and trabecular bone mass of different anti-inflammatory treatments in preadolescent children with chronic asthma. Am J Respir Crit Care Med 1996; 153:232–236.

135. Walsh LJ, Wong CA, Cooper S, Guhan AR, Pringle M, Tattersfield AE. Morbidity from asthma in relation to regular treatment—a community based study. Thorax 1999; 42:296–300.

23

Management of Severe Asthma

ANTONIO M. VIGNOLA, PASCAL CHANEZ, and JEAN BOUSQUET

University of Montpellier
Montpellier, France

I. Introduction

Asthma is a chronic inflammatory disease of the airways with variable airflow obstruction which is not always reversible under treatment (1). A subset of patients who present with severe asthma may be classified as having uncontrolled asthma despite optimal treatment. Recent published guidelines have outlined measures to control asthma and its assessment encompasses symptoms, rescue medications, pulmonary function, and quality-of-life outcomes (2,3).

Asthma responds to conventional therapy in the majority of appropriately treated patients (4). The current guidelines for treatment of chronic asthma culminate in the addition of regular oral corticosteroids after a stepwise increase in treatment. However, there are still a few patients (5 to 10% of asthmatics) whose asthma is not controlled despite such maximal conventional treatment and these patients, both children and adults, are considered to have severe (5,6) or difficult-to-treat asthma (7).

Patients with severe asthma may present severe exacerbations (unstable asthma) and/or fixed airway obstruction and/or require long-term use of oral corticosteroids to control the disease. The natural history of asthma is still poorly characterized but a small proportion of asthmatic patients develop a more severe form of the disease and need continuous long-term treatment with oral corticosteroids (8). This group of corticosteroid-dependent asthmatics is heterogeneous, since oral corticosteroids control asthma in some but not all patients.

Many drugs for the treatment of atopic diseases, including asthma, allergic rhinitis, and atopic dermatitis, are now in development. These treatments are based on improvements in existing therapies or on a better understanding of the cellular and molecular mechanisms involved in atopic diseases (9). In the present chapter, new treatments which are not used in patients are not discussed.

II. Reasons for Asthma Treatment Failure

National and international guidelines have had a profound effect on asthma deaths and hospitalizations throughout the world (10–12). Several questions need to be addressed when an asthmatic patient does not respond favorably to an optimal treatment.

First, it is important to exclude the possibility of other diagnoses, in particular for patients with an impaired fixed airflow obstruction. The distinction between asthma and COPD is notoriously difficult to ascertain in some patients (13). Other diseases such as vocal cord dysfunction may mimic asthma (14).

Second, patients do not respond equally well to treatment due to differences in pharmacogenetics (15). The β_2-adrenergic receptor is the molecular target for the β_2-agonists used in the treatment of asthma. In the human population, four polymorphisms of this receptor coding block have been found, three of which result in receptors that have different properties compared with wild type (16). Clinical studies suggest that these β_2-adrenergic receptor polymorphisms alter the asthmatic phenotype (17,18) and the response to β_2-agonist therapy (19). It is possible that, due to differences in pharmacogenetics, the long-acting β_2 agonists formoterol and salmeterol have variable effects in a subset of asthmatics (20), but the clinical demonstration is lacking (21). Moreover, tolerance to β_2-agonists is associated with β_2-adrenergic receptor polymorphism but the clinical relevance of these findings for long-acting β_2-agonists is still unclear (22). Genetic variations in the 5-lipoxygenase core promoter are involved in the response of patients to treatment with 5-lipoxygenase inhibitors (23).

Third, before consideration of true severe asthma, compliance to asthma management should be ensured (24). Underrecognition and undertreatment of asthma with appropriate amounts of inhaled steroids are major factors contributing to asthma morbidity (25) but overuse of inhaled β-agonists and underuse of inhaled corticosteroids are common in asthmatics (26,27). Moreover, it has been shown that guidelines are followed by only a few patients (28). Improvement in care for asthmatics will require greater commitment and involvement by all affected, including physicians, patients, health plan providers, and employers (29).

A key component of asthma management is education and regular medical review of the patient (2,3). A number of controlled trials have been conducted to measure the effectiveness of asthma education program. These programs improve patient knowledge, but their impact on health outcomes is less well established. At its simplest level, education is limited to the transfer of information about asthma and its causes and treatment. Although a meta-analysis of relevant studies has shown that education improves important clinical outcomes in adults with asthma (30), results are not unequivocal. A study by the Cochrane Collaboration reveals that use of limited asthma education does not appear to improve health outcomes in adults with asthma (31). However, the use of education in emergency facilities may be effective, but this needs to be confirmed. On the other hand, training in asthma self-management, which involves self-monitoring by either peak expiratory flow or symptoms coupled with regular medical review and a written action plan, appears to improve health outcomes for adults with asthma (32). Training programs which enable patients to adjust their medication based on a written action plan appear to be more effective than other forms of asthma self-management (32).

The method of inhalation should be monitored and it is surprising how often asthma control can be improved by changing the device used to administer inhaled drugs and by educating the patient.

Allergen exposure may be involved in severe asthma. There may be allergens in the home which can trigger exacerbations (33,34). Allergen avoidance may be effective in these patients. Allergen-specific immunotherapy is usually not indicated in patients with severe asthma (35). However, some patients still present uncontrolled asthma and a severe form of the disease even though all the above-mentioned features have been ruled out.

III. Therapeutic Options for Severe Asthma

Corticosteroids remain the first-line treatment of chronic asthma. However, they are not efficacious in all patients and new treatments have been proposed to improve the control of asthma.

A. Corticosteroids

Inhaled Corticosteroids

Inhaled corticosteroids offer a wide range of anti-inflammatory activity and have consistently proved to be the most effective medication for the control of asthma in children and adults. High doses of inhaled corticosteroids have an oral corticosteroid-sparing effect (36–38) and have been shown to improve severe asthma (39–44).

The administration of inhaled corticosteroids has been widely studied. Nebulized budesonide was shown to be effective in children ages 10 months to 5 years who were dependent on oral corticosteroids (45). However, even with an optimal nebulizer set-up, budesonide delivered by spacer is equipotent to that delivered by nebulizer (46) and, in practice, nebulizers are less efficient at drug deposition compared to spacers (47). For treating young children some devices such as the babyhaler are of great interest (48).

In severe asthma, the addition of long-acting β_2-agonists to inhaled corticosteroid treatment was shown to be more effective than doubling the dose of corticosteroid for both objective measures of lung function (49) and reduction in symptoms and exacerbations (50).

Systemic Corticosteroids

Some patients require short-term treatment with systemic corticosteroids, especially after an exacerbation. A Cochrane Collaboration survey showed that a short course of corticosteroids following assessment for an acute exacerbation of asthma significantly reduced the number of relapses requiring additional care and decreased β-agonist use without an apparent increase in side effects (51). Intramuscular corticosteroids appear to be as effective as oral agents.

To determine therapeutically equivalent doses of inhaled versus oral steroids for adults with chronic asthma, a Cochrane Collaboration survey was carried out (52). A daily dose of prednisolone at 7.5–10 mg/day appears to produce equivalent results to those of moderate- to high-dose inhaled corticosteroids. Side effects may be present at low doses, so if there is no alternative to oral steroids, the lowest effective dose should be prescribed.

Corticosteroid-Resistant and Corticosteroid-Dependent Asthma

In patients with severe asthma, high doses of inhaled corticosteroids in addition to long-acting β_2-agonists (53) may not be sufficient to control all patients (2). A few patients appear to be resistant to this therapy as defined by a lack of response to a short course of oral steroid treatment (54–57). Moreover, a small percentage of asthmatics who are not necessarily corticosteroid resistant develop a severe form of the disease and need continuous long-term treatment with oral corticosteroids (8,58–61). These patients are described as "corticosteroid-dependent" asthmatics.

Few studies have examined corticosteroid-dependent asthma. Clinically, these patients are highly heterogeneous, since oral corticosteroids are able to control asthma well in some patients, the best FEV_1 is highly variable, and some, but not all, patients have so-called "chaotic" peak flow charts (62). Very few studies have examined airways inflammation in corticosteroid-dependent asthmatics, but the available data suggest that eosinophils are usually in low numbers, whereas those of neutrophils are sometimes elevated (8,61,63–65). The treatment of corticosteroid-dependent asthma is usually very difficult and these patients are uncontrolled despite the use of large doses of oral corticosteroids.

If it is not possible to reduce or eliminate the use of systemic steroids, they should be given in such a way as to enhance safety. Suppression of the hypo-thalamo-pituitary-adrenal axis is lessened by taking the steroids in the morning and, if possible, on alternate days. Prednisolone tends to be used most; recent studies claim that deflazacort produces a lower incidence of steroid-induced side effects compared to prednisolone (66,67) but that the difference is not large.

B. Oral Antileukotrienes

Since the discovery of the leukotrienes and their role in asthma, there has been intense activity to produce drugs that counteract their effects (68). This has been achieved by blocking leukotriene synthesis with enzyme inhibitors (5-lipoxy-genase inhibitors, such as zileuton) or interfering with binding of leukotrienes to their receptors [leukotriene receptor antagonists (LTRA), such as montelukast, pranlukast, or zafirlukast].

Leukotriene modifiers were shown to improve severe asthma (69) and aspirin-induced asthma (70). However, in severe asthma, only a subset of patients show improvement and to date, there is no marker which can predict the efficacy of the drug. Moreover, LTRAs were shown to have a corticosteroid-sparing effect (71).

C. Anti-T-Cell Strategies

There is accumulating circumstantial evidence that the CD4+ T cell plays a central role in the pathogenesis of chronic asthma (72). Therapeutic strategies directed specifically at this cell type may offer a novel approach (73). Cyclosporin A and other immunomodulators such as FK506, rapamycin, and mycophenolic acid may be useful given their modes of action on the T lymphocyte (74). Strategies targeting T-cell costimulatory molecules and T-cell-derived cytokines may be of therapeutic utility.

Anti-CD4 Monoclonal Antibodies

A short-term trial using an anti-CD4 Mab (keliximab) to treat corticosteroid-dependent asthma was published (75). Patients given 0.5 or 1.5 mg/kg keliximab did not differ from those given placebo in change from baseline of PEF, FEV_1, or symptom score. Those given 3.0 mg/kg keliximab differed significantly from placebo recipients in change in morning and evening PEF. Symptom score showed the same pattern (though differences did not achieve significance), but there was no difference in FEV_1. There were no serious adverse effects related to treatment. Two patients had mild exacerbations of eczema and one developed a transient maculopapular rash. All doses of keliximab were associated with a reduction from baseline in CD4 count. The results were therefore modest but these findings raise the possibility that T-cell-directed treatment may be an alternative approach to the treatment of a subset of patients with severe asthma.

Oral Cyclosporin

Cyclosporin is an immunosuppressant used after organ transplantation that works by inhibiting T helper lymphocytes. The prominent role of T lymphocytes in asthma has led to trials of cyclosporin in adults which showed improved lung function (76–79) and a corticosteroid-sparing effect has been observed in some patients but not in all (80). It is always difficult to assess the corticosteroid-sparing effect of a drug, since placebo-treated patients can usually significantly reduce doses of oral and/or inhaled corticosteroids without loss of control of the disease. No randomized controlled trials have been carried out on children although its successful use in three of five children on regular oral steroids has been recently reported (81). The side effects in adults include hirsutism, parasthesia, mild hypertension, headaches, and tremor. The only concern in the pediatric report was hirsutism. There is obviously a concern about renal impairment with long-term use. Thus, a short trial with cyclosporin A may be used in some severe patients and the treatment continued under close supervision if a significant improvement has been observed.

However, nebulized cyclosporin is being tried in some posttransplant patients, and this may offer an improved risk–benefit ratio over systemic cyclosporin in asthma (82).

D. Intravenous Immunoglobulin

Intravenous immunoglobulin (IVIG) has been used for many years to treat patients with primary immunodeficiencies. More recently, IVIG has been shown to have anti-inflammatory activity when used at substantially higher concentrations (83). A number of studies have examined the efficacy of IVIG in severe allergic diseases. Although the mechanism by which IVIG may attenuate the allergic response is still undetermined, clinical studies have shown that IVIG therapy can decrease serum IgE levels and increase glucocorticoid binding affinity, while in vitro studies have shown that IVIG can decrease T-cell secretion of TH2 cytokines. Two randomized controlled studies have been carried out recently. In the first, 38 immunocompetent corticosteroid-dependent patients with severe asthma were randomly enrolled in a double-blind, placebo-controlled trial of IVIG (84) and the results showed that IVIG was safe and effective. In a second double-blind, placebo-controlled multicenter study, high doses of IVIG did not demonstrate a clinically or statistically significant advantage over placebo (albumin) infusions for the treatment of corticosteroid-dependent asthma. Subgroup analysis failed to identify markers predicting responsiveness (85). Moreover, in this study, IVIG was associated with a significant incidence of serious adverse events leading to the discontinuation of the trial.

E. Cytokine Modifiers

Over the past few decades, several key mechanisms driving asthma pathophysiology have been discovered (86). These include the roles of Th2-cytokines and, in particular, IL-5 (87) in eosinophilic inflammation. In the past few years, tools to block these have been developed. At this time, early clinical studies with neutralizing antibodies against IL-5 have been performed in asthmatics but results have yet to be published (88). The role of anti-IL-5 antibodies has been recently questioned since this antibody prevents eosinophil influx into the sputum following allergen challenge but has no effect on symptoms. Other anti-Th2 strategies are proposed but they may have some drawbacks (89).

IL-10 may be of importance as an anti-inflammatory cytokine (90,91) and has potential as a treatment in patients with severe asthma.

IL-4 mediates important proinflammatory functions in asthma, including induction of the IgE isotype switch, expression of VCAM-1 on endothelium, mucin production, 15-lipoxygenase activity, and Th2 lymphocyte stimulation leading to the secondary synthesis of IL-4, IL-5, and IL-13. Soluble recombinant human IL-4 receptor (IL-4R; Nuvance; altrakincept) inactivates naturally occurring IL-4 without mediating cellular activation. A single dose of nebulized IL-4R was found to improve asthma symptoms and pulmonary function (92). However, no study has been carried out in patients with severe asthma.

IL-13 may be of interest in the mechanisms of asthma, not only in the production of IgE but in mucus secretion and airway remodeling (93). However, strategies attempting to reduce IL-13 have not yet been tested.

IL-12 is a cytokine which potentially may counteract allergy (94), but its use is hampered by its toxic effects.

F. Anti-IgE Monoclonal Antibodies

Three companies, Genentech, Novartis Pharma AG, and Tanox Biosystems, have focused their efforts toward the strategy of anti-IgE therapy, and monoclonal antibodies against human IgE have been raised (e.g., rhu-Mab-E25 and CGP 51901). However, only one of these mAbs has been developed for the treatment of rhinitis and asthma. A monoclonal antibody was raised against the Cε3 domain of the IgE molecule (MAE11). This region of the IgE molecule is involved in the binding of IgE to its receptors (FcεRI). Complexing free IgE with MAE11 prior to its linkage with FcεRI prevents cross-linking of receptors (via antigen) and thus activation of mast cells and basophils (95). MAE11 only binds to free

IgE and does not bind to FcεRI-bound IgE. Thus, MAE11 does not activate cells bearing FcεRI, this characteristic being required to achieve a prolonged pharmacologic effect without inducing anaphylaxis (96). Hybridoma technology enables rodent monoclonal antibodies to be created but these have limited clinical utility (97). Humanized antibodies have improved pharmacokinetics and reduced immunogenicity and have already been used during clinical trials. Consequently, MAE11 was humanized and the best of several humanized variants, version 25 (Rhu-MAb-E25), was selected (95). Based on previous studies, it appeared likely that FcεRI expression on basophils and mast cells is regulated by levels of circulating IgE antibodies. Treatment with the anti-IgE mAb decreased free IgE levels to 1% of pretreatment levels and also resulted in a marked down-regulation of FcεRI on basophils (98). This effect is reversible in vitro and in vivo (99).

Rhu-Mab-E25 mAb has been tested in asthma and proof of concept was found, since rhu-Mab-E25 inhibited the late-phase allergic reaction following allergen bronchial challenge (100,101). Moreover, a recent study confirmed that rhu-Mab-E25 mAb was able to reduce oral and inhaled corticosteroids and improve the quality of life in moderate to severe asthma (102). More subjects in the two rhuMAb-E25 groups were able to decrease or discontinue their use of corticosteroids than in the placebo group, but only some of the differences were significant. After 20 weeks, serum free IgE concentrations decreased by a mean of more than 95% in both rhuMAb-E25 groups. The therapy was well tolerated. After 20 weeks, none of the subjects had antibodies against rhuMAb-E25.

Thus, a recombinant humanized monoclonal antibody directed against IgE has potential as a treatment for subjects with moderate or severe allergic asthma (103). However, there is probably a subset of severe asthmatics who will respond more favorably than others to this form of treatment and data are needed to characterize this subgroup of patients.

G. Low-Dose Oral Methotrexate

Using immunosuppressants to treat severe asthma has been proposed since the early 1960s, but was disregarded due to side effects. Within the past 15 years, however, methotrexate, an immunosuppressive and anti-inflammatory agent, has been used in cases of severe asthma (104–108) and in patients who have poorly responded to corticosteroids (109–112).

It has been proposed that the corticosteroid-sparing effect of methotrexate originates from increased sensitivity of lymphocytes to the inhibitory effects of glucocorticosteroids. The absence of an inhibitory effect on inflammatory cells in blood and mucosa suggests that this effect is achieved by modulating cell function rather than cell number (113).

It has been suggested that methotrexate is able to reduce steroid use in adults with asthma, but this is unclear (114). Moreover, methotrexate treatment is associated with several severe side effects (pulmonary fibrosis, pneumonitis, hepatic cirrhosis, and myelosuppression), and some of them have been reported in asthmatics using even low doses (115,116). Using the Cochrane collaboration, Davies et al. (117) assessed the effects of adding methotrexate to oral corticosteroids in adults with stable asthma who are dependent on oral corticosteroids. The study included 10 randomized trials (185 subjects) in which the addition of methotrexate was compared with placebo in adult steroid-dependent asthmatics. Duration of therapy needed to be at least 12 weeks. There was a reduction in oral corticosteroid dose favoring methotrexate in parallel trials (weighted mean difference −4.1 mg per day, 95% confidence interval −6.8 to −1.3) and also in crossover trials (weighted mean difference −2.9 mg per day, 95% confidence interval −5.9 to −0.2). There was no difference between methotrexate and placebo for forced expiratory volume in 1 min (weighted mean difference 0.12 L, 95% confidence interval −0.21 to 0.45). Hepatotoxicity was a common adverse effect with methotrexate compared to placebo (odds ratio 6.9, 95% confidence interval 3.1 to 15.5). The authors concluded that methotrexate may have a small steroid-sparing effect in adults with asthma who are dependent on oral corticosteroids. However, the overall reduction in daily steroid use is probably not large enough to reduce steroid-induced adverse effects. This small potential to reduce the impact of steroid side effects is probably insufficient to offset the adverse effects of methotrexate (118).

H. Colchicine

Colchicine demonstrates an array of anti-inflammatory properties which are of potential relevance to asthma. However, the efficacy of colchicine as an alternative to inhaled corticosteroid therapy for asthma is unknown. Five centers participated in a controlled trial testing the hypothesis that in patients with moderate asthma who need to use inhaled corticosteroids for control, colchicine provides therapeutic benefit as measured by maintenance of control when inhaled steroids are discontinued. In this study, colchicine was not found to be better than placebo as an alternative to inhaled corticosteroids in patients with moderate asthma (119). In another study, colchicine was unable to reduce inhaled corticosteroids (120).

I. Macrolides

Macrolide antibiotics have long been used as steroid-sparing agents in patients with severe steroid-dependent asthma (121,122). Their efficacy and their propensity to potentiate glucocorticoid adverse effects have been attributed in part to their ability to delay methylprednisone clearance (123–127). However, they are not involved in such drug interaction with other oral glucocorticosteroids such as prednisone. In vitro anti-inflammatory effects have been observed with 14-member macrolides (erythromycin and clarithromycin) but not with other macrolides (128). Clarithromycin is able to reduce eosinophil apoptosis in vitro (129).

An interesting mechanism of the anti-inflammatory properties of macrolides is associated with their action on transcription factors (130). Some macrolides such as clarithromycin (131) and roxithromycin (132,133) were shown to reduce non-specific bronchial hyperreactivity with an associated reduction in eosinophils in sputum (131) or oxygen free-radical release (133). The effects of macrolides in asthma are therefore more complex than previously thought and probably involve anti-inflammatory mechanisms. Randomized controlled trials should therefore be started in order to assess whether some macrolides may improve severe asthma with an associated reduction of inflammation (134,135).

J. Gold

The efficacy of gold salt injections in bronchial asthma was investigated in some studies. A first Japanese study showed that this treatment was effective (136). Auranofin (triethylphosphine gold), an oral gold preparation, demonstrated a steroid-sparing effect without concomitant worsening of symptoms or lung function and appeared to be more effective in corticosteroid-dependent asthmatic patients (137,138). Therefore this study has demonstrated that auranofin is useful as a steroid-sparing agent in the treatment of chronic corticosteroid-dependent asthma. The mechanisms of action are not totally clear but nonspecific bronchial hyper-reactivity 12 weeks after treatment with auranofin was decreased in a group of mild asymptomatic asthmatic patients with normal lung function (139). Side effects are described with gold therapy (140,141) but serious gold toxicity is uncommon. Many potential adverse reactions of both injectable and oral gold therapy are similar, including dermatitis, stomatitis, thrombocytopenia, leukopenia, and proteinuria, generally with increased incidence in the injectable form of treatment. Oral gold is associated with benign lower gastrointestinal side effects, including diarrhea, loose stools, and abdominal cramps that are often dose related and resolve spontaneously. The incidence of severe reactions such as thrombocytopenia, aplastic anemia, and exfoliative dermatitis is lower with oral gold than with injectable preparations.

K. Other Possible Treatments

Heparin, a glycosaminoglycan released exclusively from mast cells, also possesses anti-inflammatory actions. Its potential use in the treatment of asthma has been proposed (142,143). In one study, it was found that nebulized low-molecular-weight heparin was able to reduce asthma exacerbations (144). However, more studies are needed in patients with severe asthma. Moreover, the safety of nebulized heparin has to be assessed.

Lidocaine may also have anti-inflammatory properties (145). Inhaled lignocaine appeared to have considerable corticosteroid-sparing properties in an uncontrolled trial in 20 patients with oral-corticosteroid-dependent asthma (146). However, the results of a controlled trial are needed.

Dapsone is a potent anti-inflammatory and antiparasitic compound which is metabolized by cytochrome P450 to hydroxylamines, which in turn cause met-hemoglobinemia and hemolysis (147). Dapsone was used in corticosteroid-dependent asthma (148) but randomized controlled trials are not reported. More-over, side effects limit its use in asthma.

Other strategies may also be used but they are not validated (149).

IV. Churg–Strauss Syndrome

Churg–Strauss syndrome is an eosinophil-associated small-vessel vasculitis (150, 151). Although its pathogenesis may be distinctive and the association with se-vere late-onset asthma typical, the clinical features during the vasculitic phase widely overlap with those of the other forms of necrotizing vasculitis, and no single clinical or histologic feature is pathognomic of the condition. Renal involvement is common, although usually mild, and even when severe it tends to respond well to treatment. The prognosis for both patient and renal survival with adequate treatment is in general good. The optimal treatment strategy, how-ever, is uncertain and may differ from that for the other vasculitides. In particular, in contrast to Wegener's granulomatosis, the need for routine cyclophosphamide treatment is unconfirmed and requires further study.

The occurrence of Churg–Strauss syndrome in asthmatic patients receiving leukotriene modifiers has been widely publicized but it appears to be related to the unmasking of an underlying vasculitic syndrome that is initially clinically recognized as moderate to severe asthma and treated with corticosteroids. Anti-leukotrienes such as zafirlukast (152) and montelukast (153) do not appear to directly cause the syndrome in these patients. Moreover, the unmasking of Churg–Strauss syndrome does not appear to be associated only with antileuko-trienes. Churg–Strauss syndrome has also been observed in patients receiving inhaled corticosteroids and in whom oral corticosteroids were reduced (154).

V. Management of Patients with Severe Asthma

In patients with severe asthma whose disease is not optimally controlled with inhaled corticosteroids and long-acting bronchodilators, compliance to treatment should be carefully monitored and long-term oral corticosteroids may be neces-sary to control the disease (2) (Fig. 1). Leukotriene modifiers were shown to improve the control of asthma in some patients but reduction of oral corticoste-roids should be conducted carefully so as not to risk incurring Churg–Strauss syndrome. Long-term treatment with oral corticosteroids is not devoid of side effects and attempts to reduce the dose administered and/or to use alternate-day treatment should be regularly checked in order to attain maximal control of the disease with the fewest possible side effects.

TREATMENT: ADULTS & CHILDREN OVER 5 YEARS OLD	
Preferred treatments are in bold print.	
*Patient education is essential at every stage	
Long-Term Preventive	**Quick-Relief**
* STEP 4 **Severe** **Persistent**	Daily medications: • **Inhaled corticosteroid**, 800-2,000mcg or more, and • Long-acting bronchodilator: either **long-acting inhaled β₂–agonist** and/or sustained-release theophylline, and/or long-acting β₂–agonist tablets or syrup, and • Corticosteroid tablets or syrup long term.	• Short-acting bronchodilator: **inhaled β₂–agonist** as needed for symptoms.
* STEP 3 **Moderate** **Persistent**	Daily medications: • **Inhaled corticosteroid**, 500 mcg AND, if needed • Long-acting bronchodilator: either **long-acting inhaled β₂–agonist**, sustained-release theophylline, or long-acting β₂–agonist tablets or syrup. (Long-acting inhaled β₂–agonist may provide more effective symptom control when added to low-medium dose steroid compared to increasing the steroid dose). • Consider adding anti-leukotriene, especially for aspirin-sensitive patients and for preventing exercise-induced bronchospasm.	• Short-acting bronchodilator: **inhaled β₂–agonist** as needed for symptoms, not to exceed 3-4 times in one day.
* STEP 2 **Mild** **Persistent**	Daily medication: • Either **inhaled corticosteroid**, 200-500 mcg, or cromoglycate or nedocromil or sustained release theophylline. Anti-leukotrienes may be considered, but their position in therapy has not been fully established.	• Short-acting bronchodilator: **inhaled β₂–agonist** as needed for symptoms, not to exceed 3-4 times in one day.
STEP 1 **Intermittent**	• None needed.	• Short-acting bronchodilator: **inhaled β₂–agonist** as needed for symptoms, but less than once a week. • Intensity of treatment will depend on severity of attack (see figures on management of asthma attacks) • Inhaled β₂–agonist or cromoglycate before exercise or exposure to allergen.

Stepdown

 Review treatment every 3 to 6 months. If control is sustained for at least 3 months, a gradual stepwise reduction in treatment may be possible

Stepup

  If control is not achieved, consider stepup. But first: review patient medication technique, compliance, and environmental control (avoidance of allergens or other trigger factors).

*Dosage note: Steroid doses are for Beclomethasone Dipropionate (on the WHO list of "Essential Drugs"). Other preparations have equal effect, but adjust the dose because inhaled steroids are not equivalent on a microgram or per puff basis.

Figure 1   Asthma treatment for adults and children over 5 years of age.

Several therapeutic options such as cyclosporin A, methotrexate, colchicine, IVIG, gold, and monoclonal antibodies against IL-5 or CD4+ cells have been proposed to achieve a corticosteroid-sparing effect and an improvement of asthma control. The safety of the alternative treatments must be taken into consideration. None of these therapies have gained complete acceptance due to a usually limited clinical efficacy often associated with an appreciable rate of side effects (3). Moreover, there is large heterogeneity in severe asthma and, unfortunately, there is no phenotype of severe asthma which has been shown to respond to a particular alternative treatment when inhaled corticosteroids and long-acting bronchodilators are insufficient to control asthma. Thus, it is important to assess critically all possible interventions and to use the most appropriate remedy for each patient.

VI. Conclusions

Although patients with severe asthma represent a small percentage of asthmatics, they are at high risk for morbidity and mortality. The treatments currently available are sometimes ineffective in controlling the disease and they may induce side effects. There are therefore unmet needs in these patients. In the future, it is likely that new forms of treatment will be available and most likely these will target more specifically the immunological and inflammatory cascade of asthma. Better understanding of pharmacogenetics may help in tailoring the treatment of severe asthma to specific patients.

References

1. Bousquet J, Jeffery PK, Busse WW, Johnson M, Vignola AM. Asthma. From bronchoconstriction to airways inflammation and remodeling. Am J Respir Crit Care Med 2000; 161:1720–1745.
2. National Institutes of Health. WHO/NHLBI workshop report: Global Strategy for Asthma Management and Prevention, Publication no. 95-3659. Bethesda, MD: National Heart, Lung and Blood Institute, 1995.
3. Expert Panel Report 2: Guidelines for the Diagnosis and Management of Asthma. NIH publication no. 97-4051, April 1997.
4. Bousquet J. Global Initiative for Asthma (GINA) and its objectives. Clin Exp Allergy 2000; 30:2–5.
5. Balfour-Lynn I. Difficult asthma: beyond the guidelines. Arch Dis Child 1999; 80: 201–206.
6. Weissler JC. Syndromes of severe asthma. Am J Med Sci 2000; 319:166–176.
7. Chung KF, Godard P, Adelroth E, Ayres J, Barnes N, Barnes P, et al. Difficult/therapy-resistant asthma: the need for an integrated approach to define clinical phenotypes, evaluate risk factors, understand pathophysiology and find novel therapies.

ERS Task Force on Difficult/Therapy-Resistant Asthma. European Respiratory Society. Eur Respir J 1999; 13:1198–1208.

8. Vachier I, Chiappara G, Vignola AM, Gagliardo R, Altieri E. Terouanne B, et al. Glucocorticoid receptors in bronchial epithelial cells in asthma. Am J Respir Crit Care Med 1998; 158:963–970.

9. Barnes PJ. Therapeutic strategies for allergic diseases [in process citation]. Nature 1999; 402:B31–38.

10. Haahtela T, Laitinen LA. Asthma programme in Finland 1994–2004: report of a Working Group. Clin Exp Allergy 1996:1–24.

11. Campbell MJ, Holgate ST, Johnston SL. Trends in asthma mortality: data on seasonality of deaths due to asthma were omitted from paper but editorial's author did not know [letter]. Br Med J 1997; 315:1012.

12. Maljanian R, Wolf S, Goethe J, Hernandez P, Horowitz S. An inner-city asthma management initiative: results of an outcome evaluation. Dis Manage Health Outcomes 1999; 5:285–293.

13. Vignola AM, Gagliardo R, Guerrera D, Siena L, Chanez P, Bousquet J, et al. Are asthma and chronic bronchitis different diseases? Pro Monaldi Arch Chest Dis 1999; 54:543–550.

14. Newman KB, Mason U, Schmaling KB. Clinical features of vocal cord dysfunction. Am J Respir Crit Care Med 1995; 152:1382–1386.

15. Hall IP. Pharmacogenetics of asthma. Eur Respir J 2000; 15:449–451.

16. Liggett SB. The pharmacogenetics of beta2-adrenergic receptors: relevance to asthma. J Allergy Clin Immunol 2000; 105:S487–S492.

17. Weir TD, Mallek N, Sandford AJ, Bai TR, Awadh N, Fitzgerald JM, et al. beta2-Adrenergic receptor haplotypes in mild, moderate and fatal/near fatal asthma. Am J Respir Crit Care Med 1998; 158:787–791.

18. Taylor DR, Drazen JM, Herbison GP, Yandava CN, Hancox RJ, Town GI. Asthma exacerbations during long term beta agonist use: influence of beta(2) adrenoceptor polymorphism. Thorax 2000; 55:762–767.

19. Israel E, Drazen JM, Liggett SB, Boushey HA, Cherniack RM, Chinchilli VM, et al. The effect of polymorphisms of the beta(2)-adronergic receptor on the response to regular use of albuterol in asthma. Am J Respir Crit Care Med 2000; 162:75–80.

20. Green SA, Spasoff AP, Coleman RA, Johnson M, Liggett SB. Sustained activation of a G protein-coupled receptor via "anchored" agonist binding: molecular localization of the salmeterol exosite within the 2-adrenergic receptor. J Biol Chem 1996; 271:24029–24035.

21. Palmqvist M, Ibsen T, Mellen A, Lotvall J. Comparison of the relative efficacy of formoterol and salmeterol in asthmatic patients. Am J Respir Crit Care Med 1999; 160:244–249.

22. Lipworth BJ, Dempsey OJ. Aziz I. Functional antagonism with formoterol and salmeterol in asthmatic patients expressing the homozygous glycine-16 beta(2)-adrenoceptor polymorphism. Chest 2000; 118:321–328.

23. Silverman E. In Yandava C, Drazen JM, eds. Pharmacogenetics of the 5-lipoxygenase pathway in asthma. Clin Exp Allergy 1998; 28(suppl 5):164–170.

24. Partridge MR, Fabbri LM, Chung KF. Delivering effective asthma care—how do we implement asthma guidelines? [editorial]. Eur Respir J 2000; 15:235–237.

25. D'Souza WJ, Slater T, Fox C, Fox B, Te Karu H, Gemmell T, et al. Asthma morbidity 6 yrs after an effective asthma self-management programme in a Maori community. Eur Respir J 2000; 15:464–469.

26. Diette GB, Wu AW, Skinner EA, Markson L, Clark RD, McDonald RC, et al. Treatment patterns among adult patients with asthma: factors associated with overuse of inhaled beta-agonists and underuse of inhaled corticosteroids. Arch Intern Med 1999; 159:2697–2704.

27. Halterman JS, Aligne CA, Auinger P, McBride JT, Szilagyi PG. Inadequate therapy for asthma among children in the United States. Pediatrics 2000; 105:272–276.

28. Colice GL, Burgt JV, Song J, Stampone P, Thompson PJ. Categorizing asthma severity. Am J Respir Crit Care Med 1999; 160:1962–1967.

29. Meng YY, Leung KM, Berkbigler D, Halbert RJ, Legorreta AP. Compliance with US asthma management guidelines and specialty care: a regional variation or national concern? J Eval Clin Pract 1999; 5:213–221.

30. Devine EC. Meta-analysis of the effects of psychoeducational care in adults with asthma. Res Nurs Health 1996; 19:367–376.

31. Gibson PG, Coughlan J, Wilson AJ, Hensley MJ, Abramson M, Bauman A, et al. Limited (information only) patient education programs for adults with asthma. Cochrane Database Syst Rev 2000; 2. CD 00117.

32. Gibson PG, Coughlan J, Wilson AJ, Abramson M, Bauman A, Hensley MJ, et al. Self-management education and regular practitioner review for adults with asthma. Cochrane Database Syst Rev 2000; 2.

33. Rosenstreich DL. Eggleston P, Kattan M, Baker D, Slavin RG, Gergen P, et al. The role of cockroach allergy and exposure to cockroach allergen in causing morbidity among inner-city children with asthma. N Engl J Med 1997; 336:1356–1363.

34. Neukirch C, Henry C, Leynaert B, Liard R, Bousquet J, Neukirch F. Is sensitization to Alternaria alternata a risk factor for severe asthma? A population-based study. J Allergy Clin Immunol 1999; 103:709–711.

35. Bousquet J, Lockey R, Malling HJ. Allergen immunotherapy: therapeutic vaccines for allergic diseases: a WHO position paper. J Allergy Clin Immunol 1998; 102: 558–562.

36. Noonan M, Chervinsky P, Busse WW, Weisberg SC. Pinnas J, de-Boisblanc BP, et al. Fluticasone propionate reduces oral prednisone use while it improves asthma control and quality of life. Am J Respir Crit Care Med 1995; 152:1467–1473.

37. Nelson HS, Busse WW, de-Boisblanc BP, Berger WE, Noonan MJ, Webb DR, et al. Fluticasone propionate powder: oral corticosteroid-sparing effect and improved lung function and quality of life in patients with severe chronic asthma. J Allergy Clin Immunol 1999; 103:267–275.

38. Westbroek J, Saarelainen S, Laher M, O'Brien J, Barnacle H, Efthimiou J. Oral steroid-sparing effect of two doses of nebulized fluticasone propionate and placebo in patients with severe chronic asthma. Respir Med 1999; 93:689–699.

39. Fabbri L, Burge PS, Croonenborgh L, Warlies F, Weeke B, Ciaccia A, et al. Comparison of fluticasone propionate with beclomethasone dipropionate in moderate to severe asthma treated for one year. International Study Group. Thorax 1993; 48: 817–823.

40. Barnes NC, Marone G, Di-Maria GU, Visser S, Utama I, Payne SL. A comparison

of fluticasone propionate, 1 mg daily, with beclomethasone dipropionate, 2 mg daily, in the treatment of severe asthma: International Study Group. Eur Respir J 1993; 6:877–885.

41. Ayres JG, Bateman ED, Lundback B, Harris TA. High dose fluticasone propionate, 1 mg daily, versus fluticasone propionate, 2 mg daily, or budesonide, 1.6 mg daily, in patients with chronic severe asthma: International Study Group. Eur Respir J 1995; 8:579–586.

42. Heinig JH, Boulet LP, Croonenborghs L, Mollers MJ. The effect of high-dose fluticasone propionate and budesonide on lung function and asthma exacerbations in patients with severe asthma. Respir Med 1999; 93:613–620.

43. Pauwels RA, Yernault JC, Demedts MG, Geusens P. Safety and efficacy of fluticasone and beclomethasone in moderate to severe asthma. Belgian Multicenter Study Group. Am J Respir Crit Care Med 1998; 157:827–832.

44. Mukherjee SK. Flixotide nebules: new for chronic severe asthma. Hosp Med 1999; 60:442–443.

45. Ilangovan P, Pedersen S, Godfrey S, Nikander K, Noviski N, Warner JO. Treatment of severe steroid dependent preschool asthma with nebulised budesonide suspension. Arch Dis Child 1993; 68:356–359.

46. Bisgaard H, Nikander K, Munch E. Comparative study of budesonide as a nebulized suspension vs pressurized metered-dose inhaler in adult asthmatics. Respir Med 1998; 92:44–49.

47. Bisgaard H. Delivery of inhaled medication to children. J Asthma 1997; 34:443–467.

48. Hendriks HJ, Overberg PC, Brackel HJ, Vermue NA. Handling of a spacer (Babyhaler) for inhalation therapy in 0- to 3-year-old children. J Asthma 1998; 35:297–304.

49. Woolcock A, Lundback B, Ringdal N, Jacques LA. Comparison of addition of salmeterol to inhaled steroids with doubling of the dose of inhaled steroids. Am J Respir Crit Care Med 1996; 153:1481–1488.

50. Pauwels RA, Lofdahl CG, Postma DS, Tattersfield AE, O'Byrne P, Barnes PJ, et al. Effect of inhaled formoterol and budesonide on exacerbations of asthma. Formoterol and Corticosteroids Establishing Therapy (FACET) International Study Group. N Engl J Med 1997; 337:1405–1411.

51. Rowe BH, Spooner CH, Ducharme FM, Bretzlaff JA, Bota GW. Corticosteroids for preventing relapse following acute exacerbations of asthma. Cochrane Database Syst Rev 2000; 2.

52. Mash B, Bheekie A, Jones PW. Inhaled vs oral steroids for adults with chronic asthma. Cochrane Database Syst Rev 2000; 2. CD 002160.

53. Shrewsbury S, Pyke S, Britton M. Meta-analysis of increased dose of inhaled steroid or addition of salmeterol in symptomatic asthma (MIASMA). Br Med J 2000; 320:1368–1373.

54. Szefler SJ, Loung DY, Glucocorticoid-resistant asthma: pathogenesis and clinical implications for management. Eur Respir J 1997; 10:1640–1647.

55. Barnes PJ. Mechanisms of action of glucocorticoids in asthma. Am J Respir Crit Care Med 1996; 154:S26–S27.

56. Woolcock AJ. Corticosteroid-resistant asthma: definitions. Am J Respir Crit Care Med 1996; 154:S45–S46.

57. Demoly P, Jaffuel D, Mathieu M, Sahla H, Godard P, Michel F, et al. Glucocorticoid-insensitive asthma: a one-year clinical follow-up pilot study. Thorax 1998; 53:1063–1065.

58. Turner-Warwick M. On the observing patterns of airflow obstruction in chronic asthma. Br J Dis Chest 1977; 71:73–86.

59. Dykewicz MS, Greenberger PA, Patterson R, Halwig JM. Natural history of asthma in patients requiring long-term systemic corticosteroids. Arch Intern Med 1986; 146:2369–2372.

60. Des-Roches A, Paradis L, Bougeard YH, Godard P, Bousquet J, Chanez P. Long-term oral corticosteroid therapy does not alter the results of immediate-type allergy skin prick tests. J Allergy Clin Immunol 1996; 98:522–527.

61. Wenzel SE, Szefler SJ, Leung DY, Sloan SI, Rex MD, Martin RJ. Bronchoscopic evaluation of severe asthma: persistent inflammation associated with high dose glucocorticoids. Am J Respir Crit Care Med 1997; 156:737–743.

62. Chan MT, Leung DY, Szefler SJ, Spahn JD. Difficult-to-control asthma: clinical characteristics of steroid-insensitive asthma. J Allergy Clin Immunol 1998; 101: 594–601.

63. Tanizaki Y, Kitani H, Okazaki M, Mifune T, Mitsunobu F, Kimura I. Changes in the proportions of bronchoalveolar lymphocytes, neutrophils and basophilic cells and the release of histamine and leukotrienes from bronchoalveolar cells in patients with steroid-dependent intractable asthma. Int Arch Allergy Immunol 1993; 101: 196–202.

64. Vrugt B, Djukanovic R, Bron A, Aalbers R. New insights into the pathogenesis of severe corticosteroid-dependent asthma. J Allergy Clin Immunol 1996; 98:S33–S40.

65. Wenzel SE, Schwartz LB, Langmack EL, Halliday JL, Trudeau JB, Gibbs RL, et al. Evidence that severe asthma can be divided pathologically into two inflammatory subtypes with distinct physiologic and clinical characteristics. Am J Respir Crit Care Med 1999; 160:1001–1008.

66. Gennari C, Imbimbo B, Montagnani M, Bernini M, Nardi P, Avioli LV. Effects of prednisone and deflazacort on mineral metabolism and parathyroid hormone activity in humans. Calcif Tissue Int 1984; 36:245–252.

67. Markham A, Bryson HM. Deflazacort: a review of its pharmacological properties and therapeutic efficacy. Drugs 1995; 50:317–333.

68. Drazen JM, Israel E, O'Byrne PM. Treatment of asthma with drugs modifying the leukotriene pathway [published erratum appears in N Engl J Med 1999 Feb 25; 340(8):663]. N Engl J Med 1999; 340:197–206.

69. Kemp JP, Minkwitz MC, Bonuccelli CM, Warren MS. Therapeutic effect of zafirlukast as monotherapy in steroid-naive patients with severe persistent asthma. Chest 1999; 115:336–342.

70. Dahlen B, Nizankowska E, Szczeklik A, Zetterstrom O, Bochenek G, Kumlin M, et al. Benefits from adding the 5-lipoxygenase inhibitor zileuton to conventional therapy in aspirin-intolerant asthmatics. Am J Respir Crit Care Med 1998; 157: 1187–1194.

71. Lofdahl CG, Reiss TF, Leff JA, Israel E, Noonan MJ, Finn AF, et al. Randomised, placebo controlled trial of effect of a leukotriene receptor antagonist, montelukast,

on tapering inhaled corticosteroids in asthmatic patients. Br Med J 1999; 319:87–90.

72. Kay AB. T cells as orchestrators of the asthmatic response. Ciba Found Symp 1997; 206:56–67.

73. Kon OM, Kay AB. Anti-T cell strategies in asthma. Inflamm Res 1999; 48:516–523.

74. Corrigan CJ, Bungre JK, Assoufi B, Cooper AE, Seddon H, Kay AB. Glucocorticoid resistant asthma: T-lymphocyte steroid metabolism and sensitivity to glucocorticoids and immunosuppressive agents. Eur Respir J 1996; 9:2077–2086.

75. Kon OM, Sihra BS, Compton CH, Leonard TB, Kay AB, Barnes NC. Randomised, dose-ranging, placebo-controlled study of chimeric antibody to CD4 (keliximab) in chronic severe asthma. Lancet 1998; 352:1109–1113.

76. Szczeklik A, Nizankowska E, Dworski R, Domagala B, Pinis G. Cyclosporin for steroid-dependent asthma. Allergy 1991; 46:312–315.

77. Alexander AG, Barnes NC, Kay AB. Trial of cyclosporin in corticosteroid-dependent chronic severe asthma. Lancet 1992; 339:324–328.

78. Calderon E, Lockey RF, Bukantz SC, Coffey RG, Ledford DK. Is there a role for cyclosporine in asthma? J Allergy Clin Immunol 1992; 89:629–636.

79. Lock SH, Kay AB, Barnes NC. Double-blind, placebo-controlled study of cyclosporin A as a corticosteroid-sparing agent in corticosteroid-dependent asthma. Am J Respir Crit Care Med 1996; 153:509–514.

80. Nizankowska E, Soja J, Pinis G, Bochenek G, Sladek K, Domagala B, et al. Treatment of steroid-dependent bronchial asthma with cyclosporin. Eur Respir J 1995; 8:1091–1099.

81. Coren ME, Rosenthal M, Bush A. The use of cyclosporin in corticosteroid dependent asthma. Arch Dis Child 1997; 77:522–523.

82. Klyashchitsky BA, Owen AJ. Nebulizer-compatible liquid formulations for aerosol pulmonary delivery of hydrophobic drugs: glucocorticoids and cyclosporine. J Drug Target 1999; 7:79–99.

83. Rabinovitch N, Gelfand EW, Leung DY. The role of immunoglobulin therapy in allergic diseases. Allergy 1999; 54:662–668.

84. Salmun LM, Barlan I, Wolf HM, Eibl M, Twarog FJ, Geha RS, et al. Effect of intravenous immunoglobulin on steroid consumption in patients with severe asthma: a double-blind, placebo-controlled, randomized trial. J Allergy Clin Immunol 1999; 103:810–815.

85. Kishiyama JL, Valacer D, Cunningham-Rundles C, Sperber K, Richmond GW, Abramson S, et al. A multicenter, randomized, double-blind, placebo-controlled trial of high-dose intravenous immunoglobulin for oral corticosteroid-dependent asthma. Clin Immunol 1999; 91:126–133.

86. Wills-Karp M. Immunologic basis of antigen-induced airway hyperresponsiveness. Annu Rev Immunol 1999; 17:255–281.

87. Danzig M, Cuss F. Inhibition of interleukin-5 with a monoclonal antibody attenuates allergic inflammation. Allergy 1997; 52:787–794.

88. Lotvall J, Pullerits T. Treating asthma with anti-IgE or anti-IL5. Curr Pharm Des 1999; 5:757–770.

89. Castro M, Chaplin DD, Walter MJ. Holtzman MJ. Could asthma be worsened by

stimulating the T-helper type 1 immune response?. Am J Respir Cell Mol Biol 2000; 22:143–146.

90. Umetsu DT, DeKruyff RH. Th1 and Th2 CD4+ cells in the pathogenesis of allergic diseases. Proc Soc Exp Biol Med 1997; 215:11–20.

91. Pretolani M, Goldman M. Cylokines involved in the downregulation of allergic airway inflammation. Res Immunol 1997; 148:33–38.

92. Borish LC, Nelson HS, Lanz MJ, Claussen L, Whitmore JB, Agosti JM, et al. Interleukin-4 receptor in moderate atopic asthma: a phase I/II randomized, placebo-controlled trial. Am J Respir Crit Care Med 1999; 160:1816–1823.

93. Wills-Karp M, Luyimbazi J, Xu X, Schofield B, Neben TY, Karp CL, et al. Interleukin-13: central mediator of allergic asthma. Science 1998; 282:2258–2261.

94. Wills-Karp M. Interleukin-12 as a target for modulation of the inflammatory response in asthma. Allergy 1998; 53:113–119.

95. Presta LG, Lahr SJ, Shields RL, Porter JP. Gorman CM, Fendly BM, ed al. Humanization of an antibody directed against IgE. J Immunol 1993; 151:2623–2632.

96. Saban R, Haak-Frendscho M, Zinc M, Ridgway J, Gorman C, Presta LG, et al. Human FcERI-IgG and humanized anti-IgE monoclonal antibody MaEll block passive sensitization of human and rhesus monkey lung. J Allergy Clin Immunol 1994; 94:836–843.

97. Winter G, Harris WJ. Humanized antibodies. Immunol Today 1993; 14:243–246.

98. MacGlashan D Jr, Bochner BS, Adelman DC, Jardieu PM, Togias A, McKenzie-White J, et al. Down-regulation of Fc(epsilon)RI expression on human basophils during in vivo treatment of atopic patients with anti-IgE antibody. J Immunol 1997; 158:1438–1445.

99. Saini SS, MacGlashan D Jr, Sterbinsky SA, Togias A, Adelman DC, Lichtenstein LM, et al. Down-regulation of human basophil IgE and FC epsilon RI alpha surface densities and mediator release by anti-IgE-infusions is reversible in vitro and in vivo. J Immunol 1999; 162:5624–5630.

100. Fahy JV, Fleming HE, Wong HH, Liu JT, Su JQ, Reimann J, et al. The effect of an anti-IgE monoclonal antibody on the early- and late-phase responses to allergen inhalation in asthmatic subjects. Am J Respir Crit Care Med 1997; 155:1828–1834.

101. Boulet L, Chapman K, Côté J, Kalra S, Bhagat R, Swystun V, et al. Inhibitory effects of an anti-IgE antibody E25 on allergen-induced early asthmatic response. Am J Respir Crit Care Med 1997; 155:1835–1840.

102. Milgrom H, Fick RB Jr, Su JQ, Reimann JD. Bush RK, Watrous ML, et al. Treatment of allergic asthma with monoclonal anti-IgE antibody. rhuMab-E25 Study Group. N Engl J Med 1999; 341:1966–1973.

103. Barnes PJ. Anti-IgE antibody therapy for asthma. N Engl J Med 1999; 341:2006–2008.

104. Mullarkey MF, Blumenstein BA, Andrade WP, Bailey GA, Olason I, Wetzel CE. Methotrexate in the treatment of corticosteroid-dependent asthma. A double-blind crossover study. N Engl J Med 1988; 318:603–607.

105. Mullarkey MF, Lammort JK, Blumenstein BA. Long-term methotrexate treatment in corticosteroid-dependent asthma. Ann Intern Med 1990; 112:577–581.

106. Calderon E, Coffey RG, Lockey RF. Methotrexate in bronchial asthma. J Allergy Clin Immunol 1991; 88:274–276.

107. Guss S, Portnoy J. Methotrexate treatment of severe asthma in children. Pediatrics 1992; 89:635–639.
108. Stempel DA, Lammert J, Mullarkey MF. Use of methotrexate in the treatment of steroid-dependent adolescent asthmatics. Ann Allergy 1991; 67:346–348.
109. Coffey MJ, Sanders G, Eschenbacher WL, Tsien A, Ramesh S, Weber RW, et al. The role of methotrexate in the management of steroid-dependent asthma. Chest 1994; 105:117–121.
110. Dyer PD, Vaughan TR, Weber RW. Methotrexate in the treatment of steroid-dependent asthma. J Allergy Clin Immunol 1991; 88:208–212.
111. Erzurum SC, Leff JA, Cochran JE, Ackerson LM, Szefler SJ, Martin RJ, et al. Lack of benefit of methotrexate in severe, steroid-dependent asthma: a double-blind, placebo-controlled study. Ann Intern Med 1991; 114:353–360.
112. Shiner RJ, Nunn AJ, Chung KF, Geddes DM. Randomised, double-blind, placebo-controlled trial of methotrexate in steroid-dependent asthma. Lancet 1990; 336: 137–140.
113. Vrugt B, Wilson S, Bron A, Shute J, Holgate ST, Djukanovic R, et al. Low-dose methotrexate treatment in severe glucocorticoid-dependent asthma: effect on mucosal inflammation and in vitro sensitivity to glucocorticoids of mitogen-induced T-cell proliferation [in process citation]. Eur Respir J 2000; 15:478–485.
114. Fabbri L, Caramori G, Cosma P, Ciaccia A. Methotrexate in the treatment of systemic glucocorticoid-dependent severe persistent asthma: a word of caution. Monaldi Arch Chest Dis 1996; 51:130–137.
115. Gatnash AA, Connolly CK. Fatal chickenpox pneumonia in an asthmatic patient on oral steroids and methotrexate. Thorax 1995; 50:422–423.
116. Fertel D, Wanner A. Methotrexate: does it treat or induce asthma? [editorial]. Am Rev Respir Dis 1991; 143:1–2.
117. Davies H, Olson L, Gibson P. Methotrexate as a steroid sparing agent for asthma in adults. Cochrane Database Syst Rev 2000; 2. CD 000391.
118. Bardin PG, Fraenkel DJ, Beasley RW. Methotrexate in asthma. A safety perspective. Drug Saf 1993; 9:151–155.
119. Fish JE, Peters SP, Chambers CV, McGeady SJ, Epstein KR, Boushey HA, et al. An evaluation of colchicine as an alternative to inhaled corticosteroids in moderate asthma. National Heart, Lung, and Blood Institute's Asthma Clinical Research Network. Am J Respir Crit Care Med 1997; 156:1165–1171.
120. Newman KB, Mason UG, Buchmeier A, Schmaling KB, Corsello P, Nelson HS. Failure of colchicine to reduce inhaled triamcinolone dose in patients with asthma. J Allergy Clin Immunol 1997; 99:176–178.
121. Zeiger RS, Schatz M, Sperling W, Simon RA, Stevenson DD. Efficacy of troleandomycin in outpatients with severe, corticosteroid-dependent asthma. J Allergy Clin Immunol 1980; 66:438–446.
122. Kamada AK, Hill MR, Ikle DN, Brenner AM, Szefler SJ. Efficacy and safety of low-dose troleandomycin therapy in children with severe, steroid-requiring asthma. J Allergy Clin Immunol 1993; 91:873–882.
123. Szefler SJ, Rose JQ, Ellis EF, Spector SL, Green AW, Jusko WJ. The effect of troleandomycin on methylprednisolone elimination. J Allergy Clin Immunol 1980; 66:447–451.

124. Szefler SJ, Brenner M, Jusko WJ, Spector SL, Flesher KA, Ellis EF. Dose- and time-related effect of troleandomycin on methylprednisolone elimination. Clin Pharmacol Ther 1982; 32:166–171.

125. LaForce CF, Szefler SJ, Miller MF, Ebling W, Brenner M. Inhibition of methylprednisolone elimination in the presence of erythromycin therapy. J Allergy Clin Immunol 1983; 72:34–39.

126. LaForce CF, Miller MF, Chai H. Effect of erythromycin on theophylline clearance in asthmatic children. J Pediatr 1981; 99:153–156.

127. Fost DA, Leung DY, Martin RJ, Brown EE, Szefler SJ, Spahn JD. Inhibition of methylprednisolone elimination in the presence of clarithromycin therapy. J Allergy Clin Immunol 1999; 103:1031–1035.

128. Kohyarna T, Takizawa H, Kawasaki S, Akiyama N, Sato M, Ito K. Fourteen-member macrolides inhibit interleukin-8 release by human eosinophils from atopic donors. Antimicrob Agents Chemother 1999; 43:907–911.

129. Adachi T, Motojima S, Hirata A, Fukuda T, Kihara N, Kosaku A, et al. Eosinophil apoptosis caused by theophylline, glucocorticoids, and macrolides after stimulation with IL-5. J Allergy Clin Immunol 1996; 98:S207–S215.

130. Abe S, Nakamura H, Inoue S, Takeda H, Saito H, Kato S, et al. Interleukin-8 gene repression by clarithromycin is mediated by the activator protein-1 binding site in human bronchial epithelial cells. Am J Respir Cell Mol Biol 2000; 22:51–60.

131. Amayasu H, Yoshida S, Ebana S, Yamamoto Y, Nishikawa T, Shoji T, et al. Clarithromycin suppresses bronchial hyperresponsiveness associated with eosinophilic inflammation in patients with asthma. Ann Allergy Asthma Immunol 2000; 84:594–598.

132. Shimizu T, Kato M, Mochizuki H, Tokuyama K, Morikawa A, Kuroume T. Roxithromycin reduces the degree of bronchial hyperresponsiveness in children with asthma. Chest 1994; 106:458–461.

133. Kamoi H, Kurihara N, Fujiwara H, Hirata K, Takeda T. The macrolide antibacterial roxithromycin reduces bronchial hyperresponsiveness and superoxide anion production by polymorphonuclear leukocytes in patients with asthma. J Asthma 1995; 32:191–197.

134. Cazzola M, Salzillo A, Diamare F. Potential role of macrolides in the treatment of asthma. Monaldi Arch Chest Dis 2000; 55:231–236.

135. Avila PC, Boushey HA. Macrolides, asthma, inflammation, and infection. Ann Allergy Asthma Immunol 2000; 84:565–568.

136. Muranaka M, Miyamoto T, Shida T, Kabe J, Makino S, Okumura H, et al. Gold salt in the treatment of bronchial asthma—a double-blind study. Ann Allergy 1978; 40:132–137.

137. Nierop G, Gijzel WP, Bel EH, Zwinderman AH, Dijkman JH. Auranofin in the treatment of steroid dependent asthma: a double blind study. Thorax 1992; 47:349–354.

138. Bernstein IL, Bernstein DI, Dubb JW, Faiferman I, Wallin B. A placebo-controlled multicenter study of auranofin in the treatment of patients with corticosteroid-dependent asthma. Auranofin Multicenter Drug Trial. J Allergy Clin Immunol 1996; 98:317–324.

139. Honma M, Tamura G, Shirato K, Takishima T. Effect of an oral gold compound,

auranofin, on non-specific bronchial hyperresponsiveness in mild asthma. Thorax 1994; 49:649–651.

140. Felson DT, Anderson JJ, Mecnan RF. The comparative efficacy and toxicity of second-line drugs in rheumatoid arthritis: results of two metaanalyses. Arthritis Rheum 1990; 33:1449–1461.

141. Tozman EC, Gottlieb NL. Adverse reactions with oral and parenteral gold preparations. Med Toxicol 1987; 2:177–189.

142. Wong WS, Koh DS. Advances in immunopharmacology of asthma. Biochem Pharmacol 2000; 59:1323–1335.

143. Diamant Z, Page CP. Heparin and related molecules as a new treatment for asthma. Pulm Pharmacol Ther 2000; 13:1–4.

144. Bendstrup KE, Jensen JI. Inhaled heparin is effective in exacerbations of asthma. Respir Med 2000; 94:174–175.

145. Okada S, Hagan JB, Kato M, Bankers-Fulbright JL, Hunt LW, Gleich GJ, et al. Lidocaine and its analogues inhibit IL-5-mediated survival and activation of human eosinophils. J Immunol 1998; 160:4010–4017.

146. Hunt LW, Swedlund HA, Gleich GJ. Effect of nebulized lidocaine on severe glucocorticoid-dependent asthma. Mayo Clin Proc 1996; 71:361–368.

147. Coleman MD. Dapsone toxicity: some current perspectives. Gen Pharmacol 1995; 26:1461–1467.

148. Berlow BA, Liebhaber MI, Dyer Z, Spiegel TM. The effect of dapsone in steroid-dependent asthma. J Allergy Clin Immunol 1991; 87:710–715.

149. In 't Veen JC, Sterk PJ, Bel EH. Alternative strategies in the treatment of bronchial asthma. Clin Exp Allergy 2000; 30:16–33.

150. Masi AT, Hunder GG, Lie JT, Michel BA, Bloch DA, Arend WP, et al. The American College of Rheumatology 1990 criteria for the classification of Churg–Strauss syndrome (allergic granulomatosis and angiitis). Arthritis Rheum 1990; 33:1094–1100.

151. Eustace JA, Nadasdy T, Choi M. Disease of the month: the Churg Strauss Syndrome. J Am Soc Nephrol 1999; 10:2048–2055.

152. Wechsler ME, Garpestad E, Flier SR, Kocher O, Weiland DA, Polito AJ, et al. Pulmonary infiltrates, eosinophilia, and cardiomyopathy following corticosteroid withdrawal in patients with asthma receiving zafirlukast. J Am Med Assoc 1998; 279:455–457.

153. Wechsler ME, Finn D, Gunawardena D, Westlake R, Barker A, Haranath SP, et al. Churg–Strauss syndrome in patients receiving montelukast as treatment for asthma. Chest 2000; 117:708–713.

154. Le Gall C, Pham S, Vignes S, Garcia G, Nunes H, Fichet D, et al. Inhaled corticosteroids and Churg–Strauss syndrome: a report of five cases. Eur Respir J 2000; 15: 978–981.

24

Steroid-Resistant Asthma
New Insights and Implications for Management

DONALD Y. M. LEUNG and JOSEPH D. SPAHN

National Jewish Medical and Research Center
Denver, Colorado

STANLEY J. SZEFLER

National Jewish Medical and Research Center
and University of Colorado Health Sciences Center
Denver, Colorado

I. Introduction

Airway inflammation and immune activation play a key role in the pathogenesis of chronic asthma. Current guidelines of asthma therapy have therefore focused on the use of anti-inflammatory therapy, particularly inhaled glucocorticoids (GCs). The clinical efficacy of GCs are thought to result from a combination of effects on lung inflammation, including decreased trafficking of inflammatory cells to the lung; reduced inflammatory cell survival; diminished production of airway mucus; an inhibitory effect on inflammatory cytokine production; and other anti-inflammatory mechanisms, including the increased gene transcription of anti-inflammatory proteins (see Chapter 8 and Refs. 1,2). Asthmatics, however, vary in their responses to GCs. While the majority of patients respond to regular inhaled GC therapy, there are patients who respond poorly even when treated with high doses of oral prednisone (reviewed in Ref. 1). These patients are often referred to as ''steroid-resistant'' (SR) asthmatics and are distinguished from ''steroid-sensitive'' (SS) patients, who respond rapidly to oral corticosteroids.

GC insensitivity is likely to play a key role in the pathogenesis of severe asthma for two reasons. First, a number of studies have documented the important role of endogenous corticosteroids in modulating the magnitude of tissue allergic responses (3,4). Second, GC therapy is currently the most potent approach for treatment of airway inflammation. Failure to respond to steroid therapy results in ongoing airway inflammation, airway obstruction, and escalating use of medical resources for chronic and urgent care.

This chapter examines the role of immune mechanisms and altered GC receptors (GCR) in the pathogenesis of persistent airway inflammation in SR asthma. Understanding the mechanisms which give rise to corticosteroid resistance have important clinical implications for the management of severe asthma. It is important to evaluate these patients carefully in order to confirm the diagnosis of asthma and identify potentially correctable concomitant conditions which may confound their asthma. Once a diagnosis of SR asthma is made alternative anti-inflammatory approaches must be considered.

II. Definition of Steroid-Resistant Asthma

SR asthma is associated with several distinguishing features. These patients frequently have severe asthma characterized by persistent respiratory symptoms, nocturnal exacerbations, and chronic airflow limitation (FEV_1 <70% of predicted). Most importantly, they have a poor clinical and spirometric response to oral GC therapy (see Chapter 7). The definition of SR asthma has evolved over the past few decades as corticosteroid use has escalated with the increasing severity of asthma. SR asthma was first described in 1967 by Schwartz et al. (5), who reported six asthmatic patients with persistent eosinophilia despite treatment with 40 mg iv of hydrocortisone. In Carmichael's report in 1981 (6), their SR patients had a baseline FEV_1 of less than 60% predicted, but a 30% or greater improvement in FEV_1 following bronchodilator therapy. However, these individuals failed to increase their FEV_1's by greater than 15% after a course of prednisolone 20 mg daily for 7 days. Subsequently, in a report by Corrigan et al. in 1991 (7), SR asthma was defined as the failure to demonstrate an increase in baseline FEV_1 by greater than 15% after a course of oral prednisolone 20 mg daily for 1 week followed by 40 mg daily for a 2nd week.

The difficulty in defining SR asthma derives in part from the lack of definition of an adequate trial of systemic GC therapy. To address this issue, we studied a group of chronic asthmatics admitted to National Jewish Medical and Research Center whose morning prebronchodilator FEV_1 was <70% predicted (8). After receiving prednisone therapy consisting of a burst of at least 40 mg daily, more than 90% of patients showed a significant improvement within 7 days of initiating GC therapy. Prolongation of the course of therapy beyond 10 days did not result in significantly greater improvement in FEV_1.

Table 1 Definition of Steroid-Resistant Asthma[a]

Parameter	Steroid sensitive	Steroid resistant
Bronchodilator response	>15%	>15%
Other causes of wheezing	Ruled out	Ruled out
FEV_1/FVC	<70%	<70%
AM FEV_1	<70%	<70%
Daily prednisone dose	20 mg po b.i.d.	20 mg po b.i.d.
Treatment duration	1–2 weeks	1–2 weeks
Improvement in FEV_1	>30%	<15%

[a] This is an operational definition that may vary among investigators (see Refs. 7,9,11,19).

In a workshop on SR asthma (1), it was proposed that SR asthma be defined as the failure to improve baseline A.M. prebronchodilator FEV_1 by greater than 15% predicted following 7–14 days of oral prednisone 20 mg twice daily (Table 1). Although so-called SR asthma generally represents a relative insensitivity to GC therapy, and some patients might respond to higher doses of prednisone or its equivalent given for longer periods of time, such doses would be undesirable because of marked adverse effects associated with prolonged courses of high-dose prednisone. In a clinical setting certainly any patient not responding to prednisone 40–60 mg daily after 3 weeks is unlikely to respond to a longer course of therapy. Importantly, the diagnosis of SR asthma should be made only after an extensive evaluation to rule out other potential causes of wheezing or factors which contribute to the severity of asthma (see Chapters 11 and 13). Patients with SR asthma should fulfill the ATS criteria for diagnosis of asthma and have a bronchodilator response of greater than 15% improvement in FEV_1.

III. Immune Responses in Steroid-Resistant Asthma

A number of investigations have revealed evidence of immune abnormalities in patients with SR asthma (Table 2). Carmichael and colleagues (6) reported a defective response of peripheral blood mononuclear cells (PBMC) to GCs which correlated with clinical resistance to GC therapy. Poznansky et al. (9) reported on the phenotype and functional response of PBMC from SR asthmatics stimulated with PHA. At baseline, SS and SR asthmatics had similar proportions of T cells and monocytes. However, at doses as low as 10^{-8} M methylprednisolone, in vitro T-lymphocyte proliferation in the SS, but not the SR, asthma group was inhibited by greater than 60%.

Table 2 Immunologic Features of Steroid-Resistant Asthma

Increased levels of T-cell activation
Failure of GCs to
Inhibit PHA-induced T-cell proliferation in vitro
Decrease production of airway IL-2, IL-4 & IL-5 after GC
therapy
Reduce eosinophilia
Suppress monocyte/macrophage secretion of monokines, e.g.,
IL-8
Increased IL-2 and IL-4 gene expression in the airways
Decreased airway interferon-γ gene expression after GC

Corrigan et al. (7) found that in vitro PHA-induced proliferation and cytokine production by PBMC is inhibited by dexamethasone in SS, but not in SR, asthmatics. They also found an increased number of activated peripheral blood T cells in SR asthma (10). Cyclosporin A inhibited proliferation and cytokine production in lymphocytes in both SS and SR asthmatics. Alvarez and colleagues (11) also reported that PHA-induced proliferation of PBMC in SR asthmatics produces a reduced inhibitory response to methylprednisolone. Of note, in the presence of troleandomycin (TAO), proliferation of T lymphocytes in both SS and SR asthmatics was reduced in a dose-dependent fashion. Thus, while SR asthma is associated with refractoriness to GCs, these patients can be sensitive to other anti-inflammatory or immunosuppressive drugs.

Leung and colleagues (12) also examined bronchoalveolar lavage (BAL) cells from SS and SR asthmatics both prior to and after a 1-week course of daily high-dose (40 mg daily) prednisone. At baseline, they found no significant difference between BAL total eosinophils or numbers of activated T cells in the SR versus SS asthma group. However, after prednisone therapy, there was a significant decrease in BAL eosinophil counts and BAL activated T cells in the SS asthma group. In contrast, prednisone therapy was not accompanied by any significant changes in BAL eosinophil counts or number of BAL activated T cells in the SR asthma group. At baseline, BAL cells from patients with SR asthma compared to cells from those with SS asthma with had a significantly higher number of cells expressing mRNA for IL-2 and IL-4. However, no significant differences between these two patient populations were observed in the expression of IL-5 mRNA at baseline. After prednisone therapy, BAL cells from SS, but not SR, asthmatics demonstrated a significant decrease in the number of cells expressing IL-4 mRNA and IL-5 mRNA. Taken together, airway cells from patients with SR asthma have significantly higher levels of IL-2 and IL-4 gene expression than in SS asthma. In addition, prednisone inhibits cytokine gene expression in SS, but not SR, asthma.

IV. Mechanisms of Corticosteroid Action

GCs exert their biological effects by diffusing through the plasma membrane and binding to a specific cytoplasmic receptor, i.e., GCR-α, which belongs to the superfamily of steroid/thyroid/retinoic acid receptors that function as ligand-dependent transcription factors. The unligated, unbound GCR is thought to be a heterohexamer containing the receptor with a single steroid-binding and DNA binding subunit; two molecules of heat shock protein (hsp) 90; and one molecule each of hsp 70, hsp 56, and hsp 26 (13). The binding of GC to its receptor results in the dissociation of these molecular chaperones and translocation to the nucleus where they can activate gene transcription by binding to specific DNA sequences, called GC-responsive elements (GRE). Usually, two GRE half-sites are arranged as inverted palindromes allowing the GCR to bind the DNA as a homodimer. This generally results in increased gene transcription and protein synthesis. Anti-inflammatory effects resulting from positive gene regulation by GCs include the increased synthesis of IκB-α, an inhibitor of NF-κB (14), and increased synthesis of the anti-inflammatory cytokine IL-10 (15).

Of note, many of the inflammatory genes that are inhibited by GCs in asthmatic patients, including cytokines, chemokines, adhesion molecules, inflammatory enzymes and receptors, do not have GREs in their promoter regions and there is little evidence for the existence of negative GREs in these genes. This suggests that GCs can also cause gene repression by indirect mechanism(s). One well-characterized mechanism is protein–protein sequestration of proinflammatory transcription factors, such as AP-1 or NF-κB, directly by the GCR, thus blocking their ability to induce transcription of proinflammatory cytokine genes (16–18). Conversely, overexpression of transcription factors, such as AP-1, can also inhibit binding of the GCR to its DNA GRE recognition sites (17).

V. Glucocorticoid Receptor Abnormalities in Steroid-Resistant Asthma

Steroid resistance has been observed in a number of nonasthmatic conditions, including rheumatoid arthritis, malignancies, and chronic urticaria. The basis for steroid resistance, however, has been studied in greatest detail in familial GC resistance (19). The molecular basis for GC resistance in the various reported kindreds is heterogeneous and includes either reduced GCR numbers, decreased binding affinity for GCs, or poor DNA binding of the GCR to GRE.

Thus, it was of interest to determine whether the poor GC responses in SR asthma is due to an alteration in GCR number or binding affinity (see Table 3). In this regard, we have defined two major types of SR asthma (20). Type I is cytokine-induced or acquired. This group can further be divided into two sub-

Table 3 Clinical and Laboratory Features of Steroid-Resistant Asthma

Features	Type 1	Type II (primary)
A.M. cortisol[a]	Suppressed	No
Cause	Cytokine-induced Acquired (allergies, microbes)	Genetic
Cushingoid side effects[a])	Yes	Genetic
GCR ligand and DNA binding affinity	Reduced	Normal
GCR number	Normal or high	Low
Reversibility of GCR defect	Yes	No

[a] Characteristic observed on high-dose systemic steroids.

types: primary resistance involving immune responses that may be associated with genetic polymorphisms leading to overproduction of certain cytokines, e.g., IL-4, or various key molecules involved in alteration of GC action. Acquired GC resistance may occur as the result of allergen- or infection-induced cytokine activation or chronic exposure to medications such as β-agonists or corticosteroids. Thus, this type of GC resistance is likely to contain multiple subtypes depending on the trigger or genetic background of the host.

Clinically patients with this first type of GC resistance present as patients with SR asthma who develop severe side effects, including adrenal gland suppression from chronic treatment with systemic steroids. This is because there is only one GCR gene and these patients' GC resistance is only at the level of their immune effector cells, e.g., T cells. The rest of the tissues in their bodies are unfortunately quite sensitive to the deleterious effects of steroids and therefore susceptible to adverse systemic effects secondary to high-dose glucocorticoid therapy. Patients with this Type I form of GC resistance have poor GCR binding to corticosteroids and the DNA GRE primarily in their mononuclear cells. Their defect is reversible in vitro and in the majority of cases can be induced in their T cells by the combination of IL-2 and IL-4. Of note, monocyte GCR binding affinity can be decreased by IL-13. The difficulty in separating this group of patients into distinct subtypes, at this time, is that overproduction of cytokines such as IL-4 can occur as the result of genetic as well as environmental exposures, leading to a common final mechanism for inducing decrease of GCR binding affinity. More studies are needed to determine whether there is overlap in these various groups or whether distinct phenotypes arise that reflect reduced clinical responses to GCs.

In contrast, Type II GC resistance involves generalized primary cortisol resistance, which affects all tissues and is likely associated with a genetic mutation in the GCR (Table 3). This Type II form of SR asthma is not associated with the development of steroid-induced side effects and the GCR defect involves a low number of GCRs. It is analogous to familial cortisol resistance, which has a genetic basis as Type II SR asthma and an irreversible GCR defect that involves all cell types. It should be noted that most patients who have a provisional diagnosis of primary SR asthma are simply *not* taking their medications! As a result, they develop no side effects after being prescribed oral prednisone and they obviously derive no therapeutic effects from the steroids. When patients present with a history of primary SR asthma, it is important to confirm they are taking the oral prednisone under strict supervision and to check the A.M. serum cortisol after a course of therapy. The cytokine-induced form (Type I) accounts for >95% of SR asthma. Therefore, any patient presenting with primary SR asthma should be suspected of poor adherence to therapy until proven otherwise.

VI. Molecular Mechanisms of Steroid-Resistant Asthma

The importance of increased IL-4 production as a contributory factor to asthma severity and steroid resistance is supported by recent reports demonstrating an association between asthma severity and steroid resistance with genotypes known to enhance IL-4 production or action. In this regard, Burchard et al. (21) found an association between the IL-4 C-589T sequence variant in the IL-4 gene promoter polymorphism and decrement in pulmonary function among White asthmatic subjects. Of note, the IL-4 C-589T sequence variant is associated with increased IL-4 gene transcription. Interestingly, the frequency of this IL-4 C-589T sequence variant was significantly greater among African-American asthmatics than among White asthmatics. This observation may account for the observations in a report by Spahn et al. (22) which demonstrated that T cells from African Americans display a diminished response to GCs in vitro. Rosa-Rosa et al. (23) has also found that the R576 IL-4R-α allele associated with enhanced response to IL-4 correlates with asthma severity.

The precise mechanism by which cytokines such as the combination of IL-2 and IL-4 decrease corticosteroid responsiveness in patients with Type I SR asthma is unknown. There have been two postulated mechanisms, neither of which are mutually exclusive. The first is based on in vitro observations that cytokines induce the activation of transcription factors and that overexpression of AP-1 or other transcription factors interferes with GCR binding and function (24). Indeed, increased AP-1 expression has been reported in the PBMC of patients with SR asthma, suggesting that abnormal GCR/AP-1 interactions might contribute to corticosteroid insensitivity in asthma (25). Recently these investigators have also reported increased c-*fos* transcription rates in T cells and monocytes from SR asthmatics (26). Furthermore, pretreatment of mononuclear cells from SR asthmatics with c-fos antisense oligonucleotides enhanced GCR–DNA binding activity in SR cells. These data suggested that increased c-*fos* synthesis may act as a mechanism for the increased AP-1 and decreased GCR–DNA binding.

A second mechanism is based on studies demonstrating that alternative splicing involving exon 9 of the GCR gene gives rise to two homologous mRNAs and protein isoforms, termed GCRα and GCRβ (reviewed in Ref. 27). Both mRNAs contain the first eight exons of the GCR gene. GCRα is the classic ligand binding protein for corticosteroids which was described above. GCRβ differs from GCRα only in its carboxy terminus such that the last 50 amino acids of GCRα are replaced with a unique 15-amino-acid sequence. Several groups have shown that these differences render GCRβ unable to bind GC hormones, inhibits its ability to transactivate GC-sensitive genes, and makes it a dominant negative inhibitor of GCRα on activating GRE-containing enhancers or transrepressing NF-κB (29,30). Of note, GCRβ does not inhibit GRα-mediated transrepression of AP-1-responsive promoters (31).

Studies from our lab have demonstrated that overexpression of GCRβ in cell lines induces GC resistance, reproducing the ligand and DNA binding abnormality found in PBMC from SR asthma (32 and unpublished observations). The increased expression of GCRβ could therefore account for SR asthma. We have found that airway cells and PBMC from patients with SR asthma express significantly higher levels of GCRβ than patients with SS asthma or normal subjects (32,33). GCRβ expression was significantly higher in airway T cells than peripheral blood T cells, suggesting that the inflammatory milieu of the lung was driving the elevated GCRβ expression. Synthesis of GCR β was inducible with the combination of IL-2 and IL-4. Animal models of systemic GC resistance such as New World monkeys have approximately 10-fold higher GCRβ than GCRα levels (27). Interestingly, mice known to be extremely SS do not have GCRβ (34).

Recently Sousa et al. (35) confirmed our observations, reporting that GCRβ was elevated in their cohort of SR asthmatics previously described to have elevated cFOS expression in their mononuclear cells as a potential cause of steroid resistance (35). This raises the interesting question as to why patients with SR asthma have elevated AP-1 DNA binding activity and increased GCRβ expression. Further work is needed to establish whether increased c-FOS alters the expression of GCRβ or vice versa.

VII. Factors Contributing to Corticosteroid Resistance

Since the majority of patients with SR asthma have an acquired form of corticosteroid insensitivity induced by immune activation, it is of interest to ascertain whether factors or conditions known to contribute to poorly controlled asthma and increased corticosteroid requirements have an effect on GCR binding affinity or response to corticosteroids.

A. Allergen Exposure

We have examined whether exposure to allergens can alter GCR binding affinity in PBMC from atopic asthmatics (36). PBMC GCR binding affinity from ragweed allergic asthmatics were measured prior to, during the peak, and after ragweed season. A significant reduction in PBMC GCR binding affinity was observed during ragweed pollen season compared to before and after ragweed season. In vitro effects of allergen treatment on GCR binding affinity were also examined on PBMC from cat allergic asthmatics by incubating their cells with cat allergen. GCR binding affinity was significantly reduced after a 48-h incubation with cat allergen. These effects were allergen specific because *Candida albicans* had no effect on GCR binding affinity. Furthermore, allergen-induced reductions in GCR binding affinity were associated with significant decreases in the inhibitory effects of dexamethasone and hydrocortisone on T cells from these atopic asthmatics. The induction of GCR binding abnormalities was also found to be IL-2 and IL-4 dependent.

B. Microbial Superantigens

To further analyze the nature of T-cell activation in patients with poorly controlled asthma, we recently analyzed the T-cell receptor repertoire in poorly controlled asthmatics compared to that in well-controlled asthmatics and normal controls (37). PBMC and BAL cells from poorly controlled asthmatics (FEV_1 <75% predicted despite use of inhaled corticosteroids), well-controlled asthmatics (FEV_1 >85% predicted), and normal controls were stained for the expression of different T-cell receptor–BV regions on T cells using immunofluorescence and flow cytometry. In poorly controlled asthmatics, TCR-BV8+ (but not other TCR-BV+) T cells were significantly increased (Fig. 2). BV8 + BAL T cells were abnormally increased in both the CD4+ and CD8+ T-cell subsets of poorly controlled asthmatics, suggesting activation by a microbial superantigen (38).

To determine whether microbial superantigens could alter corticosteroid sensitivity, we assessed the capacity of 10^{-6} M dexamethasone to inhibit the stimulation of normal PBMC with a prototypic superantigen, staphylococcal enterotoxin B (SEB) versus phytohemagglutinin (PHA). As shown in Fig. 3, dexamethasone caused a 99% inhibition of PHA-induced PBMC proliferation, but only a 19% inhibition of SEB-induced PBMC proliferation (PHA vs SEB, $P <$ 0.01). Taken together, these observations suggest that bacterial or viral agents secreting superantigens may contribute to poorly controlled asthma and reduced

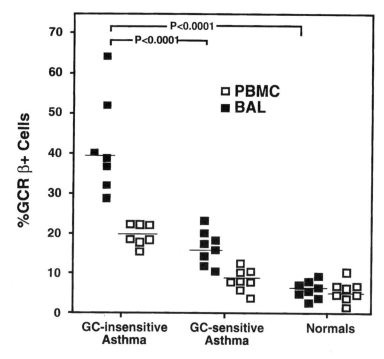

Figure 1   Percentage GRβ+ cells in freshly isolated PBMC versus BAL from steroid-resistant asthmatics versus steroid-sensitive asthmatics and control subjects. PBMC were processed and stained for GRβ immunoreactivity using an immunocytochemistry technique with a specific antibody to GRβ. (Reprinted with permission from Ref. 33.)

corticosteroid sensitivity. Interestingly, recent studies also indicate that SEB is a potent inducer of the GCRβ isoform in T cells (39).

C. Neutrophilia

Our above studies on SR asthma have generally involved patients with ongoing airway obstruction, i.e., FEV_1 <70% predicted, who were not on chronic oral corticosteroids. However, many patients with severe asthma and chronic airway obstruction are treated with prolonged courses of high-dose oral corticosteroids. Recently, Wenzel et al. (40) carried out bronchoscopic studies of the inflammatory cell infiltrate in patients with severe asthma who were dependent on high-dose oral corticosteroids (mean ± SEM FEV_1 = 58 ± 6% predicted despite daily prednisone treatment of ≥20 mg/day for more than 1 year) and compared it to

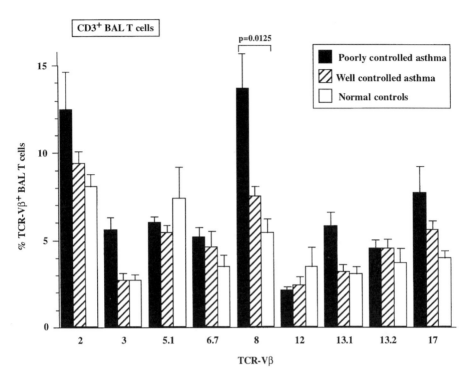

Figure 2 Percentages of Vβ+ T cells (mean ± 2 SEM) in the BAL fluid of nine subjects with poorly controlled asthma, seven subjects with well-controlled asthma, and eight normal control subjects determined with the use of nine different anti-Vβ mAbs. Subjects with poorly controlled asthma had a significantly higher (*P* = .0125) expression of Vβ8+ BAL T cells than normal control subjects. The expression of BAL T cells positive for Vβs other than Vβ8 was not significantly different among the study groups. (Reprinted with permission from Ref. 37.)

patients with moderate asthma (mean ± SEM FEV$_1$ = 65 ± 3% predicted but not requiring prednisone therapy) versus normal controls. The concentration of eosinophils in BAL fluid was highest in the moderate asthmatics not on prednisone, with little difference in eosinophils between normal controls and severe asthmatics. In contrast, the severe asthmatics demonstrated a significantly higher concentration of neutrophils in BAL than either the moderate asthmatics or the normal controls. Patients with severe asthma were also found to have significantly higher levels of leukotriene B4 and thromboxane, which respectively can induce neutrophil chemotaxis and airway hyperreactivity.

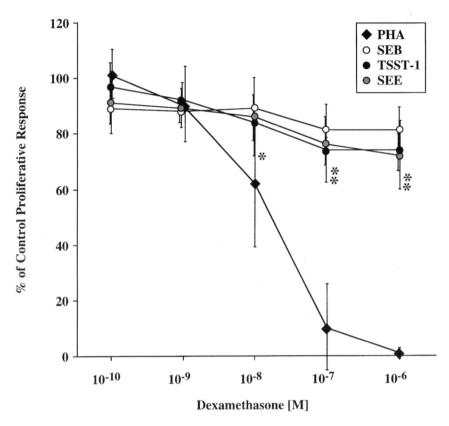

Figure 3 Effect of DEX on PBMC response to SAgs in comparison to PHA. PBMCs of seven healthy donors were incubated for 72 h with PHA (5 μg/ml) or the SAgs SEB, TSST-1, and SEE (100 ng/ml) in the presence or absence of DEX (10^{-10} to 10^{-6} mol/l). SAg-induced PBMC proliferation was significantly less sensitive to DEX than stimulation with PHA. Proliferation response under various conditions was expressed as the percentage of mitogen-induced tritiated thymidine incorporation in the absence of DEX compared with the addition of DEX. Data are expressed as mean ± SEM with a two-way repeated-measures ANOVA to determine significance (*P < .05; **P < .01). (Reprinted with permission from Ref. 39.)

These studies indicate a novel form of inflammation in severe symptomatic asthmatics despite treatment with high-dose oral corticosteroids. Importantly, it is well established that neutrophils are constitutively SR. To determine the potential mechanism of corticosteroid resistance in neutrophils, we examined relative amounts of GCRα and GCRβ in freshly isolated neutrophils (41). We observed increased GCRβ, but not GCRα, protein and mRNA expression in neutrophils at baseline and after IL-8 exposure. Thus, high constitutive expression of GCRβ by neutrophils may provide a mechanism by which these cells escape GC-induced cell death.

D. Sinusitis

Chronic sinusitis with nasal polyposis is often associated with severe asthma. Nasal polyps (NP) frequently demonstrate a poor response to treatment with intranasal steroids. We recently examined whether expression of GCRβ is increased in NP and whether its level of expression may predict GC responsiveness (42). Biopsies of the NP were obtained 1 week before and after 4 weeks of treatment with intranasal fluticasone. GCRβ expression was increased in NP inflammatory cells compared to controls. GCRβ expression in the initial NP biopsies inversely correlated with steroid responsiveness in terms of reduction in eosinophils and reduction in immunostaining for endothelial VCAM-1 and RANTES in the pre- to postbiopsies. GCRβ expression also correlated with the number of CD4$^+$ T lymphocytes in the posttreatment NP biopsies. Thus, GCRβ expression is increased in NP and is a marker of steroid resistance in this disease state.

E. Nocturnal Asthma

Recently, it has been found that PBMC from patients with noncturnal asthma exhibit reduced steroid responsiveness at 4 A.M. compared to 4 P.M. (43). To further examine the mechanism for reduced steroid responsiveness in nocturnal asthma, airway cell expression of GCRβ was examined at 4 P.M. and 4 A.M. (44). BAL lymphocytes and macrophages were incubated with dexamethasone. Dexamethasone suppressed proliferation of BAL lymphocytes similarly at 4 P.M. and 4 A.M. in both groups. However, BAL macrophages from nocturnal asthma exhibited less suppression of IL-8 and TNF-α production by dexamethasone at 4 A.M. compared to 4 P.M. whereas in the nocturnal asthma group dexamethasone suppressed IL-8 and TNF-α production equally well at both time points. GCRβ expression was increased at night only in nocturnal asthma, primarily due to significantly increased expression by BAL macrophages. IL-13 mRNA expression was increased at night, but only in the nocturnal asthma group and addition of neutralizing antibodies to IL-13 reduced GCRβ expression by BAL GCRβ macrophages. These data suggest that the airway macrophage may be the airway inflammatory cell driving the reduction in steroid responsiveness at night in NA, and this function is modulated by IL-13.

F. Fatal Asthma

Steroid resistance may be a major contributing factor to fatal asthma, since many of these patients die in the emergency room despite receiving high doses of iv corticosteroids. We have thus investigated the expression of GCRβ in large and small airways obtained from lungs from fatal asthma compared to the expression in emphysema and lungs of patients who died from nonpulmonary diseases (45). Tissue sections from airways (large and small) were obtained from seven patients who died from asthma, six patients who died from emphysema, and eight controls. There were significantly higher numbers of GCRβ immunoreactive cells in fatal asthma compared to emphysema and controls, but there was no difference in the expression of GCRβ in emphysema compared to controls. The expression of GCRβ in the small airways of asthmatics did not differ significantly from large airways. The results of this study support the association of steroid resistance and fatal asthma and provide further evidence for the role of small airways in the pathogenesis of severe asthma.

VIII. Management of Steroid-Resistant Asthma

The management of these patients poses a considerable challenge to the clinician. In a recent study we found that 25% of patients referred for severe asthma had SR asthma (46). Thus, 75% patients with severe asthma can be approached by optimizing management. A systematic, stepwise approach is important for a successful outcome (Table 4).

The first step is to obtain a thorough history, physical examination, and appropriate laboratory tests to confirm the diagnosis of asthma and rule out concomitant medical disorders which can complicate the management of chronic asthma. The diagnosis of vocal cord dysfunction, which involves abnormal vocal cord closure during inspiration, is often missed. This diagnosis can only be made by direct laryngoscopy when the patient is symptomatic and should be suspected in any adolescent or adult with recent onset of steroid-dependent asthma. Gastroesophageal reflux and/or aspiration, sinusitis, ongoing exposure to environmental allergens, or allergic bronchopulmonary aspergillosis are some of the concomitant factors that must be ruled out.

The second step is to rule out psychosocial factors affecting the illness. A large proportion of patients with apparent SR asthma have an inadequate response to therapy simply due to their noncompliance with recommended therapy. The basis for noncompliance is complex and can range from simple forgetfulness, in which case a medication diary or pill box is useful, to the inability to pay for the medications or severe psychologic problems such as depression which impair the patient's ability to function and adhere to a suggested medical regimen. Correction of these underlying problems are important to ensure adherence to therapy. In addition, it is important to keep the medication regimen as simple as possible, prioritize recommendations, educate the patient regarding their asthma

Table 4 Considerations in the Management of Steroid-Resistant Asthma

Rule out other pulmonary disorders
Concomitant medical problems affecting asthma care
  Vocal cord dysfunction
  Gastroesophageal reflux
  Chronic sinusitis or other respiratory infections
  Allergic bronchopulmonary aspergillosis
Psychosocial factors affecting self-care
  Poor adherence with medications
  Emotional factors
Inadequate technique of medication administration
Persistent inflammation due to the following chronic conditions
  Allergen exposure
  Microbial colonization
  Inadequate glucocorticoid dose/potency
  Need for combination therapy
  β-Agonist overuse
Abnormal glucocorticoid pharmacokinetics
GCR binding abnormalities
Written action plan
Alternative anti-inflammatory approach

management, and tailor the dosing to the patient's schedule. Cost of medications is also an important factor to discuss with patients.

Interestingly, psychosocial stress has been found to attenuate cortisol responses (47). This may augment underlying allergic inflammation, since cortisol secretion has been found to modulate endogenous tissue inflammation (3,4). However, the mechanisms by which stress or depressed socioeconomic factors contribute to worsening of asthma is poorly understood.

The third step is to review the patient's technique of medication administration. This should be incorporated as a routine part of the physical examination, as patients often forget proper inhaler technique. Spacer devices should be used to optimize medication delivery and reduce adverse effects of medications, especially inhaled steroids. For inhaled steroids, advise mouth rinsing and expectoration of mouth rinse to further reduce the extent of systemic steroid absorption.

The fourth step is to assure appropriate environmental control at home, at school, and at work. The focus should be on areas where the patient spends the greatest time, for example, the bedroom, or areas of high indoor allergen exposure. A number of studies have demonstrated that atopic patients who live with animals at home require higher doses of steroids to maintain control of their asthma (48). Several studies have also implicated schools as a major source of animal dander exposure (49).

The fifth step is evaluate patients for potential microbial infection of their airways. This is particularly important for patients on high doses of inhaled steroids or chronic oral steroids, as their local immune response may be compromised, thus predisposing them to colonization with opportunistic organisms, including mycoplasma and chlamydia, which can trigger inflammation (50). Such individuals may respond to a long course of clarithromycin.

The sixth step is to maximize anti-inflammatory and bronchodilator therapy for control of nocturnal exacerbations. Inhaled salmeterol administered at bedtime can be very useful in controlling nocturnal asthma. Oral theophylline can also be used as well in the treatment of nocturnal asthma. In this case, chronopharmacologic principles should be applied to optimize response to theophylline. In this regard, patients with nocturnal exacerbations may do better with a single dose of a once-daily sustained-release preparation administered in the evening compared to a standard twice-daily preparation (51). Children and rapid theophylline metabolizers appear to be prone to reduction in serum theophylline concentrations during the night (52). Occasionally theophylline pharmacokinetic studies involving 24-h monitoring of theophylline levels are needed to assist in developing individualized treatment schedules. Although there are no specific studies with leukotriene modifiers in severe asthma, available studies show an additive effect with inhaled steroids (53). Therefore, these medications may be useful in reducing the amount of steroid therapy needed to control asthma (54).

The seventh step is to modify inhaled GC therapy in an effort to reduce requirements for systemic GC therapy. One approach would be to increase the dose and frequency of inhaled GCs. This is based on the assumption that higher doses would be more effective and also that adverse effects would be less than those commonly associated with high-dose systemic GC therapy. The majority of patients with SR asthma have the acquired form, which is associated with reduced GCR binding affinity. Studies of their T cells indicate a shift to the right in their dose response to steroids rather than an absolute resistance (55). Thus, higher doses of GCs or a change to GCs with a higher binding affinity, such as fluticasone propionate, or an improved delivery system, such as a Turbuhaler for budesonide (56,57), is a reasonable initial approach to gain control of their asthma.

The eighth step is to evaluate systemic corticosteroid pharmacokinetics and receptors to maximize pulmonary function with oral corticosteroids and assess the basis of corticosteroid insensitivity in patients with poorly controlled asthma. The purpose of these studies is to determine whether there is incomplete corticosteroid absorption, failure to convert to an active form, rapid elimination, reduced

GCR number or binding affinity, or a combination of abnormalities (58,59). This evaluation is particularly important in a patient who fails to demonstrate the anticipated adverse effects of long-term, high-dose corticosteroid therapy. Measurements of plasma cortisol levels can also be used in an assessment of compliance. Patients with poor absorption of prednisone frequently respond well to oral liquid steroid preparations. In patients with rapid corticosteroid elimination, a split dosing regimen, with the second dose of the day administered in the afternoon, should be considered. In such patients, the morning dose should be titrated, the afternoon dose should be converted to a morning dose, and then an attempt should be made to reduce to alternate-day therapy.

We are also beginning to incorporate markers of inflammation, for example, exhaled nitric oxide, plasma eosinophilic cationic protein, and serum IL-2 receptors, to examine medication response (60,61). This is most useful before and after a 1- to 2-week course of oral prednisone therapy. Failure to respond with persistent elevated levels of inflammation despite treatment with high-dose prednisone provides a strong basis for incorporating alternative therapies and the diagnosis of SR asthma.

It is important to monitor patients carefully for adverse effects related to GC therapy and initiate measures to minimize their effect. For example, steroid-induced osteoporosis can be monitored with bone densitometry. Attention should be placed on providing adequate dietary calcium and vitamin D as well as other therapeutic interventions as indicated (62).

The ninth step is to develop a written action plan for acute asthma exacerbations. Emphasis should be placed on appropriate use of rescue medications such as bronchodilators and when to notify the physician. A written care plan should also be used to summarize routine prophylactic medications, including recommendations for pretreatment programs for exercise and anticipated exposure to irritants or allergens. If a patient has difficulty in following the recommendations or appears to be intentionally noncompliant, a psychological evaluation may be needed to identify psychosocial features that interfere with adherence to the treatment regimen, including learning disabilities, family dysfunction, depression, and anxiety.

The final step is to consider alternative anti-inflammatory and immunomodulator approaches. This is of particular importance in patients with the Type II or the primary form of SR asthma associated with a generalized primary GC resistance. Unfortunately, there have been no well-controlled studies of alternative therapies in SR asthma. Treatment with intravenous immunoglobulin, cyclosporine, methotrexate, and gold have been reported to have steroid-sparing effects and may be potentially useful in patients who fail steroid therapy (63–65). Limited information from in vitro studies of SR asthma suggest that T cells will respond to the immunosuppressive actions of cyclosporine, thus providing a rationale for use of this agent in the management of these patients (7). In a recent study, treatment of steroid-dependent asthma with iv IG was associated with increased GCR binding affinity (65).

To date, studies of these medications have not systematically incorporated bronchial biopsies and bronchoalveolar lavage to verify resolution of inflammation, although several case reports have now demonstrated decreased airway inflammation in SR asthmatics treated with intravenous immunoglobulin or cyclosporin (66,67). An organized program with carefully designed protocols and larger numbers of patients is needed to understand the role of these alternative anti-inflammatory therapies in the treatment of SR asthma and to identify a hierarchy of medication selection for patients with severe asthma.

In the future, more information is also needed on the pathology of severe asthma to determine whether there are ultrastructural abnormalities present that may be irreversible (Refs. 68, 69 and Chapter 5 in this volume). In this regard, it is possible that aggressive courses of anti-inflammatory or immunomodulator therapy can suppress acute inflammation, but airway remodeling may predispose the patient to residual symptoms and the development of irreversible airway disease. Of greater concern is the possibility that the persistent symptoms in certain patients could be related to noninflammatory airways hyperresponsiveness. Obviously, more effort must be placed on understanding the pathophysiology of severe asthma to refine the selection of pharmacotherapy for this challenging group of patients.

There have been no systematic studies examining the long-term prognosis of SR asthma. The major concern with this group of patients is that they are at high risk for morbidity and mortality due to asthma and the adverse effects of therapy, especially high-dose, long-term steroid therapy. During acute exacerbations of their asthma, patients with Type I SR asthma require much higher doses of intravenous corticosteroids than SS asthmatics to gain control of their inflammation. This places them at higher risk for steroid-induced side effects. In patients with Type II SR asthma, high doses of intravenous corticosteroids is also worth trying, but it is possible that they will require alternative anti-inflammatory therapy. It should be emphasized that SR asthmatics do respond to bronchodilator therapy and that such medications should be instituted early as rescue therapy. Finally, the presence of high-level persistent airway inflammation in this group of asthmatics predisposes them to the development of airway remodeling and long-term irreversible airway diseases. Thus, it is of paramount importance to treat their inflammation early and effectively.

Acknowledgments

Supported in part by NIH Grants HL36577 and HL37260 and General Clinical Research Center Grant 5 MO1 RR00051 from the Division of Research Resources.

References

1. Lee TH, Brattsand R, Leung DYM. Corticosteroid action and resistance in asthma. Am J Respir Cell Mol Biol 1996; 154(suppl):S1–S79.
2. Barnes PJ. Efficacy of inhaled corticosteroids in asthma. J Allergy Clin Immunol 1998; 102(4/1):531–538.
3. Peebles S, Togias A, Bickel CA, Diemer FB, Hubbard WC, Schleimer R. Endogenous glucocorticoids and antigen-induced acute and late phase pulmonary responses. Clin Exp Allergy 2000; in press.
4. Herrscher RF, Kasper C, Sullivan TJ. Endogenous cortisol regulates immunoglobulin E-dependent late phase reactions. J Clin Invest 1992; 90(2):596–603.
5. Schwartz HJ, Lowell FC, Melby JC. Steroid resistance in bronchial asthma. Ann Intern Med 1968; 69(3):493–499.
6. Carmichael J, Paterson IC, Diaz P, Crompton GK, Kay AB, Grant IW. Corticosteroid resistance in chronic asthma. Br Med J (Clin Res Ed) 1981; 282(6274):1419–1422.
7. Corrigan CJ, Brown PH, Barnes NC, Szefler SJ, Tsai JJ, Frew AJ, Kay AB. Glucocorticoid resistance in chronic asthma: glucocorticoid pharmacokinetics, glucocorticoid receptor characteristics, and inhibition of peripheral blood T cell proliferation by glucocorticoids in vitro. Am Rev Respir Dis 1991; 144(5):1016–1025.
8. Kamada AK, Leung DYM, Gleason MC, Hill MR, Szefler SJ. High-dose systemic glucocorticoid therapy in the treatment of severe asthma: a case of resistance and patterns of response. J Allergy Clin Immunol 1992; 90(4/1):685–687.
9. Poznansky MC, Gordon AC, Douglas JG, Krajewski AS, Wyllie AH, Grant IW. Resistance to methylprednisolone in cultures of blood mononuclear cells from glucocorticoid-resistant asthmatic patients. Clin Sci 1984; 67(6):639–645.
10. Corrigan CJ, Brown PH, Barnes NC, Tsai JJ, Frew AJ, Kay AB. Glucocorticoid resistance in chronic asthma: peripheral blood T lymphocyte activation and comparison of the T lymphocyte inhibitory effects of glucocorticoids and cyclosporin A. Am Rev Respir Dis 1991; 144(5):1026–1032.
11. Alvarez J, Surs W, Leung DYM, Ikle D, Gelfand EW, Szefler SJ. Steroid-resistant asthma: immunologic and pharmacologic features. J Allergy Clin Immunol 1992; 89(3):714–721.
12. Leung DYM, Martin RJ, Szefler SJ, Sher ER, Ying S, Kay AB, Hamid Q. Dysregulation of interleukin 4, interleukin 5, and interferon gamma gene expression in steroid-resistant asthma. J Exp Med 1995; 181(1):33–40.
13. Bloom JW. New insights into the molecular basis of glucocorticoid action. Immunol Allergy Clin N Am 1999; 19:653–670.
14. Auphan N, DiDonato JA, Rosette C, Helmberg A, Karin M. Immunosuppression by glucocorticoids: inhibition of NF-kappa B activity through induction of I kappa B synthesis. Science 1995; 270(5234):286–290.
15. John M, Lim S, Seybold J, Jose P, Robichaud A, O'Connor B, Barnes PJ, Chung KF. Inhaled corticosteroids increase interleukin-10 but reduce macrophage inflammatory protein-1alpha, granulocyte-macrophage colony-stimulating factor, and interferon-gamma release from alveolar macrophages in asthma. Am J Respir Crit Care Med 1998; 157(1):256–262.

16. Miner JN, Yamamoto KR. The basic region of AP-1 specifies glucocorticoid receptor activity at a composite response element. Genes Dev 1992; 6(12B):2491–2501.

17. Yang-Yen HF, Chambard JC, Sun YL, Smeal T, Schmidt TJ, Drouin J, Karin M. Transcriptional interference between c-Jun and the glucocorticoid receptor: mutual inhibition of DNA binding due to direct protein- protein interaction. Cell 1990; 62(6):1205–1215.

18. Schule R, Rangarajan P, Kliewer S, Ransone LJ, Bolado J, Yang N, Verma IM, Evans RM. Functional antagonism between oncoprotein c-Jun and the glucocorticoid receptor. Cell 1990; 62(6):1217–1226.

19. Chrousos GP, Detera-Wadleigh SD, Karl M. Syndromes of glucocorticoid resistance. Ann Intern Med 1993; 119(11):1113–1124.

20. Sher ER, Leung DYM, Surs W, Kam JC, Zieg G, Kamada AK, Szefler SJ. Steroid-resistant asthma: cellular mechanisms contributing to inadequate response to glucocorticoid therapy. J Clin Invest 1994; 93(1):33–39.

21. Burchard EG, Silverman EK, Rosenwasser LJ, Borish L, Yandava C, Pillari A, Weiss ST, Hasday J, Lilly CM, Ford JG, Drazen JM. Association between a sequence variant in the IL-4 gene promoter and FEV(1) in asthma. Am J Respir Crit Care Med 1999; 160(3):919–922.

22. Spahn JD, Brown EE, Covar R, Leung DYM. Do African-Americans display a diminished response to glucocorticoids (GCs)? J Allergy Clin Immunol 1999; 103 (1/2):S62.

23. Rosa-Rosa L, Zimmermann N, Bernstein JA, Rothenberg ME, Khurana Hershey GK. The R576 IL-4 receptor alpha allele correlates with asthma severity. J Allergy Clin Immunol 1999; 104(5):1008–1014.

24. Yang-Yen HF, Chambard JC, Sun YL, Smeal T, Schmidt TJ, Drouin J, Karin M. Transcriptional interference between c-Jun and the glucocorticoid receptor: mutual inhibition of DNA binding due to direct protein- protein interaction. Cell 1990; 62(6):1205–1215.

25. Adcock IM, Lane SJ, Brown CR, Peters MJ, Lee TH, Barnes PJ. Differences in binding of glucocorticoid receptor to DNA in steroid-resistant asthma. J Immunol 1995; 154(7):3500–3505.

26. Lane SJ, Adcock IM, Richards D, Hawrylowicz C, Barnes PJ, Lee TH. Corticosteroid-resistant bronchial asthma is associated with increased c-fos expression in monocytes and T lymphocytes. J Clin Invest 1998; 102(12):2156–2164.

27. Vottero A, Chrousos GP. Glucocorticoid receptor beta: View I. Trends Endocrinol Metab 1999; 10(8):333–338.

28. Bamberger CM, Bamberger AM, de Castro M, Chrousos GP. Glucocorticoid receptor beta, a potential endogenous inhibitor of glucocorticoid action in humans. J Clin Invest 1995; 95(6):2435–2441.

29. Oakley RH, Sar M, Cidlowski JA. The human glucocorticoid receptor beta isoform. Expression, biochemical properties, and putative function. J Biol Chem 1996; 271(16):9550–9559.

30. Oakley RH, Jewell CM, Yudt MR, Bofetiado DM, Cidlowski JA. The dominant negative activity of the human glucocorticoid receptor beta isoform. Specificity and mechanisms of action. J Biol Chem 1999; 274(39):27857–27866.

31. Bamberger CM, Else T, Bamberger AM, Beil FU, Schulte HM. Regulation of the human interleukin-2 gene by the alpha and beta isoforms of the glucocorticoid receptor. Mol Cell Endocrinol 1997; 136(1):23–28.

32. Leung DYM, Hamid Q, Vottero A, Szefler SJ, Surs W, Minshall E, Chrousos GP, Klemm DJ. Association of glucocorticoid insensitivity with increased expression of glucocorticoid receptor beta. J Exp Med 1997; 186(9):1567–1574.

33. Hamid QA, Wenzel SE, Hauk PJ, Tsicopoulos A, Wallaert B, Lafitte JJ, Chrousos GP, Szefler SJ, Leung DYM. Increased glucocorticoid receptor beta in airway cells of glucocorticoid-insensitive asthma. Am J Respir Crit Care Med 1999; 159(5/1): 1600–1604.

34. Otto C, Reichardt HM, Schutz G. Absence of glucocorticoid receptor-beta in mice. J Biol Chem 1997; 272(42):26665–26668.

35. Sousa AR, Lane SJ, Soh C, Lee TH. In vivo resistance to corticosteroids in bronchial asthma is associated with enhanced phosphorylation of JUN N-terminal kinase and failure of prednisolone to inhibit JUN N-terminal kinase phosphorylation. J Allergy Clin Immunol 1999; 104 (3/1):565–574.

36. Nimmagadda SR, Szefler SJ, Spahn JD, Surs W, Leung DYM. Allergen exposure decreases glucocorticoid receptor binding affinity and steroid responsiveness in atopic asthmatics. Am J Respir Crit Care Med 1997; 155(1):87–93.

37. Hauk PJ, Wenzel SE, Trumble AE, Szefler SJ, Leung DYM. Increased T-cell receptor vbeta8 + T cells in bronchoalveolar lavage fluid of subjects with poorly controlled asthma: a potential role for microbial superantigens. J Allergy Clin Immunol 1999; 104(1):37–45.

38. Kotzin BL, Leung DYM, Kappler J, Marrack P. Superantigens and their potential role in human disease. Adv Immunol 1993; 54:99–166.

39. Hauk PJ, Hamid QA, Chrousos GP, Leung DYM. Induction of corticosteroid insensitivity in human PBMCs by microbial superantigens. J Allergy Clin Immunol 2000; 105(4):782–787.

40. Wenzel SE, Szefler SJ, Leung DYM, Sloan SI, Rex MD, Martin RJ. Bronchoscopic evaluation of severe asthma. Persistent inflammation associated with high dose glucocorticoids. Am J Respir Crit Care Med 1997; 156(3/1):737–743.

41. Strickland I, Wenzel SE, Leung DYM. High expression of glucocorticoid receptor beta may provide a mechanism for neutrophil insensitivity to steroids in vivo. J Allergy Clin Immunol 1999; 103(1/2):S50.

42. Leung DYM, Hamilos DL, Thawley SE, Hamid QA. Expression of GRβ in nasal polyps (NP) and its relationship to glucocorticoid responsiveness. J Allergy Clin Immunol 1998; 101(2):196A.

43. Kraft M, Vianna E, Martin RJ, Leung DYM. Nocturnal asthma is associated with reduced glucocorticoid receptor binding affinity and decreased steroid responsiveness at night. J Allergy Clin Immunol 1999; 103(1/1):66–71.

44. Kraft M, Martin RJ, Humeston TR, Rex M, Leung DYM. Lung macrophages from nocturnal asthmatics (NA) and non-nocturnal asthmatics (NNA) exhibit differences in circadian variation in steroid responsiveness. Am J Respir Crit Care Med 1998; 157:A393.

45. Christodoulopoulos P, Leung DYM, Hamid QA. Increased expression of GRβ1 in fatal asthma. J Allergy Clin Immunol 1999; 103:890A.

46. Chan MT, Leung DYM, Szefler SJ, Spahn JD. Difficult-to-control asthma: clinical characteristics of steroid-insensitive asthma. J Allergy Clin Immunol 1998; 101(5): 594–601.
47. Buske-Kirschbaum A, Jobst S, Psych D, Wustmans A, Kirschbaum C, Rauh W, Hellhammer D. Attenuated free cortisol response to psychosocial stress in children with atopic dermatitis. Psychosom Med 1997; 59(4):419–426.
48. Murray AB, Ferguson AC, Morrison BJ. The frequency and severity of cat allergy vs. dog allergy in atopic children. J Allergy Clin Immunol 1983; 72(2):145–149.
49. Perzanowski MS, Ronmark E, Nold B, Lundback B, Platts-Mills TA. Relevance of allergens from cats and dogs to asthma in the northernmost province of Sweden: schools as a major site of exposure. J Allergy Clin Immunol 1999; 103(6):1018–1024.
50. Kraft M, Cassell GH, Henson JE, Watson H, Williamson J, Marmion BP, Gaydos CA, Martin RJ. Detection of Mycoplasma pneumoniae in the airways of adults with chronic asthma. Am J Respir Crit Care Med 1998; 158(3):998–1001.
51. Martin RJ, Cicutto LC, Ballard RD, Goldenheim PD, Cherniack RM. Circadian variations in theophylline concentrations and the treatment of nocturnal asthma. Am Rev Respir Dis 1989; 139(2):475–478.
52. Kossoy AF, Hill M, Lin FL, Szefler SJ. Are theophylline ''levels'' a reliable indicator of compliance? J Allergy Clin Immunol 1989; 84(1):60–65.
53. Tamaoki J, Kondo M, Sakai N, Nakata J, Takemura H, Nagai A, Takizawa T, Konno K. Leukotriene antagonist prevents exacerbation of asthma during reduction of high-dose inhaled corticosteroid. The Tokyo Joshi-Idai Asthma Research Group. Am J Respir Crit Care Med 1997; 155(4):1235–1240.
54. American Thoracic Society Workshop. Immunobiology of asthma and rhinitis. Pathogenic factors and therapeutic options. Am J Respir Crit Care Med 1999; 160 (5/1):1778–1787.
55. Spahn JD, Landwehr LP, Nimmagadda S, Surs W, Leung DYM, Szefler SJ. Effects of glucocorticoids on lymphocyte activation in patients with steroid-sensitive and steroid-resistant asthma. J Allergy Clin Immunol 1996; 98(6/1):1073–1079.
56. Thorsson L, Edsbacker S, Conradson TB. Lung deposition of budesonide from Turbuhaler is twice that from a pressurized metered-dose inhaler P-MDI. Eur Respir J 1994; 7(10):1839–1844.
57. Seale JP, Harrison LI. Effect of changing the fine particle mass of inhaled beclomethasone dipropionate on intrapulmonary deposition and pharmacokinetics. Respir Med 1998; 92(suppl A):9–15.
58. Hill MR, Szefler SJ, Ball BD, Bartoszek M, Brenner AM. Monitoring glucocorticoid therapy: a pharmacokinetic approach. Clin Pharmacol Ther 1990; 48(4):390–398.
59. Kamada AK, Spahn JD, Surs W, Brown E, Leung DYM, Szefler SJ. Coexistence of glucocorticoid receptor and pharmacokinetic abnormalities: factors that contribute to a poor response to treatment with glucocorticoids in children with asthma. J Pediatr 1994; 124(6):984–986.
60. Spahn JD, Leung DYM, Surs W, Harbeck RJ, Nimmagadda S, Szefler SJ. Reduced glucocorticoid binding affinity in asthma is related to ongoing allergic inflammation. Am J Respir Crit Care Med 1995; 151(6):1709–1714.
61. Lanz MJ, Leung DYM, McCormick DR, Harbeck R, Szefler SJ, White CW. Compar-

ison of exhaled nitric oxide, serum eosinophilic cationic protein, and soluble interleukin-2 receptor in exacerbations of pediatric asthma. Pediatr Pulmonol 1997; 24(5):305–311.

62. Ledford D, Apter A, Brenner AM, Rubin K, Prestwood K, Frieri M, Lukert B. Osteoporosis in the corticosteroid-treated patient with asthma. J Allergy Clin Immunol 1998; 102(3):353–362.

63. Bernstein DI, Bernstein IL, Bodenheimer SS, Pietrusko RG. An open study of auranofin in the treatment of steroid-dependent asthma. J Allergy Clin Immunol 1988; 81(1):6–16.

64. Stempel DA. Alternative anti-inflammatory and immunomodulator medications for asthma. Immunol Allergy Clin N Am 1999; 19:855–869.

65. Spahn JD, Leung DYM, Chan MT, Szefler SJ, Gelfand EW. Mechanisms of glucocorticoid reduction in asthmatic subjects treated with intravenous immunoglobulin. J Allergy Clin Immunol 1999; 103(3/1):421–426.

66. Redington AE, Hardinge FM, Madden J, Holgate ST, Howarth PH. Cyclosporin A treatment and airways inflammation in corticosteroid-dependent asthma. Allergy 1998; 53(1):94–98.

67. Vrugt B, Wilson S, van Velzen E, Bron A, Shute JK, Holgate ST, Djukanovic R, Aalbers R. Effects of high dose intravenous immunoglobulin in two severe corticosteroid insensitive asthmatic patients. Thorax 1997; 52(7):662–664.

68. Hegele RG, Hogg JC. The pathology of asthma: An inflammatory disorder. In: Szefler SJ, Leung DYM, eds. Severe Asthma: Pathogenesis and Clinical Management. New York: Marcel Dekker, 1996:61–76.

69. Minshall EM, Leung DYM, Martin RJ, Song YL, Cameron L, Ernst P, Hamid Q. Eosinophil-associated TGF-beta 1 mRNA expression and airways fibrosis in bronchial asthma. Am J Respir Cell Mol Biol 1997; 17(3):326–333.

25

Prevention of Severe Asthma
Promising Opportunities

STANLEY J. SZEFLER

National Jewish Medical and Research
  Center
and University of Colorado Health
  Sciences Center
Denver, Colorado

DONALD Y. M. LEUNG

National Jewish Medical and Research
  Center
Denver, Colorado

I. Introduction

Our first edition of *Severe Asthma*, published in 1996, was the first to focus on the topic of severe asthma as a unique feature of this disease (1). Our intention at that time was to gather the available literature for clinicians and to stimulate further research in this area. We ended the book with a chapter entitled ''Asthma Management: Past, Present, and Future.'' In that summary, we reviewed the scope of asthma management and identified critical questions that could be addressed to advance the care of asthma. Some of these questions have been answered, some partially answered, and some remain to be answered.

By 1996, we were very familiar with the concept of chronic inflammation as a feature of asthma. Attention by then had shifted to viewing inhaled steroids as the cornerstone of managing persistent asthma. As such, we began to ask questions regarding the measurement of inflammation and we also sought methods to monitor inflammation.

Shortly after publication of our book, a revised set of guidelines for the diagnosis and management of asthma were published in 1997 by the National Heart, Lung and Blood Institute National Asthma Education and Prevention Program (2). The major changes in this set of guidelines were a reclassification of

621

the levels of severity of asthma and also an update on the organization of pharmacotherapy for the respective classes of treatment. While there is considerable information on the application of treatment for controlling the symptoms related to mild intermittent, mild persistent, and moderate persistent asthma, the best steps for the management of severe asthma are not as clear. In addition, the most appropriate method to make an early diagnosis of asthma is not known. Also, the most appropriate long-term control therapy for early intervention to prevent lung deterioration associated with chronic asthma is a subject of continuing evaluation.

Since 1996, we have developed a better understanding of the features of inflammation that are associated with asthma. Inhaled steroids have been accepted as the most potent form of anti-inflammatory therapy for persistent asthma, and we now have techniques to directly and indirectly measure airway inflammation. We have now begun to appreciate the fact that chronic inflammation can lead to remodeling of the airways and a progressive decline in pulmonary function. We also have a new class of medications available, namely, the leukotriene modifiers, and we are on the brink of introducing several new classes of medications, specifically anti-IgE and cytokine modifiers. Consequently, we face the challenge of determining how these new medications will best fit into an algorithm for the treatment of asthma. This is important for establishing a unified approach to the management of asthma.

The two major questions that we should now address for severe asthma include the following: Can we reduce the prevalence of severe asthma by reversing the course once it is established? and Can we reduce the incidence of severe asthma by altering the natural course of asthma? The following discussion summarizes the insights provided by this second edition of *Severe Asthma* that will enable us to approach these two questions into the mid-2000s.

II. Can We Reverse the Course of Severe Asthma Once It Is Established?

As summarized in this book, there has been considerable insight developed into the pathology of severe asthma and the presence of airway remodeling. Chapter 5 has addressed the pathology of airway remodeling and the features that contribute to persistent inflammation. He and others have also observed that lung inflammation in asthma involves the small and large airways. The major goals of management in established severe asthma must include the arrest of inflammation and healing of the damaged airways to enable a return to near-normal pulmonary function and quality of life.

Recent observations suggest that there may be two subclasses of pathology for severe asthma: one that has a predominance of inflammatory mediators and another that is devoid of cellular features of chronic inflammation (3). In addition, it has been observed by Kraft et al. that there is a high prevalence of mycoplasma and chlamydia in biopsy specimens of patients with severe asthma (4). These observations should lead the way for further research by better categorizing the various forms in patients with severe asthma and also by identifying key driving forces for pathology.

For example, in the evaluation of the infectious component of asthma, the following questions must be addressed. Do mycoplasma and chlamydia play a role in the inflammatory nature of asthma and lead to disease persistence or progression? Can the eradication of this organism through antimicrobial therapy facilitate the improvement in pulmonary function, quality of life, and possibly remission for patients with severe asthma? Alternatively, is the organism merely a result of immune suppression secondary to aggressive anti-inflammatory therapy, specifically high-dose inhaled and systemic glucocorticoids, and of little consequence to the persistence of inflammation?

Another important area to address is the mechanisms underlying the features of steroid-insensitive asthma. Chapter 24 summarizes current knowledge of this feature of severe asthma identified in a subset of patients. In our first edition, the observation of persistent inflammation and severe asthma and the reduced binding affinity of lymphocyte glucocorticoid receptors in patients with severe asthma had been recognized. This observation, along with the recognition of increased expression of cytokine mRNA for IL-5, IL-4, and IL-2 in BALF cells of patients with severe asthma, prompted consideration for the use of high-dose, high-potency inhaled glucocorticoids in severe asthma as well as aggressive systemic glucocorticoid therapy to reduce the degree of chronic inflammation. In addition, cytokine antagonists for IL-4 and IL-5 have been developed and are currently undergoing clinical investigation. Barnes reviews the host of mediators that play a role in asthma pathology and must be considered as targets for therapeutic intervention. Any or all of these could be playing a role in persistence of severe asthma.

Subsequently, new insight into steroid-insensitive asthma has included the identification of additional cellular mechanisms that contribute to steroid insensitivity, namely the presence of elevated GCRβ and nuclear transcription factors in inflammatory cells of patients with severe asthma (5,6). Both of these components could be associated with refractoriness to high-dose steroid therapy. In addition, questions have been raised as to whether conventionally administered inhaled steroid therapy is sufficient to reduce inflammation in peripheral sites of the lung.

These pathologic features of severe asthma prompt research into the identification of methods to monitor ongoing inflammation in asthma. While bronchial biopsy is the most direct measure of the pathologic status of the airways, it has limitations. First, on a practical basis, this can only be obtained a limited number of times. Second, the small tissue specimen and the site of biopsy may not provide sufficient insight into the magnitude and nature of the inflammatory state. Promising alternatives include several noninvasive measures of airway pathology. Chapter 19 summarized available techniques to monitor inflammation and their potential application for managing severe asthma. Chapter 12 summarized the potential application of imaging techniques and the ongoing developments in this area. In addition, measurement of pulmonary function as discussed in Chapter 3 is readily available to monitor severe asthma and the impact of treatment on the course of severe asthma. Thus along with the report of symptoms, pulmonary function tests are the most readily available form of objective measurement and will remain an essential component in treatment decisions. Other techniques, such as exhaled nitric oxide if validated, will be introduced into clinical management of asthma. Attention must also be directed to diagnosing and managing concomitant disorders that frequently occur in patients with severe asthma, such as gastroesophageal reflux, reviewed in Chapter 11; vocal cord dysfunction, reviewed in Chapter 17; sinusitis, discussed in Chapter 18; sleep disorders, discussed in Chapter 14; and aspirin sensitivity, summarized in Chapter 16. In addition, controlling nocturnal asthma (Chap. 9), and using environmental control measures (Chap. 15), are essential to overall management.

Targets for future asthma management must include the prevention of progression and reversal of the course of the disease, improvement in quality of life as indicated by reduction in symptoms, and improvement in pulmonary function. A major accomplishment would be to induce remission. It is conceivable that interrupting the inflammatory process could offer this opportunity. The approaches for intervention include environmental control, if exposure to an identified environmental agent is a driving force for inflammation and amenable to avoidance, or pharmacotherapy.

In Chapter 15, on the role of allergy in severe asthma, summarizes the current understanding of the role of allergy in chronic inflammation and the specific allergens that may be important in severe asthma. Since patients with severe asthma have a high incidence of allergy and are often sensitive to multiple allergens, it will be important to identify the most relevant allergens for a specific patient and examine methods to control exposure. Given the multiple sources of allergen exposure in today's environment, it is indeed a challenging task to control exposure. Alternatives include allergen immunotherapy or some form of immunomodulation to control IgE production or another site of cellular interaction relevant to the pathogenesis of severe asthma. If there is an identifiable ingestant such as a drug, as typified by aspirin (Chap. 16), this is also a potential target for avoidance.

Chapter 6 on asthma pharmacotherapy reviews our current understanding of the role of available medications in controlling asthma. While several medications are extremely effective in reversing the symptoms of asthma and reducing the frequency of symptoms, the current search is for a medication that can modify the disease and potentially induce remission and a normalization of the airways. To date, inhaled steroids appear to offer that potential based on the results of several studies that examined airway tissue before and after inhaled steroid therapy. An evaluation of the studies that show a positive effect of inhaled steroids on reducing the thickness of collagen deposition and the number of inflammatory cells have been performed with doses of inhaled steroids exceeding 1500 μg/day. Reduction of the number of inflammatory cells and the thickness of collagen deposition are viewed as surrogate markers for airway inflammation and airway remodeling, respectively.

On the other hand, concern has been raised over the risk of high-dose, long-term inhaled steroid therapy on growth velocity, osteoporosis, and ocular disorders as discussed in Chapters 21 and 22. This apprehension has prompted a more conservative approach to the use of inhaled steroids that employs a strategy of low-dose inhaled steroid therapy combined with nonsteroid long-term control therapy. Chapter 7 reviewed the role of the newest class of treatment, namely leukotriene modifiers, as potential replacement therapy for inhaled and systemic glucocorticoids. While the application of leukotriene modifiers and other nonsteroid long-term controllers may be effective in reducing the risk for glucocorticoid adverse effects by facilitating the reduction of total glucocorticoid therapy, it is not clear whether this strategy is sufficient to alter the course of persistent inflammation. Studies are not available showing a similar effect of low- to medium-dose inhaled steroid therapy on reducing inflammation or reversing airway remodeling in patients with severe asthma.

Understanding the mechanisms of steroid resistance as summarized in Chapter 24 and the mechanisms of steroid action as summarized in Chapter 8 prompted the development of several new classes of medications, specifically cytokine antagonists and transcription factor inhibitors, that could conceivably enhance the anti-inflammatory effects of steroids. Chapter 10 discussed available alternative nonprescription therapies that patients utilize in their attempt to treat their symptoms. It will be interesting to see if the "designer" therapeutic initiatives as summarized in Chapter 23 or the complementary and alternative medicines that are utilized empirically will be the first to play a significant role in reversing the course of severe asthma. Promising new entities include anti-IgE, cytokine antagonists such as anti-IL-4, and phosphodiesterase-4 inhibitors. Each must be evaluated to determine their effect on reducing the dose of inhaled and systemic steroids necessary to control severe persistent asthma. In addition, we must develop approaches that will address the problem of psychological factors and poor medication adherence that is recognized with many severe asthma patients, as summarized in Chapter 20.

With the unfolding of the mysteries of the human genome and alterations of the genes contributing to various diseases and level of severity, it will also be important to understand the genetic features of patients with severe asthma. Chapter 2, written by leaders in this area of investigation, reviewed the potential for this new field. This information will provide not only insight for new treatments but also the potential for recognizing patients at risk for severe asthma.

III. Can We Interrupt the Course of Asthma to Halt Progression to Increasing Severity?

Our understanding of the pathogenesis of severe asthma suggests that perhaps the pathology of deposition of fibrous tissue that includes collagen, tenascin, and elastin may present a major hurdle in inducing disease remission once it has reached severe proportions. Consequently, attention should be directed toward the prevention of severe asthma in patients who have asthma and are at risk for developing a severe, life-threatening form of asthma.

There is a general feeling among asthma care specialists that early childhood asthma is underdiagnosed and undertreated. Current knowledge allows us to identify patients at high risk for asthma mortality. Information is now developing regarding patients at risk for chronic asthma, such as parental asthma, maternal smoking, atopic features and the presence of relevant allergens in the environment, and small lungs (2,7,8). While this information needs to be firmed up for application to clinical practice, we would be remiss if we did not include a risk assessment for identifying patients who go on to develop severe asthma and steroid-insensitive asthma. Perhaps it is the patients who have risk factors for asthma but are resilient to treatment with low-dose inhaled glucocorticoid therapy that are at risk for this level of severity.

As indicated in Chapter 1, one of the consequences of undertreatment may be a loss of pulmonary function (FEV_1) over time that is greater than that observed in patients without asthma and similar to that observed in chronic obstructive pulmonary disease and cystic fibrosis (9–11). It is apparent that inhaled corticosteroids are effective in controlling asthma symptoms and reducing the intensity of the inflammatory response in studies conducted in adults with asthma. Since inhaled corticosteroids reduce asthma symptoms and improve lung function, it is likely that reduction in the inflammatory response also occurs in children with asthma (Fig. 1). Unfortunately, inhaled corticosteroids do not appear to have long-lasting or disease-modifying effects. In other words, they are only effective as long as they are administered.

Two studies from the Dutch CNSLD Study Group sought to address this issue in children with moderate asthma. In the first study (12), the investigators sought to determine whether long-term budesonide therapy would result in clinical asthma remission during therapy. Of the 53 children originally randomized to receive budesonide, 60% achieved an 8-month clinical remission at some point

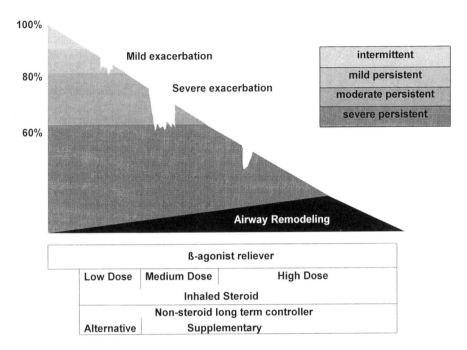

Figure 1 Conceptual model of declining lung function and airway remodeling. The lower bars depict the therapeutic intervention at each level of severity. For exacerbations of asthma β-adrenergic agonists are the medication of choice. Systemic or high-dose inhaled corticosteroids are used to resolve significant exacerbations. (Reprinted with permission from Ref. 8.)

during the 3-year study. However, only one-third were in remission upon completion of the study, and only 15% of the patients had a normal FEV_1 (>90%) and a normal PC_{20} value (>150 μg). The authors concluded that although long-term budesonide therapy improved asthma symptoms and objective measures of asthma, it did not cure the disease.

This point was strengthened in their second follow-up study (13). In this case, 28 children from the original cohort who had been on budesonide for 2–3 years were randomized to continue budesonide (8 patients; 600 μg/day) or to be completely tapered off budesonide (20 patients). All patients were followed over a 6-month period. Eight of the 20 patients tapered off budesonide had to be withdrawn during the 6-month follow-up and 5 required prednisone secondary to poor asthma control compared to none in the budesonide group. In addition, much of the gain in lung function and bronchial hyperresponsiveness that these children displayed while on 2–3 years of budesonide was lost by the end of the 6-month placebo period. Thus it appears as if inhaled corticosteroids can induce a short-lived clinical remission while on therapy. There is no known treatment that can consistently induce a lasting remission in the disease; however, inhaled corticosteroids have a relatively slow offset of effect compared to other long-term controller medications (14). Understanding the onset and progression of the inflammation, as well as its persistence, could provide insight into defining appropriate strategies for treatment depending on the stage of the disease (8).

Theories have developed that early intervention with inhaled corticosteroid therapy can be effective in preventing the progression of the disease and the risk for irreversible changes in the airways that could result in the persistence of symptoms (14–17). Thus, there appears to be a "window of opportunity" that is critical for intervention. Patients with "difficult to control asthma" have evidence of persistent inflammation (18–20). Their disease often has its onset in early childhood. Does this information suggest that children who manifest persistent inflammation in the presence of anti-inflammatory therapy could be at increased risk for disease progression? If so, it will be important to recognize these patients and provide more effective interventions at critical stages of their disease progression.

Of interest, a recent study by Sont et al. (21) evaluated the level of asthma control resulting from inhaled steroid dose adjustments using airway hyperresponsiveness as an additional guide to long-term treatment. This study used the approach of adjusting inhaled steroid dosage according to levels of clinical symptoms, bronchodilator use, peak expiratory flow variability, and FEV_1 in one group (reference group) and according to the same criteria plus the addition of another, airway responsiveness, in another (AHR-strategy group). Based on the score determined at 3-month interval evaluations, the dose could be adjusted to no inhaled steroid or low-, medium-, or high-dose inhaled steroid.

After a 2-year follow-up, the investigators made several interesting observations. First, they reported greater improvements in asthma control and pulmonary function with the AHR strategy. Second, biopsy samples obtained before and after 2-years' treatment showed significant reductions in reticular layer thickness and reduced eosinophil infiltration only in the AHR-strategy group. Finally, they observed that a higher proportion of patients in the AHR-strategy group required high- and moderate-dose inhaled steroid therapy. These observations suggest that patients with persistent asthma would receive better control and better resolution of inflammation, and the consequences of chronic inflammation, such as airway remodeling, if treatment were based on periodic measures of AHR. However, this strategy would result in treatment with higher doses of inhaled steroids, at least temporarily.

On a cautionary note, clinical experience and available literature suggest that aggressive therapy rarely normalizes AHR. At best, inhaled steroid therapy usually changes the provocative dose of methacholine and histamine by no more than twofold. Therefore, attempting to normalize AHR could result in protracted therapy and incur risk for adverse effect with little gain in response. Therefore, the application of measures of AHR needs careful consideration. Furthermore, measures of AHR are usually performed only in hospital-based specialty clinics, thus limiting access to this test. Perhaps other measures, such as sputum eosinophils or measurement of exhaled nitric oxide, or an alternative measure of ongoing inflammation or combination thereof could be included as indicators for the adjustment of inhaled steroid therapy.

It is extremely important to understand the natural history of this form of asthma to not only determine whether it can be identified by measuring pulmonary function serially over time but also to determine methods to identify patients at risk for severe asthma and subsequently signal the need for early intervention. It is also important to move toward a categorization of the various forms of severe asthma. This is not only necessary for defining appropriate inclusion/exclusion criteria for clinical research but also for communication of results and extrapolation of studies to patient care. Although this categorization could be based on the symptom complex, perhaps a better alternative is the defined pulmonary pathology, or specific measures of pulmonary function. While pulmonary function via spirometry can be reliably measured in children 5 years of age and older, techniques must be defined to measure pulmonary function in younger children to assist in early recognition of severe airway compromise or progressive deterioration in pulmonary function.

The key feature to success in this venture appears to be a focus on the individual patient. It is important to evaluate each patient presenting with asthma, to assess their risk for progression to persistent asthma, to intervene with environmental control in those patients who are sensitized and exposed to a relevant allergen, and to monitor progression of disease. Monitoring is important in characterizing the level of severity and the response to treatment. Individual monitoring could consist of a record of both mild and severe symptoms, requirement for rescue therapy, pulmonary function, and indicators of inflammation. The higher the risk, the more attention that should be paid to precise measurement of the course. This would facilitate recognition of progression of the disease by increased symptoms, decline in pulmonary function, and an increasing medication requirement for rescue and long-term control therapy. In addition, the response to an intervention could be easily assessed with a careful monitoring system. Medications that improve symptoms and alter progression could be continued and adjusted, while those having no effect on symptom control or pulmonary function could be discontinued. Alternatively, the dose of the medication could be increased if there is an identifiable dose–response relationship. This would be justified if there was a recognized reason for poor response to a conventional dose (for example, with systemic steroids); a drug interaction with an enzyme inducer such as phenytoin, persistent inflammation associated with steroid insensitivity, or poor adherence to the treatment regimen. Queries into each of these questions could be made by careful documentation of a failure to respond.

One concern is that asthma can have an early age of onset and considerable damage could be present before aggressive therapy is initiated. Since asthma has a high likelihood of onset before the age of 5 years and these patients are often initially managed by a pediatrician, it is important to reevaluate asthma management in this age group. While it is recognizably difficult to measure pulmonary function in children younger than 5 years of age, most primary care physicians and pediatricians do not incorporate pulmonary function measurements as a standard of practice even in older children and adults. This gap could be remedied by the development of pulmonary function techniques that are feasible for children younger than 5 years of age and also by strengthening the interaction of pediatrician and asthma specialist in overseeing the developmental features of severe asthma. Since severe asthma is characterized by low pulmonary function, it seems obvious that the natural history of pulmonary function should be followed in all patients with asthma to determine the rate of decline in pulmonary function for that individual patient. This is most easily monitored by following FEV_1 percentage predicted over time. Patients showing elements of progression by a decline in pulmonary function, increasing use of urgent care facilities, or an increasing medication requirement over time merit an evaluation and input from an asthma specialist. Managed care could facilitate this interaction by prompting a more organized approach to medical follow-up of the patient with asthma, especially those following a path of increasing severity.

In the coming years, the ongoing work of several high-profile asthma research networks will be presented. The National Heart, Lung and Blood Institute has sponsored three major network programs in asthma research: the Childhood Asthma Management Program (CAMP), the Asthma Clinical Research Network (ACRN), and the newly formed Childhood Asthma Research and Education (CARE) Network. In addition, several pharmaceutical research firms have initiated studies on early intervention and long-term therapy for asthma management.

The Childhood Asthma Management Program is a multicenter program that is designed to assess the effect of three different treatment strategies on lung development and the course of asthma (22,23). In 1993 over 1000 children between the ages of 5 and 12 years with mild to moderate asthma were enrolled and randomly assigned to either inhaled nedocromil, inhaled budesonide, or placebo groups. The subjects were carefully followed for symptoms, pulmonary function, body development, and need for additional therapy. The treatment phase came to a close in 1999 and was followed by a 4-month wash-out phase. The key observations in this recently reported study included the following important observations (24). First, inhaled steroid at a dose of 400 µg/day of budesonide via

Turbuhaler provided significantly better asthma control as indicated by reduced hospitalization rate, emergency room visits, and need for prednisone intervention for acute exacerbations as well as a reduced requirement for supplementary medications compared to inhaled nedocromil and placebo. Second, reassuring information was provided regarding the safety of long-term inhaled steroid therapy. The previously reported effect of inhaled steroids on reducing growth velocity is limited to the first year of treatment and does not progress with continued treatment. Final adult height for the inhaled steroid group is projected to be comparable to the patients in the other two study groups. Third, there is no evidence for concern regarding risk for reduction in bone density or sexual development in the age group treated in this study. Fourth, the significant reduction in airway responsiveness noted in the inhaled steroid group at the end of the long-term treatment course was lost within only 4 months of discontinuation of treatment and was comparable to the other two study groups.

A curious observation in this study was the failure of the inhaled steroid course to have a significant effect on lung growth as measured by postbronchodilator FEV_1 percentage predicted over time. While there was an initial increase in FEV_1 shortly after beginning treatment, it gradually declined over the remaining period of treatment and was comparable to the inhaled nedocromil and placebo group at the end of the study. This would suggest that continuous inhaled steroids do not affect lung growth in patients with well-established mild to moderate persistent asthma. This population of patients had a mean duration of asthma of 5 years. Perhaps intervention was not initiated soon enough or the subgroup of patients with severe asthma are the subpopulation of patients subject to a more rapid decline in pulmonary function over time, a specific study of therapeutic intervention in this group is needed.

The CAMP subjects will now be followed for an additional 4–5 years to determine the impact of the aggressive course of treatment on long-term outcomes such as final adult height and lung function. In addition, the data will be further analyzed to gain additional insight into features that determined medication response versus failure by incorporating data from measures on patient adherence, family dynamics, markers of inflammation, and pharmacogenetics. This study will impact the way we manage asthma in children and the way we examine the effect of treatment over at least the first decade of the 2000s. Of great significance is that CAMP provides a method to obtain a "profile of performance" for long-term therapy and sets the standard for comparison. At the present time, inhaled steroids remain the preferred treatment for mild to moderate persistent asthma. Other long-term therapies, such as the leukotriene modifiers, and newly introduced treatments, such as anti-IgE, should be assessed for comparative or greater effects on the various measures of effect examined in CAMP.

Another cooperative study program, the Asthma Clinical Research Network, was formulated in 1993 and has taken a lead role in investigating major issues around the pharmacotherapy of asthma. To date, the ACRN has provided information on the effects of regular β-adrenergic agonist therapy on asthma control, the lack of beneficial effect of colchicine in persistent asthma, and the role of long-acting β-adrenergic agonists as steroid-reducing agents in moderate persistent asthma and as monotherapy for persistent asthma (25–27). This network is currently completing work on the development of models to compare the beneficial and systemic effects of the various inhaled glucocorticoids (28). The large database compiled in this study allows this network to conduct studies on the genetics of asthma (genotype) with a carefully characterized asthma population (asthma phenotype) as well as on their responses to medications. The Network is now conducting a long-term study to examine the relative beneficial effects of an inhaled glucocorticoid and a leukotriene antagonist on altering the decline in pulmonary function associated with persistent asthma.

The recently formed Childhood Asthma Research and Education (CARE) Network has selected the evaluation of early intervention with inhaled glucocorticoid on the natural history of asthma to be among its initial studies. Another study will characterize the features that are associated with response or lack of response to an inhaled glucocorticoid and a leukotriene antagonist. The Network will also evaluate methods for measuring pulmonary function in children and define techniques suitable for application in clinical research and clinical practice.

It is important to remember that an attempt to study the genetics of asthma and responses to treatment is multifaceted. It requires an examination of the genetics associated with the disease presentation, the genetics associated with medication response or failure to respond, and the genetics of predisposition toward adverse effects of a medication (29). All of these are exciting areas and needed for clinical care. For example, if genetic analysis could provide the necessary information to determine the likelihood of a patient developing severe asthma, having a poor response to a medication such as an inhaled glucocorticoid, and having a predisposition to adverse effects of glucocorticoid therapy, the focus of management could shift earlier to alternative anti-inflammatory and immunomodulator therapies for that patient.

This work is especially important as we develop new medications and attempt to identify their niche in asthma management. The concept of disease modifiers has been raised but now must be defined. It would seem that a disease modifier should not only reduce inflammation but also alter disease progression, for example, prevent airway remodeling, halt the decline in pulmonary function, and significantly reduce morbidity and mortality associated with asthma. Selection of the relevant disease category, the identification of medications most likely to alter the course of the disease, and monitoring response to treatment would appear to offer the opportunity to significantly impact the progression to severe asthma and thus reduce the incidence of severe asthma.

IV. Summary

The second edition of *Severe Asthma* has assimilated the current information on the diagnosis, pathology, and management of severe asthma. Significant opportunities are available to reverse the course of the disease and to prevent its development. Advances in management will require continued research on the natural history of severe asthma, pathogenesis, application of markers of inflammation, and pharmacogenetics and likely continuing development of new medications to fill unmet needs. Success in these target areas should lead to a reduction in the incidence and prevalence of severe asthma and overall improvement in outcomes for asthma patients as well as a reduction in the allocation of health care dollars dedicated to the management of severe asthma.

Acknowledgments

Supported in part by Public Health Services Research Grants 1NO1-HR-16048; HL36577, HL 37260, and HL 51834; General Clinical Research Center Grant 5 MO1 RR00051 from the Division of Research Resources; and the NICHHD Pediatric Pharmacology Research Unit Network Grant 1-U01-HD37237.

References

1. Szefler SJ, Leung DYM, eds. Severe Asthma: Pathogenesis and Clinical Management. New York: Marcel Dekker, 1995.
2. National Asthma Education and Prevention Program Expert Panel Report 2: Guidelines for the Diagnosis and Management of Asthma. Pub. No. 97–4051, 1997.
3. Wenzel SE, Schwartz LB, Langmack EL, Halliday JL, Trudeau JB, Gibbs RL, Chu HW. Evidence that severe asthma can be divided pathologically into two inflammatory subtypes with distinct physiologic and clinical characteristics. Am J Respir Crit Care Med 1999; 160(3):1001–1008.
4. Kraft M, Cassell GH, Henson JE, Watson H, Williamson J, Marmion BP, Gaydos CA, Martin RJ. Detection of Mycoplasma pneumoniae in the airways of adults with chronic asthma. Am J Respir Crit Care Med 1998; 158:998A.
5. Leung DYM, Hamid Q, Vottero A, Szefler SJ, Surs W, Minshall E, Chrousos GP, Klemm DJ. Association of glucocorticoid insensitivity with increased expression of glucocorticoid receptor beta. J Exp Med 1997; 186(9):1567–1574.
6. Hamid QA, Wenzel SE, Hauk PJ, Tsicopoulos A, Wallaert B, Lafitte JJ, Chrousos GP, Szefler SJ, Leung DYM. Increased glucocorticoid receptor beta in airway cells of glucocorticoid-insensitive asthma. Am J Respir Crit Care Med 1999; 159(5/1): 1600–1604.
7. Warner JO, Naspitz CK. Third International Pediatric Consensus statement on the management of childhood asthma: International Pediatric Asthma Consensus Group. Pediatr Pulmonol 1998; 25(1):1–17.

8.   Szefler SJ. Asthma: The new advances. In: Barness L, ed. Advances in Pediatrics.
     St. Louis: Mosby, 2000:283–304.
9.   Peat JK. Asthma: a longitudinal perspective. J Asthma 1998; 35(3):235–241.
10. Weiss ST. Early life predictors of adult chronic obstructive lung disease. Eur Respir
     Rev 1995; 31(5):303–309.
11. Lange P, Parner J, Vestbo J, Schnohr P, Jensen G. A 15-year follow-up study of
     ventilatory function in adults with asthma. N Engl J Med 1998; 339(17):1194–
     1200.
12. van Essen-Zandvliet EE, Hughes MD, Waalkens HJ, Duiverman EJ, Kerrebijn KF.
     Remission of childhood asthma after long-term treatment with an inhaled corticoste-
     roid (budesonide): can it be achieved?: Dutch CNSLD Study Group. Eur Respir J
     1994; 7(1):63–68.
13. Waalkens HJ, Van Essen-Zandvliet EE, Hughes MD, Gerritsen J, Duiverman EJ,
     Knol K, Kerrebijn KF. Cessation of long-term treatment with inhaled corticosteroid
     (budesonide) in children with asthma results in deterioration: The Dutch CNSLD
     Study Group. Am Rev Respir Dis 1993; 148(5):1252–1257.
14. Haahtela T, Jarvinen M, Kava T, Kiviranta K, Koskinen S, Lehtonen K, Nikander
     K, Persson T, Selroos O, Sovijarvi A, et al. Effects of reducing or discontinuing
     inhaled budesonide in patients with mild asthma. N Engl J Med 1994; 331(11):700–
     705.
15. Agertoft L, Pedersen S. Effects of long-term treatment with an inhaled corticosteroid
     on growth and pulmonary function in asthmatic children. Respir Med 1994; 88(5):
     373–381.
16. Selroos O, Pietinalho A, Lofroos AB, Riska H. Effect of early vs late intervention
     with inhaled corticosteroids in asthma. Chest 1995; 108(5):1228–1234.
17. Overbeek SE, Kerstjens HA, Bogaard JM, Mulder PG, Postma DS. Is delayed intro-
     duction of inhaled corticosteroids harmful in patients with obstructive airways dis-
     ease (asthma and COPD)?: The Dutch CNSLD Study Group. The Dutch Chronic
     Nonspecific Lung Disease Study Groups. Chest 1996; 110(1):35–41.
18. Leung DYM, Martin RJ, Szefler SJ, Sher ER, Ying S, Kay AB, Hamid Q. Dysregula-
     tion of interleukin 4, interleukin 5, and interferon gamma gene expression in steroid-
     resistant asthma. J Exp Med 1995; 181(1):33–40.
19. Wenzel SE, Szefler SJ, Leung DYM, Sloan SI, Rex MD, Martin RJ. Bronchoscopic
     evaluation of severe asthma: persistent inflammation associated with high dose glu-
     cocorticoids. Am J Respir Crit Care Med 1997; 156(3/1):737–743.
20. Vrugt B, Wilson S, Underwood J, Bron A, de Bruyn R, Bradding P, Holgate ST,
     Djukanovic R, Aalbers R. Mucosal inflammation in severe glucocorticoid-dependent
     asthma. Eur Respir J 1999; 13(6):1245–1252.
21. Sont JK, Willems LN, Bel EH, van Krieken JH, Vandenbroucke JP, Sterk PJ. Clini-
     cal control and histopathologic outcome of asthma when using airway hyperrespon-
     siveness as an additional guide to long-term treatment: The AMPUL Study Group.
     Am J Respir Crit Care Med 1999; 159(4/1):1043–1051.
22. The Childhood Asthma Management Program (CAMP): design, rationale, and meth-
     ods: Childhood Asthma Management Program Research Group. Control Clin Trials
     1999; 20(1):91–120.
23. Zeiger RS, Dawson C, Weiss S. Relationships between duration of asthma and

asthma severity among children in the Childhood Asthma Management Program (CAMP). J Allergy Clin Immunol 1999; 103(3/1):376–387.

24. The Childhood Asthma Management Program Research Group. Long term effects of budesonide or nedocromil in children with asthma. N Engl J Med 2000; 343(16): 1054–1063.

25. Drazen JM, Israel E, Boushey HA, Chinchilli VM, Fahy JV, Fish JE, Lazarus SC, Lemanske RF, Martin RJ, Peters SP, Sorkness C, Szefler SJ. Comparison of regularly scheduled with as-needed use of albuterol in mild asthma. Asthma Clinical Research Network. N Engl J Med 1996; 335(12):841–847.

26. Fish JE, Peters SP, Chambers CV, McGeady SJ, Epstein KR, Boushey HA, Cherniack RM, Chinchilli VM, Drazen JM, Fahy JV, Hurd SS, Israel E, Lazarus SC, Lemanske RF, Martin RJ, Mauger EA, Sorkness C, Szefler SJ. An evaluation of colchicine as an alternative to inhaled corticosteroids in moderate asthma: National Heart, Lung, and Blood Institute's Asthma Clinical Research Network. Am J Respir Crit Care Med 1997; 156:1165–1171.

27. Israel E, Drazen JM, Liggett SB, Boushey HA, Cherniack RM, Chinchilli VM, Cooper DM, Fahy JV, Fish JE, Ford JG, Kraft M, Kunselman S, Lazarus SC, Lemanske RF, Martin RJ, McLean DE, Peters SP, Silverman EK, Sorkness CA, Szefler SJ, Weiss ST, Yandava CN. The effect of polymorphisms of the beta(2)-adrenergic receptor on the response to regular use of albuterol in asthma. Am J Respir Crit Care Med 2000; 162(1):75–80.

28. Szefler SJ, Martin RJ, and the National Heart, Lung and Blood Institute Asthma Clinical Research Network. Evaluation and comparison of inhaled steroids. In: Schleimer RP, O'Byrne PM, Szefler SJ, Brattsand R, eds. Airway Activity and Selectivity of Inhaled Steroids in Asthma—Mechanisms, Models of Evaluation and Clinical Impacts. In press.

29. Roses AD. Pharmacogenetics and future drug development and delivery. Lancet 2000; 355:1358–1361.

AUTHOR INDEX

C

SUBJECT INDEX

A

Acetaminophen, aspirin-sensitive respiratory disease, 371–372
Activator protein 1, glucocorticoid interaction with, 179–181
Acupuncture, 228–230
Adenosine, 70–71
Adherence to treatment regimen, 484–488
Adolescence, diagnosis in, 9–10
Adulthood,
  early, diagnosis in, 10–12
  late, diagnosis in, 12–14
Age,
  airway responsiveness, 41–42
  diagnosis of asthma, 5–14
    adolescence, 9–10
    early adulthood, 10–12
    early childhood, 5–9
    late adulthood, 12–14
    late childhood, 9–10
Agricultural workers, 398
Air pollutants, 45, 396–399
Airflow resistance, 50–52
  with sleep disorders, 328–332
Airway hyperresponsiveness,
  gastroesophageal reflux, 249
  monitoring, 459–460

Airway inflammation measurement, 460–464
  bronchoalveolar lavage, biopsy, 464
  exhaled gases, 463–464
  induced sputum examination, 460–463
Airway obstruction and asthma, distinguishing in imaging, 296
Airway remodeling, 89–124
  cartilage changes, 107–108
  effect of treatment on, 108
  epithelial damage/desquamation, 90
  goblet cells, 90–91
  inflammation, 101–107
  smooth muscle hypertrophy/hyperplasia, 91–93
  somatic components of asthma, 90–108
  subepithelial fibrosis, 93–101
    basement membrane, 95
    collagens, 96
    fibronectin, 96–97
    matrix metalloproteinases, 97–100
    myofibroblasts, 100–101
    proteoglycans, 97
    tenascin, 97
  vascular changes, 107
Airway resistance, 51–52
  nocturnal asthma, 203–205

659